Oncology Nursing in the Ambulatory Setting

Issues and Models of Care

SECOND EDITION

Patricia C. Buchsel, RN, MSN, FAAN
Clinical Faculty
University of Washington, School of Nursing
Seattle, WA

Chief Operating Officer
Creative Cancer Concepts, Inc.
Dallas, TX

Connie Henke Yarbro, RN, MS, FAAN
Clinical Associate Professor
Division of Hematology/Oncology

Sinclair School of Nursing
Editor, *Seminars in Oncology Nursing*
University of Missouri-Columbia
Columbia, MO

JONES AND BARTLETT PUBLISHERS
Sudbury, Massachusetts
BOSTON   TORONTO   LONDON   SINGAPORE

World Headquarters
Jones and Bartlett Publishers
40 Tall Pine Drive
Sudbury, MA 01776
978-443-5000
info@jbpub.com
www.jbpub.com

Jones and Bartlett Publishers Canada
2406 Nikanna Road
Mississauga, ON L5C 2W6
CANADA

Jones and Bartlett Publishers International
Barb House, Barb Mews
London W6 7PA
United Kingdom

Library of Congress Cataloging-in-Publication Data
Oncology nursing in the ambulatory setting : issues and models of care /
[edited by] Patricia Buchsel, Connie Yarbro.-- 2nd ed.
    p. ; cm.
Includes bibliographical references and index.
  ISBN 0-7637-1474-7 (paperback)
  1. Cancer--Nursing. 2. Ambulatory medical care.
  [DNLM: 1. Ambulatory Care--organization & administration. 2.
Oncologic Nursing--organization & administration. WY 156 O5754 2004]
  I. Buchsel, Patricia Corcoran. II. Yarbro, Connie Henke.
  RC266.O56 2004
  616.99'40231--dc22
                        2003025162

Production Credits
Aquisition Editor: Kevin Sullivan
Production Manager: Amy Rose
Editorial Assistant: Amy Sibley
Production Assistant: Tracey Chapman
Cover Design: Anne Spencer
Marketing Manager: Ed McKenna
Manufacturing and Inventory Coordinator: Amy Bacus
Composition: AnnMarie Lemoine
Printing and Binding: Malloy, Inc.
Cover Printing: Malloy, Inc.

Printed in the United States of America
08 07 06 05 04   10 9 8 7 6 5 4 3 2 1

To oncology nurses who remain true to their calling in offering excellence and enduring care to patients and their families throughout the continuum of care.

Contributors

Susan Weiss Behrend, RN, MSN, AOCN©
Clinical Nurse Specialist
Fox Chase Cancer Center
Philadelphia, PA

Dawn Camp-Sorrell, MSN, FNP, AOCN©
Oncology Nurse Practitioner
Chelsea, AL

Laura M. Chisholm, RN, MSN
Warren Grant Magnuson Clinical Center
National Institute of Health
CDR, USPHS, Nurse Corps
Bethesda, MD

Cathy Coleman, RN, OCN©
Coleman Breast Center Consultation Services
Tiburon, CA

Carol P. Curtiss, RN, MSN
Curtiss Consulting
Clinical Nurse Specialist Consultant
Greenfield, MA

Georgia Cusack, RN, MSN
Clinical Nurse Specialist
Outpatient Cancer Center
Warren Grant Magnuson Clinical Center
National Institutes of Health
Bethesda, MD

Georgia M. Decker, MS, RN, CS-ANP,
  AOCN©, CNS
Integrative Care
Albany, NY

Sharon Elad, DMD
Oral Medicine Specialist
Lecturer, Oral Medicine Department
Hadassah-Hebrew University School of
  Dental Medicine
Jerusalem, Israel

Joel B. Epstein, DMDC, MSD, FRCD©,
  FCDS (BC)
Professor and Head
Department of Oral Medicine and Diagnostic
  Services
College of Dentistry
University of Illinois
Director of Interdisciplinary Programs in Oral Cancer
College of Medicine
Chicago, IL

Carmen P. Escalante, MD
The University of Texas MD Anderson Cancer
  Center
Department of General Internal Medicine
Ambulatory Treatment and Emergency Care
Houston, TX

Catherine Glennon, RN, CAN, MHS, OCN©
Oncology Services DUMC
Duke University Medical Center
Durham, NC

Elizabeth Gomez, RN, MSN
Newtonnet Publications
Ridgefield, CT

Rebecca Hawkins, MSN, ACP, AOCN©
Oncology Nurse Practitioner
St. Mary Regional Cancer Center
Pendleton, OR

Antoinette Jones, RN, BSN
Nurse Manager
Warren Grant Magnuson Clinical Center
National Institutes of Health
Bethesda, MD

Linda U. Krebs, RN, PhD, AOCN©
Associate Professor
University of Colorado School of Nursing
Denver, CO

Kim K. Kuebler, MN, RN, ANP-CS
Adjuvant Therapies LLC
Palliative Care Practice/Consultation and Research
Atlanta, GA

Mary Dee McEvoy, PhD, AOCN©, RN
Director, The Joseph F. Cullman Jr. Institute for
  Patient Care
The Mount Sinai Hospital
New York, NY

Cyril Meyerowitz, DDS, MS
Professor & Chair, Eastman Department of Dentistry
Director, Eastman Dental Center
University of Rochester Medical Center
New York, NY

Randi Z. Moskowitz, RN, MPH, MBA
Joseph Aprile Cancer Institute
Saint Vincent Catholic Medical Centers
New York, NY

Barbara J. Murphy, RN, MN, AOCN©
Oncology Nurse Educator
Ashburn, VA

Lillian M. Nail, PhD, RN, FAAN
Professor of Nursing
Oregon Health and Science University
Portland, OR

Betsy Patterson, RN, MSN, ACNP, AOCN©
Independent Educator and Consultant
Inman, SC

Douglas E. Peterson, DMD, PhD
Professor and Head
Department of Oral Diagnosis
School of Dental Medicine
Associate Director
Cancer Center
University of Connecticut Health Center
Farmington, CT

Christine Rimkus, RN, MSN, AOCN©
Oncology Clinical Nurse Specialist, Consultant
St. Louis University Hospital
St. Louis, MO

Kim Schmit-Pokorny, RN, MSN, OCN©
Manager/Case Manager
Oncology/Hematology Section
University of Nebraska Medical Center
Omaha, NE

Mark M. Schubert, DDS, MSD
Professor
Department of Oral Medicine
Director of Oral Medicine
University of Washington School of Dentistry
Seattle Cancer Care Alliance
Seattle, WA

Kathleen M. Shuey, MS, RN, CS, ACON©
Manager, Nurse Education and Admixture Training
Pharmacy Services
Albuquerque, NM

Anna L. Schwartz, RN, PhD
Research Associate Professor
School of Nursing
University of Washington
Seattle, WA

Rosalie U. Valdres, RN, MSN, FNP, CNS
Advanced Practice Nurse
Department of General Internal Medicine,
Ambulatory Treatment and Emergency Care
University of Texas MD Anderson Cancer Center
Houston, TX

Valorie Wilkins
Department of Pharmacy
Stevens Hospital
Edmonds, WA

Contents

PREFACE   XV

Chapter 1   *Ambulatory Care Administrative*
               Concepts: An Overview *1*

PATRICIA BUCHSEL AND CATHERINE GLENNON

Introduction   1
History of Ambulatory Care Nursing   1
Trends Supporting the Shift to Ambulatory Care   2
Ambulatory Care Defined   6
New Issues in Ambulatory Care   7
Facility Planning and Space Use: Function and Form   23
Future Trends   26
Appendix A   27

Chapter 2   *Economic Issues in Ambulatory Care* *33*

CATHERINE GLENNON AND MARY DEE McEVOY

Introduction   33
Inflow   35
Outflow   43
Patient Costs   45
Conclusion   46

Chapter 3 *The Internet and Ambulatory Oncology Nursing Care* 49

ELIZABETH G. GOMEZ

Introduction	49
The Start of Something Big	49
In the Clinic	51
A Familiar Role: The Trusted Patient Guide	51
At Your Service: The Personal Digital Assistant	54
Shall We Talk? Or Type? Patient Communication	57
E-Consults for the "E-Patient"	58
In The Waiting Room	58
Can't Get Out? We'll Come to You. Web-Based Learning Opportunities for the Ambulatory Oncology Nurse	59
Distance Education	60
A Matter of Trust	61
Conclusion	62

Chapter 4 *Role of the Advance Oncology Nurse Practitioner* 65

DAWN CAMP-SORRELL AND REBECCA HAWKINS

Introduction	65
History of the Oncology NP	65
Job Settings for the Oncology NPs	66
Reimbursement Issues	69
Prescriptive Authority	72
License and Certification to Practice	74
Future Issues	78

Chapter 5 *Current Models of Physician Office Practices* 81

KATHLEEN M. SHUEY

Introduction	81
History of Ambulatory Clinics in Oncology	81
Ambulatory Practice Settings	82
Evolving Role of the Oncology Office Nurse	83
Patient Classification Systems	89
Practice Economics and Reimbursement	90
Practice Setting Trends and the Nursing Shortage	92
Conclusion	95

Chapter 6   Oncology Infusion Centers *99*

LAURA M. CHISHOLM, GEORGIA CUSACK, AND ANTOINETTE JONES

Introduction	99
Overview of Outpatient Cancer Care	99
ICs	100
Planning an IC	100
Services Provided	104
Practice Models	106
Workload Analysis	107
Nursing Roles	108
Managers and Administrators	108
Clinical Nurse	109
Unlicensed Assistive Personnel	110
Recruitment and Retention	111
Current Issues	112

Chapter 7   Outpatient Surgery in the Oncology Setting *115*

RANDI Z. MOSKOWITZ

Introduction	115
Historical Perspectives	115
Trends in Ambulatory Surgery	116
Advantages of Ambulatory Surgery	117
Types of Ambulatory Surgery Facilities	118
Patient Care Issues	121
Planning and Developing an Ambulatory Surgery Center	129
Example of an Oncology Ambulatory Surgery Center	133
Future Trends	135

Chapter 8   Radiotherapy Treatment Centers/ Ambulatory Dimensions *139*

SUSAN WEISS BEHREND

Introduction	139
Radiation Treatment Centers: Ambulatory Oncology Models	141
Past Present Future Settings	142
Operational Structures of Radiation Oncology Centers	144
The Multidisciplinary Team	150
Ambulatory Radiation Oncology/Trajectory of Patient Care	179
Patient Education	187

Active Clinical Treatment/Special Considerations
  in Radiation Oncology   188
Conclusion   198
Appendix A   204

**Chapter 9   Hematopoietic Stem Cell Transplant
                 Outpatient Models** *211*

KIM SCHMIT-POKORNY

Introduction   211
Models of Outpatient Transplantation   212
Advantages and Disadvantages of Outpatient
  Transplantation   216
Patient Eligibility   217
Care Partner Selection   217
Patient and Care Partner Education   217
The Outpatient Program   218
Outpatient Transplant Process   220
Outcomes   224
Alternatives to Outpatient Transplantation:
  Cooperative Care   226
Conclusion   227

**Chapter 10   The Breast Cancer Clinic:
                 Yesterday, Today, and Tomorrow** *231*

CATHY COLEMAN

Introduction   231
Overview   231
Yesterday: The Courage to Change   232
Today: Getting Started, Staying Focused,
  and Achieving Growth   234
Tomorrow: The Courage to Lead   243

**Chapter 11   Managing Pain in Ambulatory
                 and Home Care** *247*

CAROL P. CURTISS

Introduction   247
Managing Pain in Ambulatory Care   248
Integrating Pain Management into Clinical Care   249
Pain Clinics, Centers, and Services   254
Conclusion   258

Chapter 12 **Palliative and Hospice Care Issues and Concepts in the Ambulatory Care Setting** *263*

KIM K. KUEBLER

Introduction	263
How Americans Are Dying	263
The Evolution of Palliative Care	265
Integrating Palliative Care	266
Palliative Care Assessment Tools	269
Hospice Care	271
Continuity and Coordination of Care	273
Conclusion	275

Chapter 13 **Oral and Dental Management for Cancer Patients** *279*

SHARON ELAD, JOEL B. EPSTEIN, CYRIL MEYEROWITZ, DOUGLAS E. PETERSON, AND MARK M. SCHUBERT

Introduction	279
The Treatment Team	279
Patient Care	280
Patient Evaluation and Assessment	281
Patient Education	287
Mucositis	291
Salivary Gland Dysfunction	298
Infection	299
GVHD	301

Chapter 14 **Pharmacy Issues in Ambulatory Oncology** *309*

VALORIE WILKINS

Introduction	309
The Role of the Pharmacist	309
Drug Distribution	313
Clinical Services	316
Evaluation of Pharmacy Services and Pharmaceutical Care	319
Conclusion	320
Appendix A	321
Appendix B	322
Appendix C	323

Chapter 15 Research and Clinical Trials in
Ambulatory Oncology Care 327
LINDA U. KREBS

Introduction   327
Historical Issues and Milestones   328
Overview of Clinical Research   328
Issues in Clinical Trial Participation   334
Nursing Roles and Responsibilities   342
Conclusion   346

Chapter 16 Symptom Management Programs: The Role of
the Nurse in Ambulatory Care 351
ANNA L. SCHWARTZ AND LILLIAN M. NAIL

Introduction   351
History   352
Issues in Developing Nurse-Run Symptom-Focused
   Clinics   352
The Future of Ambulatory Cancer Care   353

Chapter 17 Integrating Complementary and Alternative
Medicine Therapies into an Oncology
Practice: A Short History of Medicine 355
GEORGIA DECKER

Introduction   355
Strategies for CAM Program Development   361
Presenting Your CAM Proposal   373

Chapter 18 Community-Based Survivorship Programs 377
BARBARA J. MURPHY, CHRISTINE RIMKUS, AND BETSY PATTERSON

Impact of Cancer Diagnosis   378
History of Cancer Survivor Support Groups   379
Effectiveness of Support Groups   380
Emergence of Support/Survivor Groups   381
What Is a Support Group?   382
What Is a Survivor Group?   383
Types of Groups   383
Special Populations   387
Psychological Effects of Survivorship   390
Economic Issues   391
Insurance Coverage   392
Spirituality   392

Quality of Life 393
How to Establish a Survivor Group 393
The Internet as a Resource 397
Survivorship Issues 399
Late Effects of Cancer Treatment 399
Cardiac Effects 401
Reproductive Effects 402
Fatigue 404
Thyroid Dysfunction 404
Secondary Malignancies 405

Chapter 19   The Building of a Cancer-Related
Fatigue Clinic *413*

CARMEN P. ESCALANTE AND ROSALIE U. VALDRES

Introduction 413
CRF Clinic Objectives 414
CRF Clinic Profile 414
CRF Clinic Framework 414
CRF Clinic Patient Selection 416
CRF Clinic Assessment Packet 416
CRF Clinic Operations 417
CRF Clinic Wisdom 419

Chapter 20   The Future of Ambulatory Nursing in the
Oncology Setting *423*

CATHERINE GLENNON

Introduction 423
Aging 424
Generation Mix 424
Diversity 424
Terrorism 425
Impact on Oncology Nursing 425
Future 426
Nursing Shortage 426
Conclusion 429

INDEX 430

Preface

More than ten years ago, we published the first edition of *Oncology Nursing in the Ambulatory Setting*. That effort was written to guide oncology nurses and health care providers through the mazes of shifting care from the hospital setting to the outpatient area. That historic transition of care was sparked by efforts to lower health care costs by shortening or avoiding hospitalizations and by the increased ability to deliver sophisticated treatment outside of the hospital setting. The transition has now occurred as documented in that 90% of oncology care is delivered in the ambulatory care setting. The number of professional nurses working in this environment is growing accordingly, but at a time of the most critical nursing shortage in our nation's history. The economic and technical issues of several years ago remain constant today but are complicated by new social demographics, institution of evidence-based practice guidelines, and new generations of pharmaceutical agents.

Our nation's social demographics are now widely diversified, practice guidelines are more sophisticated and demanding, and research endeavors have developed novel agents to cure or extend a good life for survivors of cancer. We are an aging nation as well. Caring for an aging population having cancer as a chronic disease is now compounded with associated comorbid conditions such as cardiac, pulmonary, and other functional disorders, making increasing demands on professional health care givers. These patients comprise the largest population requiring health care. This number will escalate as aging "baby boomers" place further monetary constraints on an already challenged health care system. Health care goals now reach beyond the ultimate goal of cure to one of offering patients an extended quality of life that is acceptable to the patient. Our nation has also realized a marked increase in the diversity of cultures of Mexican, African, Latin American, and Asian origins. The impact of such diversification implies not only language barriers but communication styles, personal space issues, and unique cultural beliefs. All of these factors are now intergrated into an ambulatory care area that represents over 90% of oncology care given nationwide.

The skills demanded of the oncology nurse practicing in today's multidisciplinary setting barely resemble that of a decade ago and so it is that we offer a vastly revised second edition of our book. The first part of our book discusses administrative issues and resources to direct the nurse administrator to structure efficient, fiscally sound, and clinically relevant practice patterns. Included in these discussions are numerous strategies and skills to mirror today's ambulatory care setting. Information on harnessing the power of electronic resources to provide accurate and rapid information on administrative and clinical concepts is woven throughout the chapters.

Career options have emerged in concert with the changing face of ambulatory care oncology settings. To address the issues and challenges inherent in keeping pace with these new venues, chapters are included on instituting, developing, and utilizing these roles to their maximum potential. The roles of the advanced nurse practitioner/clinical nurse specialist and the triage nurse, although relatively new, are expanding at an exponential rate. A growing number of oncology nurses are now consultants to clinical settings, the pharmaceutical industry, and the legal system. They offer their skills in specific areas of disease or symptom management, particularly pain and fatigue. These issues are attended to in a number of chapters.

New clinical sites dedicated to specialty areas such as pain, fatigue, breast health, and symptom management have emerged. For example, our original chapter written on the practice of an oncology nurse in the physician's office bears no resemblance to today's fast-paced outpatient clinic administrator who may orchestrate the care for hundreds of patients a day. Infusion centers, day surgeries, radiation centers, and hematopoetic clinics are updated in this book. The concepts of hospice care and palliative care are now being recognized as similar entities that demand a chapter on creating outpatient care consistent with current thinking. The recognition of legitimate complementary and alternative approaches to cancer and its treatment prompted us to include a chapter on this subject. Finally, because we are a nation of a growing number of cancer survivors, a discussion on this important aspect of care has also been added.

It is our hope that we have provided a comprehensive and enduring guide and reference for oncology nurses and related cancer health care professionals to pursue excellence in oncology care.

Patricia C. Buchsel, RN, MSN, FAAN
Connie Henke Yarbro, RN, MS, FAAN

Chapter 1

Ambulatory Care Administrative Concepts: An Overview

Patricia Buchsel

Catherine Glennon

Introduction

It is estimated that 80 to 90% of care given to patients with cancer is delivered in the ambulatory care setting. The percentage of revenue generated by the traditional hospital setting has been reduced from 85% of total revenue to less than 50%, whereas ambulatory care revenues have in many settings risen to 50% or more of historical total revenue (Chitnis, 2001). Accordingly, there has been a shift of oncology nursing staff from the acute care setting to the ambulatory setting. Although the exact number of oncology nurses practicing in the outpatient setting is unknown, the Oncology Nursing Society (ONS) reports that almost 25% of its membership identify themselves as ambulatory care nurses (Bruce, 2003).

The shift of patient care from the inpatient to the ambulatory care setting has been spurred by economic, technological, and social shifts, all influencing diverse models of outpatient care. These shifts, with their inherent problems, have changed the way that administrators think and respond to developing new paradigms of practice. This chapter defines ambulatory care vis-a-vis the most pressing issues that administrators need to incorporate in developing, maintaining, or improving ambulatory care for patients with cancer.

Subsequent to a brief history of ambulatory care nursing, this chapter offers an overview of the current and future economic, technological, and social factors shaping the nation's burgeoning outpatient populations. The second part discusses emerging issues that successful oncology administrators needs to address for oversight of their respective outpatient areas. Finally, the third part offers an overview of the generic characteristics of the physical layout and accruements needed in the outpatient setting. The authors of other chapters in this book discuss their respective specialty areas relative to clinical practice and, where appropriate, their architectural requirements.

History of Ambulatory Care Nursing

The first professional nurses to care for patients with cancer in an ambulatory care setting were probably among those pioneers in the early part of the 20th century. Most nurses during 1900 and 1913 practiced as trained nurses for the wealthy or were public health nurses in settlement houses among the thousands of poor immigrants who were pouring into America. As these early nurses proved their worth in decreasing public health problems, administrative organizations began to flourish. The first public health nursing and visiting nurse associations were established in 1890; medical and nursing societies operated registries. In 1890, the first industrial nurses were employed by chocolate factories to assess "candy girls" for vermilion poisoning. Nurse leaders demanded organizations to establish consistent standards of practice in nursing school entry requirements, lengthened study programs; and raised the standards of nursing education. The next decades brought mandatory licensure laws, a Nurse Practice Act, and a National Council of State Boards of Nursing (Schorr & Kennedy, 1999).

The role of the oncology nurse changed radically during the later part of the 20th century. No more was the office-based nurse limited to welcoming patients and families to clinics, scheduling appointments, and changing the paper on examination tables (Nevidjon, 1993). As safer treatment agents and more effective supportive measures became available, the oncology nurse in ambulatory care became challenged with managing dramatically increasing numbers of patients with acute or chronic cancer. This era saw the traditional role of administering toxic chemotherapy and radiation, once reserved for the hospital setting, shift to the ambulatory care setting. The most challenging hurdle in developing and maintaining outpatient centers was the dearth of information that was available to build their programs. Those charged with creating these care settings worked in isolation because few guidelines or standards of care existed. Clinical guidelines, practice standards, billing systems, medical records organization, after-hours care, and any other issues were created on shifting inpatient practice guidelines to the ambulatory care setting. Challenges of retrofitting ambulatory care units from pre-existing unused buildings or hospital space to efficient, cost-effective areas to accommodate escalating numbers of patients called for creativity and a common-sense approach.

The emergence of ambulatory oncology care in the late 1990s led the ONS to publish results of national surveys of salary, staffing, and professional practice patterns in ambulatory care settings. These surveys provided oncology nurse administrators with the first meaningful data to use as a benchmark in creating ambulatory care administrative and practice issues (ONS, 1990, 1991, 1992). Concomitantly, the American Academy of Ambulatory Care Nurses (AAACN) was founded in response to the need to define nursing role dimensions in promoting wellness, preventing illness, and managing acute and chronic disease to affect the most attainable positive health status along the life span. The AAACN outlined the first conceptual framework to guide professional nurses in ambulatory settings (Hass, 1998).

Unlike those early administrators, current managers can make use of national guidelines and numerous resources to guide them in their pursuit of excellence in ambulatory care. For example, members of the National Comprehensive Cancer Center have collaborated on best practice standards; the Foundation for the Accreditation of Hematopoietic Cell Therapy (2002), has defined transplantation administrative and clinical practice issues and the Association of Community Cancer Centers (2002) has established over 25 standards for cancer programs. Professional nursing organizations such as the ONS (Itano & Taoka, 1998) and the American Academy of Ambulatory Nursing (Robinson, 2001) have outlined optimal care for the patient with cancer and his or her family in the ambulatory care setting (**Figure 1.1**) (ONS, 2002a).

Trends Supporting the Shift to Ambulatory Care

Economic Trends

Significant economic issues surrounding healthcare have led to the mass exodus from inpatient to outpatient settings. The economic or financial burden to meet the healthcare needs of our nation

Figure 1.1 ONS POSITION STATEMENT ON ONCOLOGY SERVICES IN THE AMBULATORY PRACTICE SETTING

It is the position of the ONS that

- Regardless of setting (i.e., clinic, office, or home) or intervention, patient safety must be the priority in planning and providing quality cancer care.
- Consent is obtained after patients are informed of the risks and benefits for all interventions and their impact on quality of life, including financial implications.
- Quality care for individuals with cancer is best accomplished by registered nurses who have been educated and certified in the oncology specialty.
- Patients and caregivers are given written and oral instructions and access to resources for self-care in preventing and managing side effects from cancer and/or its treatment.
- The patient–staff mix promotes a hazard-free, safe, and therapeutic environment.
- Personnel are responsible for documenting the care provided and processing accurate codes for services rendered.
- Use of medication and chemotherapy requires that
  - Personnel prepare and handle all antineoplastic medications in accordance with ONS and Occupational Safety and Health Administration guidelines. Personnel who administer chemotherapy and biotherapy should successfully complete the ONS Chemotherapy Course.
  - An appropriate emergency response can be readily activated, and all clinical staff are certified in basic life support.
  - Emergency medications (e.g., epinephrine, atropine, diphenhydramine) are readily available for use.
  - Guidelines appropriate for providing quality oncology nursing care are written and followed for the management of cardiac/respiratory arrest, anaphylactic reaction, fluid overload, hypertension and hypotension, seizures, extravasations, chemical spills, and other emergency sequelae that may occur.
  - Before infusion of medication, a registered nurse who has demonstrated competency in oncology nursing assesses patients and family members for
    o Their ability to identify and report untoward or adverse effects
    o Their provision of self-care
    o Their willingness to participate in and follow the treatment plan
  - Patients receiving continuous infusion therapy have a vascular access device in place and either are under the care or supervision of a home infusion service that follows these guidelines or have 24-hour access to ambulatory/office professional staff.
- Use of conscious sedation requires that
  - Written guidelines and policies are followed.
  - State, governmental, and Joint Commission on Accreditation of Healthcare Organization (2002) regulations are enforced. Only practitioners who have demonstrated competency may administer conscious sedation.
  - Oxygen and reversal medications (e.g., naloxone) are readily available for use. Monitoring of the patient is done before, during, and after the procedure and are documented. Education is provided to the patient and family, and discharge occurs when specific written criteria are met.
  - Ongoing assessment is closely maintained by registered nurses who have demonstrated competency.
  - When state regulations have not been developed to guide staff mix, advanced cardiac life support certification is the preferred level of emergency competencies.

Procedures and/or interventions not listed require strict adherence to policy, procedure, and guidelines that are in agreement with the standards of ONS.

ONS Position Statement on Oncology Service in Ambulatory Practice Setting, 2002. Reprinted with permission.
http://www.ons.org/xp6/ONS/Information.xml/journals_and_positions.sml/ambulatorypractice.xml.

has given rise to the creation of novel care settings to lessen the costs of care. The nature of our current healthcare system is one of insufficient funding to deliver affordable heathcare to a large number of U.S. citizens. It is estimated that by the year 2008 our country's healthcare spending will surpass $2.3 trillion, representing 15% of the nation's gross domestic product (Heffler et al., 2001). Currently, $115 billion is spent annually in the care of the cancer patient, and $4 billion is spent annually for research (National Coalition in Cancer Research, 2004). In spite of this stupendous dollar amount, almost 41-million individuals in the nation's population have no insurance coverage (National Coalition in Cancer Research, 2004).

Technological Advances

Changes in treatment and supportive care therapies have contributed significantly to burgeoning outpatient numbers. Revolutionary advances in biotechnology have created novel approaches to cure cancer or extend quality of life years to thousands of patients. Cancer vaccines, targeted therapies, and oral chemotherapies are now in clinical trials and in standard practice, allowing treatment to be given almost exclusively in outpatient settings; however, these shifts present conflicting dilemmas for the outpatient administrator. There may be a reduction of nursing time to administer targeted oral chemotherapies, but the management of dose-dense chemotherapy protocols requires intensive nursing time. For example, gefitinib is a new oral agent that isolates and destroys selected epithelial tumors while sparing healthy tissue. Adverse effects are minimal, and patients are assessed monthly in the clinic and monitored in their homes via telephone consultation. In contrast to targeted therapies, patients receiving dose-dense therapies treatment require concentrated nursing time for patient education, chemotherapy administration, symptom management, and follow-up care by telecommunications.

Improvements in supportive care agents include granisetron for nausea, darbepoetin alfa for cancer-related anemia, and pegfilgrastim for prevention and treatment of infection; a further decrease in nursing time. As technology becomes even more sophisticated, outpatient arenas will continue to serve all but the most critical patients.

Social Shifts

AN AGING POPULATION

America is an aging nation, leading to a new profile of cancer patients and their family caregivers. The increasing number of patients living with cancer as a chronic disease has been a driving force in increasing the need for outpatient space. The average life expectancy increased by more than 30 years in the 20th century. Currently, people over 65 years of age account for the largest growing population. By 2050, people older than 80 are expected to make up 36% of the population (Holmes & Muss Hyman, 2003; Mafrica et al., 2002). Over 1 million American's are diagnosed with cancer, and over 500,000 will die of this disease annually. Most of these older citizens with cancer, as well as with other healthcare diseases, will swell the ranks of an already overflowing and understaffed healthcare system. Older patients often have comorbid diseases that exacerbate their cancer symptoms. Dodd, Miaskowski, West, Paul, and Lee (2002) studied oncology outpatients to determine the prevalence of pain, fatigue, and sleep disturbances and to determine the prevalence of a higher number of comorbid conditions. In addition to cancer symptom clusters, outpatients reported comorbid conditions such as back problems (65.2%), allergies (58.5%), headaches (50.5%), hemorrhoids (46.3%), arthritis (33.3%), and hypertension (30.4%) (Dodd et al., 2002). Caregivers, who are essential to the success of outpatient programs, are often afflicted with chronic disease themselves. For example, treatment protocols such as the "mini" transplant, which is given almost exclusively in outpatient settings, are designed for patients who cannot tolerate high doses of chemotherapy and irradiation. Caregivers are responsible for a large part of patients care, including symptom management, medication administration, and physical care. Donors are also often older, thus requiring additional care than those in the myeloablative setting. Oncology nurses who are practicing in these areas now manage general disease entities such as diabetes and cardiovascular, pulmonary, and orthopedic diseases that are often seen in the older person (Chouinard, 2003; Groff, 2004; Schmit-Pokorny, Franco, Frappier, & Vyhlidah, 2003). To address some of these issues, the ONS has recently updated their position on care of the older population (**Figure 1.2**).

Perhaps one the most unanticipated changes in the healthcare industry is the impact of the shift-

ing cultural profile of the nation's population. For example, in 2000, approximately 12.5% of the total U.S. population was comprised of Hispanics. Approximately 67,000 new cancer cases are expected to be diagnosed among Hispanics in 2003 (O'Brien et al., 2003); and providing culturally sensitive healthcare to diverse groups is a growing mandate for healthcare workers that will significantly impact the care provided by ambulatory care nurses. The demographics of the U.S. population have realized a marked increase in the diversity of cultures of Mexican, African, Latin American, and Asian origins. Not only do language barriers exist among nationalities, but cultural phenomena, barriers to healthcare, time and environmental control, communication style, per-

---

Figure 1.2 ONCOLOGY NURSING SOCIETY AND GERIATRIC ONCOLOGY CONSORTIUM: JOINT POSITION ON CANCER CARE IN THE OLDER ADULT

It is the position of ONS and the Generic Oncology Consortium (GOC) that care of older adults with cancer requires the following:
- Elimination of ageism in research, education, care, and public policy, as it stands against core American values of autonomy and choice
- Education of students and practicing clinicians across health disciplines in both oncology and older person care on the unique physiological, developmental, psychological, emotional, social, and spiritual needs of older adults with cancer and their families
- Incorporation of measurement of age beyond chronological to include biological, functional, and personal dimensions
- Acknowledgment of and assessment for risks related to declining functional reserve as part of normal aging
- Redefinition of optimal outcomes to extend beyond disease-free survival and to include comorbidity, function, and quality of life
- Full and equal access to cancer care across the trajectory (e.g., screening, diagnosis, treatment, rehabilitation, palliative care, survivorship, and wellness care)
- Interdisciplinary teams and comprehensive geriatric assessment to optimize treatment planning, access, and resulting outcomes
- Integration of geriatric oncology care within and across care settings and delivery systems, including primary care, acute and critical care, and long-term institutional and home care and hospice
- Increased funding for basic, clinical, and translational research in aging and cancer.
- Improved education, outreach, and incentives for older adults to participate in clinical research
- Advocacy, policy, and legislation that recognizes the demographic implications of aging and cancer and mandates necessary research and development of appropriate health and social services

Used with permission. ONS (in press). Oncology Nursing Society and Geriatric Oncology Consortium Joint Position on Cancer Care in the Older Adult.

sonal space issues, and social organization also exist (Itano, 1998). As these and more culturally diverse patients demand care for their cancers, outpatient areas will need to accommodate multi-lineage nurses.

THE NURSING SHORTAGE

Ambulatory administrators, until recently, have faired better than their inpatient counterparts relative to staff recruitment and retention. Oncology nurses view the ambulatory setting to be as challenging but not as stressful as inpatient units. As the nursing shortage worsens, ambulatory care settings are being faced with vacant positions. Administrators need to lobby for improving work environments that will not only recruit but also retain qualified nurses by ensuring them a quality work life. Providing flexible work schedules, ensuring safe practice areas, and offering onsite child care, exercise programs, onsite continued certification education programs, competitive salaries, and re-entry programs for those nurses who have not practiced in the work place over a period of time are essential. Administrators can insist that mandatory overtime is not required, that lunch and break time are honored, and that a voice in decisions concerning the provision of care in the workplace is heard. The ONS has issued a position statement on the impact of the nursing shortage that administrators can use as a framework for insisting on sufficient budgetary allotments for quality care and quality of life for nurses (**Figure 1.3**) (ONS, 2002b). Because ambulatory care in the oncology setting has matured, it is now possible to characterize the scope of nursing practice.

Ambulatory Care Defined

Historically, ambulatory care is defined as a clinic or office practice setting and is most often affiliated with regional cancer centers or large hospitals (Hass, 1998). Chapter 6 also offers an overview on ambulatory care sites and nursing practice. Once reserved for stable patients with little symptomatology and for those requiring little supportive care, ambulatory care has now emerged as a dynamic, fast-paced, comprehensive system, once reserved for the hospital setting that has the organizational, professional, and clinical competencies to care for patients and their families. In addition to the changing pace of ambulatory care settings, the nature of the oncologic services rendered has expanded to highly specialized settings such as the following:

- Surgical oncology
- Radiation oncology
- Prevention and early detection of cancer
- Cancer risk assessment, screening, and diagnosis
- Specific cancer centers (i.e., breast health, prostate cancer)
- Hematopoietic stem cell transplantation
- Long-term follow-up
- Genetic counseling
- Psychologic oncology
- Nutrition clinics
- Dental clinics
- Nurse-managed clinics

The defining characteristics of current oncology outpatient settings are those with the following:

- High patient volume to nurse ratios
- A high volume of patient phone calls
- High numbers of procedures or treatments
- Increased 24-hour responsibility for after-hours care
- Coordination of consultations with multiple clinicians
- Difficulty in determining staffing hours and patient ratios
- Increased need for patient education within a limited timeframe
- Multiple interactions among diverse healthcare settings, such as readmission to inpatient services, skilled care, home care, hospice care, and multidiscipline collaboration

- New nursing roles (i.e., triage nursing, research protocol coordinators) (Hass, 1998)

Chapters 6 and 8 have a more complete discussion of these issues.

New Issues in Ambulatory Care

Nursing administrators in ambulatory care units have long been challenged by traditional issues of space requirements, escalating patient populations, staffing issues, and economic survival. A growing body of literature addresses classic management concerns and considerations (Buchsel & Whedon, 1995; Buchsel & Yarbro, 1993; Mayer, Madden, & Lawrenz, 1990). This section of the chapter emphasizes the current needs that man-

date critical attention and timely solutions to escalating healthcare issues. These include establishing programs that not only focus on the bricks and mortar of ambulatory care but incorporate new mandates aimed at economic survival, management of new technology, and patient safety and patient education, all attended to in a healthcare environment of a major nursing shortage. Economic constraints caused by the overall cost of cancer care demand a new approach to capturing revenues for nursing services that were heretofore denied. Examples of nursing services that consume hours that are not reimbursed by third-party payers are patient education programs and follow-up care such as patient compliance.

A recent survey that the ONS conducted sought to identify current nursing issues in ambulatory care. Respondents were asked to

---

Figure 1.3 THE IMPACT OF THE NATIONAL NURSING SHORTAGE ON QUALITY CANCER CARE

It is the position of the ONS that
- The shortage of nurses seriously jeopardizes quality cancer care, to which all citizens have a right.
- Professional nursing organizations should enact programs individually and collectively to address the nursing shortage.
- ONS will actively contribute to building the long-term infrastructure for nursing by taking specific actions to attract people to and retain them in nursing. Such actions include participation in the Nurses for a Healthier Tomorrow (2001) program (a campaign launched by a coalition of 24 nursing and healthcare organizations to attract people to the nursing profession) and internship programs as well as seeking appropriate legislation.
- The ONS will work to attract nurses to oncology nursing by providing opportunities to learn more about oncology nursing, by completing research studies that examine the oncology nursing workforce, and by providing job shadowing and mentoring opportunities.

Legislation
- The employment of immigrant nurses may be regarded as one of many solutions to the nursing shortage problem, provided that immigrant nurses meet U.S. standards, that we do not disadvantage their countries of origin by employing them, and that the country builds an infrastructure to supply nurses within the United States to meet the growing demand.
- Federal programs, such as loan repayments and tax incentives, should be created to provide people with motivation to enter the nursing profession, to reimburse them for doing so, and to require them to work in geographic areas with underserved populations.
- Federal and state legislation enacting loan repayment programs is needed to fund scholarships for those currently in nursing who wish to advance their levels of education.

(continues)

Figure 1.3 THE IMPACT OF THE NATIONAL NURSING SHORTAGE ON QUALITY CANCER CARE (CONT'D)

- Nursing schools must receive adequate funding to recruit and retain faculty so that qualified applicants will not be denied admission because of a lack of faculty or space.
- Innovative legislation must ensure that the reimbursement model applied to graduate medical schools is applied to public and private graduate nursing schools.
- Direct Medicare and Medicaid reimbursements and reimbursements by private payors and Health Maintenance Organizations should be made for advanced-practice nursing services whether they are provided within an outpatient or inpatient care setting.

Education
- Programs should be developed and funded to encourage young people and minorities to enter the nursing profession. One such program could be an initiative to produce public-service announcements that accurately and positively portray the profession of nursing.
- Innovative programming should be initiated at primary and secondary school levels to encourage nursing as a career choice.
- More oncology content should be incorporated into nursing-school curricula, and more creative ways are needed to educate nurses, such as distance learning.
- Academic and healthcare institutions should collaborate on initiatives, such as innovative internship and mentorship programs, to help resolve the nursing shortage.

Workplace Environment
- Improvements in the work environment are needed to ensure a quality work life for nurses. Such improvements include providing nontraditional and flexible work schedules, ensuring ergonomically acceptable work environments, making on-site child care available to accommodate evening shifts, and establishing reentry programs for nurses who have been out of the workforce.
- Healthcare institutions should address and resolve stressful, negative workplace issues, such as mandatory overtime, inadequate salaries, and nurses' lack of voice in decisions concerning the provision of care.
- Research grants should be created to assess model programs that restructure the current healthcare environment, to make the most efficient use of all healthcare professionals' skills, and to evaluate nursing contributions to health care in general and cancer care specifically.
- Systems should be developed to routinely monitor outcomes of hospital patient care that are sensitive to nursing and nurse staffing.

Reprinted with permission. Oncology Nursing Society, 2002. The Impact of the National Nursing Shortage on Quality Cancer Care.

describe their responsibilities and key concerns related to their practice (**Tables 1.1** and **1.2**). Based on these concerns, oncology nurses may find several tools that may help them in their daily practice. A heightened awareness of the ONS position statement such as **Figure 1.5** and knowledge of published ambulatory care staffing tools (**Figures 1.6** and **1.7**) can provide support to the oncology nurses seeking solutions to critical issues in their practice setting. Additional areas of support from ONS and other educational venues

include information on new cancer therapies, evidence-based guidelines, and practice standards. Not surprising, the nurses requested the ONS to provide educational programs about new cancer therapies, evidence-based guidelines and practice standards, and assistance with the issues of the nursing shortage.

Patient Safety

One of the most sensitive areas of concern in today's healthcare setting is patient safety.

Table 1.1 Issues in Ambulatory Oncology Nursing Practice

	N (%) Respondents
Clinical Care	
Practiced across state lines	19%
Routinely mixed chemotherapy agents	40%
Transcribed handwritten chemotherapy orders from physicians	63%
Telephone Triage	
Utilized an assessment guide	19%
Utilized a telephone documentation form	93%
Patient Education	
Have primary responsibility for patient education for disease process,	96%
procedures, treatment and side effects, and symptom management.	84%
Primary responsibility for orientation of patients to clinic	
Billing for the patient education was not supported in their practice	75%
Physician Delegation	
RN administered intrathecal chemotherapy	11%
RN performed invasive procedures	5%
Palliative Care	
MD or PA had primarily responsible for transferring and managing	60%
patients to palliative care	
Viewed palliative care as an RN responsibility	70%
Staffing	
Lacked staffing tools	80%
Clinical Trials	
Involved in clinical trials	86%
Employed clinical trial nurses	75%
Reimbursement	
Involved in billing	74%
Obtained drugs for indigent patients	49%
Reviewed patient charges for accuracy	39%
Legislative Issues and Policies	
Had no involvement with legislative issues	39%
Nursing Shortage	
Hired less experienced nurses	50%
Had open positions available	47%
Nursing Role in Outcomes	
Stated that their interventions frequently prevented hospital admissions	64%
Stated they frequently decreased cost of care	62%
Frequently improved patient's quality of life	84%
Frequently improved quality of care	88%
Frequently increased patient and family satisfaction	92%
Frequently increased their own job satisfaction	80%

Data reprinted with permission from the Oncology Nursing Society, "ONS Ambulatory/Office Nurse Survey Steering Council Report" – Internal Document – September 2002. ONS retains the copyright for the information included in this table.

Table 1.2 KEY AREAS TO IMPROVE WITHIN AMBULATORY ONCOLOGY NURSING PRACTICE

	N (%) Respondents
More time for patient education	59%
Salary and benefits	47%
Professional development	45%
Staffing	37%
Recognition of the importance of patient education	36%
Support for the expanded role of the ambulatory nurse	31%
Lack of standardized documents across practice settings	31%
Duplication of documentation	27%
Aspects of care delegated from MD to nurse	13%
Aspects of care delegated to Licensed Practical Nurses and unlicensed personnel	8%

Data reprinted with permission from the Oncology Nursing Society, "ONS Ambulatory/Office Nurse Survey Steering Council Report" – Internal Document – September 2002. ONS retains the copyright for the information included in this table.

Patients are entitled to safe environments that protect them from medical errors and from harm caused by a lack of a physically safe environment, such as poorly working medical equipment. Patients being cared for in ambulatory care settings are at great risk for numerous factors that effect patient safety. Those who are at risk are those who are older, those with declining cognitive status, and those with physiologic functional and nutritional impairment. Those who are receiving or who have received chemotherapy agents such as vincristine, vinblastine, taxanes, cisplatin iphosphamide, high-dose cytarabine, and high cyclophosphamide may have neurotoxic symptoms, predisposing them to falls (Holley, 2002). Pain and its accompanied distresses have been shown to have a negative impact on patients receiving care in ambulatory care clinics. Wells, Murphy, Wujcik, and Johnson (2003) examined the unique and combined effects of pain intensity, pain-related distress, analgesic prescription, and negative mood on interference with daily life and noted that ambulatory care patients experienced not only pain but also pain-related distress. The researchers noted the important role of ambulatory care nurses to search for methods to alleviate

pain-related stressors. Research in the area of designing safe and efficient clinics for patients with pain is essential to the well-being of thousands of patients with cancer.

Recent reports have raised the awareness of the growing number of medication errors in hospital settings, but few studies have illustrated the scope and impact of medical errors occurring in ambulatory care settings. Gandhi et al. (2003) performed a prospective cohort study at four adult primary care practices involving 1,202 outpatients. Of the 661 patients who responded to the survey, 162 had adverse drug events, with a total of 181 events. Twenty-four of the events were serious. Fifty-one were ameliorable, and 20% were preventable. Of the 51 ameliorable events, 32 were noted to be the physician's failure to respond to medication-related symptoms and 10 to the patient's failure to inform the physician of adverse symptoms. The researchers concluded that monitoring by healthcare providers could greatly reduce this number of errors.

The Institute of Medicine recently published the results of a study examining the role of nursing in medication errors. This report, "Keeping Patient Safe: Transforming the Work Environment of the Nurse," expands on previous Institute of Medicine reports aimed at improving patient safety. The study committee was composed of experts in patient safety, nursing, healthcare quality, engineering, operations research, multidisciplinary team practices, human factors, industrial psychology, and communications. The study found that nurses, who now constitute 54% of the nation's health providers, may make fewer errors in medicine management if their work environment was improved. A major finding was that nurses who work over 12 consecutive hours were at risk for making medical mistakes related to fatigue. Further advantages of reducing nurse's hours are increased in patient safety and patient education programs (2003).

Thus, the key to today's challenges is for nurse leaders to work with their hospital administrative colleagues to bring about an environment that fosters quality nursing leadership, includes nursing as an integral part of the executive management team, designs policies and programs that involve nurses in shared decision making, improves quality outcomes, and places the necessary high value on nurses as essential to the health and well-being of the patient and the community (Rutledge, 2004). Nurses, when empowered and properly supported, can ensure the safety of the work environment, not only for patients under their care, but also for the entire healthcare team. The report also stresses the importance of leadership and the need for directed resources to support the educational and training needs of the nursing staff. Recommendations particular to improving ambulatory nurses' working conditions and patient safety included the following:

1. Establish policies to prevent nurses who provide direct patient care from working longer than 12 hours in a 24-hour period and more than 60 hours per 7 days.
2. Schools of nursing, state boards of nursing, and healthcare organizations should educate nurses about the threat to patient safety that fatigue causes.

3. Redesign of nursing workplaces to create time-saving measures and maximum efficiency.
4. Place nurse leaders/managers in executive decision-making positions that can represent the interest of nursing staff and improve communication between nurses, physicians, and other healthcare professionals.

Other organizations are addressing the issue of patient safety. In January 2003, all Joint Commission of Association of Hospital Organizations (JCAHO)-accredited healthcare organizations began to be surveyed for implementation of the specific recommendations, or acceptable alternatives, in ambulatory care settings (**Table 1.3**) (**Figure 1.4**) (ONS, 2002c).

One of the most crucial administrative responsibilities in patient and staff safety is to define institutional responsibilities relative to the preparation, administration, and disposal of antineoplastic agents. The ONS has written a position statement to guide administrators on educating the professional nurse who administers chemotherapy or biotherapy (**Figure 1.5**) (ONS, 2002d). Chapter 11 offers a thorough discussion of administrative considerations when planning chemotherapy infusion space and implementing practice considerations (**Figure 1.8**).

Patient/Caregiver Education

Patient education and patient safety are the cornerstones of achieving excellence in patient outcomes. One does not exist independent of the other. The ultimate goal of patient education is to assure safe, positive clinical outcomes while minimizing stress for the family and assuring the cost-effectiveness of the educational programs (Bodenheimer, Lorig, Holman, & Grumbach, 2003). Without adequate patient education, hospital admissions are increased, and clinical staff is overextended; patients view their treatment as unsuccessful and fear the economic sequelae.

Table 1.3 JOINT COMMISSION OF ACCREDITATION HOSPITAL ORGANIZATION SAFE PRACTICE STANDARDS FOR AMBULATORY CARE

Improve the accuracy of patient identification.

1. Use at least two patient identifiers whenever taking blood samples or administering medications or blood products.

2. Before the start of any surgical or invasive procedure, conduct a final verification process, such as a "time out," to confirm the correct patient, procedure, and site, using active communication techniques.

Improve the effectiveness of communication among caregivers.

1. Implement a process for taking verbal or telephone orders that require verification "read back" of the complete order by the person receiving the order.

2. Standardize the abbreviations, acronyms, and symbols used throughout the organization, including a list of abbreviations, acronyms, and symbols.

Improve the safety of using high-alert medications.

1. Remove concentrated electrolytes (including, but not limited to, potassium chloride, potassium phosphate, sodium chloride of more than 0.9%) from patient care units (JCAHO safety goals).

2. Standardize and limit the number of drug concentrations available in the organization.

Improve the safety of using infusion pumps.

1. Ensure free-flow protection on all general-use and patient-controlled analgesia intravenous infusion pumps used in the organization.

Improve the effectiveness of clinical alarm systems.

1. Implement regular preventive maintenance and testing of alarm systems.

2. Assure that alarms are activated with appropriate settings and are sufficiently audible with respect to distances and competing noise within the unit.

© *Joint Commission on Accreditation of Healthcare Organizations, 2004. Reprinted with permission.*

Finally, the cost of care to the institution escalates. Careful planning with the healthcare team is essential to have meaningful and seamless programs that embrace these critical components. Strategies to assure quality education programs include detailed orientations of how to use the resources of the clinic and implementation of patient education programs that are aimed at self-care.

Patient and family orientation to outpatient functions can set the tone of the patient's entire clinical experience. Orientation to the physical layout of the clinic removes some stress from an already overwhelmed patient. Gallant and Coutts (2003) evaluated a new patient orientation program in a cancer center to determine the extent to which the orientation program was successful.

The education program was designed to provide patients with information about the centers' facilities and procedures, to offer opportunities to ask questions, and to discuss their personal concerns. The objectives of the study were to determine whether patients valued the orientation program and to judge whether the program altered the patients' self-reported emotional state. A total of 213 of 330 questionnaires (64.5%) were completed and returned. Study results showed that the patients were extremely satisfied with the program because it assisted them in being able to deal with their first visit and increased their feeling of relaxation and comfort. The researchers determined that the use of information and support interventions could improve cancer care

---

Figure 1.4 ONS POSITION ON THE PREVENTION AND REPORTING OF MEDICATION ERRORS

It is the position of the ONS that
* Institutions and state and national organizations must provide ongoing education to employees and members regarding medication errors and ways known to prevent errors.
* Nursing licensing and certifying bodies must incorporate questions on their licensing and certification exams to ensure professional competencies related to the prevention of medication errors.
* Healthcare facilities and agencies must provide education for the public regarding the role of the patient in preventing medication errors. Each institution also should inform the public of the programs that it has in place to prevent errors.
* Computerized technology related to medication ordering, dispensing, and administration must be developed that addresses the unique needs of the patient with cancer. Continued monitoring of the use of such technology in preventing errors must be maintained.
* Oncology care settings must standardize the kinds of equipment used for the administration of medications to patients with cancer (e.g., volumetric infusion pumps). In addition, equipment with safety features must be used (e.g., free-flow prevention).
* Pharmacists must be consulted for their valuable expertise and should be included in patient care rounds.
* Patient information must be available at the site of patient care.
* Healthcare practitioners and institutions must develop systematic processes for identifying and reviewing medication errors. These processes must be supported from the practitioner caring for patients to the top administrator. Punitive actions within these processes must be eliminated to allow the openness of discussion regarding the errors, with the ultimate goal of establishing the safest system possible.
* Systems for analyzing medication errors must be established within each healthcare institution and care setting at the state and national levels. Collaborative efforts between institutions, states, and agencies should be maximized to optimize this analysis process and to develop comprehensive systems for preventing errors.
* Voluntary error reporting must be established as the national standard. This system must be nonpunitive, focus on the prevention of medical errors, and establish confidentiality as an absolute standard. The primary goal of such a system should be the improvement and enhancement of patient safety.
* Federal protections of individuals reporting medication errors would strengthen the ability to collect a comprehensive and solution-oriented database. Federal law, although necessary to ensure protection associated with national reporting systems, should not preempt state evidentiary laws that provide greater protections.
* Research related to measures to reduce medication errors effectively must be supported, with the ultimate goal of fostering improvement in patient safety.

ONS Position Statement on the Prevention and Reporting of Medication Errors (2002).

(2003). Printed educational resources are available and should be used (Yarbro, Frogge, & Goodman, 2004) (**Figure 1.9**). An example of a patient self-care teaching tool on ascites for the patient with fluid and electolyte imbalances. The ONS also provides the patient information and educational resources on the ONS web page (2004).

Patient compliance with self-care is largely dependent on the family or friend of the patient,

---

Figure 1.5 ONS POSITION STATEMENT ON THE EDUCATION OF THE PROFESSIONAL REGISTERED NURSE WHO ADMINISTERS AND CARES FOR THE INDIVIDUAL RECEIVING CHEMOTHERAPY AND BIOTHERAPY

Specialized preparation of the professional registered nurse can ensure a safe level of care for the individual receiving chemotherapy. This statement defines the position of the ONS regarding the preparation of the professional registered nurse who administers chemotherapy and cares for these patients.

The 2001 ONS Chemotherapy and Biotherapy Guidelines and Recommendations for Practice describes basic didactic content and clinical experiences necessary for the preparation of the professional registered nurse to care for individuals across treatment settings. Course content includes the following:

- A cancer review covering tumor cell kinetics and angiogenesis
- The drug development process
- Principles of cancer chemotherapy, biotherapy, and immunotherapy
- Pharmacology of cytotoxic agents
- Drug administration, as well as administration schedule, dose determinations, drug response, and drug delivery systems
- Administration procedure
- Safe practice considerations
- Mixing, storage, and labeling of chemotherapeutic agents
- Side effects, as well as principles of management and patient education

Educational courses, such as the ONS Chemotherapy and Biotherapy Course, that meet these requirements prepare professional registered nurses to perform behaviors that can then be evaluated.

It is the position of the ONS that

The use of the contents of this publication will provide the necessary didactic information to administer cytotoxic drugs safely and competently. Successful completion of the didactic portion must be followed by the successful completion of a clinical practicum under the auspices of the nurses' institution or sponsoring agency.

ONS Board of Directors Approved 1992, July 1997, June 1999, November 2002.

---

particularly in the ambulatory care setting. Although the patient is often the focus of the healthcare provider, the family caregivers are at risk for physical and emotional sequela resulting from caregiver burden. As the number of accessible caregivers dwindles because of their own chronic illness, economic burdens, and family and workplace demands, oncology outpatient facilities need to provide access to appropriate, timely, and ongoing education and training so that caregivers can fulfill their responsibility and be advocates to their loved ones.

Evidence-Based Practice: A Must

The best practice guidelines are rapidly becoming a standard of care in the healthcare setting. These standards are based on treatment models that use evidence-based medicine, evidence-based practice, or research use. Evidence-based medicine is the "conscientious, explicit, and judicious use of current best evidence in making decisions about care of individual patients" (Sackett & Rosenberg, 1995). DePalma (2003) defined evidence-based practice as "a total process beginning with knowing what clinical questions to ask, how to find the best practice, and how to critically appraise the evidence for validity and applicability to the particular care situation." Research use refers to the review and critique of scientific research, and then the application of the findings to clinical practice. Evidence-based models have been created by the National Comprehensive Cancer Center and other notable cancer centers. Several Internet evidence-based models are available and have search capabilities and extensive annotated links/lists of other resources (DePalma, 2003).

To improve patient care further, the ONS is embarking on the concept of nursing-sensitive outcomes. Nursing-sensitive outcomes are those that are significantly impacted by nursing interventions. The interventions need to be within the scope of nursing practice and an integral of the process of nursing. Nursing-sensitive outcomes address symptoms, psychologic distress, function, and economics of specific outcomes. These may include but are not limited to fatigue, insomnia, nausea, constipation, anorexia, breathlessness, diarrhea, altered skin/mucous membranes, and neutropenia (Given et al., 2003). Administrators in an ambulatory care setting need to keep pace with this evolution and begin to incorporate nursing-sensitive outcomes in their clinics. If successful in improving patient care while being economically sound, they may assist with reimbursement fees that are not currently recognized.

Effective Triage Nursing

The growth of ambulatory care has created new roles and responsibilities for oncology nursing. A prime example is the role of the triage nurse who has become responsible for directing escalating numbers of patients with numerous symptoms and treatments to appropriate supportive care. Triaging of patients for medical care is an age-old practice. The word triage is derived from the French *trier*, meaning "to sort." The triage nurse may be dedicated to assessing patients during clinic hours by phone or assessing those who arrive without appointments. The concept of pri-

oritizing medical attention to those most likely to survive was practiced in France in the early 1800s but now extends to disasters such as war, earthquakes, battlefield settings, and large-scale accidents. The role of the triage nurse is now extended to patient education and follow-up care. The AAACN has outlined expectations for the triage nurse (Espensen, 2001).

1. Confers with patient on creating plans of care
2. Assessment performed through telecommunication in lieu of a physician assessment
3. Gives guidance to the patient or patient caregiver
4. Educates the patients on care issues
5. Evaluates patient's knowledge and ability to carry out instructions
6. Uses the nursing process for assessments
7. Understands the triage guidelines and algorithms
8. Can direct the patient to the correct treatment setting (inpatient services, emergency room care, next-day clinic appointment, etc.)
9. Evaluates plan of care

Cost-Effectiveness

The healthcare program that goes forth without critical attention to cost-effectiveness is rare. Although oncology nurses know that they contribute to the cost-effectiveness of patient care, few data exist to support this theory. A recent telephone survey to oncology centers to query reimbursement practices for triage or patient education found that of those surveyed, none were able to charge for the oncology nurse's time for triage or patient education time (Susan Newton, personal communication, February 4, 2004).

A growing number of companies now market triage programs to healthcare providers. Initially, these commercial entities developed services to assist large health maintenance organizations and other health plans. These systems usually rely on computers with huge medical information databases to guide nurses, provide consistency, and standardize quality (Derlet, 2003). Because of the specialty of oncology practice, nursing administrators considering commercial entities are challenged to scrutinize the clinical experiences, level of nursing expertise, liability components, and procedures of these programs.

Legal Issues

The scope of patient acuity in the ambulatory oncology setting requires 24-hour responsibility with legal issues that are consistent with hospital settings. A discussion of the myriad of legal issues in the ambulatory arena is beyond the scope of this chapter. Perhaps the most worrisome legal issue is the documentation of triage and after-hours care. Careful documentation, particularly with triage content, must be concise and accurate and must conform to the institution's standards of care. Adherence to written standards of care is a nursing responsibility and can be used in a court of law if needed (Anastasia, 2002).

Nursing Leadership

Leadership skills in the ambulatory setting are critical, as the nurse manager/leader oversees the care of increasing volumes of patients and families. Positive changes in patient flow and patient care are impacted by the leader's knowledge of program planning, evaluation, inquiry, and research. In addition to the knowledge, skills for implementation of evidence-based research and best practices are required. Collaboration is a key element of leadership. Collaboration occurs with many different constituents at multiple levels and about multiple issues within and outside the organization. Three specific roles have been identified as critical components of nursing leadership. These are an organization/systems role, a professional role, and a clinical nursing role. Responsibilities identified under each role are as follows (Hass, 1998):

Organization/Systems Role:
1. Practice/office support
2. Fiscal management
3. Communication, collaboration, and conflict management
4. Informatics
5. Context of care delivery models
6. Care of the caregiver
7. Priority management/delegation/supervision
8. Cross-cultural competencies
9. Entrepreneurial skills
10. Building customer-focused systems
11. Meeting workplace regulatory compliance
12. Advocacy in the organization and in the community
13. Legal issues
14. Workload

Professional Role:
1. Evidence-based practice
2. Leadership inquiry and research use
3. Clinical quality improvement
4. Staff development
5. Regulatory compliance
6. Patient self-care
7. Ethics

Clinical Nursing Role:
1. Patient education
2. Advocacy
3. Care management
4. Assess, screen, triage
5. Telephone nursing practice
6. Collaboration/resource identification and referral
7. Clinical procedures, independent/interdependent/dependent
8. Primary, secondary, and tertiary prevention
9. Communication/documentation
10. Outcome management
11. Protocol development usage

The oncology administrator can use this comprehensive blueprint along with the standards and guidelines outlined by other professional organizations cited in this chapter to organize, implement, and direct the ambulatory care center's mission, vision, and operational plan.

Many leadership theories also exist that can guide the leader in the ambulatory setting. Newer leadership theories assume situational instability and focus on the human relationship building process to provide stability. Transformational leadership theory is aimed at congruence between the vision and agenda of the leader, as well as the followers. No prescribed set of actions exists. Instead, the focus is on the goals, and proper actions to achieve these goals are defined; however, the actions may be constantly changing. Trust is a constant in this leadership theory and includes trust in the organization as well as mutual trust between the leader and followers (Robinson, 2001). The ambulatory care nurse leader has many resources available to guide him or her, as discussed here. This is critical to ensure quality in practice as the leader continually assesses, plans, implements, and evaluates the increasingly complex needs of the outpatient setting.

Clinical Trials

Oncology research studies were once limited to clinical trials in hospital settings. With the large number of outpatients being placed on a growing number of research protocols, recruitment and data collection have increased the responsibilities of outpatient nurses. Large community practice settings may have dedicated oncology nurses or research program coordinators to manage study protocols. More often, it is the responsibility of an already overburdened oncology nurse to collect research data. It is common practice for the pharmaceutical industry to want to conduct phase IV trials in the community setting. The purpose of phase IV trials is to collect new information about benefits, risks, and side-effects of medications or medical devices not previously identified in earlier trials. These studies, like all research studies, can pose hidden obstacles that are not immediately apparent. Pharmaceutical companies may offer physicians up to $5,000 per patient enrolled in a clinical trial, and often, input from nursing managers is not sought before study commitments. Recruitment, data collection, patient education, tracking missed appointments, and reporting adverse effects often fall to the oncology nurse. In these instances, some oncology managers have negotiated a shared benefit of the financial gains garnered from heavily underwritten studies. These benefits include funding for educational programs and textbooks. Nursing managers need to be intimately involved in the feasibility of all research to determine the true cost and ethics (Martin & Xistris, 2000). Chapter 16 gives a complete discussion of research issues in ambulatory care settings. The ONS has crafted a position statement designed to guide researchers in conducting sound and ethical clinical trials (**Figure 1.10**) (ONS, 2002f).

Informatics

Oncology in the ambulatory setting is constantly evolving to encompass the best practice. One area deserving much attention is informatics. Nurses are continuously assessing ways to enhance practice via technology. Many areas of opportunity exist to upgrade or incorporate the latest technology, such as medical records, billing, chemotherapy and radiation oncology order entry systems, physician order entry, nursing documentation, and telecommunications such as paging and phone systems. Each requires assessment of the integrity of the system, patient confidentiality implications, enhancement of productivity, and financial implications.

Nursing has incorporated technology into practice to the level that it is considered a specialty field in nursing. The American Nurses Association has defined nursing informatics (NI) as "the specialty that integrates nursing science, computer science, and information science in identifying, collecting,

Figure 1.6 Treatment Levels for Infusion Log

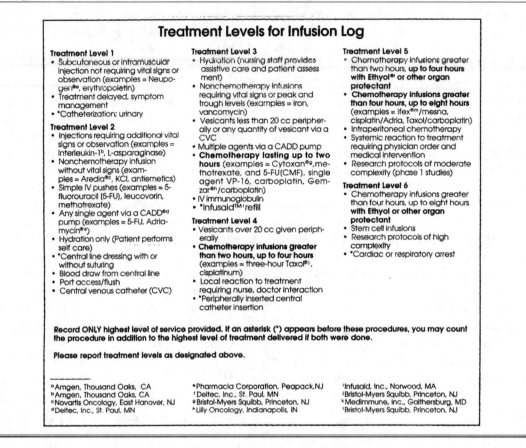

Treatment Levels for Infusion Log

Treatment Level 1
- Subcutaneous or intramuscular injection not requiring vital signs or observation (examples = Neupogen[a], erythropoietin)
- Treatment delayed, symptom management
- *Catheterization; urinary

Treatment Level 2
- Injections requiring additional vital signs or observation (examples = Interleukin-1[b], L-asparaginase)
- Nonchemotherapy infusion without vital signs (examples = Aredia[c], KCl, antiemetics)
- Simple IV pushes (examples = 5-fluorouracil (5-FU), leucovorin, methotrexate)
- Any single agent via a CADD[d] pump (examples = 5-FU, Adriamycin[e])
- Hydration only (Patient performs self care)
- *Central line dressing with or without suturing
- Blood draw from central line
- Port access/flush
- Central venous catheter (CVC)

Treatment Level 3
- Hydration (nursing staff provides assistive care and patient assessment)
- Nonchemotherapy infusions requiring vital signs or peak and trough levels (examples = iron, vancomycin)
- Vesicants less than 20 cc peripherally or any quantity of vesicant via a CVC
- Multiple agents via a CADD pump
- **Chemotherapy lasting up to two hours** (examples = Cytoxan[e], methotrexate, and 5-FU(CMF), single agent VP-16, carboplatin, Gemzar[h]/carboplatin)
- IV immunoglobulin
- *Infusaid[i] refill

Treatment Level 4
- Vesicants over 20 cc given peripherally
- **Chemotherapy infusions greater than two hours, up to four hours** (examples = three-hour Taxol[i], cisplatinum)
- Local reaction to treatment requiring nurse, doctor interaction
- *Peripherally inserted central catheter insertion

Treatment Level 5
- Chemotherapy infusions greater than two hours, up to four hours with Ethyol[i] or other organ protectant
- **Chemotherapy infusions greater than four hours, up to eight hours** (examples = Ifex[m]/mesna, cisplatin/Adria, Taxol/carboplatin)
- Intraperitoneal chemotherapy
- Systemic reaction to treatment requiring physician order and medical intervention
- Research protocols of moderate complexity (phase 1 studies)

Treatment Level 6
- Chemotherapy infusions greater than four hours, up to eight hours with Ethyol or other organ protectant
- Stem cell infusions
- Research protocols of high complexity
- *Cardiac or respiratory arrest

Record ONLY highest level of service provided. If an asterisk (*) appears before these procedures, you may count the procedure in addition to the highest level of treatment delivered if both were done.

Please report treatment levels as designated above.

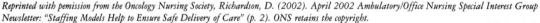

[a] Amgen, Thousand Oaks, CA
[b] Amgen, Thousand Oaks, CA
[c] Novartis Oncology, East Hanover, NJ
[d] Deltec, Inc., St. Paul, MN
[e] Pharmacia Corporation, Peapack, NJ
[f] Deltec, Inc., St. Paul, MN
[g] Bristol-Myers Squibb, Princeton, NJ
[h] Lilly Oncology, Indianapolis, IN
[i] Infusaid, Inc., Norwood, MA
[j] Bristol-Myers Squibb, Princeton, NJ
[k] Medimmune, inc., Gaithersburg, MD
[l] Bristol-Myers Squibb, Princeton, NJ

Reprinted with permission from the Oncology Nursing Society, Richardson, D. (2002). April 2002 Ambulatory/Office Nursing Special Interest Group Newsletter: "Staffing Models Help to Ensure Safe Delivery of Care" (p. 2). ONS retains the copyright.

processing and managing data and information to support nursing practice, administration, education, research and the expansion of nursing knowledge." The core product of nursing is patient care, and NI, like the other practice areas of nursing research, education, and administration, exists to support the highest possible technology (International American Medical Informatics Association, 2003).

A subset of this group, the Nursing Informatics Working Group, was designed to promote the advancement of NI within the larger multidisciplinary context of health informatics. The working group represents the interests of NI for members in the working group and American Medical

Informatics Association, and provides member services and outreach functions (International American Medical Informatics Association, 2003).

The Healthcare Information and Management Systems Society (HIMSS) is the healthcare industry's membership organization that is exclusively focused on providing leadership for the optimal use of healthcare information technology and management systems for the betterment of human health. As the largest and only dedicated global healthcare information and management systems association, HIMSS serves more than 14,000 individual members in the United States and internationally, 42 state and regional chap-

Figure 1.7 INFUSION LEVELS REPORT

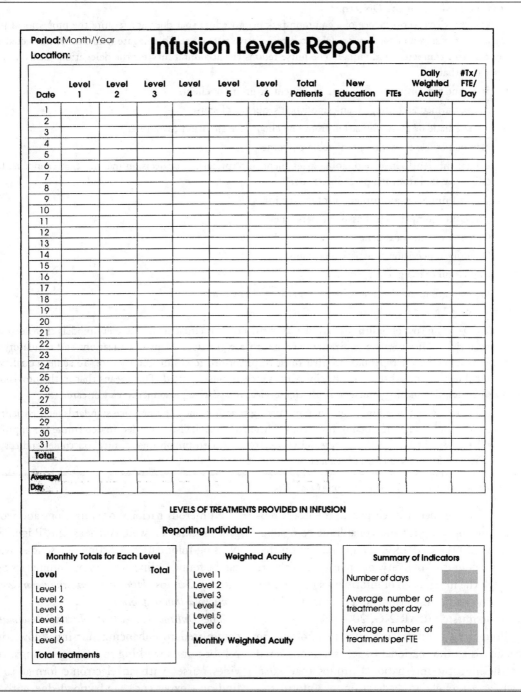

Figure 1.8 THE USE OF ASSISTIVE PERSONNEL IN CANCER CARE

It is the position of the ONS that

The repetitive performance of a common task or procedure that does not require the professional judgment of a registered nurse may be delegated to assistive personnel. To delegate is to tranfer a selected nursing task to a competent individual. The nurse retains the accountability for the delegation. Tasks may be delegated that

- Frequently recur in the daily care of a client or group of clients
- Are performed according to an established sequence of steps
- Involve little or no modification from one client care situation to another
- May be performed with a predictable outcome
- Do not inherently involve ongoing assessment, interpretation, or decision making that cannot be logically separated from the procedure(s) itself

Registered nurses maintain accountability for

- Validating competency of assistive personnel
- Ongoing client assessment
- Ongoing supervision of assistive personnel
- Evaluation of the client's response to care
- Interpretation and decision making regarding client care

Background

The growing cost of healthcare has increased the need for efficient care delivery models that decrease the financial risk for healthcare organizations and healthcare practices. Many organizations and regulatory agencies are evaluating the types of work that must be performed to ensure quality care. To achieve quality care, the ONS understands that a multidisciplinary approach must be used. This means that in the provision of nursing care, the oncology nurse will use the services of assistive personnel in cancer care.

Issues that affect licensure, regulation of nursing practice, oncology practice standards, and patient care outcomes require ongoing nursing research. Additional research also is needed to determine the appropriate provider mix and to define cancer care delivery systems that ensure optimal clinical outcomes and cost-effective care for individuals with cancer.

Reprinted with pemission from the Oncology Nursing Society, 2002.

ters, and more than 150 corporate members representing top supplier and consultant companies (HIMSS, 2004). CARING is an organization that is advancing the delivery of quality healthcare through the integration of informatics in practice, education, administration, and research with a focus on nursing (CARING, 2004).

Promoting informatics and technology in nursing is an international issue, as demonstrated by the multiple international groups that exist, such as the Belgian Federation of Informatics Associations (2004) and the Australian Nursing Informatics Special Interest Group (2004).

Numerous national organizations and working groups exist as well, such as the Puget Sound Nursing Informatics. A listing of resources available can be found online at Nursing Infomatics Special Interest Groups *(http://www.nursing.umaryland.edu/ ~snewbold/skngroup.htm).*

The *OnLine Journal of Nursing Informatics* is committed to enhancing nursing knowledge on NI for nurses working in diverse settings. It provides nurses with an electronic format to share findings, experience, and knowledge with nursing colleagues involved in all facets of NI.

Figure 1.9 Patient Education Tool for Patient Self-Care Teaching Tool for Patients with Fluid and Electrolyte Imbalances

Ascites

Patient Name _____

This guide will help you to know how to live with the fluid in your abdomen. You will learn how to handle pain if it occurs.

Symptom and Description

Ascites is a symptom that occurs when large amounts of fluid pool in your abdomen. The fluid can cause a sense of fullness and make your clothes fit tightly. The effects of the fluid can be managed with the care outlined in this guide.

Management

1. *Diet:* There are no limits to your diet. Try to eat foods that are high in protein and calories. Small, frequent meals (up to 6 meals a day) may be easier for you to eat.

2. *Pain control:* Rate your pain daily using a scale of 0 to 10 in which 0 equals no pain and 10 equals the worst pain that you can imagine. Select the number that best describes your level of pain.

0   1   2   3   4   5   6   7   8   9   10

no pain   worst
                                           pain

3. *Activity:* There are no limits to your activities. You should do what you feel like doing. Rest periods may be helpful. Elevate your feet/legs when sitting.

4. *Diary:* Keep a record of your daily pain rating and activity level on the patient data record included. Bring this with you when you come for your next visit with your nurse or doctor.

Follow-up

Call your nurse or doctor if any of the following occurs:

A weight gain so that your clothes do not fit

Trouble breathing or shortness of breath

Nausea or vomiting

An increase in pain rating to above 4 for 2 days in a row

Phone Numbers

Nurse: _____   Phone: _____

Physician: _____   Phone: _____

Other: _____   Phone: _____

Comments _____

_____

_____

Patient's
Signature: _____   Date _____

Nurse's
Signature: _____   Date: _____

Source: Winkelman, W. A., (2003). Ascites, in C. H. Yarbro, M. H. Frogge M. Goodman (Eds.): Cancer Symptom Management (ed. 3, pp. 401–421) Sudbury, MA: Jones and Bartlett Publishers.

As outlined, the oncology nurse has not only ample resources available to evaluate technology and informatics as they strive to improve patient care through professional practice, education, and research, but he or she also has numerous opportunities to immerse himself or herself professionally in this unique area that has a drastic impact on the oncology patients and professional population's quality of care (American Nursing Association Scope and Standards of Practice, 2004). The Scope and Standards of Nursing Informatics Practice was developed by the American Nursing Association as a resource and guide for informatics educational programs, NI practitioners, employers, research and funding agencies, and others needing to understand informatics in the profession of nursing. For the oncology nurse, there are numerous nursing organizations, groups and journals, and the Symposium on Computer Applications in Medical Care. The 3,200 members of AMIA include physicians, nurses, computer and information scientists, biomedical engineers, medical librarians, and academic researchers and educators. The AMIA is the official United States representative organization to the quality of care (American Nursing Association Scope and Standards of Practice, 2004). The American Nursing Informatics Association provides networking, education, and information resources that strengthen the roles of nurses in the field of informatics. The field of NI includes domains of clinical information, education, and administrative decision support (International Medical Informatics, 2003).

The AMIA was formed in 1990 by the merger of three organizations—the American Association for Medical Systems and Informatics, the American College of Medical Informatics, and the American Nursing Informatics Association. They are devoted to serving as a professional network and forum for the development and advancement of nurses working in healthcare informatics and to assessing measures and systems impacting patient care.

Maintaining Standards for Other Disciplines

Two important clinical disciplines that are essential to the care of the ambulatory oncology patient are discussed here.

NUTRITION

In 2001, the Joint Commission on Accreditation of Hospital Organizations (JCAHO) published nutrition standards that require an ambulatory care organization to use clinical practice guidelines to evaluate and treat patients with specific diagnoses, conditions, or symptoms. JCAHO mandates clearly states that nutritional care must be provided across the cancer continuum of prevention, medical care, survival, and palliation and that the patient and family are included in assessment and management of the plan. The American Dietetic Association, the National Comprehensive Cancer Network, and the Association of Community Cancer Centers have developed their individual standards of care. In March 2000, the Association of Community Cancer Centers issued standards to direct administration in designing interdisciplinary programs that meet the needs of patients with cancer and their families. These standards, now being used in over 680 medical centers nationwide, can be used as a guideline for those developing or maintaining outpatient centers.

Standard I. A specially trained nutritionist in dietary counseling must be available to work with patients who are at risk for dietary problems and their families. The nutritionist should be available to medical and nursing staff to assure assessment and referral of patients.

Standard II. A multidisciplinary team, including the patient and family, is required to work with the nutritionist in nutrition and hydration.

Standard III. The nutritionist can provide dietary guidelines on reducing cancer risk through community education (Association of Community Cancer Centers, 2002; Gabbard, Luthringer, & Eldridge, 2002).

PSYCHOSOCIAL SERVICES

The emotional burden associated with cancer, its diagnosis, treatment, outcomes, and long-term effects includes a wide range of emotions. Although surveys show that between 20 to 40% of patients demonstrate significant levels of distress, fewer than 10% of them are referred for psychosocial assistance. Some of the barriers to receiving psychosocial care are the cost of mental health services, cultural attitudes, and stigma attached to seeking psychosocial support (Matthews, Corrigan, & Rutherford, 2003). Many outpatient administrators struggle to find strategies to integrate psychosocial care into the oncology clinics. LaRue (2002) suggested a framework to integrate psychosocial care into the oncology clinic. The components are as follows (LaRue, 2002):

1. Integrate psychosocial services as part of the oncology team
2. Make psychosocial services easily accessible
3. Remove stigma of receiving psychosocial care
4. Include a staff support program with weekly team case conferences
5. Debrief staff on the occasion of an emotional or physical traumatic death
6. Have memorial services or remembrance ritual to provide formal closure after patients' deaths
7. Assist staff in separating cancer care from personal time

Facility Planning and Space Use: Function and Form

Function

The steps to planning an outpatient facility follow a classic sequence and are dependent on the mission, values, visions, and economic resources of the organization. The planning committee needs to represent the scope of services and departments who support the delivery of the product line. A multidisciplinary team of knowledgeable, dedicated professionals who are committed to integration of these concepts into current and future goals of the organization is indispensable for a timely and financially sound process (Buchsel & Whedon, 1995; Lamkin, 1993). Without this cooperation, personal department agendas delay timelines, add to potential cost overruns, and team tension. Planning teams include the following:

- A member of the institution's board of directors
- An administrative officer
- A medical, nursing, dietary, and mental health director
- Plan operations
- Housekeeping
- An infectious disease consultant
- Administrative supportive services
- Materials supply
- Pharmacy

The institution's mission statement is to create a strategic plan, develop goals, and define operational considerations and will serve as a guide to the planning process. Large cancer centers often have a master plan to guide the location and building design. As part of the planning, each department head is asked to submit a request for space, personnel, and equipment. It is sometimes referred to as a "wish list."

Space Requirement

The minimal square footage for patient care areas depends on institutional, local, federal, and JCAHO requirements and on space constrictions; however, the planning team can benefit by knowing established generic space requirements that can serve as a baseline for preliminary discussion. Chapter 7 offers a full discussion of space require-

---

Figure 1.10   ONS POSITION ON CANCER RESEARCH AND CANCER CLINICAL TRIALS

It is the position of the ONS that

- Federal funding for all levels of cancer research must be significantly increased.

- All clinical trials must be peer reviewed, include participant informed consent, and have been approved through an institutional review board process.

- Every person diagnosed with cancer must have the right to participate in a clinical trial if medically indicated.

- Individuals at high risk for cancer or those who wish to change behaviors that increase cancer risk must be offered the opportunity to participate in cancer-prevention trials. The goal of these trials is to reduce cancer incidence and mortality.

- All barriers to participation in clinical trials, including both recruitment and retention, must be abolished.

- Participation in clinical trials must be a standard benefit of all health insurance plans, and legislation must be adopted to prohibit denials of trial-associated patient care reimbursement costs.

- Content related to cancer research and clinical trials must be incorporated into basic educational curricula of healthcare professionals and fostered through continuing education.

- More effective strategies to promote public awareness and understanding of cancer research and clinical trials must be devised, implemented, and evaluated.

- Improved strategies to facilitate the participation of underrepresented populations must be devised, implemented, and evaluated.

- Concepts of quality cancer care, as defined by the ONS in its position on "Quality Cancer Care," must be incorporated into the planning and coordination of clinical trials.

- Coordination of clinical trials (e.g., coordination of clinical sites, development of standardized treatment orders, symptom management, patient education and advocacy, facilitation of informed consent, assistance with participant accrual and retention) is best accomplished by registered nurses who have been educated and certified in oncology nursing.

- Nurses design, initiate, and facilitate clinical research studies to address quality-of-life issues for people with cancer. The goal of quality-of-life research is to improve the lives of those who have been affected by cancer.

- Continuing informed consent must be assured for all individuals considering or participating in clinical trials.

- Solutions or innovative strategies to decrease financial burdens associated with institutional participation in clinical trials must be devised.

ONS Position on Cancer Research and Cancer Clinical Trials (2002).

ments. An example of a creative solution to using restrictive space is evidenced in the new Sloan Kettering Cancer Center in New York City. Architects have constructed a 55,000-ft^2 five-story addition above a pre-existing pavilion (Memorial Sloan Kettering Cancer Center Newsletter, 2003).

Advanced medical technology and equipment are major considerations in space design. In addition to the space requirements for such technology and equipment, electrical requirements, weight load, and other physical plant accommodations are to be considered. Most architects recommend an additional 10 to 15% allocation "pocket" or extra space for future requirements.

Form

The design of an ambulatory care center can improve patient outcomes, enhance staff satisfactions, create operational savings over the life of a building, and be a marketing strategy to attract patients. Design requirements and applications vary among organizations and are shaped by organizational missions, disease product lines, site considerations, and operational philosophies and practices. An expert on architect design has coined the term "evidence-based design," which is seen as a creation of functional environments that help patients cope with the stresses of cancer treatment. Researchers have established scientific evidence that environmental characteristics can influence patient-care outcomes. Studies have shown how well-designed environments can reduce anxiety, lower blood pressure, and lessen pain. Conversely, other studies have shown how poorly designed environments contribute to depression and a greater need for pain medication (Weiner, 2003). The trend today is to create a wellness rather than illness atmosphere. Creating an environment to support a sense of control, promote privacy, encourage social support, and provide access to nature and other positive distractions is now encouraged (Weiner, 2003). Some professional organizations offer "healing" designs that use functional and ergonomic approaches. A Midwest cancer center created a spirituality and healing center that offers a range of complementary healthcare services from acupuncture to Chinese herbal medicine, to healing touch therapy to chiropractic and massage. One of the approaches used in creating the center was Feng Shui, to arrange workspace to promote inner harmony for unimpeded flow of chi, or life energy (Shlesinger, 2003). Other approaches that offer patients and their families comfort are listed in **Table 1.4**.

Choosing an architectural firm that is expert in healthcare facilities is critical, and considerable research is needed to determine the optimal organization. Architects, in addition to having building skills, need expert communication tactics to interact with both professional and non-

---

Table 1.4 PATIENT AMENITIES FOR AMBULATORY CARE CENTERS

Located in close approximation of acute care center

Transportation provided if on a large campus

Overnight accommodations with a restaurant for the patient's family

Convenient access to food, telephones, and restrooms

Easy to read and accurate signage

Accessible waiting areas

Adequate space between patients in waiting rooms

Designated family lounge spaces

Educational and learning center space for patients and family members

Access to electronic educational materials

Natural light

Noise reduction using sound adsorbing carpeting, white noise

Artwork

Plants (artificial for the immunosuppressed patient)

Separate staff areas from patient areas

Patient-controlled chair or bed

Headphones and handsets for music and to manage the television/DVD player

professional staff. Without the expertise of various healthcare staff intimately familiar with the nuances of their jobs, the best of architects fail. The American Institute of Architects for Health Care Academy consists of architects from the private and public sectors, with a particular interest and/or expertise in the design of health facilities. Consultation with these sources can guide the oncology administrator in making the best selection for his or her facility.

Future Trends

The future of ambulatory care nursing is one of increasing growth, vitality, and change as the 21st century evolves, but not without its challenges. Technology is moving at such a rate that by 2007, most of what was done in the hospital setting will be done in ambulatory care (Porter-O'Grady, 2001). Less invasive, short-term cancer treatments such as cancer vaccines, dose-dense combination therapy, and targeted therapy will overtake familiar chemotherapy and radiation. Alternative therapies will become more seamlessly integrated into cancer care. Oncology nurses will experience the challenge of new information technology systems. Computerized provider (or physician) order entry and barcode-enabled point-of-care medication management systems will be installed in the ambulatory care setting to improve efficiency and decrease medication errors. Handwritten orders will be rare. The application of real-time imaging, robotic technology, telemetry, and voice response, have significant ramifications. Telecommunications using reactive response systems will enhance patient education, compliance, and improved clinical outcomes.

As the older portion of the population grows, cancer will be the primary chronic disease in America. Cancer prevention programs will proliferate in efforts to teach persons to avoid the known risk factors such as tobacco use and encourage them to adopt healthy diets, exercise,

and stress management. Furthermore, it is believed that information technology will help consumers to make better choices about healthcare, thus getting more value-added services. Use of healthcare websites by consumers tripled in 2002 as individuals spent more time exploring their options before making healthcare decisions. Oncology nurses will spend an increasing amount of time helping patients to sort creditable information about disease, diagnostic tests, and treatment options. Those without a healthcare background can have difficulty sorting sound and evidenced information from less reliable sources. Nurses practicing in outpatient settings will require comprehensive but diverse educational programs to assure and enhance their critical thinking skills, independent clinical judgment, management and organization skills, leadership abilities, and understanding of diverse cultural approaches to healthcare (Mafrica, 2002). The impact of the nursing shortage, although not fully realized, will forever change the type and deliverer of oncology supportive care.

Appendix A

SURGICAL SERVICES

Title	Salary	Location	Total beds	OR Suites	Cases/year
Director	$90,000	Dallas, Texas	225	9	5,000
Director	$125,000	East Central Texas	350	13	6,000
Director	$70,000	South Carolina	50	2	700
Director	$75,000	Columbus, Nebraska	68	3	3,000
Director	$80,000	Central Kansas	150	6	
Director	$90,000	Billings, Montana	268	11	18,000
Director, Surgery/ Ambulatory	$70,000 to $75,000	Vermont	75	3	2,300
Manager	$85,000	Northern California	80	5	
Manager	$70,000	Indianapolis, Indiana	247	11	8,000
Manager	$85,000 to $95,000	Southwest Connecticut	425	12	7,000
Manager	$60,000	Southwest Iowa	54	2	633
Manager	$90,000	Boston, Mass.	134	6	5,000
Manager, PACU/Day Surgery/Endo	$85,000	Minnesota	275	12-bed PACU	
Manager of Cardiac Surgery	$70,000 to $80,000	Central New York State	352	2	500
Manager of GI	$75,000	Central New York State	352		6,750

EMERGENCY SERVICES

Title	Salary	Location	Total beds	Visits/year
Director	$85,000	Clearwater, Florida area	300	16,000
Director - Level I	$100,000	Pittsburgh, Pennsylvania	836	60,000
Director	$100,000	Western Texas	342	50,000
Director - Level I	$90,000	Columbia, Missouri	233	30,000
Director - Level II	$85,000	Central Illinois	309	30,000
Manager	$75,000	Oklahoma City, Oklahoma	650	25,000
Manager	$75,000	Oklahoma City, Oklahoma	650	33,000
Manager - Level II	$60,000 to $65,000	Central Kansas	125	15,000

LABOR AND DELIVERY

Title	Salary	Location	Total beds	Births/year
Director, Family Birthing Center	$95,000	Central California	395	3,000
Director of Women's Services	$84,000	Butte, Montana	100	500
Manager	$70,000	Northeast Pennsylvania	258	800
Manager	$85,000	Central Ohio	800	7,000

MEDICAL/SURGICAL

Title	Salary	Location	Total beds	Unit size
Director	$90,000	Oklahoma City, Okla.	900	60-beds
Manager	$85,000	Las Vegas, Nevada	715	2 36-bed units
Manager Med/ Surg/Oncology	$80,000	Boston, Mass.	234	37-beds
Manager	$70,000	Northeast Pennsylvania	258	

CRITICAL CARE/TELEMETRY

Title	Salary	Location	Total beds	Unit size
Manager, Critical Care	$80,000	Tacoma, Washington area	225	8-bed ICU 16-bed telemetry
Manager, Telemetry	$100,000	Southern California	175	36-beds

CARDIOVASCULAR SERVICES

Title	Salary	Location	Total beds
Director	$95,000	South central Missouri	120

ONCOLOGY

Title	Salary	Location	Total beds
Administrator, Medical/Cancer Services	$85,000	Cedar Rapids, Iowa	350
Director	$120,000	Omaha, Nebraska	500
Manager	$70,000	Northeast Pennsylvania	258

Published with permission from Peter Benson, Executive Research Consultant.

References

American Nursing Association Scope and Standards of Practice. (2004). Retrieved February 8, 2004 from *http://nursingworld.org/books/pdescr.cfm?cnum=15.#NIP21*

Anastasia, P. J. (2002). Telephone triage and chemotherapy symptom management in the ambulatory care setting. *Oncology Supportive Care Quarterly, 1*, 40–55.

Association of Community Cancer Centers. (2002). Retrieved March, 2004 from *http://www.accc-cancer.org*

Australian Nursing Informatics Special Interest Group. (2004). Retrieved February 8, 2004 from *http://littlefish.com.au/anisig/anisighome.htm*

Belgian Federation of Informatics Associations. (2004). Retrieved February 8, 2004 from *http://www.bfia.be/#ecdl*

Bodenheimer, T., Lorig, K., Holman, H., & Grumbach, K. (2003). Patient self-management of chronic disease in primary care. *JAMA, 288*, 2469–2475.

Bruce, S. D. (2003). Ambulatory/office setting offers nurses new rewards. . . and new challenges. *ONS News, 18*, 1–5.

Buchsel, P. C. & Whedon, M. B. (Eds.). (1995). *Bone Marrow Transplantation: Administrative and Clinical Strategies*. Sudbury, MA: Jones and Bartlett Publishers.

Buchsel, P. & Yarbro, C. H. (Eds.). (1993). *Oncology Nursing in the Ambulatory Care Setting: Issues and Models of Care*. Sudbury, MA: Jones and Bartlett Publishers.

CARING. (2004). Retrieved February 8, 2004 from *http://www.caringonline.org/*

Chitnis, S. P. (2001). Ambulatory care: The inevitable future. *Health Care Management*. Retrieved July 27, 2003 from *http://www.expresshealthcaremgmt.com/20010831/editorial2.htm*

Chouinard, M. (2003). Non myeloablative hematopoietic transplantation. In P. C. Buchsel & P. M. Kapustay (Eds.), *Peripheral Stem Cell Transplantation: A Clinical Text Book*, supplement 3.

DePalma, J. (2003). Evidence based practice. Retrieved March 1, 2004 from *http://onsopcontent.ons.org/toolkits/ebp/definition/definition.htm*

Derlet, R. (2003). Triage. Retrieved March 1, 2004 from *http://www.emedicine.com/emerg/topic670.htm#*

Dodd, M. J., Miaskowski, C., West, C., Paul, S., & Lee, K. (2002). The prevalence of symptoms clusters and comorbidity in oncology outpatients. *Oncology Nursing Forum, 29*, 340 (abstract 35).

Espensen, M. (2001). Telehealth nursing practice. In J. Robinson (Ed.), *Core Curriculm for Ambulatory Care Nurses* (pp. 389–405). Philadelphia: W.B. Saunders Company.

Foundation for the Accreditation of Hematopoietic Cell Therapy. (2002). Standards for hematopoietic progenitor cell collection, processing & transplantation. Foundation for the Accreditation of Hematopoietic Cell Therapy (FACT) 2nd Edition. Omaha, NE: Medical Center.

Gabbard, D., Luthringer, S., & Eldridge, B. (2002). Integrating nutrition into your cancer program. Retrieved December 14, 2003 from *http://www.accc-cancer.org/publications/Standofcare.pdf*

Gallant, M. D. & Coutts, L. M. (2003). Evaluation of an oncology outpatient orientation program: Patient satisfaction and outcomes. *Supportive Care in Cancer, 11*, 800–805.

Gandhi, T. K., Weingart, S. N., Borus, J., Seger, A. C., Peterson, J., Burdick, E. et al. (2003). Adverse drug events in ambulatory care. *New England Journal of Medicine, 348*, 1556–1564.

Given, B., Beck, S., Etland, C., Homes Gobel, B. H., Lamkin, L., & Marsee, V. (2003). *ONS Sensitive Outcomes Definition*. Pittsburgh, PA: Oncology Nursing Society.

Groff, P. (2004). The role of the donor in hematopoietic stem cell transplantation. In P. C. Buchsel & P. M. Kapustay (Eds.), *Peripheral Stem Cell Transplantation: A Clinical Text Book*, supplement 3.

Hass, S. (1998). Ambulatory care nursing conceptual framework. *American Academy of Nursing Viewpoint, 20*, 16–17.

Healthcare Information and Management System Society. (2004). Retrieved February 8, 2004 from *http://www.himss.org/asp/index.asp*

Heffler, S., Levit, K., Smith, S., Smith, C., Cowan, C., Lanzenby, H. et al. (2001). Health spending growth up in 1999; faster growth expected in the future. *Health Affairs, 20*, 193–203.

Holley, S. (2002). A look at the problem of falls among patients with cancer. *Clinical Journal of Oncology Nursing, 6*, 193–197.

Holmes, C. E. & Muss Hyman, H. (2003). Diagnosis and treatment of breast cancer in the elderly. *CA: A Cancer Journal for Clinicians, 53*, 227–244.

Institute of Medicine. (2003). A Shared Destiny: Community Effects on Uninsurance. Washington, DC: National Academies Press.

International American Medical Informatics Association. (2003). Retrieved February 8, 2004 from *http://www.amia.org/working/ni/main.html*

International Medical Informatics. (2003). Retrieved February 8, 2004 from *http://www.ania.org/aboutAnia.asp*

Itano, J. K. (1998). Cultural issues. In J. K. Itano & K. N. Taoka (Eds.), *Core Curriculum for Oncology Nursing* (3rd ed., pp. 60–76). Philadelphia: W.B. Saunders Company.

Itano, J. K. & Taoka, K. N. (Eds.). (1998). *Core Curriculum for Oncology Nursing* (3rd ed.). Philadelphia: W.B. Saunders Company.

Lamkin, L. (1993). The new oncology clinic. In P. C. Buchsel & C. H. Yarbro (Eds.), *Oncology Nursing in the Ambulatory Setting* (pp. 107–132). Sudbury, MA: Jones and Bartlett Publishers.

LaRue, L. J. (2002). Integrated psychosocial care of patients with cancer in the ambulatory care setting. *Oncology Supportive Care Quarterly, 1,* 7–18.

Mafrica, L., Ballon, L. G., Culhane, B., McCorkle, M., Murphy, M. M., & Worrall, L. (2002). Oncology Nursing Forum 29. Retrieved February 29, 2004 from *http://www.ons.xp/ONS_Publications.xml/ONF.xml/ONF2002/*

Martin, R. V. & Xistris, D. (2000). Ambulatory care. In C. H. Yarbro, M. H. Frogge, M. Goodman, & S. L. Groenwald (Eds.), *Cancer Nursing Principles and Practice* (5th ed., pp. 574–578). Sudbury, MA: Jones and Bartlett Publishers.

Matthews, A. K., Corrigan, P. W., & Rutherford, J. L. (2003). Mental illness stigma as a barrier to psychosocial services for cancer patients. *Journal of the National Comprehensive Cancer Network, 1,* 375–379.

Mayer, G. G., Madden, M. J., & Lawrenz, E. (1990). *Patient Care Delivery Models.* Rockville, MD: Aspen Publications.

Memoral Sloan Kettering Cancer Center Newsletter. (2003). Retrieved January 18, 2004 from *http://www.mskcc.org/annual/building*

National Coalition in Cancer Research. (2004). Retrieved March 1, 2004 from *http://www.cancercoalition.org/faq.html*

Nevidjon, B. M. (1993). The changing role of oncology nursing in ambulatory care settings. In P. C. Buchsel & C. H. Yarbro (Eds.), *Oncology Nursing in the Ambulatory Care Setting: Issues and Models of Care* (pp. 21–34). Sudbury, MA: Jones and Bartlett Publishers.

Nursing Informatics Special Interest Groups. (2004). Retrieved February 8, 2004 from *http://www.nursing.umaryland.edu/~snewbold/skngroup.htm*

O'Brien, K., Cokkinides, V., Jemal, A., Cardinex, C. J., Murry, T., Samuels, A. et al. (2003). Cancer statistics for Hispanics, 2003. *CA: A Cancer Journal for Clinicians, 53,* 209–226.

Oncology Nursing Society. (1990). The national survey of salary, staffing, and professional practice patterns in office-based nursing. Pittsburgh: Oncology Nursing Press.

Oncology Nursing Society. (1991). The national survey of salary, staffing, and professional practice patterns in radiation therapy-based oncology. Pittsburgh: Oncology Nursing Press.

Oncology Nursing Society. (1992). The national survey of salary, staffing, and professional practice patterns in infusions suites. Pittsburgh: Oncology Nursing Press.

ONS Position Statement on Ambulatory Care. (2002a). Retrieved March 1, 2004 from *http://www.ons.org/Positions/oncology_services.pdf*

ONS. (2002b). A Position Statement on the Impact of the Nursing Shortage on Quality of Care.

ONS Position Statement on The Prevention and Reporting of Medication Errors. (2002c). Retrieved February 29, 2004 from *http://www.ons.org/Positions/medication_errors.pdf*

ONS Position Statement on Education of the Professional RN Who Administers and Cares for the Individual Receiving Chemotherapy and Biotherapy. (2002d). Retrieved March 2, 2004 from *http://www.ons.org/xp6/ONS/Information.xml/Journals_and_Positions.xml/ONS_Positions.xml/EducationofProfessionalRN.xml*

ONS Position Cancer Research and Cancer Clinical Trials. (2002e). Retrieved February 29, 2004 from *http://www.ons.org/xp6/ONS/Information.xml/Journals_and_Positions.xml/ONS_Positions.xml/CancerResearch.xml*

ONS Patient Information and Education Resource. (nd). Retrieved March 1, 2004 from *http://www.ons.org/xp6/ONS/Education.xml/PIER.xml*

Porter-O'Grady, T. (2001). Profound change: 21 century nursing. *Nursing Outlook, 49,* 182–186.

Robinson, J. (2001). Ambulatory care nursing administration and practice standards, *Core Curriculum for Ambulatory Care Nursing* (2nd ed.). Philadelphia: W.B. Saunders Company.

Rutledge, D. (2004). What are healthcare organizations doing to promote patient safety in medication administration? *ONS News 19,* 4–9.

Sackett, D. L. & Rosenberg, W. M. (1995). On the need for evidence-based medicine. *Journal of Public Health Medicine, 3,* 330–334.

Schlesinger, M. (2003). Retrieved March 1, 2004 from *http://www.lightyears2.com/HealingEnvironments.html*

Schmidt-Pokorny, K., Franco, T., Frappier, B., & Vyhlidal, R. G. (2003). The cooperative model: An innovative approach to deliver blood and marrow stem cell transplant care. *Clinical Journal of Oncology Nursing, 7,* 509–556.

Schorr, T. M. & Kennedy, M. S. (1999). *100 Years of American Nursing: Celebrating a Century of Caring.* Philadelphia: J.B. Lippincott.

Weiner, M. (2003). Hospital design trends: Responding positively to the needs of the health care environment. *http://www.chicagohospitalnews.com/Archives/06June03/060307Design.htm*

Yarbro, C. H., Frogge, M. H., & Goodman, M. (2004). *Cancer Symptom Management* (3rd ed.). Sudbury, MA: Jones and Bartlett Publishers.

Wells, N., Murphy, B., Wujcik, D., & Johnson, R. (2003). Pain-related distress and interference with daily life of ambulatory patients with cancer and pain. *Oncology Nursing Forum, 30*, 977–984.

Chapter 2

Economic Issues in Ambulatory Care

Catherine Glennon

Mary Dee McEvoy

Introduction

The care of oncology patients in the ambulatory setting can be an intensely rewarding experience for the nurse. Patients look to the nurse for expert knowledge, as well as emotional support and compassion. The nurse is honored to provide such care. Oncology nurses enjoy learning about new therapies and the application of those therapies to the patients they serve. Satisfaction is found in understanding the patient's experience of care, in assisting patients and families as they move through the cancer trajectory, and in finding the right intervention for a specific symptom. Alleviating pain and managing symptoms are hallmarks of the oncology nurse's repertoire of skills.

Although an issue that is not often viewed as rewarding, the economics of cancer can also be seen as a symptom in need of management. Often the financial aspects of any life situation such as making a major purchase, including buying a house or a car or financing an education can be frustrating. Consider then the even greater frustration when patients and families thoughts and concerns are centered on management of disease and its attendant treatment. Initially, when faced with a cancer diagnosis, families will often say that they

are not worried about the cost of care; their only interest lies in obtaining the best possible medical care. Nevertheless, sooner or later, the cost of care will have to be managed. It is in the best interest of the patient and family that the nurse has some understanding of the financial issues embedded in a cancer diagnosis, as well as the financial issues facing the institution in which they work. Indeed, the ambulatory care nursing conceptual framework that Haas delineated identifies healthcare fiscal management as one of the components of the organizational/systems role of the ambulatory care nurse (Haas, 1998). The other two roles include that of clinical nursing and professional roles. This chapter reviews the cost of healthcare in the United States and the cost of cancer care specifically. Economic issues will be presented from the institutional perspective, followed by the perspective of the individual patient.

Healthcare costs are rising at unprecedented rates. According to the Centers for Medicare and Medicaid Services, in 2001, healthcare spending grew over 8.7% to over 1.4-trillion dollars, with the cost of healthcare predicted to double to $3.1 trillion or 18% of the gross domestic product through 2012 (Heffler et al., 2003). Each individual in the United States personally understands rising healthcare costs. Those employed experience this as they confront the reality of their weekly or monthly paycheck. Employers are paying less for health insurance as the rates continue to skyrocket. As employers pay less, employees must pay more. The choice that each person faces is whether to have less coverage or to continue the same coverage at increased rates, thus realizing that less money is available for daily living. Those who are not employed may have their insurance covered through the government-sponsored programs of Medicare and Medicaid. However, Medicare and Medicaid have limits to their coverage as well. In today's economic environment, some physicians are choosing not to accept patients with Medicare coverage, as Medicare does not fully cover the cost of the care provided. Those physicians view patients who have only Medicare as a liability to the financial stability of their practices. Finally, of great concern are the "working poor," those people who make too high of a salary to be eligible for government-sponsored programs but make too little to afford insurance. A recent Institute of Medicine report indicated that more than 80% of children and adults who were uninsured lived in working families (Institute of Medicine, 2001). Poverty guidelines are used to determine eligibility for some federal assistance programs. According to poverty guidelines (Table 2.1), a family of two would need to make less than $11,940 to qualify for some federal assistance programs. Recent data show that approximately 15% of Americans under the age of 65 years do not have health insurance, and Medicare covers only 25% of the older population. Among people who do not have a regular source of healthcare, 5.7% claim that the cost is the greatest barrier to obtaining healthcare (American Cancer Society, 2002).

Correspondingly, the cost of cancer care is also rising. According to the National Institutes of Health, the estimated cost of cancer for the year 2001 was $156.7 billion. Approximately 10% of the cost relates to lost productivity because of illness and approximately 50% of the cost is the cost of lost productivity because of premature death (American Cancer Society, 2002).

There are numerous approaches that could be presented regarding economic issues associated with cancer care from an institutional perspective. The framework chosen for this chapter is presented in **Figure** 2.1. Simply stated, the financial issues associated with ambulatory care relate to inflow and outflow. Inflow is the amount of money that comes into the ambulatory care center through patient revenues. There are, of course, additional sources of inflow, such as contributions, grants, and endowments; however, these are added on benefits and should not be depended on to support the overall care delivery system. The second major concept to understand is outflow, which is the money that flows out of the system

Table 2.1   2003 FEDERAL POVERTY GUIDELINES

Size of Family Unit	48 Contiguous States and Washington, D.C.	Alaska	Hawaii
1	$8,980	$11,210	$10,330
2	$12,120	$15,140	$13,940
3	$15,260	$19,070	$17,550
4	$18,400	$23,000	$21,160
5	$21,540	$26,930	$24,770
6	$24,680	$30,860	$28,380
7	$27,820	$34,790	$31,990
8	$30,960	$38,720	$35,600
For each additional person, add	$3,140	$3,930	$3,610

Source: Federal Register, 68, 26, 6456–6458.

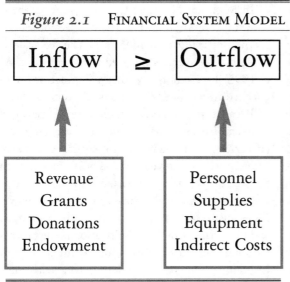

Figure 2.1 FINANCIAL SYSTEM MODEL

as a result of the cost of providing care. Outflow includes such areas as the cost of personnel, the cost of supplies and equipment, and the overhead costs. Conceptually, inflow should at the minimum equal outflow and should ideally be greater than outflow. However, a steady state in this system model is rarely achieved, as there are factors that are continually impacting inflow and outflow. The revenues received from patients are under a constant state of flux because of changes in regulations and payment systems. Changes in regulations can be instituted retroactively so that the money expected in January of a budget year would not be actualized until later in the year and may even be actualized at a lesser amount than originally anticipated. Correspondingly, outflow is also in a constant state of flux because of variables such as rising supply costs and rising salaries needed to retain qualified personnel.

Inflow

Patient revenues are the predominant source of revenue in ambulatory care and arise from three systems: an insurance system, a government-sponsored system, or private pay. The majority of people in the United States belong to employee-sponsored insurance programs; however, there are

also a smaller number who pay privately for their healthcare insurance. In the past, the predominant type of insurance was fee-for-service. In the fee-for-service system, the patient chooses a healthcare provider from a wide range of providers. Specialists were allowed at the desire of the insured. The insured had a wide range of options available. Insurance programs require that a deductible be paid before the insurance; program pays for services. The amount of the deductible is related to the cost of the insurance that is, insurance plans with high deductibles usually cost less per month than plans with lower deductibles. Additionally, a copay is required, which is the amount that the insured must pay at each provider visit. The copay was instituted as an incentive to limit the number of healthcare visits to those situations in which it was truly needed. In other words, it was felt that if the patient were required to pay a portion of each visit, they would visit the physician only when truly warranted.

Managed-care programs began to develop as an alternative to fee-for-service programs, which were thought to be expensive insurance programs. Managed care is a system of healthcare delivery that achieves both cost-effective and quality healthcare through an emphasis on prevention, case management, and medically necessary appropriate care. Different from the fee-for-service system, managed care is financed through methods called prepaid health insurance and capitation. In prepaid health insurance, a managed-care contractor pays a fixed fee to the provider for each enrollee for specific services regardless of the service provided. The provider is then responsible for delivering all of the services defined in the managed-care contract. Because the physician receives a fixed fee regardless of the number of services provided, a concerted effort is made to be efficient in the use of resources, to coordinate care carefully, and to define patient outcomes specifically.

There are numerous types of managed-care models in existence, each with a slightly different method of defining the components of capitation.

Some examples of managed-care plans include Preferred Provider Organization (PPO), Point of Service (POS), Health Maintenance Organization (HMO), Independent Practice Association (IPA), Physician Hospital Organization (PHO), and Medicare Managed Care.

In the PPO, a contract exists between the health plan and providers, with an emphasis on discounted fees. Providers in the PPO are in-network providers, that is, those who have a contract with the PPO. Patients are permitted to use both in-network and out-of-network providers for their care. However, if an in-network provider is seen, a reduced copayment is required. Although patients have the option of using out-of-network providers, when done so, the patient incurs a higher cost through a higher copayment. Thus, the plan gives incentives for the patients to use the in-network providers as opposed to nonparticipating out-of-network providers. In the POS, there is flexibility to choose a provider at the point of service. The chosen provider could be a primary-care provider or a specialist; however, once again, the insured pays a higher copayment with more out-of-pocket expenses.

The most popular type of managed care is the HMO, in which a patient chooses a primary-care provider who is the primary physician as well as the "gatekeeper" of services. The provider is responsible for all aspects of care and must authorize a referral to other providers if necessary. Currently, many HMO plans allow patients to see specialists without the primary care physicians' authorization as long as the specialist is within the network of the HMO. One of the disadvantages of HMO plans is that the provider runs the risk of not being paid if predefined outcomes are not met and unnecessary services are delivered.

In the IPA, the independent physicians or group of physicians within a practice enroll patients to the IPA and contract with HMOs to provide the care. In the PHO, physicians and hospitals contract with HMO plans and provide care to a defined population of patients.

In Medicare Managed Care, reimbursement is paid in capitation rather than a fee-for-service method of traditional Medicare. The fee scale is based on the average adjusted per capita cost. As of 1998, 17.2% of the Medicare populations were enrolled in managed-care plans (Barton, 1999).

Because the underlying premise of managed care emphasizes both quality of care and cost effectiveness, mechanisms to ensure quality of care must be developed. These mechanism become of increasing importance to the public as the topic of medical errors continues to evolve. Mechanisms to control cost include capitation and precertification. Precertification is the process of obtaining authorization or permission from insurance companies for referrals and costly procedures to ensure payment. Some mechanisms to ensure quality include the Health Plan Employer Data and Information Set, which acts like a report card and ensures quality management, reports physician's credentials, delineates member's rights and responsibilities, defines preventative health services, reports utilization management, and reviews medical records. Measures to control both cost and quality include a concurrent review of the care delivered to hospitalized patients. Concurrent review is meant to manage costly cases with respect to length of stay and discharge. In addition, nurses perform disease management, health promotion and education, and case management for specific populations in order to manage chronic diseases more efficiently, to promote healthier lifestyles, and to decrease the costs by early detection of disease.

Medicare and Medicaid are government-sponsored insurance programs. The largest payer group for healthcare is the government (Finkler & Kovner, 2000). Medicare was initiated in 1965 through Title 18 of the Social Security Act and is an insurance program for the older population and disabled. Medicare Part A covers hospitalizations, and Part B covers physician fees. Medicare is administered by the Health Care Financing Administration (HCFA), now called the Center for Medicare and Medicaid Services (CMS). To qualify for Medicare, a specific age and number of years worked as "Medicare-covered employment" is required. Medicare Part A is available without premiums for those who are greater than 65 years of age and who have worked 10 years in "Medicare-covered employment." Beginning in 2003, Medicare Part B carried a monthly premium deducted from the social security payment (Centers for Medicare and Medicaid, Medicare Amounts, 2003).

Medicaid is an insurance program for the indigent population in the United States. Individual states administer Medicaid. As state budgets vary widely, the services that are available to the indigent also vary widely. In times of budget deficit, the services are always in constant threat of elimination.

The Center for Medicare and Medicaid Services, in its role as payer of Medicare and Medicaid programs, sets numerous regulations that other insurers then follow. If an institution wished to receive payment through Medicare and Medicaid, it must then follow the rules. Through the Omnibus Budget Reconciliation Act of 1968, the HCFA was mandated to develop a prospective payment system for outpatient services, replacing the previous cost-based system of payment. Before this ruling, hospital-based ambulatory care services were reimbursed by Medicare based primarily on cost. The prospective payment system pays hospital ambulatory settings a predetermined rate. Originally called Ambulatory Payment Groups, they were developed for ambulatory services delivered in a hospital setting including surgery, emergency room, and outpatient clinic settings. In 1968, Ambulatory Payment Groups were modified to form Ambulatory Payment Classifications (APCs) (Health Systems Management Network, 2002). Some form of APCs will be required for all states. Each APC is assigned a weight based on the median cost of the service within a geographic area. Payment rates are nationally determined, but payment varies by

geographic area because the cost of the service varies by geographic area (CMS). For example, generally, a service provided in New York City will cost more than the same service provided in a city in the Midwest. Many oncology services find the payment under the APC system insufficient to cover the cost of providing the service. Physician fees are paid separately and are based on three factors: a nationally uniform relative value for the service, a geographic adjustment factor, and a national conversion factor that converts the relative weights to payment amounts (Centers for Medicare and Medicaid Services: Federal Registrar, 2002).

In the absence of a national coverage policy, Medicare carriers are responsible for determining regional coverage based on the advice and input of medical and specialty societies and a review of current medical practice. Medicare is administered through local medical review policies (LMRPs), which are guidelines explaining how the Medicare Program pays the claims (Health Care Financing Administration, 2002). Each policy contains International Classification of Diseases diagnosis codes, addition or deletion of diagnosis, and replacement procedure codes.

To help process Medicare claims, the HCFA contracts with private insurance companies, referred to as carriers, intermediaries, and program safeguard contractors. These entities are called "Medicare contractors." Medicare contractors review and adjudicate claims for services to assure that Medicare payments are made only for services that are covered under Medicare Part A or Part B. In the absence of a specific national coverage decision, local contractors may make coverage decisions at their own discretion. Contractors may publish LMRPs to provide guidance to the public and medical community within a specific geographic area. These LMRPs explain when an item or service will be considered covered (including when it is "reasonable and necessary") and how it should be coded. If a contractor develops an LMRP, its LMRP applies only within the area it serves. Although another contractor may come to a similar decision, he or she is not required to do so. The CMS does not approve LMRPs but may review them to ensure that they do not conflict with national coverage decisions.

An LMRP may not conflict with a national coverage decision once the national coverage decision is effective. If a national coverage decision conflicts with a previously developed LMRP, the contractor must change the LMRP to conform to the national coverage decision. A contractor may, however, make an LMRP that supplements a national coverage decision. The HCFA requires that all contractors make their LMRPs available to the public on their contractor Website. Providers may submit requests for new or revised national coverage decisions to the HCFA. All contractors LMRPs are gathered on a monthly basis and listed on the Internet at *http://www.lmrp.net*.

A contractor's LMRP development process is required to be open to the public. This includes first developing a draft LMRP, making it available to the public, and soliciting comments on it. Beginning January 1, 2001, each contractor began listing their draft LMRPs on their contractor Websites and allowed electronic comments (Center for Medicare and Medicaid Services, 2002). CMS has activated a Website for users to browse and search a list of titles for all new LMRP (*www.draftlmrp.net*).

Before payment can be received, of course, bills must be generated and sent. Current procedural terminology is a systematic listing and coding of procedures and services that physicians perform (Anderson, Beebe, & Dalton et al., 2001). Each procedure or service is identified with a five-digit code. The purpose of the terminology is to provide a uniform language that will accurately describe medical, surgical, and diagnostic services and will thereby provide an effective means for reliable nationwide communication among physicians, patients, and payors. Current procedural terminology is the most widely accepted nomenclature for the reporting of physician procedures and services.

Physicians are required by law to submit a diagnosis code for every disease in order to receive Medicare reimbursement. The International Classification of Diseases is based on the official version of the World Health Organizations Ninth Revision (Hart & Hopkins, 2001). It is readily apparent from the previous discussion that billing in ambulatory care is very complex and must be completed thoroughly to maximize reimbursement. At the same time, there are rules governing provider visit types and the components of each visit type. If these rules are not followed correctly, practices can be charged with Medicare fraud and suffer financial penalties. In the recent past, a number of ambulatory practices have been charged with Medicare fraud, such as the Clinical Practices of the University of Pennsylvania (Bunch & Flannery, 1995). At issue was the billing for patient visits that physicians in training conducted. The Clinical Practices of the University of Pennsylvania settled with Medicare for $30 million. In order to bill for Medicare, an attending physician must see all patients. This regulation has been interpreted in a number of ways, but the interpretations have not been consistent with the intent of the regulation. For example, oncology physicians in training often see patients as part of their training and attending physicians supervise them. The nature of the supervision is specifically identified along with the guidelines for billing and can be found in the Medicare Carriers Manual. These guidelines are in constant flux, and compliance offices monitor them closely in most institutions. In the case of the University of Pennsylvania, huge fines were levied, and reimbursement to Medicare was required. In truth, many billing errors relate to poor systems and a lack of knowledge of the regulations. Although a painful example, this occurrence brought many teaching institutions to re-evaluate how patients were seen, and billing processes changed to accommodate the Medicare rules.

Although the regulations set forth regarding payment for services often make one feel like

Alice slipping through the rabbit hole, it is important for providers to understand the rules and regulations in order to maximize payment. Payment policies of Medicare are set forth in the Federal Register. Maximizing payment means assuming responsibility for not only delivering care but also assisting in assuring that the care is billed correctly. Nurses must have a general understanding of the regulations set forth for payment. Most ambulatory oncology practices have billers, supervisors, and regulatory experts that keep abreast of the changing rules and regulations and assure that the bills are correct and sent out in a timely manner. However, nurses as the frontline caregivers should review the payment ticket or charge master to be sure that all that was done for the patient is checked appropriately. This includes being sure that the patient identification information is correct, that the diagnosis is correct, that the visit type is correct, and that all of the interventions delivered are billed for. It is also essential that documentation matches the payment ticket. **Table 2.2** lists steps for the nurse to take to maximize payment for services. Changing rules and regulations are the responsibility of the supervisor assigned to billing; in some cases, this

might be a business manager, but in others, it might be a nurse. The supervisor will keep the staff abreast of changes that the CMS and other insurance agencies make. It is important for the nurse to understand that patients are often responsible for the portion of the bill that insurance does not cover. Making sure that payment from the insurance company is maximized is essential for the benefit of the institution as well as the patient.

Ten steps for billing under APCs have been published by Bowers et al. (2003). These include the following:

- Know your charges, revenues, and expenses.
- Bill for each service to which you are entitled. APCs allow special billing if care is provided and documented by an interdisciplinary team.
- Track payment denials and act on them quickly.
- Keep abreast of changes in billing and coding.
- Ensure communication among departments.
- Update information technology.
- Build a charge master.
- Use modifiers correctly.
- Verify and update diagnosis codes.
- Educate and keep close tabs on your pharmacy.

Although nurses as direct caregivers are not responsible for many of the components listed previously, they do have a direct impact on several of them, such as knowing the charges, revenues, and expenses for the care that they provide and ensuring communication among departments.

Regulations set forth by CMS affecting Medicare reimbursement are not always in the patient's best interest but must be followed for reimbursement to occur. For example, in order to be reimbursed by Medicare for injections of hematopoetic growth factors, the drug must be administered in the ambulatory care setting;

Table 2.2 **Steps to Maximize Payment for Services**

1. Assure completion of the "charge slip."
   - Name, address, social security information
   - Diagnosis
   - Date and level of visit
2. Check all interventions completed.
   - Blood draws
   - Intravenous fluids
   - Infusions
   - Procedures/tests
3. Assure all medications administered listed.
   - Chemotherapy
   - Premedications
4. Assure physician signature.
5. Assure that documentation reflects services provided.

patients cannot self-inject it. This poses operational problems for programs in that they often must make arrangements to be open during the weekend to administer these subcutaneous injections, and it is also burdensome for the patient who must come to the setting. Nevertheless, for payment to be received, the guidelines that the payor set forth must be followed.

Changes in regulations fill the daily newspapers and are actively followed by many lay advocate groups, such as the American Association of Retired Persons. The American Association of Retired Persons magazine lists proposed changes in legislation and encourages its members to comment on the changes. Many nurses are not interested in following changes in proposed legislation, but it is to their benefit and the benefit of their patients that they do so. One can see from the discussion thus far that federal and state legislation governs payment for cancer care. Nurses can be powerful voices for changes in legislation that will benefit patients and families. One association that monitors legislation related to healthcare economics is Volunteers in Healthcare. Their Website provides information on legislation that is under consideration as well as provides a link to state legislation. **Table 2.3** lists a sampling of legislation that should be of interest to the oncology nurse.

In addition, professional organizations are advocates for quality cancer care, including access to affordable treatment. The Oncology Nursing Society (ONS), representing over 29,000 nurses, published their call for "Comprehensive Legislation and Regulatory Action to Win the War on Cancer" in June 2001. This was included in the Health Policy Agenda for the ONS annual meeting. Not only does ONS support access to cancer care but also to clinical trials, specialists, and prescription drug coverage for senior citizens. The ONS Website (*www.ons.org*) has a "Capital Hill Electronic Advisory Report" under the "News" section that updates all viewers on recent legislative effort. A recent review includes an update on the "Access to Cancer Therapies Act," as well as a link to information on "Oral Anti-Cancer Therapies" (retrieved February 7, 2003, from *http://www.ons.org*). The "Access to Cancer Therapies Act" (HR1624/S 913) provides Medicare coverage for oral anticancer drugs. Information given on this act includes the current status of the bill, as well as a list of those legislators who are in support of the bill. Thus, the oncology nurse is armed with the information needed to take action in support of the proposed legislation. In addition to providing information, meeting with congressional leaders is a legislative effort that the society and other professional cancer organizations perform. This meeting has a tremendous impact on the financial climate of cancer care. Supporting these legislative endeavors is an important part of the advocacy role of the oncology nurse.

Pharmaceuticals are a major component of the expense of oncology care and, as such, a major focus of reimbursement. An institution that is unable to maximize billing for pharmaceuticals is destined to be unsuccessful in maintaining financial integrity.

Billing for drugs is complicated in the oncology setting in that they may be delivered off-label (i.e., for a disease not originally approved by the Federal Drug Administration or in a dosage or method not normally used). The drug package insert provides the information on use of the drug. Other sources of information on drug usage include drug evaluations by the American Medical Association, American Hospital Formulary Drug Information, and the United States Pharmacopoeia Drug Information. If the usage of the drug appears in one of the three sources listed previously, if is supported by published scientific data, or if it is medically accepted, the Medicare Cancer Coverage Improvement Act of 1993 mandates financial coverage. However, the definition of "medically accepted" is clearly open to interpretation. Thus, off-label use often requires negotiation with the patient's insurer in order to assure pay-

Table 2.3 SELECTED FEDERAL LEGISLATION RELATED TO ECONOMICS OF CARE

S 812 HR 1862	Greater Access to Affordable Pharmaceuticals Act of 2001	Amends the Food, Drug, and Cosmetic Act to provide greater access to affordable pharmaceuticals. An amendment would permit commercial importation of prescription drugs from Canada.
S 2536	Rx Flexibility for States Act	Clarifies that a state is not prohibited from entering into drug rebate agreements.
S 2244 HR 4614	Prescription Drug Price Parity for Americans Act	Permits the commercial importation of prescription drugs from Canada.
S 2042	Access to Affordable Health Care Act	Expands access to affordable healthcare and strengthens the safety net in rural and underserved areas.
HR 2635	To amend Welfare Reform	Allows states to provide primary and preventative care to all individuals.
S 1177	Access to Affordable Rx Drug Act of '01	Approves the continuation of demonstration projects that would expand access to prescription drugs under the Medicaid program.
HR 16	National Health Insurance Act	To provide a program of national health insurance.

Retrieved from the World Wide Web, 2/19/03, http://www.volunteersinhealthcare.org.

ment. In some instances, nurses can be effective in the negotiation process. However, at times, the physician's voice is needed. Documentation of the use through scientific articles is often needed. Nurses and physicians will often complain that negotiating with insurance companies on treatments should not be a part of their responsibilities. If the insurance does not pay for the service, the burden of payment falls on the patient and family, adding to an already stressful time.

Payment for pharmaceuticals under the APC system uses "J" codes for billing. J codes are billed as units of the drug, with each drug having a specific definition of 1 U per a specified milligram of drug. Units are rounded up to the highest whole number. Waste should also be included in the billing. Close relationships with the pharmacy are essential for maximizing payment.

Every pharmaceutical company has systems in place to accommodate those who are not insured and who are unable to pay for the drug recommended. **Figure 2.2** lists the services that each pharmaceutical company provides. This listing must be readily available to those who care for oncology patients. In some instances, a social worker may be able to initiate the paperwork necessary; in other instances, it must be the patient himself or herself. Although a clear benefit to patients, the paperwork required can be overwhelming and at times represent a stigma for the patient. Information relating to the patient's insurance, economic situation, and assets is often required. The nurse's role is to assist the patient through this process with dignity and respect. Viale and Mister (2001) reported on their experience in creating a "Medication Assistance Program" in their public teaching facility. Designed as a method to save money, a full-time coordinator for the program was employed by the Department of Pharmacy. The coordinator tracked patients in the clinic, worked with patients to complete the paperwork, if eligible, and developed relationships with the pharmaceutical companies. During the first fiscal year, the Medication

Figure 2.2 SELECTED MEDICATION ASSISTANCE PROGRAMS AVAILABLE TO ONCOLOGY CARE

Amgen: Safetynet Program for Neupogen
800-272-9376
Eligibility is based on the patient's insurance status and income level.

AstraZeneca Foundation Patient Assistance Program
800-424-3727
Eligibility is based on income level and lack of any other means to pay for medication.

Aventis Oncology PACT Program
800-996-6626
Provides Taxotere and Gliadel to patients. Eligibility is based on their lack of insurance.

Anzemet Hotline
800-996-8607
Eligibility is based on the patient's insurance status and lack of eligibility for government-assisted programs.

Lovenex
888-632-8607
Eligibility depends on patients meeting financial criteria; however, no tax return is needed.

Bristol-Meyers Squibb Oncology/ Immunology Access Program
800-272-4878
Eligibility is based on household size, income, self-paid expenses, and prescription coverage for assistance.

Eli Lilly and Company Gemzar Patient Assistance Program
888-4-GEMZAR (888-443-6927)
Eligibility is based on income, a lack of medical insurance, and ineligibility for any programs with drug benefit provision.

Genentech, Inc. Uninsured Patient Assistance Program
800-879-4747
Eligibility is based on the patient's inability to receive public or private insurance reimbursement. This program is for Activase or Rituxan. Genentech will provide replacement of the amount of product used to treat the patient.

Genetics Institute Neumega Access Program
888-638-6342 (888-NEUMEGA)
Eligibility is based on the uninsured or underinsured patient who has limited financial resources.

Glaxo Wellcome, Inc. Patient Assistance Program
800-722-9294
Eligibility is based on multiples of the federal poverty level adjusted for household size. Income documentation is required after 90 days of coverage. This program is for Zofran and Zyban.

GlaxoSmithKline Reimbursement Hotline
800-699-3806
Eligibility is based on an annual household income of less than $25,000, a lack of medical insurance, and an inability to participate in government-sponsored programs covering cost of pharmaceuticals. This program is for Hycamtin.

Janssen Pharmaceutical Patient Assistance Program
800-652-6227
All of Janssen's prescription products, including fentanyl transdermal, will be free to those who meet eligibility program criteria.

Novartis Oncology Assistance Hotline
800-282-7630 (for Aredia)
Eligibility is based on household income and lack of prescription coverage.
877-GLEEVEC (for Gleevec).
Eligibility is based on a lack of insurance or pharmacy benefit coverage.

Ortho Biotech, Inc. Procritline Program
800-553-3851
Eligibility is based on meeting specific medical criteria and the lack of financial resources or third-party coverage.

Pfizer, Inc., Diflucan and Zithromax Patient Assistance Program.
800-869-9979
Eligibility is based on a lack of insurance or third-party coverage, with income less than $25,000 per year without dependents or less than $40,000 with dependents.

Pharmacia & Upjohn, Inc. RxMAP Prescription Assistance Program.
800-242-7014
Eligibility is based on federal poverty level and a lack of prescription drug coverage.

Roche Oncoline and Helpline
800-443-6676
Income criteria is not required for the Oncology Medical Needs Program for Kytril.
Eligibility is based on income and requires submission of a 1040 tax return and documentation of no insurance coverage for medications. This program is for Xeloda, Vesanoid, and FuDR.

Reprinted with permission from, Viale, P. & Mister, S. (2001). Utilization of medication-assistance programs for medically uninsured patients: One public teachers hospital's experience. Journal of clinical Onocology, 5, p. 249. Updated March 2003.

Assistance Program (MAP) program captured $1,450,000 in received medications, 30% of which were related to oncology (Viale & Mister, 2001, p.251.)*

The cost of drugs is often unknown to the nursing staff. Drug information articles rarely include the cost of specific drugs. Instead, common elements of drug information include classification, indication, action, metabolism, excretion, half-life, adverse reactions, interactions, route and dosage, nursing implications, and patient teaching. Although all of these components are essential to

* *Additional resources regarding medication assistance programs include the Red Book (Cardinale, 2001) and the Website of the Pharmaceutical Research and Manufacturers of America organization at www.prma.org. This Website has a special area on Patient Assistance Programs.*

nursing care, information on cost is important for the financial issues for the patients. Recently, Wilkinson (2001) and Dolbey (2002) have included a reference to the associated pharmacy-assistance programs for the drugs discussed in their articles. This practice will be helpful as nurses continue to learn about the cost of cancer treatments.

Outflow

Outflow is defined as the expenses that must be managed in the ambulatory care of cancer patients. Outflow includes such areas as personnel, supplies, equipment, and overhead costs.

Personnel is one of the most expensive costs of caring for cancer patients, with nursing being one of the most expensive professionals involved in the care. Medical care is also expensive, but medical care is directly billable; thus, the associated cost of medical care is not often viewed in a negative light. In the constant attempt to manage costs, a reduction in personnel or a change in the skill mix of personnel is often contemplated. However, a changing skill mix in oncology practices is difficult because of the administration of chemotherapy. Nurses with expertise in administering chemotherapy, managing the side effects of treatment, and educating patients about their disease and treatment are essential for delivery of quality patient care. In addition, consumers are becoming more informed on what comprises quality cancer care and are looking for nurses who are expert in the delivery of care. Financial prudence requires that the right nurses be hired to provide the correct care at the correct time. This requires that nurse executives understand the delivery of care in the outpatient setting and the timing of patient visits.

The nursing shortage of today impacts the delivery of cancer care, as well as the satisfaction of the nursing staff. Many factors contribute to the current shortage, including the aging of the nursing workforce, more career options available to women resulting in fewer young people choosing careers in nursing, and high dissatisfaction among healthcare workers. With the current nursing shortage, recruitment and retention of nurses will continue to be foremost on the agenda of the nurse manager or director in oncology ambulatory practices. The latest summary of the registered nurse population reported by the U.S. Department of Health and Human Services (USDHHS, 2001) reflected that of the 2,201,813 registered nurses in the United States, 81.7% are employed in nursing (USDHHS, p. 22). Twenty-eight percent or 625,139 of the employed nurses are working on a part-time basis, with the highest percentage of part time nurses working in ambulatory care settings (USDHHS, p. 23). The American Hospital Association investigated the healthcare worker shortage as it applies to hospitals and commissioned a report entitled "In Our Hands" (American Hospital Association, 2002). The Bureau of Health Professions projects that by 2010, 3.1-million new jobs will exist in addition to 2.2-million replacement jobs (AHA, 2002, p. 9). Strategies recommended to address the current shortage include fostering meaningful work, improving the workplace partnership, broadening the base of healthcare workers, and building a societal support. The American Hospital Association's outlined recommendations apply to the ambulatory care setting, as well as the inpatient hospital setting.

Although these recommendations do not address salary, there is little doubt that the earnings of registered nurses impact an individual's desire to pursue a career in nursing. The United States Department of Health and Human Services reported data on the registered nurse population in the United States. The average annual earnings of full-time employed nurses is $46,782, which represents a 2.7% increase on an annual basis between 1996 and 2000 (USDHHS, 2001, p. 27). The average annual earnings for full-time status varies by geographic settings, with those in the West North Central area earning $36,958 compared with those in the Pacific area earning $49,825 (USDHHS, p. 36). Wages are sited as a dissatisfier for nurses; thus, as the nursing shortage continues, demands for higher wages and better benefits will be made. Settings where registered nurses earned less than the overall average included ambulatory care at $45,256. Job satisfaction declines with age, with the exception of those working in ambulatory care. This suggests that the conditions in ambulatory care settings may accommodate older workers better than other settings.

Cancer care, although rewarding, can also be very taxing, as nurses experience stress over the high volume of patients that are cared for in 1 day and the complex treatments that are delivered in the outpatient settings. A national survey commissioned by the Oncology Nursing Society in 2001 (Lamkin, Rosiak, Buerhaus et al., 2001) indicated that nurses in the outpatient setting report providing care for a range of from 3–60 patients in 1 day, with the majority reporting caring for a range of 5–20 and a mean of 16.34 patients in 1 day. Sixteen patients and families to care for in 1 day can be extremely stressful. Sixty-five percent of the respondents report caring for more patients than they feel is appropriate. Stress and dissatisfaction with work contribute to high turnover of staff. Expenses associated with recruitment of staff are very high and demand that retention become a major initiative in every healthcare setting. A savvy administrator will realize this and develop strong relationships with the staff in order to identify and improve working conditions, thus contributing to a satisfying work experience.

Numerous organizations are investigating the nursing shortage and the work that must be done now to accommodate the even worse shortage projected in the future. Along with 18 other nursing organizations, the ONS worked together to develop a strategic plan called Nursing's Agenda for the Future (retrieved from the Internet, *http:// www.nursingworld.org/naf* on April 2002). These organizations represent the ability

of this shortage to break down the barriers between organizations to work for a common societal good.

Nursing is becoming maturer as a profession in the work of documenting the outcomes of care and the financial impact of nursing care specifically. Ritz et al. (2000) reported on a randomized clinical trial investigating the effect of advanced nursing care on quality of life and cost of women diagnosed with breast cancer. They based this study on the landmark work of Brooten et al. (1986) who investigated the outcomes of care that advanced practice nurses provided for low birth weight infants. Ritz et al. pointed out the difficulty of examining cost data because often costs such as lost income and additional expenses incurred by the patient and family are not easily available or known to the subject. Cost data included in her study were charges and reimbursements. Provider fees were not available. The Mischel Uncertainty in Illness Scale, Profile of Mood States, and the Functional Assessment of Cancer Therapy measured quality of life. Quality of life, as evidenced by uncertainty, was significantly different in the intervention group compared with the control group. Mood disturbance decreased significantly in unmarried women in the control group compared with the intervention group, but not in the entire group. There was no change in the Functional Assessment of Cancer Therapy scores. The results of the financial analysis reported no significant difference in the costs associated with the intervention group compared with the control group. Discussion of the findings indicated that the outpatient visits were often for treatment-related purposes such as chemotherapy or radiation therapy and may not be impacted by the intervention of advanced practice nurses.

The study by Ritz et al. (2000), however, similar to the one by Brooten et al. (1986) is an important example of the work that must be done to differentiate the care that is provided by nurses, as well as document the financial impact of the care. This work will have significant impact on how nursing care is valued and structured in the future. An important study by Needleman (Needleman et al., 2001) identified outcomes in hospitalized patients that were impacted by nurse staffing and staffing mix. Although related to inpatient hospital care, studies similar to the work of Needleman et al. will need to be developed for the ambulatory care setting.

Efficient scheduling is also required for efficient use of staff and to enhance patient satisfaction. Without an efficient scheduling system, patients or staff will be left waiting. Patients may end up arriving all at the same time and thus have to wait for their treatment. At the same time, nurses will be left waiting for patients to arrive with no one to treat at any given time. When patients do arrive, they want to be treated in a timely manner. Waiting causes an increase in anxiety for the patient and an increase in stress for the nurse, as well as the pharmacists and other healthcare professionals involved in the care. Several institutions have attempted to define scheduling systems that are designed to maximize efficiency of staff and reduce wait times for patients. Managers of ambulatory care should give them careful attention so that scarce resources are not wasted.

Supplies and equipment are also major sources of outflow for ambulatory care services. As in inflow, the major cost of supplies is pharmaceuticals. Although maximizing reimbursement is the strategy of choice in the area of inflow, the correct use of drugs is the strategy of choice in outflow. Often drug choice is based on habit or convenience; however, clinical evidence should be the driving aspect of the decision on which drug to recommend for a specific situation. Engstrom, Hernandez, Haywood, and Lilenbaum (1999) reported on an important study of the efficacy and cost effectiveness of the use of antiemetic drug therapy. This team sought to define guidelines for antiemetic use that were appropriate as well as cost effective. One aspect of their success likely relates to the fact that they used an interdisciplinary team of a nurse practitioner, nurse specialist, clinical pharmacist, and physician for the development and implementation of their plan. The purpose of the study was to develop consistent guidelines relating to antiemetic use, to increase patient compliance, to optimize nurse and pharmacy time, and to deliver medications in a cost-effective manner. Specifically, they were interested in replacing costly intravenous drugs with oral drugs when possible. The results demonstrated that oral antiemetic guidelines were safe and effective when targeted to the emetic potential of each drug. In addition, $17,591 was saved during the first 9 months of the study. This study is important in that it demonstrates the financial impact of targeted treatments. Studies such as this could be replicated by institutions to obtain financial savings as well as obtain buy-in for changes needed.

Additional supplies include the cost of intravenous therapies, tubing, dressings, as well as other additional medical surgical supplies. Nurses must be vigilant in managing these costs while providing quality care to patients. Each caregiver has a responsibility to be prudent in their use of supplies.

Overhead costs are not visible, but are included in the management of ambulatory care. Overhead includes such aspects as rent and utilities such as heat and electricity. Overhead costs generally cannot be impacted by efficiencies of care. Still, it is important for nurses to understand that the cost of providing care to patients is all encompassing.

Patient Costs

Discussion of the economics of ambulatory care would not be complete without a discussion of economics from the view of the patient and family. This topic is usually referred to as out-of-pocket expenses but can also include the stress related to lost wages for both the patient and the caregiver of the patient. Patient costs include such items as transportation costs, childcare, clothing costs. Shelby, Taylor et al. (2002) reported on a two-phase investigation to identify the role of community-based organizations in meeting the needs of cancer patients. Phase I involved collecting information on nonprofit organizations serving cancer patients and phase II involved identifying the reported needs of breast and prostate cancer patients. Among patients with prostate cancer, the five most reported needs included personal adjustment to illness (37.5%), home care (22.2%), financial assistance (19.1%), transportation (13%), and communication with health professionals (8.1%). Breast cancer patients identified these same categories, however, with a different order and percentage. For breast cancer patients, personal adjustment to illness was also the first at 45.1%, followed by financial assistance (20.8%), transportation (14.2%), home care (14.1%), and communication with healthcare professionals (5.9%). This study clearly emphasizes the important role that financial assistance plays in the well-being, or lack thereof, of cancer patients and their families.

Given et al. (1994) studied out-of-pocket expenses of patients with breast cancer, finding that those who died between the first interview and the six month period incurred mean costs of $7,290 (SD = $3,904), and those who survived the same time period mean incurred costs of $2,983 (SD= $3,368). More (1998) studied out-of-pocket expenses in outpatients receiving chemotherapy. Five categories of expenditures were used, including clinic visits, symptoms and side effects, support/assistance, administrative costs, and quality-of-life costs. She found that total expenditures ranged from $12–$3,130 with a mean monthly expenditure of $741. There are not many people in the United States who can easily spend an additional $700 per month. Of particular note are the additional stories of patients that were not reflected in the amounts that were quantified. These include one person who owed $15,000 in medical bills for which he was awaiting reimbursement decisions by his insurance company, two subjects who could no longer afford their rent and were forced to move in with their relatives, and one person who was unable to seek employment because of the fatigue associated with treatment and was forced to return to a public assistance program. Because there were only 20 subjects in this study, these stories are particularly compelling and cause one to reflect on the possible magnitude of financial issues in cancer care for the individual patient and family.

Given this evidence of financial concerns for patients and families, the very minimum of quality of care demands that institutions provide information for assistance programs for patients and their families. **Table 2.4** lists a number of Internet resources for financial assistance. Nurses must be attune to any indication that a patient is experiencing difficulty with finances. Such cues might be coming late to treatment because of transportation problems, a move to a different address, references to unpaid bills, and any indication of additional anxiety. These may be easy to overlook in the busy ambulatory care setting; however, it is essential that nurses are sensitive to these cues and assist with follow through as needed.

Conclusion

In summary, this chapter has focused on the economic issues relating to caring for cancer patients in the ambulatory setting. Financial issues were analyzed from the perspective of inflow and outflow as well as from the individual patient and family perspective. Nurses must keep informed of financial issues that impact care and develop programs to assist patients and families as they experience the trajectory of cancer.

Table 2.4 SELECTED INTERNET RESOURCES FOR FINANCIAL ASSISTANCE

Cancer Care	www.cancercare.org 800-813-HOPE	Provides free professional help through counseling, education, information, and direct financial assistance. The Website lists a range of over 20 organizations that offers financial assistance.
American Cancer Society	www.cancer.org	A complete listing of disease-specific organizations and their Internet link is available on the Website of ACS. Many of the specific organizations offer a variety of financial assistance programs.
Avon	www.avoncrusade.com	Sponsors specific programs for breast cancer, with a special assistance fund for underserved women entitled the "AVONCares Program for Medically Underserved Women." It provides financial assistance, education, and support services to low income, uninsured, and underinsured women.
Patient advocate foundation	www.patientadvocate.org	A national nonprofit organization that serves as a liaison between patients and their insurer to resolve insurance issues.

References

2003 HHS Poverty Guidelines. (2003). *Federal Register*, 68, 6456–6458.

American Cancer Society. (2002). *Cancer Facts and Figures*. New York: American Cancer Society.

American Hospital Association Commission on Workforce for Hospitals and Health Systems. (2002). *In Our Hands*. American Hospital Association.

Barton, P. (1999). *Understanding the US Health Services System*. Chicago: Health Administration Press.

Anderson, C., Beebe, M., Dalton, J., Duffy, C., Evans, D., & Glenn, R. (2001). *Current Procedural Terminology* (Professional Edition). Chicago: AMA Press.

Bowers, M., Wade, S., & Travers-Currie, C. *10 Steps to Better Billing Under APCs*. Retrieved February 21, 2003 from *http://www.assoc-cancer-ctr.org/publications/journaljuly01*

Bunch, W. & Flannery, M. (1995). Feds to cough it up! A bitter pill to swallow for Penn Hospital Docs must pay $30 mil for Medicare billings. *Philadelphia Daily News*. December 13, 1995.

Brooten, D., Kumar, S., Brown, L., Butts, P., Finkler, S., Bakewell-Sachs, S. et al. (1986). A randomized clinical trial of early hospital discharge and home follow-up of very low birth weight infants. *New England Journal of Medicine, 315*, 934–939.

Cardinale, V. (Ed.). (2001). *2001 Drug Topics Red Book* (105th ed.). Montvale, NJ: Medical Economics.

Centers for Medicare and Medicaid Services. (2003). *Medicare Amounts for 2003*. Retrieved February 21, 2003 from *http://www.medicare.gov/basics/amounts2003.asp*

Centers for Medicare and Medicaid Services. (2002). Local medical review policy. Retrieved July 10, 2002 from *http://www.hcfa.gov/medicare/mr/lmrp.htm*

Centers for Medicare and Medicaid Services. (2002). *Federal Register December 31, 2002*. Department of Health and Human Services.

Dolbey, C. (2002). Epirubicin Hydrochloride. *Clinical Journal of Oncology Nursing, 6*, 247–248.

Engstrom, C., Hernandez, I., Haywood, J., & Lilenbaum, R. (1999). The efficacy and cost effectiveness of new antiemetic guidelines. *Oncology Nursing Forum, 26*, 1453–1458.

Finkler, S. & Kovner, C. (2000). *Financial Management for Nurse Managers and Executives*. (2nd ed.). Philadelphia: W.B. Saunders Company.

Given, B., Given, C., & Stommel, M. (1994). Family and out-of-pocket costs of women with breast cancer. *Cancer Nursing, 2*, 187–193.

Hart, A. & Hopkins, C. (2001). *ICD-9-CM: Expert for Physicians* (6th ed.). West Valley, UT: Ingenix, Inc.

Health Care Financing Administration. (2002). Local Medical Review Policy. Retrieved July 10, 2002 from *http://www.hcfa.gov/medicare/mr/lmrp.htm*

Health Systems Management Network. (2002). Ambulatory patient classifications. Retrieved July 25, 2002 from *http://www.hssm.com/hsmntxt/ambulatory-payment-classifications-review.htm*

Heffler, S., Smith, S., Keehan, S., Clemens, M. K., Won, G., & Zezza, M. (2003). Health spending projections for 2002–2003. Health Affairs. Retrieved February 7, 2003 from *http://healthaffairs.org*

Institute of Medicine. (2001). Coverage matters: Insurance and health care. Retrieved December 16, 2002 from *http://www.iom.org*

Lamkin, L., Rosiak, J., Buerhaus, P., Mallory, G., & Williams, M. (2001). Oncology nursing society workforce survey part II: Perceptions of the nursing workforce environment and adequacy of staffing in outpatient and inpatient oncology settings. *Oncology Nursing Forum, 29*, 93–100.

More, K. (1998). Out-of-pocket expenditures of outpatients receiving chemotherapy. *Oncology Nursing Forum, 25*, 1615–1621.

Needleman, J., Buerhaus, P., Mattke, S., Stuart, M., & Zelensky, K. (2001). Nurse staffing and patient outcomes in hospitals. US Department of Health and Human Services, Bureau of Health Professions, Division of Nursing. Retrieved October 10, 2001 from *http://www.bhpr.hrsa.gov/dn/staffstudy.htm*

Viale, P. & Mister, S. (2001). Utilization of medication assistance programs for medically uninsured patients: One public teaching hospitals experience. *Clinical Oncology Nursing, 5*, 247–253.

US Department of Health and Human Services, Health Resources and Services Administration, Bureau of Health Professions. (2001). The Registered Nurse Population, March 2000. Retrieved August, 2003 from *http://www.bhpr.hrsa.gov/healthworkforce/reports/rhproject/report.htm*

Ritz, L., Nissen, M., Swenson, K., Farrell, J., Sperduto, P., Sladek, M. et al. (2000). Effects of advanced nursing care on quality of life and cost outcomes of women diagnosed with breast cancer. *Oncology Nursing Forum, 27*, 923–932.

Shelby, R., Taylor, K., Kerner, J., Coleman, E., & Blum, D. (2002). The role of community-based and philanthropic organizations in meeting cancer patient and caregiver needs. *A Cancer Journal for Clinicians, 52*, 229–246.

Wilkenson, K. (2001). Irinotecan Hydrochloride. *Clinical Journal of Oncology Nursing*, 179–180.

Chapter 3

The Internet and Ambulatory Oncology Nursing Care

Elizabeth G. Gomez

Introduction

The Internet has revolutionized the communications world like nothing before. Its predecessors—the telegraph, telephone, radio, television, and computer—set the stage for this revolution. The Internet is simultaneously a worldwide broadcasting system, a mechanism for information dissemination, and a medium for collaboration that exists without regard for geographic location or time. It is not an exaggeration to state that no other industry has felt its impact more than healthcare (Beyea, 1997; Anonymous, 1998; Newbold, 2003).

All oncology healthcare professionals working in ambulatory settings find the Internet (and very often an Intranet) a silent, present partner in delivering quality cancer care (Gomez & Clark, 2001). The Internet and the myriad of wireless devices that can be attached to it are helping to reduce administrative expenses, are ensuring safer drug delivery, and are freeing ambulatory oncology nurses from administrative tasks (Clark, 1999). The Internet is also allowing busy ambulatory care nurses to stay abreast of changes in cancer information through a variety of distance education and electronically enhanced learning programs (Blum, Kramer, & Johnson, 2001;

Cameron, 2003). This chapter outlines Internet-based technologies and programs that can be deployed in an oncology ambulatory setting.

The Start of Something Big

The Internet is so ubiquitous that it strange to think that it has been around for only a few years. In the early 1990s with the advent and acceptance of the World Wide Web, a revolution in healthcare was born. Since that time, an overwhelming abundance of cancer information, much of it formerly locked away in medical libraries, has became a searchable part of the public domain (Kane, Rothman, & Catton, 2001; Oermann, Lesley, & Koefler, 2002). Access to the many cancer websites that are available has enabled a generation of healthcare consumers to be better informed and active participants in the decision-making process. In turn, this has raised the bar for nursing and patient education.

In a nutshell, the Internet is a very general infrastructure that allows computers to link together. It uses standardized protocols (mainly transport layer protocol/internet protocol) that allow computers of different shapes and sizes and those using different software to communicate seamlessly (Coiera,

1996). It is the Hypertext Mark-Up Language (HTML) developed by Tim Berners-Lee, that allows any document on the World Wide Web to be connected or "linked" to any other document. For the nurse and the patient searching the Internet for credible cancer information, these links can be both a blessing and a curse. The Internet is the network of computers that allows these documents to be transmitted (Gomez & Clark, 2001; Gomez, King, & DuBois, 1998; Newbold, 2003) (**Figure 3.1**).

Technology has long been a driver of change and a critical tool for success in the healthcare arena. Thus, it is not surprising that cancer information has been available since the nascent days of the Internet. Early websites dedicated to cancer included the following: Oncolink (now available at *www.oncolink.com*), which was started at the Radiation Oncology Department at University of Pennsylvania, the National Cancer Institute Website, ONS Online (now the ONS Website), and the American Cancer Society Website (*www.cancer.org*). There were also a host of commercial sites, such as *Oncology.com*, *Lifespire.com*, and WebRN with resources dedicated to the oncology nurse (Gomez et al., 1998). The Internet is by its very nature transient and at times unreliable. Many of the early oncology websites (circa 1996–1997) have merged with larger sites or have disappeared completely. This fact is presented as a cautionary note. Despite its great growth and potential, "here today, gone tomorrow" remains de rigueur when it comes to Internet-based sources of healthcare information (Gomez & Clark, 2001; Newbold, 1997).

Figure 3.1 INTERNET INFRASTRUCTURE

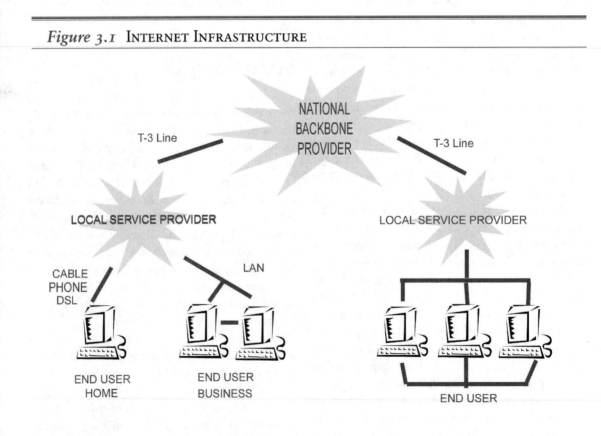

In the Clinic

This section focuses on how the Internet impacts ambulatory oncology nurses in their clinical settings.

A Familiar Role: The Trusted Patient Guide

From the infusion suite to the examination room, access to the Internet improves the delivery of quality cancer care. Recent studies report that most oncology nurses view its impact positively (Dixon, Horderm, & Armstrong, 2001; Taylor et al., 2001). Perceived advantages of using the Internet include speed of information delivery, convenience, privacy, information currency, and the ability to seek diverse points of view about a clinical topic. It is almost impossible to conceive managing a busy outpatient clinic without computers and wide area information systems.

Patients report that they do not fully trust the information that they find on the Internet and seek corroboration of their "research" from other sources, especially their oncology nurse. When an ambulatory nurse can corroborate the information a patient finds on the Internet, particularly at the time of diagnosis, it not only validates his or her expertise but also is very often the beginning of the therapeutic relationship (Clark & Gomez, 2001; Oermann et al., 2002; Pemberton & Goldblatt, 1998).

Patients need this type of guidance. For all of its good points, the Internet still has its drawbacks. Patients commonly site the following negatives when it comes to using the Internet: its impersonal nature, the amount of time it takes to find information, the lack of access to a "fast" computer, and the sheer abundance of cancer information available (Davey, Butow, & Armstrong, 2003). Managing information overload is inherent in the ambulatory oncology nurse's role. As a trusted patient guide, the Internet is one tool that the ambulatory oncology nurse has at his or her disposal to educate patients about their cancer (Biermann, 2003).

Access to medical databases such as Medline, CINHAL, and TOXNET is no longer restricted to the healthcare professional, and it is not uncommon for the ambulatory nurse to feel that the "patient knows more than they do" about his or her particular cancer. Accept that a patient may have information that the nurse has not yet come across (Pemberton & Goldblatt, 1998). This is especially true when it comes to rarer cancers or when a nurse is "covering" another clinic or when he or she is changing careers. Increased Internet use by patients and their families should not be viewed as a problem but as an opportunity for patients and their treatment team to work together. Even if one's knowledge of a particular topic is limited, a general knowledge of what constitutes a credible cancer website will go a long way in ensuring that the patient has been properly educated. For example, simply pointing them to an online support group will help them realize that they are not alone in the fight against cancer (Clark & Gomez, 2001; Metz, 2002; Pemberton & Goldblatt, 1998). (**Tables 3.1** and **3.2** show a list of credible cancer websites).

Although the Internet is never a substitute for one-on-one patient teaching, it can greatly enhance it. Nurses working in freestanding or satellite outpatient clinics can print all of the patient education materials that they need right from the Internet or from the hospital Intranet. Some never even "stock" paper copies of patient education materials anymore. Printing out "new" copies (from trusted sources) ensures that the information is the most up to date available.

Another advantage on the Internet-based system is "customability." Some online patient education tool creators (e.g., Cancer Source's Patent Education Wizard) allow a nurse to enter the patient's age, stage, prior treatments, and other variables to create a customized printable education document. Patients can also receive a document that has instructions on how to access the education plan via the web, and nurses can create a document for the chart containing the patient's information and the content selected for the plan.

Table 3.1   CREDIBLE TUMOR-SPECIFIC WEBSITES

Consider this list of websites when connecting to the Internet from a hospital or when setting up a media room. They are longstanding and meet accepted standards for credibility: authorship, privacy, and disclosure.

Brain cancer

American Brain Tumor Association	http://www.abta.org/
National Brain Tumor Foundation	http://www.braintumor.org/
National Library of Medicine: Tutorial on Brain Cancer	http://www.nlm.nih.gov/medlineplus/tutorials/braincancer.html

Breast cancer

BreastCancer.Net	http://www.breastcancer.net/
Breast Cancer Online	http://www.bco.org/
Komen Breast Cancer Foundation	http://www.komen.org/
National Alliance of Breast Cancer Organizations	http://www.nabco.org/

Colorectal cancer

Colon Cancer Alliance	http://www.ccalliance.org/
Colorectal Cancer Network	http://www.colorectal-cancer.net/

Eye cancer

Eye Cancer Network	http://www.eyecancer.com/

Head and neck cancer

Let's Face It	http://www.faceit.org/
International Association of Laryngectomees	http://www.larynxlink.com/index.html
Support for People with Oral and Head and Neck Cancer	http://www.spohnc.org/index.html

Kidney cancer

Association of Online Cancer Resources—Kidney Cancer	http://listserv.acor.org/archives/kidney-onc.html
Kidney Cancer Association	http://kidneycancerassociation.org/default1.html
MedlinePlus: Kidney Cancer	http://www.nlm.nih.gov/medlineplus/kidneycancer.html

Liver cancer

Liver Tumor.org	http://www.livertumor.org/

Table 3.1 CREDIBLE TUMOR-SPECIFIC WEBSITES (CONT'D)

Lung cancer

Lung Cancer.org	http://www.lungcancer.org
Lung Cancer Online	http://www.lungcanceronline.org/
National Library of Medicine tutorial on lung cancer	http://www.nlm.nih.gov/medlineplus/tutorials/lungcancer.html

Lymphoma and leukemia

Childhood Leukemia Center	http://www.patientcenters.com/leukemia/index.html
Leukemia and Lymphoma Society of America	http://www.leukemia.org/hm_lls
Lymphoma Information Network	http://www.lymphomainfo.net/

Melanoma

Melanoma Patients' Information Page	http://www.mpip.org/
Melanoma Research Foundation	http://www.melanoma.org/

Multiple myeloma

International Myeloma Foundation	http://www.myeloma.org/myeloma/home.jsp
Multiple Myeloma Research Foundation	http://www.multiplemyeloma.org/
National Library of Medicine: Multiple Myeloma	http://www.nlm.nih.gov/medlineplus/tutorials/ multiplemyeloma.html

Oral cancer

Oral Cancer Foundation	http://www.oralcancerfoundation.org/

Ovarian cancer

FORCE: Facing Our Risk of Cancer Empowered	http://www.facingourrisk.org/index.php
International Ovarian Cancer Connection	http://www.ovarian-news.com/
Ovarian Cancer National Alliance	http://www.ovariancancer.org/
National Ovarian Cancer Coalition	http://www.ovarian.org

Pancreatic cancer

Pancreatic Cancer	http://www.healthyfoundations.com/pancreatic/
Pancreatic Cancer Action Network	http://www.pancan.org/
Pancreatica.org	http://www.pancreatica.org/

Prostate cancer

National Library of Medicine: Prostate Cancer	http://www.nlm.nih.gov/medlineplus/tutorials/ prostatecancer.html
National Prostate Cancer Coalition	http://www.4npcc.org/
Phoenix5	http://www.phoenix5.org/
US TOO International Prostate Cancer	http://www.ustoo.com/

Table 3.2 CREDIBLE GENERAL CANCER WEBSITES

American Cancer Society
http://www.cancer.org/docroot/home/index.asp

American Society of Clinical Oncology
http://www.asco.org/

American Society of Pediatric Hematology and Oncology
http://www.aspho.org/

American Association Cancer Research
http://www.aacr.org/

Association Cancer Online Resources
http://www.acor.org/

American Academy of Ambulatory Care Nursing
http://aaacn.inurse.com/

Association of Pediatric Oncology Nurses
http://www.apon.org/

Cancer 411
http://www.cancer411.com/index.asp

Food and Drug Administration: Approved Cancer Drugs
http://www.fda.gov/cder/cancer/approved.htm

Food and Drug Administration's Oncology Reference Tools
http://www.fda.gov/cder/cancer/index.htm

InteliHealth: Genetic Testing Guide
http://www.intelihealth.com/IH/ihtIH/WSIHW000/32193/32193.html

National Cancer Institute: CancerNet
http://cancer.gov/cancerinformation

National Comprehensive Cancer Network
http://www.nccn.org/

National Center for Complementary and Alternative Medicine
http://www.nccam.nih.gov/

Oncology Nursing Society
http://www.ons.org

Ten years ago, customized patient education seemed like a pipe dream. It simply would not have been feasible to develop print pieces to cover every situation. A creative use of the Internet handles this problem nicely. Mass distribution of patient education materials via the Internet or Intranet also allows for some degree of uniformity in the patient education delivered across settings (Clark, 1999; Gomez & Clark, 2001; Metz, 2002). Everyone, literally, is on the same page.

At Your Service: The Personal Digital Assistant

Hand-held computing is the next "big thing" for the ambulatory oncology nurse. Data capture and retrieval using a personal digital assistant (PDA) is enhancing the delivery of quality cancer care and improving its efficiency dramatically. The

---

Table 3.3 SUGGESTED GUIDELINES WHEN COMMUNICATING WITH PATIENTS
VIA E-MAIL

Consider these general principles when communicating with patients via e-mail.

- Ask patients what method of communication they prefer and document that preference in a patient's chart.
- Establish up front the topics (e.g., prescription refills, appointment scheduling) that will be permitted via e-mail. Ultrasensitive topics, such as health status, HIV status, and mental illness, should never be discussed in e-mail.
- Instruct patients to use specific subject lines in their messages. Suggested titles include prescription question, appointment change, and billing question.
- Teach patients that neither doctors' offices nor healthcare organizations are liable for information lost during technical failures or power outages.
- Instruct patients to include their first and last name and patient identification number in the body of the message.
- Request that patients use their autoreply feature to acknowledge that they received the e-mail.
- Never use e-mail for urgent matters. Examples of urgent matters include life-threatening blood counts, test results that require immediate follow-up, and responses to anyone who is suicidal.
- Establish a turnaround time for messages. For example, state that all nonurgent e-mail will be answered within 36 hours. Develop a quality assurance system to monitor compliance.
- Follow the HIPPA guidelines. In particular, patients should be aware if anyone other than the sender will see the e-mail.
- Inform the patient about who will answer e-mail when the primary nurse is on vacation or out sick for an extended period of time.
- Make weekly backups of messages and develop an archive in each practice setting.
- As a general rule, e-mail messages should be included as part of the medical record, even if this means printing them out and inserting them in the chart. Include any replies and confirmation of receipt.
- Configure an automatic reply to acknowledge receipt of messages from patients. Use the autoreply to instruct patients on where to call for emergencies.
- Maintain a mailing list of patients, but as a general rule, do not send group mailings. Use the blind copy feature in software if sending a group e-mail.
- As with all e-mail communications, avoid joke telling or libelous references.

---

migration of healthcare informatics to mobile devices is no longer part of the "long-term plan." It is here today and arrived earlier than anyone would have predicted. PDAs are currently used for research, clinical data collection, prescribing, capturing patient charges, some forms of patient education, and scheduling. A host of clinical and reference tools is available for the PDA (Beyea, 1997; Suszka-Hildebrandt, 2001; Terry, 2002).

PDAs have come a long way from their introduction almost a decade ago. Sluggish and bulky products such as Apple's "Newton" hand-held computer have evolved into smaller, quicker devices than contain a significant amount of computing power (Ebell, 1995; Schneider, 2001; Smith, 2002). Over time, the software for the PDA has also improved, and the number of choices has increased exponentially. There is very little a PDA cannot do when compared with its older cousin, the desktop PC (**Table 3.4**).

The following is a list of the types of applications that ambulatory oncology nurses are loading into their PDA.

- Drug reference programs. Looking up drug information remains the most popular use of the PDA in the ambulatory setting (Newbold, 2003; Schneider, 2002; Smith, 2001). These drug guides provide up-to-date information on dosages, delivery, and cost. They let the prescriber know whether there is a generic equivalent available. If the drug database is integrated with a suite of other clinical management tools, it can often highlight potential interactions and contraindications.

- E-prescribing programs. Prescription errors put not only patients at risk, but are extremely time consuming for the ambulatory care nurse when they result in call-backs to either the patient or the pharmacist (Newbold, 2003). By using a PDA, the prescriber can write the order electronically and send it directly to the pharmacy. Programs integrated in a suite of clinical applications can even "precheck" the formulary, notify the prescriber of potential drug interactions, and check the patient's insurance coverage.

- Billing applications. PDAs provide the ideal way to track billable information. Many of these programs have the billing codes embedded, eliminating the cumbersome process of looking them up after the fact (Newbold, 2003). Another advantage is that billing data can be transferred directly to an institutional mainframe computer so that all changes are accounted for properly and transcription errors are minimized. Programs such as these are favorites for oncology nurse practitioners.

- Medical calculators. What a timesaver! The PDA can quickly perform many essential medical calculations such as IV drip rates, analgesic conversions, body surface area, and creatinine clearance. Ambulatory nurses in infusion centers have put down their charts and picked up their PDAs for the calculator function alone.

- Medical reference libraries. Because most PDAs can easily fit into a laboratory coat, they make the ideal repository for reference material, surpassing bulky books for usefulness. There are dozens of PDA titles specific to oncology and nursing. These programs have replaced the "cheat sheets" or index cards once commonly found in laboratory coats a mere 3 years ago.

- Patient tracking. These programs allow ambulatory nurses to maintain profiles of individual patients. It is important to remember that almost all of these profiles include personal and demographic information (Blum et al., 2001). These profiles, like the medical record, are subject to the Health Insurance Portability and Accountability Act (HIPAA). HIPPA was designed to standardize the way that all healthcare organizations electronically exchange patient data and to protect patients from unauthorized disclosure of their medical records. HIPAA regulations require healthcare organizations to formalize a plan that complies with auditability, security, privacy, and transaction exchange standards. In this context, they protect patient confidentiality. It is recommended that ambulatory nurses use only the programs and secure systems provided by their institution for patient tracking (Pancoast, Patrick, & Mitchell, 2003).

As mentioned previously, literally hundreds of programs are available that would be of interest to the oncology ambulatory nurse, and they are far too numerous to list here. These two websites—Palm One: Health Care (available at *http://palmone.com/us/solutions/healthcare/*) and the PDA Cortex (available at *http://www.pda cortex.com/*)—both review and sell most of these products.

Shall We Talk? Or Type? Patient Communication

The telephone triage process is a large component of the ambulatory nurse's role. Some nurses dedicate an entire workday each week just to returning phone calls. Using a self-documenting tool such as e-mail to communicate routine items such

---

Table 3.4 TIPS FOR CHOOSING A PDA

Devices in the handheld computer category offer a very broad range of functionality. Consider these factors when selecting a PDA:

Color.	Do you need it? Probably, yes, especially if your work requires looking at a lot of images. Color screens offer a clearer display, and this can improve readability. One notable disadvantages of a color screen is the decreased battery life.	**Software.**	Currently more medical software is available for the Palm OS. The software library for Pocket PC is slowly increasing, and many popular applications originally written for the Palm OS now have a Pocket PC counterpart.
Memory.	Having enough memory is critical. Without it, the number of programs available will be limited. Palm OS devices usually have 8 to 16 MB of memory, and Pocket PCs usually have 32 to 64 MB of memory. As a general rule, Palm OS applications typically use less memory than the Pocket PC version of the same product. Can more memory be added? Is the devise expandable? Virtually all devices (with the exception of very low-end models) accept memory cards or sticks.		Popular programs for ambulatory oncology nurses, such as databases, drug guides, and calculators, are generally available on both platforms.
		Battery life.	A simple monochrome (black and white) PDA will last longer on battery power than a color PDA. A wireless connectivity feature is also a drain on battery power.
Operating system.	Operating systems come in two flavors: Pocket PC, created by Microsoft, and the Palm OS, from Palm Computing. The most important aspect of the operating system is not who makes it but the amount of software that has been written for it. Windows users may find the Pocket PC interface more familiar.	**Percentage of market share.**	Currently, there are many more Palm OS devices then Pocket PC devices. Software developers are more likely to write applications for the Palm OS. It is important that one's PDA be compatible with that of their colleagues and the institution's network because that is where most data sharing will take place.
		Price.	PDAs generally range anywhere from $100 to $350. As a rule, Pocket PCs are slightly more expensive than Palm devices. Look for sales. Many refurbished products with guarantees are also available.

as appointments, schedules, and prescriptions has saved many oncology ambulatory nurses countless hours (Ferguson, 2002; Gomez & Clark, 2001).

Patient e-mail, defined as "computer-based communication between clinicians and patients within a contractual relationship in which the healthcare provider has taken on an explicit measure of responsibility for the client's care," is an entirely different type of communication (Kane & Sands, 1998). It, too, has advantages, such as a reduction in nonurgent telephone calls and pages, increased patient satisfaction and participation, and improved record keeping of all patient communications (eRisk Working Group on Healthcare, 2002; Ferguson, 2002).

Nurses, pharmacists, and physicians should communicate with e-mail with great care. There are various national guidelines (none of which are legally binding) and institution-specific guidelines to bear in mind when communicating in this way (Kane & Sands, 1998) (see **Table 3.3** for more detailed guidance).

American Medical Informatics Association (AMIA) recommends that healthcare providers maintain a mailing list of their patients, but they state that doctors should never send group e-mails where other recipients are listed. Additionally, a patient's e-mail address should not be shared with marketers or even family members (Kane & Sands, 1998).

E-Consults for the "E-Patient"

Despite the many innovations in telepathology and teleradiology, it remains impossible for the healthcare professional to examine a patient virtually. Those who offer healthcare advice or services via the Internet directly to patients must rely on the "e-patient" and the information that they provide (or withhold). Deprived of the rich information resources such as physical exams, personal communication, pathology samples, and the complete medical record, the healthcare professional offering a clinical opinion is operating at a disadvantage. Although the technology is sure to improve, today's healthcare professional must compensate for this lack of information by limiting advice to generalities. At this time, direct communication with the e-patient is not recommended.

The online consultation that is given in exchange for direct patient payment introduces an additional risk. Payment for an e-consult implies that the healthcare provider will assume the same responsibility for the e-patient's care as they would for the "real" patient sitting in the waiting room. It is imperative that all e-consults include an explicit follow-up plan and that the plan be clearly communicated to the patient (Orlick, 2003).

Models for e-consultation systems are being developed. Successful programs focus on peer-to-peer interaction, with physicians and nurse practitioners acting on behalf of their patients who are seeking specialty advice or second opinions. There is a notable program at the Dana Farber Cancer Institute in Boston. Their system makes it easy to receive a specialist's consultation while not disrupting the patient's relationship with his or her current healthcare team. The patient's care remains local. The primary healthcare provider who knows the patient the best can incorporate the specialist's advice into the overall treatment plan.

In The Waiting Room

The Internet has become a valued source of cancer patient education because millions of people now use the Internet as their primary source in gathering health information (Gomez & Clark, 2001). An increasing number of patients and their families are using the Internet for health-related "research" through websites, newsgroups, chat rooms, and listservs. Many report that the ability to seek out information on their own can be "empowering" (Ahmann, 2000).

What setting could be better than the patient waiting room to begin that search? It seems ideal. The patients have time, are interested in the topic, and have a healthcare professional steps away to help them clarify any questions. A networked computer in a waiting room may be significantly faster than the computer that the patient has at home, or it may be their only access to a computer. The benefits of translation software cannot be understated. In theory, patients who have access to the Internet should enter the actual examination room for consultation and treatment more informed and less anxious.

Offering this type of service requires some planning. Simply connecting a computer and giving patients "free reign" will not do. The goal is to make the clinic experience more efficient, not less. Backed up clinic schedules will occur if patients have downloaded reams of information for the nurse to review while they were waiting (Ahmann, 2000; Clark, 1999; Clark & Gomez, 2001). Here are five "S's" to consider when setting up a waiting room computer:

- **Security.** Computers are expensive. Bolt the computer, keyboard, and mouse to a large, bulky stand, preferably one on wheels. Make the computer as difficult to steal as possible. Lock it up at night.
- **Screen size.** Size and clarity matter. A desktop computer with a 15- to 17-inch screen is recommended. This will allow patients with poor vision to enlarge the text on the page. In general, laptops should be avoided.
- **Sound.** Many excellent patient education programs are available via streaming video, and the bulk of these have an audio component. The waiting room computer should be enabled with a piece of hardware called a "sound card." Provide headsets, as not everyone in the waiting room will want to hear the program.
- **Staff.** Collaboration with the information technology (IT) department is essential when placing a computer in a patient area. They must address all technical questions according to the institution's policy on computer use. Day-to-day maintenance is also the responsibility of IT department. When staffing allows, having a nurse, a dedicated media specialist, or a medical librarian in the waiting room can help to assist patients. Some institutions offer computer orientation and training classes.
- **Selection.** Be proactive! Preselect 5 to 10 websites that offer credible cancer information and ask the IT department to bar access to any others. If the outpatient setting is dedicated to a specific type of cancer, select even more disease-specific sites. Patients should be taught to be skeptical and to approach all other cancer information cautiously. There are several online "sitecheckers" (e.g., the well-established Health Information Technology Institute IQ Tool) [Rippen et al., 1999] which can be applied to help patients evaluate quality. (See **Tables 3.1** and **3.2** for lists of credible websites).

Can't Get Out? We'll Come to You. Web-Based Learning Opportunities for the Ambulatory Oncology Nurse

Old Reliable: The Listserv Option

A mailing list group (also commonly known as a listserv) is a type of global participation journal. It is one of the most enduring web applications (Baxter, 1997; Chappell, 1999).

This is how it works:

- The user subscribes to the list or group of their choice (subscriptions are usually free).

- All messages posted to the group are sent to everyone subscribed. Users can receive messages individually or in one long e-mail (called the "digest") at the end of the day. The digest mode can be very helpful for large lists that have many messages.
- The user can reply to any of the messages or send an entirely new message or topic (called a thread).

The task of keeping track of subscribers and making copies of messages is automated by a software program called "ListServ," hence the name (Baxter, 1997).

Lists can be moderated, but for the most part, they are unmoderated. On unmoderated lists, all messages posted to the group's address are automatically sent to the group; thus, nurses are advised to review their posts carefully before sending and to avoid "flaming" or speaking negatively about others. This is a handy way to get answers to clinical questions and hear diverse opinions (Baxter, 1997; Chappell, 1999). There are many listserv e-mail groups for ambulatory oncology nurses (see **Table 3.5** for some of the most active).

Distance Education

Distance education has gained acceptance as a method for delivering healthcare education across the many specialties that contribute to the delivery of quality cancer care. Nurses, oncologists, surgeons, pharmacists, physician assistants, radiation therapists, phlebotomists, and administrative and support staff are all using the Internet to keep their oncology knowledge current (Berke & Wiseman, 2003; Dixon et al., 2001; Taylor et al., 2001).

Many accredited schools of nursing now offer instruction via distance education in their degree programs. Once impossible to imagine, it is now entirely feasible to achieve a basic or advanced degree in nursing without ever stepping foot on a campus (Bentley, 2003; Schuster, 2003). This new form of education is radically different from the traditional lecture and clinical experience format. Delivering formal nursing education via distance education is raising many questions among nursing educators. Topics currently being studied are the impact of distance education on professionalism, role development, and the establishment of a nursing identity (Taylor et al., 2001).

Ambulatory oncology nurses can now take full advantage of a myriad of continuing education opportunities via the Internet. Attending a meeting in a distant city to earn continuing education credits is no longer required (Shuster, 2003). Professional organizations, such as the Oncology Nursing Society, the Association of Pediatric Oncology Nurses, and the Association of Ambulatory Care Nurses, offer many continuing education credits in a distance education format. Their offerings are becoming more varied and sophisticated. Like their physician colleagues, oncology nurses are now able to access "virtual sessions" from major cancer nursing meetings. The "virtual" option has even affected the nurse attending the meeting "live." Oncology nurses are choosing to attend other sessions knowing that they can "come back" to a competing session via the Internet (Dixon et al., 2001; Kane et al., 2001).

The Association of Critical Care Nurses has taken the distance education-based continuing education a step farther. For a fee, they offer a complete orientation to critical care nursing. This highly successful program, entitled "Essentials of Critical Care Orientation: An Introduction to Critical Care," is based on a series of modules that nurse experts developed and it uses a variety of technologies. A high-speed Internet connection is required to participate in the program (American Association of Critical Care Nurses, 2003). The program has been implemented by over 250 hospitals nationwide and has become a cornerstone in institution-specific critical care nursing orientation programs. Many residents are also using the program. Nurses can review the modules alone or in groups and are given a timeframe to complete the program. It is innovative programming such

Table 3.5 LISTSERV E-MAIL GROUPS FOR THE AMBULATORY ONCOLOGY NURSE

To join any of these listservs send a message to the e-mail address listed with the word "subscribe" (no quotes) in the message line.

alert@listserv.acor.org
Cancer Legislative Alert System

biotherapyandimmunotherapy@lists.cancersource.com
CancerSource.com Biotherapy and Immunotherapy Mailing List

breast-onc@listserv.acor.org

cancer-fatigue@listserv.acor.org
Fatigue Associated with Cancer and Cancer Treatments

cancer-fertility@listserv.acor.org
Fertility Issues Associated with Cancer

cancer-hospice@listserv.acor.org
Cancer-Hospice

cancer-l@listserv.wvnet.edu
CANCER-L: Support for People with Cancer

cancer-pain@listserv.acor.org
Pain Associated with Cancer and Cancer Treatments

colon@listserv.acor.org
Colon Cancer Discussion List

hipaa-regs@list.nih.gov
Notification of Regulation Publication

jnci-l@webber.oup.co.uk
Oxford Journals: Journal of the National Cancer Institute

as this that will propel nursing distance education to an even higher level.

A Matter of Trust

Trust is the cornerstone of the therapeutic nurse–patient relationship. To receive appropriate care, patients must reveal private information. They depend on their nurse to keep this information safe and confidential. They also depend on their nurse to provide accurate information about their particular cancer (Gomez & Clark, 2001; Holmes, 2003). The Internet, for all of its advantages, has made it more difficult for the ambulatory oncology nurse to establish a trusting patient relationship.

How can you trust someone you may have never met or do not know very well? In the impersonal and anonymous environment of the Internet, nurse experts who field questions from patients in "Ask the Expert" e-mail systems, in chat rooms, or on message boards are cautioned to remember that anyone participating in an online forum is able to present himself or herself as a patient. Ambulatory oncology nurses must also bear in mind that just about anyone who has access to a computer, an Internet connection, basic web-publishing software, and small amount of technical knowledge can set up a professional-looking website (Ferguson, 2002; Oermann, 2002).

Trust is becoming more difficult to establish even with one's "own" patients. With more patient contact shifting to e-mail, the number of personal encounters has decreased. A timely phone "call back," even one for a routine matter, indicates a certain level of care and concern. It may also provide the patient with an opportunity to mention another issue. In general, e-mail communication does not allow for this type of disclosure. Ending the e-mail with a phrase such as "please contact me if anything should come up between now and our next appointment" can facilitate meaningful communication. It is imperative that ambulatory nurses answer their e-mail in a timely way, just as they would a phone call.

There are other ways to establish trust. Unlike traditional healthcare, the Internet is not restricted by geographic or political boundaries. Patients are able to search for cancer information, products, and treatments on a worldwide network. Ambulatory nurses must counsel patients that different laws govern how healthcare professionals are licensed, how cancer treatments are advertised and sold, and most importantly, how their private information will be treated from country to country. Helping the patient determine which existing national, state, or local laws apply to online practices is yet another opportunity to develop a trusting relationship.

Would you trust someone who gave you bad information? Recognizing that patients are going to use the Internet to obtain cancer information, it is critical that ambulatory nurses provide them with the knowledge to sort out the "wheat from the chaff." As discussed previously here, "presurfing" the Internet and selecting credible sites for patients are ways to do this (Gomez & Clark, 2001). For the most part, however, patients will be searching without a nurse by their side. Once a patient "strays" from the preselected sites, and inevitably they will, they need the tools to decide what is good information and what is bad (Clark & Gomez, 2001; Rippen et al., 1998).

Currently, there is not a uniformly recognized "seal of approval" for cancer websites. Most, such as the long-standing Health on the Net (1999) program, are voluntary programs that are self-

policing (Oermann, 2002). This is sure to change in the near future. Leading the charge are accrediting bodies such as the Utilization Review Accreditation Commission (URAC), an independent, nonprofit healthcare organization that established a set of web quality standards and a "check-up" service to measure compliance with them.

All systems that are striving to define "quality" for Internet-based healthcare information have these important criteria in common: determining credible authorship, ensuring the confidential handling of private information, and full disclosure of the resources used to develop the site (Clark, 1999; Gomez & Clark, 2001). Ambulatory nurses who teach their patients to look beyond the "bells and whistles" and focus instead on these three criteria can be counted among the most trustworthy of all.

Conclusion

Ambulatory nursing practice is unique in the numerous ways addressed by the contributors of this book. As stated, these nurses function autonomously and may be working miles away from their main hospitals. They increasingly are using telehealth and web-based applications and some version of a personal digital assistant. As technology becomes even more sophisticated and oncology nurses continue to be in short supply, electronic communication in clinical, educational research, consulting, and patient education will become even more important.

References

Ahmann, E. (2000). Supporting families' savvy use of the Internet for health research. *Pediatric Nursing, 26,* 419–423.

American Medical Informatics Association. (1998). White Paper: Guidelines for the clinical use of electronic mail with patients [electronic version]. *Journal of the American Medical Informatics Association, 5,* 1–12. Retrieved December 10, 2003 from *http://www.amia.org/pubs/other/email_guidelines.html*

Anonymous. (1998). Nursing sites to showcase Nightingale Tracker. *Interactive Healthcare Newsletter, 14,* 4.

Anonymous. (2000). PDAs help nurses improve care and save time. *Healthcare Benchmarks & Quality Improvement, 9,* 44–46.

Baxter, B. (1997). Using e-mail and listservs. *Nursing, 27,* 21–22.

Bentley, G. (2003). RN to BSN program: Transition from traditional to online delivery. *Nurse Educator, 28,* 121–126.

Berke, J. & Wiseman, T. L. (2003). The e-learning answer. *Nursing Management, 10,* 2609.

Beyea, S. (1997). Connecting points: Personal computers: Me and my palm pilot. *Computers in Nursing, 15,* 183–184.

Biermann, J. S. (2003). Cancer websites you can recommend to your patients. *Oncology, 17,* 322–324, 328–329.

Blum, J., Kramer, J., & Johnson, K. (2001). The palm as a real-time wide-area data-access device. *Journal of the American Medical Informatics Association, 8,* 52–56.

Cameron, S. (2003). Clinical calculators for hand-held computers. *Canadian Family Physician, 49,* 1152–1153.

Chappell, S. (1999). Internet tools for gastroenterology nurses and associates. *Gastroenterology Nursing, 22,* 214–216.

Clark, P. (1999). How can we coach patients to become critical consumers of information they find on the Internet? *ONS News, 14,* 8.

Clark, P. M. & Gomez, E. G. (2001). Details on demand: Consumers, cancer information, and the Internet. *Clinical Journal of Oncology Nursing, 5,* 19–24.

Coiera, E. (1996). The Internet's challenge to health care provision. *British Medical Journal, 312,* 3–4.

Dixon, H., Hordern, A., & Borland, R. (2001). The breast cancer distance education program: Development and evaluation of a course for specialist breast care nurses. *Cancer Nursing, 24,* 44–52.

Davey, H. M., Butow, P. N., & Armstrong, B. K. (2003). Cancer patients' preferences for written prognostic information provided outside the clinical context. *British Cancer Journal, 89,* 1450–1456.

Ebell, M. H. (1995). Hand-held computers for family physicians. *Journal of Family Practice, 41,* 385–392.

eRisk Working Group on Healthcare. (2002). Guidelines for Online Communications. Retrieved November 16, 2003 from *http://www.medem.com/*

Ferguson, T. (2002). From patients to end users. *British Medical Journal, 324,* 555–556.

Health On the Net Foundation. (2000). HON code of conduct. Retrieved November 27, 2003 from *http://www.hon.ch/HONcode/*

Holmes, B. (2003). Elderly consumers: Wired and tapping into online health content. Consumer Technographics Brief. Forrester Research Group. Retrieved November 16, 2003 from *http://www.forrester.com/*

Gomez, E. & Clark, P. M. (2001). The Internet in oncology nursing. *Seminars in Oncology Nursing, 17,* 7–17.

Gomez, E., King, C., & DuBois, K. (1998). Improving oncology nursing practice through understanding and exploring the Internet. *Oncology Nursing Forum, 10,* (Suppl), 4–10.

Kane, B. & Sands, D. Z. (1998). Guidelines for the clinical use of electronic mail with patients. *Journal of the American Medical Informatics Association, 5,* 104–111. Retrieved December 10, 2003 from *http://www.jamia.org/cgi/reprint/5/1/104*

Kane, G. M., Rothman, A., & Catton, P. (2001). Staying up-to-date through distance education: The radiation therapy perspective. *Journal of Cancer Education, 16,* 205–208.

Metz, J. M. (2002). A multi-institutional study of Internet utilization by radiation oncology patients. *International Journal of Radiation Oncology and Biology Physics, 56,* 1201–1205.

Newbold, S. K. (1997). Update on virtual nursing informatics organizations. *Computers in Nursing, 15,* 122–125.

Newbold, S. K. (2003). New uses for wireless technology. *Nursing Management, 22,* 30–32.

Oermann, M. H., Lesley, M., & Kuefler, S. F. (2002). Using the Internet to teach consumers about quality care. *Joint Commission Journal of Quality Improvement, 28,* 83–89.

Orlick, R. (2003). Malpractice liability for informal consultations. *Family Medicine, 35,* 476–481.

Pancost, P. E., Patrick, T. B., & Mitchell, J. A. (2003). Physician PDA use and the HIPAA Privacy Rule. *Journal of the American Medical Informatics Association, 10,* 611–612.

Pemberton, P. J. & Goldblatt, J. (1998). The Internet and the changing roles of doctors, patients, and families. Retrieved November 27, 2003 from *http://www.mja.com.au/public/issues/xmas98/pemberton/pemberton.html/*

Rippen, H., Guard, R., Kragen, M., Byrns, P., Silber, S., & Buckovich, S. (1999). Criteria for assessing the quality of health information on the Internet [Policy paper]. Retrieved November 27, 2003 from *http://hitiweb.mitretek.org/iq/*

Schneider, T. (2001). Easy access to a world of information: Using a handheld computer. *Journal of Emergency Nursing, 27,* 42–43.

Schuster, G. (2003). A strategy for involving on-campus and distance students in a nursing research course. *Journal of Continuing Education Nursing, 34,* 108–115.

Smith, J. P. (2002). Travel nursing: Welcome to the wireless world: Essentials for a traveling nurse? Staying connected and staying organized. *Nursing, 36,* 20–22.

Suszka-Hildebrandt, S. (2001). Handheld computing: The next technology frontier for school nurses. *Journal of Scholarly Nursing, 17,* 98–102.

Taylor, J., Hobbie, W., Carlino, H., Deatrick, J., Fergusson, J., & Lipman, T. (2001). Describing the value of specialized distance education in pediatric oncology nursing. *Journal of Pediatric Oncology Nursing, 18,* 26–36.

Terry, K. (2002). Beam it up, doctor. *Medical Economics, 12,* 34–36.

Chapter 4

Role of the Advance Oncology Nurse Practitioner

Dawn Camp-Sorrell

Rebecca Hawkins

Introduction

The nurse practitioner's (NP) role in oncology, although relatively new, is emerging and expanding at an expeditial rate. NP positions within oncology are being developed in a variety of settings with a wide range of responsibilities and role diversities. The role of the NP requires astute clinical skills, critical thinking ability, and a high level of decision making. Often there are few role models, and the job can lead to feelings of isolation (Koelbel, Fuller, & Misener, 1991). This chapter explores the role of the NP, the issues surrounding the role, and future issues in oncology.

History of the Oncology NP

The development of the NP role in a large part was in a response to a need for additional healthcare providers as a way to increase patient access to healthcare. Academic NP programs began in the 1960s in response to the shortage of primary healthcare physicians. The NP's role was to assist patients with healthcare needs by complementing the physician's role. Initially, the role emerged in rural and occupational settings with emphasis on

primary care (Kelly & Mathews, 2001). The initial role of the NP was designed to meet the needs of children by establishing the pediatric NP. The first NP program was designed by Loretta Ford, EdD, PNP, FAAN, and Henry Silver, MD, FAAP, at the University of Colorado (Ford & Silver, 1967) to prepare pediatric NPs.

Initially, organized nursing did not support this nursing role and referred to this advanced nurse as a "physician substitute" (Murphy-Ende, 2002). Because of the lack of funds and the poor perception of the NP role, most NP programs were offered through continuing educational programs or as certificate programs instead of formal nursing programs. By 1974, the American Nurses Association (ANA) defined and supported the NP role for pediatrics and adult populations. Numerous studies have been conducted that support the competence of NPs, the cost effectiveness of NP services, and patient satisfaction with NPs as providers (Bryant & Clark, 2002; Cole, Mackey, & Lindenberg, 2001; Feldman, Ventura, & Crosby, 1987; Knudtson, 2000; Molde & Diers, 1985)

In 1975, Masters of Science in Nursing (MSN) programs became available based on the medical model for preparing the NP. For the past 30 years, NPs have made significant contribution to quality healthcare (Wyatt, 2001). There are approximately 20 programs that offer an NP Masters of Science in Nursing with an emphasis in oncology (Brown & Hinds, 1999). Educational programs for NPs in oncology nursing continue to change to meet the current healthcare needs. Each program varies in which oncology content is included in the curricula. The program may offer specialization in a specific patient population, such as adult versus pediatric. Other programs may offer specialization in the clinical area of oncology.

Job Settings for the Oncology NPs

Numerous barriers continue to block the full potential on the oncology NP (ONP) as a healthcare provider. Barriers include legislative restrictions of reimbursement, a lack of full prescriptive authority, a lack of support from physicians, a lack of administrative support, a lack of public knowledge, and role ambiguity (Pearson, 2002). The NP was once thought to function in the outpatient setting, but today the role boundaries are limitless. Currently, ONP's work in multiple settings, including hospitals, clinics, hospice, home care, and long-care facilities. Different patient populations are being served by the ONP, including the terminally ill, patients under active treatment and entered on clinical trials, cancer survivors, and those individuals requiring screening and detection or genetic counseling (Bush & Watters, 2001). Each setting and patient population provide the NP with a variety of opportunities, despite different rules, regulations, and barriers.

The American Academy of Nurse Practitioners has developed a framework for the ONP practice, including obtaining histories, performing physical examinations, ordering and interpreting diagnostic tests, and planning treatments, patient education, and counseling (Kinney, Hawkins, & Hudman, 1997) (**Table** 4.1). The goals and expectations of the NP and the organization are important in the success of the role (Bush & Watters, 2001). In private practice, collaboration between the NP and physician is key for success. Collaboration has been defined as an interpersonal process and commitment between two or more professionals to solve problems based on identified goals, purpose, or outcomes (Bush & Watters). Medicare requires NPs to collaborate with physicians to meet reimbursement requirements. Physicians manage patient's care in a systematic approach. If the system is broken, the system is fixed. Once the problem is fixed, there is no need to search for another problem. NPs practice from a holistic approach. The NP has the insight to look toward potential problems such as long-term chemotherapy or radiation-induced side effects.

Numerous issues must be considered when negotiating for a job, including the NP's scope of practice, annual evaluations, practice guidelines, job description, documentation procedures, role responsibilities, professional development opportunities, and procedures expected to be performed (Shay, Goldstein, Matthews, Trail, & Edmunds, 1996). One of the most important considerations of a NP is the acquisition of a caseload. How will patients become part of the NP practice? Will the physicians decide who and how many patients the NP sees? Will performance be based on the number of patients seen?

Challenges for role implementation will be determined by the ONP's experience, knowledge base, clinical experience, and competence (Bush & Watters, 2001). NPs need to accept and understand professional responsibility of patient care and acknowledge situations that the NP is not equipped to handle. Physicians need to appreciate the level of expertise of the NP and not have unrealistic expectations.

Another important consideration is to whom the NP will report for problems and annual evaluations. Each reporting structure has benefits and drawbacks for each particular institution.

Table 4.1 EXAMPLES OF ONP CLINICAL PRACTICE

NP Role	Components
History Taking	Patient's chief complaint: reason for the encounter
	History of presenting illness: chronologic description of the complaint, including location, quality, severity, timing, context, modifying factors, and associated symptoms
	Past medical history: prior illnesses, hospitalizations, or surgeries
	Medications: current, allergies
	Social history: marital status; living arrangements; current job status; use of illicit drugs, alcohol, and tobacco; education level; sexual history
	Family history: health status or cause of death of grandparents, parents, siblings, children with specific disease related to the presenting problem(s) or hereditary problems placing the patient at risk
	Review of systems: identify signs and symptoms being experienced<ul><li>General: weight change, fever, night sweats, fatigue, behavior change</li><li>Diet: 24-hour recall, restrictions, likes, dislikes</li><li>Skin, hair, nails: skin disease, pigment or color changes, mottling, change in mole, pruritus, rash, lesion, easy bruising, petechiae, easy bleeding</li><li>Musculoskeletal: joint pain, stiffness, edema, limitation of weakness, back pain</li><li>Head and neck: headache, dizziness, limitation of movement, stiffness</li><li>Endocrine: excessive hunger or thirst, frequent urination</li><li>Lungs: cough, wheezing, shortness of breath</li><li>Heart: dyspnea on exertion, limitation of activity, palpitations, tachycardia</li><li>Breasts: performance of self-examination, lumps, tenderness, edema, dimpling, retraction</li><li>Hematologic/lymphatic: edema or tender lymph nodes, excessive bleeding, excessive bruising</li><li>Gastrointestinal: pain, nausea, vomiting, diarrhea, constipation, rectal bleeding, anal itching</li><li>Genitourinary: painful urination, polyuria, oliguria, penile or testicular pain, discharge, edema, rash</li><li>Neurologic: numbness, tingling, altered sensation, altered mobility, confusion</li><li>Emotional status: support systems, recent losses, coping skills</li></ul>

(continues)

Table 4.1 EXAMPLES OF ONP CLINICAL PRACTICE (CONT'D)

NP Role	Components
Physical Examination	Methods of examination: inspection, palpation, percussion, and auscultation • Constitutional: vital signs, weight, height, general appearance of patient • Integument, hair, nails: texture, temperature, color, distribution, lesions • Head: configuration, scalp tenderness, masses • Eyes: visual acuity, extraocular movement, visual fields, conjunctivae, sclerae, lids, PERRLA (pupils equal round reactive to light and accommodation), funduscopic exam • Ears: external structure, auditory acuity, otoscopic exam • Nose: external structure, nasal mucosa, septum, turbinates • Mouth: lips, tongue, teeth, gingiva, buccal mucosa, pharynx • Neck and axilla: symmetry of neck, thyroid gland, carotid pulses and bruits, lymph node, trachea, jugular venous distention, neck distention • Chest: symmetry, lung sounds, heart sounds, breast exam, respiratory effort • Abdomen: bowel sounds, bruits, pulsations, hernias, striae, hepatomegaly, splenomegaly, lymph nodes • Extremities: evaluate skin, muscles, joints, and range of motion; pulses, deep tendon reflexes, sensation, strength, gait • Male and femal genitalia • Neurologic: orientation, alertness, cranial nerve assessment
Diagnostic Tests	Laboratory Radiologic: X-rays, computed tomography scans, magnetic resonance imaging, position emission tomography (PET) imaging Specialized and invasive testing: such as bone marrow aspiration, nerve conduction studies, colonoscopy (tests are ordered from basic to complex to invasive)
Planning Treatment	Collect all pertinent data Develop differential diagnosis Plan appropriate treatment: nonpharmacologic or pharmacologic Provide patient education Provide counseling
Referral	Out of NP scope of practice, specialized problem, required specific diagnostic testing
Follow-up	Short- and long-term to evaluate treatment, make changes, evaluate compliance, provide maintenance

AMA, 2002; ASCO, 2000; Camp-Sorrell & Hawkins, 2000.

Understanding the politics and level of support for an advanced practice role within the area of practice will help to determine the level of support for the NP role. It is useful to prepare the team members for the NP role by educating them. Handouts explaining the NP's role, in-service education, and informal conversations are useful for staff to become familiar with the role (Bonnel, Belt, Hill, Wiggins, & Ohm, 2000).

Clinical practice guidelines are often used to guide the NP in making clinical decisions (Camp-Sorrell & Hawkins, 2001; Goolsby, 2001). Guidelines should discuss the clinical problems for the identified populations in which exceptions can be made in its application. Guidelines cannot be applied if the patient's actual condition is not within the suggested recommendations. Guidelines can only be beneficial when the NP can accurately assess the patient's presenting complaint and make a correct diagnosis. NPs must stay abreast of changes and developments in clinical practice considering that guidelines are usually updated every five years (Goolsby). Guidelines should not be rigid formulas that cannot be varied but are meant to provide information to make a decision and individualized to each patient setting. **Table 4.2** provides Websites for clinical practice guidelines.

Reimbursement Issues

Knowing the regulations and requirements for the state of practice regarding reimbursement is essential for the NP position. In 1998, federal legislation allowed NPs to apply for direct reimbursement for services under Medicare Part B. NPs can be reimbursed at 80% of the lesser charge or 85% of the fee schedule amount for the same service when provided by a physician (Camp-Sorrell & Spencer-Cisek, 1995). NPs are allowed to make an independent evaluation of each patient without the physician having to see the patient. According to Medicare policy, NPs are viewed as midlevel practitioners (American Medical Association [AMA], 2002). Although physicians do not have to be onsite for reimbursement, the law requires the NP to work in collaboration with a physician. NPs must have documentation of this collaborative process with the physician (i.e., a policy outlining how the physician and NP collaborate on patients).

Although the Centers for Medicare & Medicaid Services (CMMS), formerly the Healthcare Financing Administration (HCFA), makes national Medicare policy, local carriers such as Blue Cross Blue Shield process Medicare claims in a designated geographic area. Other local carriers have been designated by Medicare to process claims for durable equipment, nutritional supplies, orthotics, prosthetics, and oral chemotherapy (AMA, 2002; American Society of Clinical Oncology [ASCO], 2000). A number of national policies have been established by the CMMS of services that are or are not covered by Medicare. Local carriers have authority to determine whether a particular item or service is covered. For instance, a chemotherapy agent may be covered by one state for a certain cancer but not in another. If allowed by state law, Medicare allows NPs to supervise chemotherapy and biotherapy

---

Table 4.2 GUIDELINES WEBSITES

- Agency for Healthcare Research and Quality National Guideline Clearinghouse at http://www.guidelines.gov
- Cancer Net PDQ Cancer Information Summaries at http://cancernet.nci.nih.gov/pdqfull.html
- Medical Matrix at http://www.medmatrix.org/_Spages/Practice_Guidelines.asp
- Medscape Multispecialty Practice Guidelines at http://www.medscape.com
- American Medical Association Code Guidelines at www.ama-assn.org/cpt

administration without the presence of a physician (ASCO). Although the NP would be reimbursed for the patient visit at 85% of the physician schedule for the current procedural terminology (CPT) level, the chemotherapy and biotherapy agents would be reimbursed at 100% because drugs are not paid according to the physician schedule (ASCO).

Reimbursement laws are regulated by federal and state programs to reimburse NPs for services provided. Unfortunately, these services are compared with physician's reimbursement (AMA, 2002). Under Medicare law, NPs are authorized to be reimbursed for Medicare services provided to patients regardless of the setting under their own Medicare billing number. Therefore, Medicare reimburses NPs when services are provided in nursing homes, rural healthcare settings, rural health clinics, health maintenance organizations (HMOs), federally qualified health centers, and ambulatory settings. With all "incident to" services billed, the physician must be present in the clinical setting for services to be covered by Medicare. The " incident to" provision means that an NP must collaborate with the physician when conducting the initial visit and developing the treatment plan. In subsequent patient visits for the same problem, the NP can see the patient independently under the NP's provider number.

CMMS develops and implements the rules and regulations regarding Medicare reimbursement. NPs must follow the rules, regulations, and documentation guidelines (Buppert, 2001). Medicare law requires NPs who see Medicare patients to have a provider number for each site practice. Forms can be obtained from each state Medicare local carrier provider. After January 2003, NPs must have a master's degree if first applying, must be certified by a national certifying body, and must meet the state requirements for NP practice.

NPs continue to be the backbone of Medicaid primary services across the United States. Medicaid is a federal–state program for individuals who cannot afford healthcare (AMA, 2002).

Each program is managed by each state's Medicaid agency. Medicaid programs pay directly to the provider as payment in full; therefore, the patient cannot be billed.

Tricare is insurance provided by the Department of Defense to certain categories of civilians such as military personnel dependents. This program is similar to Medicare in physician fee schedule (ASCO, 2000). Indemnity insurance is the traditional form of coverage in which the insurer can select any healthcare provider such as Blue Cross Blue Shield. The preferred provider organization (PPO) provides coverage for physicians and hospitals designated by the PPO. Outside the PPO, the insurer would have to pay an increased amount. The HMO provides healthcare coverage to a patient for a fixed payment. Different models exist such as a staff physician who works directly for HMO, a group physician who has a contract with the HMO, and a network in which the physician provides care to more than one HMO. Reimbursement for NP services varies state to state with each of the previously mentioned private insurance plans.

The Office of the Inspector General and the Department of Health and Human Services investigate Medicare abuses, including money paid for services not provided, medically unnecessary service, incorrectly coded services, noncovered services, and miscellaneous errors (Buppert, 2001). If the Office of the Inspector General is successful in proving fraud, the consequences of committing a fraud may include the following: (1) a fine that may have to be paid, (2) mandated continuing education, (3) mandated compliance program with reports to supervision agency, (4) scheduled or random auditing, (5) a loss of NP license, or (6) criminal prosecution with possible jail sentencing and a loss of Medicare billing ability.

Auditors may request visit notes for a particular patient for a particular day (Buppert, 2001). Poor documentation of services rendered is often where the provider fails to support services provided. **Table 4.3** outlines information required to

Table 4.3 CRITERIA FOR DOCUMENTING CODES FOR ESTABLISHED PATIENT OFFICE VISIT

	Level 1	Level 2	Level 3	Level 4	Level 5
History	Minimal with one line explaining nature of visit (can be performed by registered nurse)	Problem focused HPI: one to three elements ROS: positive or negative responses for one system related	Expanded problem focused HPI: one to three elements status of three or more or inactive conditions to the problem	Detailed HPI: four or more elements or the status of three or more chronic ROS: positive or negative responses for two to nine systems FH/SH: one item	Comprehensive HPI: four or more elements or inactive conditions ROS: positive or negative responses for 10 or more systems FH/SH: one item
Examination	Minimal	One to five elements	Six to 12 elements	Twelve to 18 elements	Minimum of 18 elements in at least nine organ or body systems
Decision-Making	Minimal	Straight forward	Low complexity Two or more self-limiting problems or one stable chronic illness, or one acuteuncomplicated illness	Moderate complexity One chronic illness with mild exacerbation or progression, or treatment side effect; Two stable chronic illnesses; new problem with uncertain diagnosis, acute illness with systemic manifestations	High complexity One chronic illness with severe exacerbation; acute or chronic illness posing threat to life or bodily function
Time (usually)	Five minutes	Ten minutes	Fifteen minutes	Twenty-five minutes	Forty minutes
Example	Visit for growth factors	Chemotherapy visit with symptoms such as nausea or vomiting	Patient on treatment for breast cancer, fatigue, growth factors	History of breast cancer with new brain metastasis, ataxia	History of prostate cancer with a 3-month history of fatigue, weight loss, anorexia, bone pain, incontinence

HPI - history of presenting illness; ROS - Review of systems; FH - family history; SH - social history.
See Table 4.1 for detailed information on the components of HPI, ROS, FH, SH, and PMH.

bill for each level of service provided, including history taken, physical examination, decision making, and time spent with the patient. If the record does not support the CPT code billed, the Medicare carrier may decline to reimburse or may ask for a previous reimbursement be repaid. Codes must be used to bill for the NP services. There is no limitation on CPT codes for NPs who are seeing patients within their own scope of practice. By understanding the principles of coding, an NP in private practice can bring in more money. It is important to learn when to use modifiers, when to bill under NP's own provider number, when to use "incident to" billing, and requirements for billing new versus established patients.

International Classification of Diseases, 7th edition, Clinical Modification (ICD-9-CM) codes for various diagnosis is used when submitting insurance claims (AMA, 2002). Which CPT code to submit for services is based on three key factors: (1) the nature of the history taken, (2) a physical examination, and (3) the complexity of

decision making involved in the patient's care (**Table 4.1**). Decision making is further classified into three parts: (1) the extent to which there are multiple diagnosis or treatment options, (2) the complexity or amount of data that must be considered, and (3) the risk involved in making the decision.

Prescriptive Authority

The United States government recognizes two classes of drugs, including over-the-counter drugs and legend drugs, which require a prescription from a licensed healthcare provider. Initially, prescriptive authority was largely limited to physicians and osteopaths. In recent years, the right to prescribe has changed to include different healthcare providers such as NPs (Lofholm & Katzung, 1998). The primary organizations controlling the privilege of prescribing in the United States are the state medical boards under the powers delegated to them by the state legislatures.

Table 4.4 CLASSIFICATION OF CONTROLLED SUBSTANCES

	Potential for Abuse	Comments
Class 1 (e.g., heroin, cocaine)	High	No accepted medical use in United States
Class 2 (e.g., morphine, codeine)	High	Accepted medical use with abuse may lead to physical or psychologic dependence
Class 3 (e.g., butabarbital, benzphetamine)	Less than 1 or 2	Accepted medical use with moderate or low potential for physical or psychologic dependence
Class 4 (e.g., alprazolam, diazepam)	Less than 3	Accepted medical use with limited potential for dependence
Class 5 (e.g., diphenoxylate hydrochloride, cough syrup with codeine)	Less than 4	Accepted medical use with limited dependence possible

One barrier for NPs' practice is prescriptive authority and the inability in many states to prescribe controlled substances (**Table** 4.4). Most states have a protocol with a formulary of drugs commonly prescribed. All states have some type of prescriptive authority (**Figure** 4.1). This authority varies from state to state with the major discrepancies of prescribing narcotics. Several states enforce the authority to dispense controlled substances through independent Drug Enforcement Agency registrations (McDermott, 1995). A key component of the NPs role is prescriptive authority, and the lack there of is a barrier to many.

One study demonstrated that NPs given prescriptive authority practice safely and consistently in their scope of practice (Hamric, Worley,

---

Figure 4.1 SUMMARY OF ADVANCED PRACTICE NURSE LEGISLATION: LEGAL AUTHORITY AND SCOPE OF PRACTICE

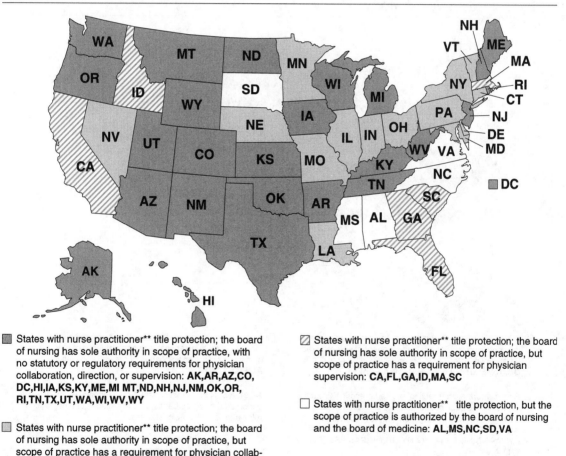

▓ States with nurse practitioner** title protection; the board of nursing has sole authority in scope of practice, with no statutory or regulatory requirements for physician collaboration, direction, or supervision: **AK,AR,AZ,CO, DC,HI,IA,KS,KY,ME,MI MT,ND,NH,NJ,NM,OK,OR, RI,TN,TX,UT,WA,WI,WV,WY**

▒ States with nurse practitioner** title protection; the board of nursing has sole authority in scope of practice, but scope of practice has a requirement for physician collaboration: **CT,DE,IL,IN,LA,MD,MN,MO,NE ,NV, NY,OH,PA,VT**

▨ States with nurse practitioner** title protection; the board of nursing has sole authority in scope of practice, but scope of practice has a requirement for physician supervision: **CA,FL,GA,ID,MA,SC**

☐ States with nurse practitioner** title protection, but the scope of practice is authorized by the board of nursing and the board of medicine: **AL,MS,NC,SD,VA**

[Washington, D.C., is included as a state in this table.]

KEY: * This table provides a state-by-state summary of the degree of independence for all aspects of NP scope of practice, including diagnosing and treating (except prescribing). See table: Summary of APN Legislation: Prescriptive Authority for a state-by-state analysis of NP prescriptive authority.
** This information may apply to other APNs (clinical nurse specialists, nurse midwives, and nurse anesthetists). See State Summary for details.
Stae with APRN Board.

Lindebak, & Jaubert, 1998). This study has been a stimulus to support legislative efforts to expand prescriptive authority to qualified NPs in the United States. Additionally, this study demonstrated the benefits that NPs have to patients by being able to prescribe medications to meet the patient's needs.

License and Certification to Practice

Currently the American Nurses Credentialing Center offers NP certification in family, adult, pediatric, geriatric, school nurses, and acute care. The Oncology Nursing Certification Corporation

---

Figure 4.2 SUMMARY OF ADVANCED PRACTICE NURSE LEGISLATION: PRESCRIPTIVE AUTHORITY

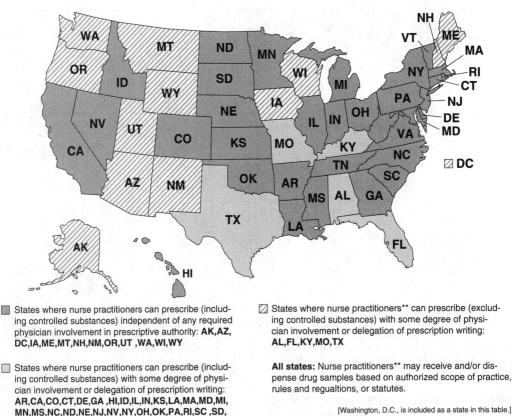

▓ States where nurse practitioners can prescribe (including controlled substances) independent of any required physician involvement in prescriptive authority: **AK,AZ, DC,IA,ME,MT,NH,NM,OR,UT ,WA,WI,WY**

☐ States where nurse practitioners can prescribe (including controlled substances) with some degree of physician involvement or delegation of prescription writing: **AR,CA,CO,CT,DE,GA ,HI,ID,IL,IN,KS,LA,MA,MD,MI, MN,MS,NC,ND,NE,NJ,NV,NY,OH,OK,PA,RI,SC ,SD, TN,VA,VT,WV**

▨ States where nurse practitioners** can prescribe (excluding controlled substances) with some degree of physician involvement or delegation of prescription writing: **AL,FL,KY,MO,TX**

All states: Nurse practitioners** may receive and/or dispense drug samples based on authorized scope of practice, rules and regualtions, or statutes.

[Washington, D.C., is included as a state in this table.]

KEY: * This table provides a state-by-state analysis of NP prescriptive authority. For analysis of other aspects of the NP scope of practice (including diagnosing and treating), see table: Summary of APN Legislation: Legal Authority for Scope of Practice
  ** This information may apply to other APNs (clinical nurse specialists, nurse midwives, and nurse anesthetists). See State Survey for details.
  Schedule IV and/or V controlled substance only.
  Nurse practitioners do not have written prescribing or dispensing authority; the process falls under delegated medical authority.

offers an advanced certified nurse program; however, this is not specific to NPs. **Figure** 4.2 provides a summary of each state's advanced practice legal authority for scope of practice, which varies among states. The NP scope of practice is defined by federal regulations, state nursing practice acts, and organizational guidelines. The American Nurses Association, the Oncology Nursing Society, and the National Council of State Board of Nursing have different types of scopes of practices developed. These scopes of practice may be useful guidelines to develop job descriptions (**Figure** 4.3).

Figure 4.3 ONP JOB DESCRIPTION

Introduction to Job Description
This Job Description for Oncology Nurse Practitioners was developed by the Nurse Practitioner Special Interest Group (SIG) of the Oncology Nursing Society in 1996. It is a compilation of many ONP job descriptions and it is intended to be used only as a template for developing a personal job description, not in its entirety.

I. Administrative
    A. Establishes goals and objectives for his/her area in congruence with the assigned department's goals and objectives on an annual basis. Target dates for implementation and evaluation of goals are established.
    B. Participates in review and revision of job descriptions, policies, and procedures.
    C. Ensures that developmental and intradepartmental policies, procedures, and standards of care are maintained and assists in interpreting these for patients and visitors.
    D. Promotes philosophy of employer and acts as a role model and resource person for staff.
    E. Ensures and maintains patient/family confidentiality at all times.

II. Clinical
    A. Assesses the physical and psychosocial status of clients by means of interview, health history, physical examination, and diagnostic studies.
    B. Recognizes deviations from normal in the physical assessment. Works in collaboration with a physician in formulating treatment plans for health problems and follow-up.
    C. Writes prescriptions for medication, blood products based upon laboratory results, routine diagnostic and follow-up studies, therapeutic measures, and post-discharge care in accordance with written practice protocols.
    D. Determines eligibility of patients for entry into clinical trials based on findings.
    E. Requests written consultation from physicians and other healthcare professionals to ensure appropriate and quality patient care.
    F. Interprets and evaluates findings of studies/tests.
    G. Relays appropriate information regarding patient care to the collaborating physician.
    H. Administers therapeutic measures and obtains specimens as prescribed.
    I. Evaluates the quality of care provided and recommends changes for improvement.
    J. Initiates appropriate actions to facilitate the implementation of therapeutic plans that are consistent with the continuing healthcare needs of the client.
    K. Dictates follow-up letters to referring physicians with summaries of treatment, response, and plan.
    L. Maintains provision of preventive health services (e.g. screening, risks assessment, immunizations, PAP smears, self-breast exam).
    M. Dictates or writes patient history, admissions, care plans, progress, and discharge notes.
    N. Interacts with program assistants and data managers for optimal patient care.
    O. Assists in the management of family dynamics and coping mechanisms during acute and chronic phases of patient care.
    P. Conducts or participates in daily multidisciplinary rounds and ensures appropriate and quality care for assigned patient.
    Q. Provides on-call coverage.
    R. Triage patients determines the urgency of physician's evaluation.

(continues)

Figure 4.3 ONP JOB DESCRIPTION (CONT'D)

III. **Skills Required**
   A. Effective verbal and written communication skills to communicate with diverse populations, including physicians, employees, patients, and families.
   B. Leadership skills to direct others toward the successful treatment of patients.
   C. Analytical skills to evaluate patient status and healthcare procedures/techniques and to monitor quality of care.
   D. Fiscal skills to monitor and control costs and revenue.
   E. Willingness to learn and remain flexible in the changing healthcare environment.
   F. Ability to assist staff in times of crisis or emergency.
   G. Ability to conceptualize, develop, and implement new ideas or systems.
   H. Ability to exercise sound judgement and discretion while performing duties.
   I. Ability to meet with the public outside the institution and efficiently market and promote cancer treatment.
   J. Ability to determine work priorities, assign work, and insure proper completion of work assignments.

IV. **Communication**
   A. Establishes relationships with professional and/or other health-related groups within the community.
   B. Shares clinical expertise with professional and supportive personnel.
   C. Documents and reports care in an accurate, timely manner using appropriate forms and records.
   D. Works effectively with others. Collaborates with other health disciplines to ensure continuity and quality of care.
   E. Uses interpersonal skills to work productively with all levels of hospital personnel.

V. **Self-Development and Professional Responsibility**
   A. Makes a significant and sustained contribution to the nursing profession through publishing, committee involvement, educational media development or scientific inquiry, or use of creative approaches to enhance quality of care.
   B. Demonstrates professionalism and accountability.
   C. Maintains clinical and administrative expertise through formal and informal programs.
   D. Demonstrates expertise in patient care.
   E. Maintains current knowledge of healthcare techniques and practices by participating in workshops, seminars, and professional organizations.

VI. **Research**
   A. Applies current concepts and findings from research and/or studies to practice.
   B. Initiates change in clinical practice based on current concepts and findings.
   C. Participates in multidisciplinary research activities.
   D. Functions as a principal investigator or coinvestigator for nursing research protocols.
   E. Participates in journal club.

VII. **Continuous Quality Improvement**
   A. Identifies, analyzes, and resolves patient care problems to foster significant improvement in patient care.
   B. Participates in intradisciplinary continuous quality improvement activities on an ongoing basis.
   C. Demonstrates a commitment to improving the quality of care provided to clients.

Figure 4.3 ONP JOB DESCRIPTION (CONT'D)

VIII. Qualifications
   A. License and current registration to practice in state.
   B. Graduate from a registered NP program.
   C. Master's degree in nursing.
   D. One full-time year of post-licensure clinical nursing experience.
   E. Privileges or eligibility to apply.

IX. Education
   A. Patient
      1. Educates patients and families about the disease process and treatment.
      2. Provides information to patients and families related to symptom management and psychosocial response to the diagnosis of cancer and related treatment.

   B. Staff/Student
      1. Identifies the learning needs of nursing/medical staff and students and implements appropriate educational programs.
      2. Provides formal and informal education to staff in oncology care.
      3. Uses local, regional, and national forums to educate other professionals about advanced practice roles and issues-related care.
      4. Precepts graduate nursing students.
      5. Participates in the development of educational materials for patients and healthcare providers.

   C. Community
      1. Provides consultation to lay groups and other healthcare professionals in the community.

X.   Reimbursement
   A. Varies per institution and state.

XI. Case Management
   A. Leads family conferences.
   B. Coordinates care for complex patients through multidisciplinary team.
   C. Coordinates, attends, and positively endorses cancer rehabilitation meetings.

XII. Policy Adherence
   A. Adheres to standard policies for infection control, fire, and safety departments.
   B. Attends mandatory in-services related to hospital and departmental policies and conforms to state and federal regulations.
   C. Complies with the hospital attendance guidelines regarding timeliness of notification, and promptness in reporting for duty.
   D. Practices within the legal boundaries of nurse practitioner. Understands responsibilities, communication, and authority lines.
   E. Composes standard policies/procedures for specialty areas and uses standardized procedure guides to practice.

> The Oncology Nursing Society (ONS) does not assume responsibility for the opinions expressed and information provided by authors or by Special Interest Groups (SIGs).

Note: From Nurse Practitioner Special Interest Group Newsletter, 11(1), (pp. 2–3), 2000, Oncology Nursing Society. Copyright 2000 by Oncology Nursing Society. Reprinted with permission.

Future Issues

There are several issues that the ONPs will face in the future. Active participation by all NPs is essential to help build and further develop the role. Quality of care is an issue that is of interest to patients, third-party payers, and providers. There is little research that evaluates the quality of care provided by NPs (Bryant & Clark, 2002) and none that is specific to the care provided by ONPs. Patient satisfaction with the care provided by the NP is one measure of quality of care. To date, little has been done to demonstrate patient satisfaction of the care that NPs provide. It would be useful to have a standardized approach in measuring this aspect of quality of care and to publish the results for documentation and justification of the role. In addition to quality of care, the NP must document as a unique healthcare provider by demonstrating the impact the role has on patient outcomes. These two areas are examples of the need for research and documentation as it relates to the role of the ONP. Many areas of research and documentation are needed in the literature to help strengthen the role and support its place in the healthcare arena.

It is also crucial that NPs become involved in the political environment to assist with legislative passage of healthcare bills that involve NP practice (Hawkins, 1995). For example, the lack of consistency between states in the scope of practice and prescriptive authority for NPs makes passage of national laws difficult. Although small, a movement is afoot to help expand the services of the NP. Legislation has been drafted to make it possible for home health agencies and hospice agencies to accept NP referrals. Other legislation has been proposed to expand reimbursement for NP services provided. However, expansive legislation is needed that will allow NPs in all states to provide services in a variety of settings, unrestricted prescriptive authority, and proper reimbursement to meet the needs of oncology patients.

Escalating healthcare costs and access issues give NPs new opportunities to meet changing healthcare needs. Many barriers to NPs' practice are disappearing, primarily because of economic reasons. The traditional healthcare system is no longer affordable, and NPs are shown to be cost-effective to their physician counterparts. NPs will need to continue to influence changes in healthcare through the political arena. NPs should be familiar with the state legislative environment and educate the public and legislators about the NP role and function.

References

American Medical Association. (2002). *Current Procedural Terminology: CPT 2002*. Chicago: AMA Press.

American Society of Clinical Oncology. (2000). *Practical Tips for the Practicing Oncologist*. Alexandria, Virginia: American Society of Clinical Oncology.

Bonnel, W., Belt, J., Hill, D., Wiggins, S., & Ohm, R. (2000). Challenges and strategies for initiating a nursing facility practice. *Journal of the American Academy of Nurse Practitioners, 12*, 353–359.

Brown, J. K. & Hinds, P. (1999). Assessing master's programs in advanced practice oncology nursing. *Oncology Nursing Forum, 26*, 1371–1380.

Bryant, R. & Clark, M. C. (2002). Advance practice nurses: A study of client satisfaction. *Journal of the American Academy of Nurse Practitioners, 14*, 88–92.

Buppert, C. (2001). Avoiding Medicare fraud. *The Nurse Practitioner, 26*, 70–75.

Bush, N. J. & Watters, T. (2001). The emerging role of the oncology nurse practitioner: A collaborative model within the private practice setting. *Oncology Nursing Forum, 28*, 1425–1431.

Camp-Sorrell, D. & Hawkins, R. (2000). *Clinical Manual for the Oncology Advanced Practice Nurse*. Pittsburgh: Oncology Nursing Press.

Camp-Sorrell, D. & Spencer-Cisek, P. (1995). Reimbursement issues for advance practice. *Oncology Nursing Forum, 22* (Suppl.), 31–34.

Cole, F. L., Mackey, T. A., & Lindenberg, J. (2001). Wait time and satisfaction with care and service at a nurse practitioner managed clinic. *Journal of the American Academy of Nurse Practitioners, 13*, 467–472.

Feldman, M., Ventura, M., & Crosby, F. (1987). Studies of nurse practitioner effectiveness. *Nursing Research, 36*, 303–308.

Ford, L. C. & Silver, H. K. (1967). The expanded role of the nurse in childcare. *Nursing Outlook, 15*, 43–45.

Goolsby, M. J. (2001). Evaluating and applying clinical practice guidelines. *Journal of American Academy of Nurse Practitioners, 13*, 3–6.

Hamric, A. B., Worley, D., Lindebak, S., & Jaubert, S. (1998). Outcomes associated with advanced nursing practice prescriptive authority. *Journal of the American Academy of Nurse Practitioners, 10*, 113–118.

Hawkins, R. (1995). Concluding remarks: Window to the future of advance practice in oncology nursing. *Oncology Nursing Forum, 22* (Suppl.), 43–44.

Kelly, N. R. & Mathews, M. (2001). The transition to first position as nurse practitioner. *Journal of Nursing Education, 40*, 156–162.

Kinney, A. Y., Hawkins, R., & Hudman, K. S. (1997). A descriptive study of the role of the oncology nurse practitioner. *Oncology Nursing Forum, 24*, 811–820.

Knudtson, N. (2000). Patient satisfaction with nurse practitioner service in a rural setting. *Journal of the American Academy of Nurse Practitioners, 12*, 405–412.

Koelbel, P., Fuller, S., & Misener, T. (1991). Job satisfaction of nurse practitioners: An analysis using Herzbeg's theory. *Nurse Practitioners, 16*, 43–56.

Lofholm, P. W. & Katzung, B. G. (1998). Rational prescribing and prescription writing. In B. G. Katzung (Ed.), *Basic & Clinical Pharmacology* (7th ed., pp. 1041–1050). Stamford: Appleton & Lange.

McDermott, K. C. (1995). Prescriptive authority for advance practice nurses: Current and future perspectives. *Oncology Nursing Forum, 22* (Suppl.), 25–30.

Molde, S. & Diers, D. (1985). Nurse practitioner research: Selected literature review and research agenda. *Nursing Research, 34*, 362–367.

Murphy-Ende, K. (2002). Advanced practice nursing: Reflections on the past: Issues for the future. *Oncology Nursing Forum, 29*, 106–112.

Pearson, L. (2002). Fourteenth annual legislative update. *The Nurse Practitioner, 27*, 10–52.

Wyatt, J. S. (2001). Continuing the discussion of advanced practice in acute care: Past and future. *Pediatric Nursing, 27*, 419–421.

Chapter 5

Current Models of Physician Office Practices

Kathleen M. Shuey

Introduction

Historically, the role of the office or clinic nurse has been to assist the physician at his practice (Martin & Xistris, 2000). The nurse's tasks included managing the flow of patients, answering the phone, and completing paperwork. Nurses were viewed more as an assistant or handmaiden of the physician than as an independent healthcare practitioner. Technical skills were not perceived as essential. A lower salary reflected the perks of having Monday through Friday business hours and an undemanding, nonclinical job. Here the role of the oncology nurse in an ambulatory setting, skills sets used in ambulatory care, and issues unique to the setting are discussed.

History of Ambulatory Clinics in Oncology

During the 1800s, care of the sick moved from the home to the hospital setting, where trained assistants cared for the ill (Lynaugh, 1990). As nursing began to develop into a profession in the United States, student nurses were trained and later employed in the hospital setting. Early on, students provided the bulk of the clinical work-

force in the hospital. As healthcare began to evolve from reacting to illness to developing initiatives focusing on health, the role of the nurse also evolved. Ambulatory care nursing can actually be traced back to 1893 when New York City set up milk stations to educate mothers on infant feeding (Igen & Taylor, 1912).

The evolution of oncology practice from an academic setting to a community-based specialty began about 30 years ago, in the early 1970s (Association of Community Cancer Centers, 2003a). As physicians moved their practices to community settings, they searched for nurses who were knowledgeable of the cancer experience and associated treatments to care for their patients. These nursing professionals became part of multidisciplinary, hospital-based teams. Over the next two decades, our understanding of cancer, expanding treatment options, and improved management of toxicities allowed patients to be treated in a variety of settings: hospital, clinic, home, and hospice.

In the 1980s with escalating healthcare costs, implementation of a diagnostic related group-based system of reimbursement, and the advent of managed care, physicians and nurses were challenged to evaluate alternate settings for the delivery of oncology care. Over a 10-year period, the number of available hospital beds and inpatient admissions declined (Prescott & Soeken, 1996). Care moved from inpatient hospital systems to outpatient hospital and physician office settings. Approximately 80% to 90% of all oncology care is now delivered in ambulatory settings (Harris & Bean, 1991). With increased availability of these facilities, it is now possible for patients to maintain a somewhat normal lifestyle (Moskowitz, 1990).

Ambulatory Practice Settings

Ambulatory care offers a diverse set of treatment locations for patients. In the general medical setting, treatment centers include physician- and managed-care practices, publicly funded facilities such as county health departments and rural health clinics, specialized treatment facilities (drug and alcohol treatment, cardiac rehabilitation), school and work settings, and senior citizen and childcare centers (Bellack, 1998). Oncology treatment can occur in all of these locations (Table 5.1).

University hospital outpatient departments were developed to fulfill the mission of academic health centers (Hackbarth, Haas, Kavanagh, & Vlasses, 1995; Haas & Hackbarth, 1995a; Haas & Hackbarth, 1995b; Haas, Hackbarth, Kavanagh, & Vlasses, 1995c). In addition, these facilities provided learning experiences for medical students and residents who staffed the clinic.

Table 5.1   OUTPATIENT AMBULATORY CLINIC SETTINGS

University hospital outpatient departments

Community hospital outpatient centers

Federal health systems

Community and freestanding centers

Medical group practices

Bellack, 1998; Hackbarth et al., 1995; Haas et al., 1995a; Haas et al., 1998; Haas et al., 1995b; Haas, 2001.

Depending on the mission of the facility and funding, services might include primary healthcare, specialty care, or tertiary treatment. Nurses in university or academic outpatient departments were among the first to begin to describe the role of the nurse in ambulatory care (Browne, 2001). Community hospital outpatient centers may be part of non-profit (or not-for-profit) organizations or for-profit ventures. Originally developed to provide charitable services to the community, today these clinics provide services, on a smaller scale, that are similar to those found in the university setting (Hackbarth et al., 1995; Haas et al., 1995a; Haas et al., 1995b; Haas et al., 1995c). Depending on the focus of the community hospital outpatient department, registered nurses may serve more in management roles, whereas ancillary staff delivers care. In high-tech programs (dialysis center, cancer center), more professional nursing staff are employed (Hackbarth et al., 1995; Haas et al., 1995a; Haas et al., 1995b; Haas et al., 1995c). Federal health systems provide healthcare to specific patient populations. Examples include the Department of Defense programs for military personnel, the Veteran's Administration, and Indian Health Services. Again, based on available funding, services are similar to university and community outpatient centers. Community and freestanding clinics provide specialty-type services, such as dialysis or rehabilitation. These clinics may be part of local health departments, extensions of university or community hospital outpatient centers, or for-profit ventures.

Medical group practices range from single-physician practices to large multiphysician group practices. Single-physician practices, however, have decreased significantly over the past decade (Stackhouse, 1998). Group practices allow physicians to consolidate resources. The scope of services is dependent on the practice focus. Some practices offer a multitude of services (managed-care treatment facilities), whereas others are specialty focused (cancer centers). Components of the nursing role in this setting include triage, management and coordination of patient care, support for clinical procedures, and patient education (Hackbarth et al., 1995; Haas et al., 1995a; Haas et al., 1995b; Haas et al., 1995c).

Patients that are seen in the ambulatory treatment setting have a diverse set of care needs and may require complex treatment regimens. With increasing availability of information over the Internet and synopses of emerging treatments seen on the local nightly news, patients and their families may present to the outpatient setting well informed about their treatment options (Haas, 2001). Services offered in ambulatory oncology treatment settings now include prevention, traditional clinical services, and support services. **Table 5.2** lists services that are available to oncology patients in ambulatory settings. Depending on the services available at the clinic, multiple healthcare disciplines, in addition to nursing, may be available to augment the patient experience (**Table 5.3**). Accessibility of services and availability of professional nursing care have enhanced and promoted ambulatory clinic settings as viable options for the treatment of cancer.

Evolving Role of the Oncology Office Nurse

Office-based oncology nursing is multifaceted. In addition to traditional hospital-type clinical skills, nurses are required to deliver care within a finite time frame, obtain a comprehensive nursing and medical history; assess, plan, and educate the patient and his or her family; deliver complex chemotherapy treatments; plan appropriate symptom-management interventions; facilitate research; and sometimes provide managerial assistance to the practice. Nurses in an ambulatory setting must respond rapidly to patient needs within a short time frame (Haas, 2001). Patients in this setting are sicker and require more care than a few years ago because of changes in hospital length of stay and intensive treatments that

Table 5.2 SERVICES AVAILABLE IN AMBULATORY SETTINGS

Screening	Prevention and early detection
	Genetic screening and counseling
Diagnostic	Radiology
	Laboratory services
Procedures	Biopsies
	Bone marrow aspiration
	Colposcopy
	Lumbar puncture
	Management of Omaya reservoir
	Paracentesis
	Placement of long-term intravenous access devices
Treatment	Outpatient surgery
	Radiation therapy
	Chemotherapy
	Bone marrow/stem cell transplant
	Transfusion services
	Symptom management
	Antibiotic therapy
	Physical therapy/rehabilitation
Support	Patient/family education
	Counseling
	Nutritional counseling
	Survivor services

are now available in the outpatient setting. This is far removed from perceptions of 10 to 15 years ago that office nurses fulfill only clerical and assistive functions, direct traffic, answer the telephone, and order supplies (Tighe, Fisher, Hastings, & Heller, 1985). Although these functions are still part of the day-to-day life, an office nurse must be an independent decision maker with a comprehensive understanding of cancer, its treatment, and side-effect management (Harris & Bean, 1991; Tighe et al., 1985).

Characteristics of ambulatory care settings include high-volume, time-sensitive encounters, based on a set appointment schedule (Mastal, 2001). Patient encounters are in minutes and

Table 5.3   ADDITIONAL CLINIC HEALTHCARE RESOURCES

Discipline	Role
Dietician	Nutritional screening and assessment Patient education on nutrition therapy
Licensed vocational/practical nurse	Rooming patients Shot clinic
Pharmacist	Preparation of cytotoxic agents Patient education on chemotherapy regimens Drug inventory management Facilitate charge capture process
Pharmacy/admixture technician	Drug admixture/preparation of cytotoxic agents Drug inventory management
Psychologist	Identify and treat patients requiring intense mental health treatment
Social worker	Psychosocial assessment Ongoing counseling Consultant to healthcare team
Unlicensed assistive personnel (medical assistant)	Laboratory procedures Rooming patients

Browne, 2001; Fountain, 1993; Lamkin, 1994.

hours instead of days and weeks. The registered nurse may be working alone in the ambulatory setting or may be supported by additional nursing staff and unlicensed assistive personnel (UAP). Fewer traditional resources, nursing administration support, clinical nurse specialist, pharmacy, and even supplies may be available (Bellack, 1998).

Patient visits (or encounters) in the ambulatory setting are episodic and may occur as a single encounter or over a period of days, weeks, months, or years (Martin & Xistris, 2000). These encounters may be face to face or via telephone. In some instances, electronic communication (e-mail) may be used. Types of patient encounters include new patient and return/follow-up visits, treatment visits, and education or counseling visits (Haas & Hastings, 2002). In addition to scheduled encounters, unscheduled walk-in visits occur. The nature of unscheduled visits can vary from emergent situations to minor treatment (such as injections or prescription refills). Efficient scheduling

will enhance the use of clinic services. The quality of patient care provided in clinic settings is not dependent on only the clinical skills of the staff but also on the soundness of supports such as scheduling (Angiulo & Dickey, 2001). Clinic wait time causes patient dissatisfaction. In some clinics, the majority of patient treatments occur between 10 a.m. and 3 p.m. To facilitate patient flow and prevent treatment backlogs, clinics may schedule certain activities, such as shots, for a predefined time. Additionally, extended evening hours for treatment and having weekend treatment and shot clinics can prevent appointment schedule compression.

Factors that can impact the efficiency of services and care delivered include flow through the facility, volume of patients seen, number of treatments delivered, and physician practice styles. Use of midlevel providers (such as advanced practice nurses and physician assistants), availability and competency of UAP, and availability of additional clinical services such as laboratory, radiology, and pharmacy are additional factors to consider (Haas & Hastings, 2002).

As in the hospital setting, registered nurses assess patients, develop and implement nursing care plans, evaluate care, and maintain medical records (Bureau of Labor Statistics, 2002; Bureau of Labor Statistics, 2000; Reville & Almadrones, 1989). Patients present with a diverse set of care requirements: education, intravenous access and pump management, treatment delivery, toxicity management, and support (related to physical, psychosocial, and financial needs). Because of the intensity of patient needs and complex issues related to cancer treatment, oncology nurses must have a comprehensive and current knowledge base, must function independently, and must be self-directed (Price & Frank-Lightfoot, 2000; Lin, Aiken, Bailey et al., 1993).

The Oncology Nursing Society, the Association of Community Cancer Centers, and the American Academy of Ambulatory Care Nursing have published standards related to the practice of oncology ambulatory nursing. Key tenets of the standards are as follows: (1) Registered nurses with specialized knowledge and skill in oncology and who are certified in the oncology specialty accomplish the best care. (2) Preparation and handling of medications are in accordance to Occupational Safety and Health Administration guidelines. (3) Emergency response is readily available. (4) An experienced oncology nurse who has the appropriate level of education, management, and leadership skills directs the leadership of the oncology staff. (5) An appropriate clinical nursing expert is available on a consultant basis (Haas et al., 1995b; Haas & Hastings, 2002; Angiulo & Dickey, 2001; Association of Community Cancer Centers, 2003b; Oncology Nursing Society, 2001). In addition to following published standards, individual clinics should contemplate implementing specific clinical competencies for nursing staff. Suggested areas for demonstration of competency include admixture, chemotherapy administration (initial and annual assessment of

skill), and management of extravasations, central lines, and implanted pumps. Documentation of competency should be maintained in the employee file. Continuing education activities may be designed to promote competency and development of the nursing staff. Provisions must also be made to develop all staff at the clinic, including clerical, UAP, and other available healthcare resources (Haas et al., 1995b).

Actual nursing responsibilities vary office to office. Office structure can vary from a small, one-physician practice with minimal clinic staff to a freestanding cancer center that includes medical oncology, transplantation services, an onsite pharmacy and laboratory, and radiation therapy. Even though the size of the clinic may vary, elements of the nursing role are similar. These elements can be categorized into nine core dimensions: enabling operations, technical procedures, nursing process, telephone communication, advocacy, teaching, high-tech procedures, care coordination, and community outreach (Bellack, 1998) (**Table 5.4**). Nursing process and care coordination remain the same regardless of practice location: hospital, ambulatory clinic, or home care/hospice. The registered nurse assesses, plans, implements, and evaluates patient care. Coordination of services ensures continuity of care between multiple sites of service and disciplines. Referrals for additional services are often initiated

Table 5.4 CORE DIMENSIONS OF THE OFFICE NURSE ROLE

Enabling operations
Technical procedures
Nursing process
Telephone communication
Advocacy
Teaching
High-tech procedures
Care coordination
Community outreach

Bellack, 1998.

and managed by nurses. Coordination of care between multiple settings (hospital, clinic, or home care/hospice) requires that the oncology nurse actively participate in treatment planning.

Enabling Operations

Enabling operations are those functions that support the daily operation of the clinic. Tasks consist of unskilled activities that require little professional judgment (Hackbarth et al., 1995), for example, maintaining a safe and secure environment to meet patient needs, providing a safe work environment, and obtaining medical records are examples of enabling operations (Bellack, 1998). Supplying rooms, keeping inventory control, selecting, purchasing, and maintaining equipment and supplies, scheduling appointments, and billing of chemotherapy administration are nonclinical responsibilities of the nurse (Hackbarth, Haas, Kavanaugh et al., 1995; Angiulo & Dickey, 2001). Except for verification of chemotherapy-related billing, these functions may be delegated to UAP. This allows the nurse to focus directly on the patient and his or her needs.

Technical Procedures

Technical procedures include preparing the patient for encounters with the physician, chaperoning physician visits, and assisting with procedures and specimen collection (**Table 5.5**).

Technical procedures may also be delegated to UAP who have demonstrated competency in the specific skill.

Telephone Communication

Telephone communication primarily involves the triage of patient- or family-initiated phone calls. Communications between practitioners, alternate settings (such as the hospital or home care), and insurance providers are also elements of telephone communication. Telephone triage will vary among clinics. At some clinics, a triage nurse is assigned. This could be a permanent position or a position that is rotated among existing staff on a daily or weekly basis. At other clinics, each nurse may handle the phone calls of patients that he or she is treating or a particular physician with whom he or she is working. Regardless of how the individual practice assigns staff, office-based oncology nurses manage a high volume of telephone calls on a variety of clinical problems. The ability to triage the calls appropriately and efficiently is mandatory for nurses in this setting. Research has shown that office nurses spend more time receiving and returning phone calls from patients and families than on any other task (Hagan, Morin, & Lepine, 2000; Chahl, 1997; Greenberg, 2000).

Telephone calls may cover a broad range of clinical and nonclinical problems, including symptom complaints, clarification of informa-

---

Table 5.5   ONCOLOGY TECHNICAL PROCEDURES

Assisting with medical procedures

Assisting with biopsy (cervical, endometrial, vulvar)

Assisting with bone marrow aspiration

Assisting with colposcopy

Assisting with loop electrosurgical excision procedure

Assisting with lumbar puncture

Assisting with a papanicolaou test/smear

Assisting with paracentesis

Assisting with Omaya reservoir

tion, prescription refills, resource referral, reimbursement issues, bereavement counseling, crisis management, and interpretation of laboratory test and diagnostic exam results. The office nurse must have effective communication skills, physical and psychosocial assessment skills, and access to pertinent health records to facilitate triage decision making. Telephone calls should be prioritized based on the urgency of the problem. Complete and accurate information is needed to assist in disposition of the call. Development of protocols that are linked to a complaint or condition, potential assessment questions, and nursing interventions allow for consistent follow-up by all nurses in the practice (Giarelli, Gholz, Haisfield-Wolfe, Mitchell, & Smith, 2001). Documentation should include the date and time of the original phone call, the date and time of the return phone call, the physician, the reason for the call, the action taken and/or the instructions given, and name of the nurse (American Academy of Ambulatory Care Nursing, 2003) (**Figure 5.1**).

Advocacy

Patient advocacy no longer consists of serving solely in the conventional role of patient advocate and facilitating patient–physician communication or assisting the patient through the treatment process. With changes in healthcare reform, promoting public relations and keeping patients informed of the changing healthcare environment are also part of this role. Nurses are working with legislators on issues of reimbursement and nursing shortage. Today, the nurse must balance the needs of the patient and those of the clinic.

Patient Education

Teaching or patient education is one of the key components of the clinic nurse role. Education promotes and supports patient recovery and enables the patient to make informed healthcare decisions (Standards of Oncology Education, 1995). Although treatment visits are for defined time frames, return visits allow the nurse the opportunity to assess the patient's readiness to

Figure 5.1   TELEPHONE TRIAGE FORM

Date/time of call:	Date/time call returned:
Patient name:	Medical record #:
Relationship to patient:	Phone number:
Reason for call:	Action taken/instructions:
Referrals:	
Physician:	RN signature:

learn, to tailor information to fit the needs of the individual patient and family, and to assess comprehension (Browne, 2001) (**Table 5.6**).

Educational sessions may be individual or group and may focus on one or multiple educational needs. Areas of patient education include cancer diagnosis, the clinical/treatment process (i.e., what happens while in the clinic), the goal of treatment, chemotherapy/immunotherapy agents and treatment schedule, common side effects, self-care behaviors, nutrition, sexuality, safe handling/exposure issues, management of equipment and supplies (central lines, implanted pumps), emergency call information, and follow-up appointment information. Classes on the general principles of chemotherapy and management of central lines lend themselves to group formats.

Adequate resources must be available to facilitate the education process. Resources include print material and videotapes/DVD/audiocassettes. Additionally, a private or quiet area for educational sessions and materials for return demonstration (for injections and catheter care) are needed. Print materials reinforce teaching sessions and provide reference materials for later review. Educational materials can be obtained from a variety of sources (e.g., the National Cancer Institute, the American Cancer Society,

the National Coalition of Cancer Survivors, and pharmaceutical or product companies). When evaluating materials for use, review content for appropriateness and impartiality.

After completion of the session, patient understanding should be evaluated. This can be assessed by verbalization of understanding or return demonstration depending on the material presented. Documentation should reflect all of the elements of the session: assessment of readiness to learn, identified barriers to learning, teaching method and materials used, and understanding of information. Complete documentation will facilitate follow-up by other clinical staff when the patient returns to the office.

High-Tech Procedures

High-tech procedures are related to treatment administration of chemotherapy and immunotherapy, management of supportive care regimens (antiemetic therapy, growth factors, bisphosphonates), and occasional blood product administration or monitoring requirements of the specific therapy (Bellack, 1998). Management of central lines and implanted pumps also requires skilled oncology nursing assessment and intervention. Specific activities involved in the care and management of central lines consist of preventative

---

Table 5.6   ELEMENTS OF THE PATIENT EDUCATION PROCESS

Assess for readiness to learn and/or barriers to learning

Emotional barriers	Body image change
Culture values	Age
Language	Intellectual/educational level
Religious beliefs	Physiological state (sensory deficits, anxiety, depression)
Personal motivation/attitude	Environment in which learning is to occur

Assess knowledge of disease process and treatment plan

Assess past experience with cancer

Assess level of anxiety

Educational activities should be modified based on patient's readiness to learn and identified barriers

Education may include a variety of methods and tools (including but not limited to verbal, written, visual, auditory, tactile tools)

Assess for understanding

catheter maintenance, sterile dressing changes, management of persistent-withdrawal occlusion, insertion, and catheter repair (see **Table 5.7** for a list of nursing procedures).

Community Outreach

The last dimension, community outreach, includes activities that are geared toward education of the community and profession. To accomplish community outreach-related goals, the nurse must have an understanding of programs that are available in the community. Participating in health fairs and community education (i.e., I Can Cope, Look Good Feel Better), precepting students, and providing educational offerings to other healthcare professionals are a few examples of community outreach.

Documentation

Several documentation styles can be used in the clinic setting. Some clinics use a flow sheet or chart format to record data. Narrative notes may be used alone or to supplement information provided in a flow sheet or chart format (Behrend, 1994). Charting by exception entails defining a care plan and then documenting any unexpected response to that plan. Documentation should include nursing assessment and interventions, procedures, drug therapy, telephone communication, and teaching provided. Documentation provides written verification of services rendered. If services provided are not documented adequately, payment reversal (request from insurer for return of payment) can occur. Remember that if it was not documented, it was not done.

Patient Classification Systems

Over the last two decades, as patients have moved from the hospital setting to ambulatory care to home care settings, patient acuity has increased. The implementation of a DRG-based reimburse-

Table 5.7   ONCOLOGY HIGH-TECH PROCEDURES

Intravenous access
  Management of peripheral intravenous
    access devices
  Management of central access devices
  Insertion of peripheral access devices
    (peripheral intravenous, midline, peripherally
    inserted central catheter)
  Use of intravenous pump (stationary or
    ambulatory)
  Managing an implanted pump

Chemotherapy
  Administration
  Bladder instillation
  Intralesional administration
  Management of chemotherapy spills
  Management of extravasation
  Management of hypersensitivity reaction
  Peritoneal infusion

Miscellaneous treatments
  Antibiotic therapy
  Antifungal therapy
  Bisphosphonates
  Blood and related product administration

Clinic procedures
  Conscious sedation
  Pulse oximetry
  Therapeutic phlebotomy

ment system and managed care has also played a role in the changing patient care setting and increased acuity. In the hospital setting, patient classification systems serve as a means of determining staffing requirements (Medvec, 1994). As in hospital settings, a variety of classification systems are available to measure acuity in ambulatory care. Systems may evaluate staffing or intensity or a combination of the two. Staffing classification systems examine the evaluation and assessment of patient needs, determination and provision of the appropriate number and mix of staff, and evaluation of outcomes (Haas & Hastings, 2002). Staffing needs will vary based on the patient appointment and treatment load for the day. The appointment schedule can assist in predicting workload. However, walk-ins, urgent visits, no shows, and overbooking practices can impede this process (Haas, 2001). Nursing intensity classification systems evaluate the complexity of nursing care (Haas & Hastings, 2002). In the ambulatory care setting, intensity may vary because of the episodic nature of patient visits.

In the 1960s, hospitals began using patient classification systems to monitor workload and to determine staffing (Bellack, 1998). Hospital patient classification systems do not translate to ambulatory care settings because of the nature of the care delivered in that setting. Most patient classification systems that have been developed for use in the outpatient arena have been created from a medical perspective to capture use of physician resources (Bellack, 1998) (see **Table 5.8** for a list of patient classification systems that have been developed for use in the ambulatory care setting). Most of the available systems are task based and do not evaluate the complexity of care delivered. The ideal patient classification system will evaluate complexity of care (intensity), tasks, resources, time required to deliver care (workload), and patient outcome. The tool would also have established validity and reliability.

Practice Economics and Reimbursement

In addition to the clinical aspects of oncology care, nurses in the ambulatory setting must be attuned to the financial impact of care that is delivered in this setting. In the hospital setting, many costs are bundled in the room charge, including nursing services (Bowker, Star, & Spasser, 2001). Information from the inpatient unit is sent to the billing office, and limited contact exists between clinical departments and billing. In the ambulatory setting, nurses are directly involved with charging for services and verifying the accuracy of the information required

for billing purposes. Nursing not only provides information directly to the billing department but also serves as a check to verify that the clinical information submitted is accurate.

The charges submitted by the billing department for a service hopefully cover the actual cost of the service plus a degree of profit for the practice. Cost of service can be divided into direct and indirect costs. Direct costs are related to the actual service provided: nursing time (translated to salary), supplies, and medications (Noa & D'Angelo, 2001). Indirect costs are not related to the specific service delivered. Examples of indirect cost include salary of business office employees, rent, and office equipment such as computers (Noa & D'Angelo, 2001). These costs are used to determine the practice fee schedule or service charge. The charge or fee often does not reflect what is collected from Medicare, Medicaid, insurance plans (HMO, PPO, indemnity), or the patient.

Coding

The Centers for Medicare and Medicaid Services, formerly the Health Care Financing Administration, determine the rules for reporting healthcare services. In 1992, a resource-based relative value system was implemented to determine physician payment for Medicare provided services. Relative value units, which include work, practice expense, and malpractice expense, were established for clinical services. Each relative value unit is then multiplied by a regional price index to determine the reimbursement rate for the service (Noa & D'Angelo, 2001).

Coding is a method that is used to report patient services to Medicare, Medicaid, and private insurance plans. Correct coding of services can expedite reimbursement. Current Procedural Terminology codes are the recognized coding system for reporting of professional services, procedures, and supplies used to Medicare, Medicaid, and other insurance providers (American Medical Association, Current Procedural Terminology,

Table 5.8 CLASSIFICATION SYSTEMS

System	Characteristics
Medical approaches	
Diagnostic cluster	Based on medical diagnosis made during ambulatory encounter; grouped into one of 110 groups or clusters of similar diagnoses.
Ambulatory visit groups	Groups are formed from the major diagnostic categories.
Products of ambulatory care	Includes labor and ancillary services typically delivered during an ambulatory visit. System is not dependent on patient diagnosis.
Ambulatory care groups	Consists of 51 categories based on demographics and disease patterns. Formed by grouping ICD-9 diagnoses and the number of ambulatory care visits made during a year's time (used in HMO setting for utilization review).
Ambulatory severity index	Measures severity of illness by two major dimensions: biophysical—related to number and type of diagnoses—and behavioral—includes physical and psychosocial functioning, social factors, and patient compliance. Rating is completed by the provider at the time of the visit.
Nursing approaches	
Factor classification tools	Uses a scoring system—individual patient care requirement is given a score. Scores are totaled for each patient, and the patient is then categorized according to the numerical value.
Hoffman and Wakefield	Developed set of nursing care factors for classifying patients in an ambulatory care. Self-reports by office staff were used to establish initial estimates of time and frequency parameters for tasks.
Johnson	Combination of physician driven, dependent nursing activities, and independent care needs (including nurse-initiated psychosocial support and patient teaching).
Kirsch	Department specific approach to outpatient and short-stay patient classification. Time is related to patient descriptors through relative value units.
PINAC	Evaluates severity of illness, complexity of care, psycho-social needs of the patient. Also looks at type of visit (scheduled, telephone, emergency visit, etc.).
PINI (Patient Intensity for Nursing Index)	Patient is scored from 1 (independent and fully mobile) to 5 (immobility and dependence on nursing to accomplish mobility functions). Produces a mobility score that can be used to assess the patient's need for care and to determine limitations before and after interventions.
Prototype classification tools	Compares the patient's condition with categories containing broad descriptions of care requirements.

(continues)

Table 5.8   CLASSIFICATION SYSTEMS (CONT'D)

System	Characteristics
Richards and Tracy	Evaluated nurse staffing patterns in a single setting. Nursing time was associated with direct patient care activities. Three phases were evaluated: checking in, examination room functions, and checking out.
Verran	Evaluated six areas of responsibility, which included 44 representative nursing activities. Time and complexity were associated with activities.

Huffman & Wakefield, 1986; Johnson, 1989; Kirsch & Talbott, 1990; Prescott, Phillips, Ryan, & Thompson, 1991; Richards & Tracy, 1984; Verran, 1986a; Verran, 1986b.

2002). Three levels of codes are used. Level I codes consist of a five-digit code used for reporting services that the physician provided or that are under the direct supervision of the physician. Office visits (Evaluation and Management codes classifying the type of physician visit and intensity of the visit), therapeutic or diagnostic infusions, and chemotherapy administration are examples of level I codes (**Table 5.9** and **Table 5.10**). Level II codes provide more detailed information on the service provided or supply used. These codes consist of one alphabetic character followed by four digits. Examples include J-codes (J9000-J9999: chemotherapy drug codes) and Q-codes (temporary codes for procedures, services, or supplies). Level III codes are assigned by individual state Medicare carriers and vary from state to state. These codes are used to describe new procedures that have not yet been assigned a level I or level II code. In addition to CPT codes, ICD-9 (International Classification of Disease, 9th revision) codes are used to describe the clinical diagnosis or patient diagnosis that the physician is managing. Information documented in the medical chart, surgical pathology, extent of disease, or symptoms are used to determine the ICD-9 code that is then placed on the claim and submitted by the practice.

Nursing must assist in providing accurate coding information to the billing office on services delivered and drugs administered. Correct coding will prevent having to refile inaccurately submitted claims and facilitate timely reimbursement to the practice.

Practice Setting Trends and the Nursing Shortage

No discussion of nursing would be complete without addressing the issue of nursing shortage. Every four years, the Department of Health and Human Services (DHHS) surveys a sample of registered nurses drawn from active practitioners in each of the 50 states (Spratley, Johnson, Sochalski,

Table 5.9   HCPCS CODING LEVELS

Level	Code	Purpose
I	CPT	Reporting of services performed by healthcare providers
II	HCPCS national codes	Reporting of medical services and supplies provided to Medicare and Medicaid patients
III	HCPCS local codes	Assigned and maintained by individual state Medicare carriers

American Medical Association, HCPCS Level II, 2002.

Table 5.10   OUTPATIENT CODES

Reason for Visit	Codes
Evaluation and management codes	
New patient	99201, 99202, 99203, 99204, 99205
Established patient	99211, 99212, 99213, 99214, 99215
Therapeutic or diagnostic infusions	
Intravenous infusions for therapy/diagnosis	90780
Each additional hour (up to eight hours)	90781
Chemotherapy administration	
Subcutaneous or intramuscular with or without local anesthesia	96400
Intralesional	96405
Intralesional (more than seven lesions)	96407
Intravenous push	96408
Infusion, up to one hour	96410
Infusion, one to eight hours	96412
Initiation of prolonged infusion	96414
Intra-arterial, push technique	96420
Administration into pleural cavity	96440
Administration into peritoneal cavity	96445
Administration, via reservoir	96452
Administration into central nervous system	96520
Maintenance of portable pump	96530

American Medical Association, CPT, 2002.

Fritz, & Spencer, 2000). This intensive survey evaluates trends in practice setting, salary, level of education, and overall satisfaction. Although hospitals remain the major employer of registered nurses, movement of nursing staff into other practice settings is occurring. Approximately 0.5 million more registered nurses were employed in hospital settings in 2000 compared with 20 years earlier (Spratley et al., 2000). However, the percentage of nurses in hospital settings compared with the total percentage of working registered nurses has declined. This decline has been offset by increases in employment in the areas of public health, community health, and ambulatory care (**Table 5.11**). The Bureau of Labor Statistics predicts a 24% increase in the number of registered nurses working in the physician office setting between 1994 and 2005 (Bellack, 1998).

Salary changes have also occurred in practice settings. In 1988, only 25% of office nurses earned more than $10 per hour, and less than 10% earned more than $15 per hour (Barhamand, 1991). This translated to annual earnings of approximately $20,800 to $31,200. In 1992, the average annual earnings for an ambulatory care nurse were $27,949 (Moses, 1997). Numbers available from DHHS demonstrate that ambulatory nursing salaries now approximate those of nurses in the hospital setting (Spratley et al., 2000) (**Table 5.12** and **Table 5.13**).

Information from DHHS indicates that the average age of a registered nurse, regardless of practice setting in March 2000, was 43.3 (Spratley et al., 2000). Hospital-employed registered nurses compared with registered nurses in an ambulatory care setting were 41.8 and 44.3, respectively. Breakdown by age and setting indicates that most employed nurses, regardless of setting, are 40 to 54 years old (**Table 5.14**).

Table 5.11   REGISTERED NURSE EMPLOYMENT SETTINGS

Employment Setting	Estimated Percentage
Hospital	59.1%
Nursing home/extended-care facility	6.9%
Nursing education	2.1%
Hospice	0.9%
Ambulatory care setting	9.5%
Solo practice (physicians)	1.1%
Solo practice (registered nurses)	0.1%
Partnership mixed professional group	1.1%
Freestanding clinic (physicians)	0.3%
Ambulatory surgery center (nonhospital based)	1.2%
Dialysis unit	0.7%
Dental practice	0%
Home Health Service/HHS	0.5%
Other ambulatory setting	0.9%

Spratley et al., 2000.

Table 5.12   2002 MEDIAN SALARY: REGISTERED NURSES

Median Annual Salary in Industries Employing Registered Nurses	Median Earnings
Personnel supply services	$46,860
Hospitals	$45,780
Home healthcare services	$43,640
Offices and clinics of medical doctors	$43,480
Nursing and personal care facilities	$41,330

Bureau of Labor Statistics, 2002.

Table 5.13   2002 MEDIAN SALARY: CLINIC SETTINGS

Setting	Mean Annual Salary
Offices and clinics—overall	$47,230
Offices and clinics—MD	$47,240
Offices and clinics—DO	$40,620

Bureau of Labor Statistics US Department of Labor, 2002.

Registered nurses under the age of 30 represent only 10% of the total working population (American Nursing Association, 2001).

The average age of registered nurses is projected to peak at 45.5 in 2010 (Hal, 2001). As the average age increases, the need for registered nurses is also expected to increase. The Department of Labor predicts that employment for registered nurses will grow faster than average for all other occupations through 2010 (Bureau of Labor

Table 5.14   EMPLOYED REGISTERED NURSES BY SETTING AND AGE GROUP

Employment Setting	Percentage by Age									
	< 25	25–29	30–34	35–39	40–44	45–49	50–54	55–59	60–64	> 65
Hospital	4%	9%	12%	16%	19%	18%	11%	7%	3%	1%
Nursing home, extended care facility	2%	8%	8%	12%	15%	17%	14%	11%	5%	5%
Nursing education	0%	2%	3%	8%	15%	20%	22%	17%	9%	3%
Community public health	1%	6%	9%	14%	17%	20%	15%	10%	5%	3%
Student health service	1%	2%	8%	11%	20%	20%	17%	10%	6%	4%
Occupational health	2%	5%	9%	8%	20%	20%	14%	9%	6%	5%
Ambulatory care setting	1%	5%	9%	14%	19%	21%	16%	8%	4%	2%
Other	0%	3%	7%	12%	18%	21%	18%	11%	4%	4%

Spratley et al., 2000.

Statistics, 2002). Nursing is 1 of 10 occupations projected to have the largest number of new jobs. Increased employment needs will be seen in all sectors, including office-based nursing. As the nursing profession evaluates strategies to recruit and retain nurses into the workforce, special attention should be paid to the needs of the office-based oncology setting. As the pool of experienced oncology nurses decreases through attrition and retirement, less experienced nurses will fill the void. Strategies such as public service announcements promoting oncology nursing, incentive programs to retain existing staff, mentoring programs focusing on elementary, junior, and senior high school students, and promotion of education (advanced degrees, licensed vocational nurse (LVN) to registered nurses, loan forgiveness based on service to underserved areas) will recruit and ultimately retain nurses in the profession (Woelkers, Jamieson-Baker, Hammon, & Einstein, 2002).

Conclusion

The number of cancer cases is expected to double by 2050 (Woods, 2003). In addition to an increased population of oncology patients, an increasing number of high-tech procedures and treatments are being delivered in the ambulatory care setting. Nursing in this setting is multifaceted and includes traditional nursing care and administrative, clerical, and ancillary duties. Nurses and physicians work closely together to deliver appropriate, high-quality, state-of-the-art cancer care. Nurses choose to work in ambulatory care for a variety of reasons, including the challenging nature of the job, the ability to work closely with patients and see the impact of nursing/medical interventions, and the flexible scheduling options (Hackbarth et al., 1995).

References

American Academy of Ambulatory Care Nursing. (2003). Telehealth Nursing Practice and Administration Standards. *American Academy of Ambulatory Care Nursing* [On-line]. Retrieved February 13, 2004 from *http://www.aacn.org/resource/telephone.htm*

American Medical Association. (2002). *Current Procedural Terminology: CPT 2003*. Chicago, IL: American Medical Association.

American Medical Association. (2002). *HCPCS Level II* (14th ed.). Salt Lake City: Ingenix.

American Nursing Association. (2001). Policy Statement from Tri-Council members: Strategies to reverse the new nursing shortage. *Nursing World* [On-line]. Retrieved February 13, 2004 from *http://www.ana.org*

Angiulo, C. & Dickey, E. (2001). Practice/office support. In J. Robinson (Ed.), *Core Curriculum for Ambulatory Care Nursing* (pp. 70–83). Philadelphia, PA: W.B. Saunders Company.

Association of Community Cancer Centers. (2003a). *Association of Community Cancer Centers: First 25 Years. Association of Community Cancer Centers* [On-line]. Retrieved February 13, 2004 from *http://www.accc-cancer.org*

Association of Community Cancer Centers. (2003b). Standards for cancer programs. *Association of Community Cancer Centers* [On-line]. Retrieved February 13, 2004 from *http://www.accc-cancer.org*

Barhamand, B. A. (1991). A survey of the role, benefits, and realities of the office-based oncology nurse. *Oncology Nursing Forum, 18*, 31–37.

Behrend, S. W. (1994). Documentation in the ambulatory setting. *Seminars in Oncology Nursing, 10*, 264–280.

Bellack, J. P. (1998). Changing roles, responsibilities, and employment patterns of registered nurses in ambulatory care settings. In E. O'Neil & J. Coffman (Eds.), *Strategies for the Future of Nursing* (pp. 113–142). San Francisco, CA: Dussey-Bass Publishers.

Bowker, G. C., Star, S. L., & Spasser, M. A. (2001). Classifying nursing work. *Online Journal of Issues in Nursing* [On-line]. Retrieved February 13, 2004 from *http://www.nursingworld.org/ojin*

Browne, R. (2001). Ambulatory care team. In J. Robinson (Ed.), *Core Curriculum for Ambulatory Care Nursing* (pp. 55–69). Philadelphia: W.B. Saunders Company.

Bureau of Labor Statistics. (2000). *2000 National Occupational Employment and Wage Estimates*. Washington, DC: U.S. Government Printing Office.

Bureau of Labor Statistics. (2002). *Occupational Outlook Handbook, 2002–2003 Edition, Registered Nurses*. Washington, DC: U.S. Government Printing Office.

Chahl, H. M. (1997). Identifying nursing roles, responsibilities, and practices in telehealth/telemedicine. *Healthcare Information Management, 11*, 5–13.

Fountain, M. J. (1993). Key roles and issues of the multidisciplinary team. *Seminars in Oncology Nursing, 9*, 25–31.

Giarelli, E., Gholz, R., Haisfield-Wolfe, M. E., Mitchell, A., & Smith, A. M. (2001). SNAP-shots: Scenes from nursing action plans—the cultivation of leadership in oncology nursing. *Oncology Nursing Forum, 28*, 883–893.

Greenberg, M. E. (2000). The domain of telenursing: Issues and prospects. *Nursing Economics, 18*, 201, 220–222.

Haas, S. (2001). Ambulatory care nursing specialty practice. In J. Robinson (Ed.), *Core Curriculum for Ambulatory Care Nursing* (pp. 3–15). Philadelphia: W.B. Saunders Company.

Haas, S. & Hastings, C. (2002). Staffing and workload. In J. Robinson (Ed.), *Core Curriculum for Ambulatory Care Nursing* (pp. 133–147). Philadelphia: W.B. Saunders Company.

Haas, S. A. & Hackbarth, D. P. (1995a). Dimensions of the staff nurse role in ambulatory care: Part III—Using research data to design new models of nursing care delivery. *Nursing Economics, 13*, 230–241.

Haas, S. A. & Hackbarth, D. P. (1995b). Dimensions of the staff nurse role in ambulatory care: Part IV—Developing nursing intensity measures, standards, clinical ladders, and QI programs. *Nursing Economics, 13*, 285–294.

Haas, S. A., Hackbarth, D. P., Kavanagh, J. A., & Vlasses, F. (1995c). Dimensions of the staff nurse role in ambulatory care: Part II—Comparison of role dimensions in four ambulatory settings. *Nursing Economics, 13*, 152–165.

Hackbarth, D. P., Haas, S. A., Kavanagh, J. A., & Vlasses, F. (1995). Dimensions of the staff nurse role in ambulatory care: Part I—Methodology and analysis of data on current staff nurse practice. *Nursing Economics, 13*, 89–92.

Hagan, L., Morin, D., & Lepine, R. (2000). Evaluation of telenursing outcomes: Satisfaction, self-care practices, and cost savings. *Public Health Nurse, 17*, 305–313.

Hal, K. (2001). Testimony of the American Nurses Association on the nursing shortage and its impact on America's health care delivery system before the Subcommittee on Aging Committee on Health, Feb. 1, 2001. *Nursing World* [On-line]. Retrieved February 13, 2004 from *http://www.ana.org*

Harris, M. G. & Bean, C. A. (1991). Changing the role of the nurse in the hematology-oncology outpatient setting. *Oncology Nursing Forum, 18*, 43–46.

Huffman, F. & Wakefield, D. S. (1986). Ambulatory care patient classification. *The Journal of Nursing Administration, 16*, 2–30.

Igen, P. V. & Taylor, P. E. (1912). New York Association For Improving the Condition of the Poor. Committee for the Reduction of Infant Mortality. Retrieved on March 28, 2004 from *http://medcat.wustl.edu/cgi/ecd.cgi?0:WUM:ECDZR:694179*

Johnson, J. M. (1989). Quantifying an ambulatory care patient classification instrument. *The Journal of Nursing Administration, 19*, 36–42.

Kirsch, E. & Talbott, J. (1990). Outpatient and short-stay patient classification systems. *Nursing Management, 21*, 118–122.

Lamkin, L. (1994). Outpatient oncology settings: A variety of services. *Seminars in Oncology Nursing, 10*, 229–236.

Lin, E. M., Aikin, J. L., Bailey, W., Fitzgerald, B., Mings, D., Mitchell, S. et al. (1993). Improving ambulatory oncology nursing practice. An innovative educational approach. *Cancer Nursing, 16*, 53–62.

Lynaugh, J. E. (1990). Debate: Is there anything new about the nursing shortage. In J. C. McCloskey & H. K. Grace (Eds.), *Current Issues in Nursing* (3rd ed., pp. 169–179). St. Louis, MO: C. V. Mosby Company.

Martin, V. R. & Xistris, D. (2000). Ambulatory Care. In C. H. Yarbro, M. H. Frogge, M. Goodman, & S. H. Groenwald (Eds.), *Cancer Nursing: Principles and Practice* (pp. 1641–1660). Sudbury, MA: Jones and Bartlett Publishers.

Mastal, M. (2001). Context of ambulatory care. In J. Robinson (Ed.), *Core Curriculum for Ambulatory Care Nursing* (pp. 31–54). Philadelphia: W.B. Saunders Company.

Medvec, B. R. (1994). Productivity and workload measurement in ambulatory oncology. *Seminars in Oncology Nursing, 10*, 288–295.

Moses, E. B. (1997). *The Registered Nurse Population: Findings from the National Sample Survey of Registered Nurses, March 1996*. Rockville, MD: U.S. Department of Health and Human Services.

Moskowitz, R. (1990). New trends in ambulatory oncology care. In P. Ashwanden, A. E. Belcher, E. A. H. Mattson, R. Moskowitz, & N. E. Riese (Eds.), *Oncology Nursing: Advances, Treatments, and Trends into the 21st Century* (pp. 259–275). Rockville, MD: Aspen Publications.

Noa, C. & D'Angelo, L. (2001). Ambulatory care nursing specialty health care fiscal management. In J. Robinson (Ed.), *Core Curriculum for Ambulatory Care Nursing* (pp. 84–95). Philadelphia: W.B. Saunders Company.

Oncology Nursing Society. (2001). Oncology Nursing Society Position Statement: Oncology services in the ambulatory setting. *Oncology Nursing Forum, 28*, 14.

Prescott, P. A., Phillips, C. Y., Ryan, J. W., & Thompson, K. O. (1991). Changing how nurses spend their time. Image: *Journal of Nursing Scholarship, 23*, 23–28.

Prescott, P. A. & Soeken, K. L. (1996). Measuring nursing intensity in ambulatory care. Part I: Approaches to and uses of patient classification systems. *Nursing Economics, 14*, 14–21, 33.

Price, S. A. & Frank-Lightfoot, L. (2000). Evolving roles and professional practice models for nursing. In C. F. Chang, S. A. Price, & S. K. Pfoutz (Eds.), *Economics and Nursing: Critical Professional Issues* (pp. 243–273). Philadelphia: F.A. Davis Company.

Reville, B. & Almadrones, L. (1989). Continuous infusion chemotherapy in the ambulatory setting: The nurse's role in patient selection and education. *Oncology Nursing Forum, 16*, 529–535.

Richards, J. & Tracy, R. (1984). An assessment process for nursing staff patterns in ambulatory care. *The Journal of Ambulatory Care Management, 7*, 69–79.

Spratley, E., Johnson, A., Sochalski, J., Fritz, M., & Spencer, W. (2000). Findings from the national sample survey of registered nurses. Washington, DC: U.S. Department of Health and Human Services, Health Resources and Service Administration.

Stackhouse, J. C. (1998). *Into the Community: Nursing in Ambulatory and Home Care*. Philadelphia: J.B. Lippincott.

Standards of Oncology Education. (1995). *Standards of Oncology Education: Patient/Family and Public*. Pittsburgh, PA: Oncology Nursing Press.

Tighe, M. G., Fisher, S. G., Hastings, C., & Heller, B. (1985). A study of the oncology nurse role in ambulatory care. *Oncology Nursing Forum, 12*, 23–27.

Verran, J. A. (1986a). Testing a classification system for the ambulatory care setting. *Research in Nursing and Health, 9*, 279–289.

Verran, J. A. (1986b). Patient classification in ambulatory care. *Nurse Economic$, 4*, 247–251.

Woelkers, J. F., Jamieson-Baker, P. A., Hammon, D. K., & Einstein, A. B. (2002). Effective strategic planning in clinical cancer services: A road map to success. *Oncology Issues, 17*, 22–28.

Woods, H. R. (2003). Side effects. *Nurse Week*, 9–10.

Chapter 6

Oncology Infusion Centers

Laura M. Chisholm

Georgia Cusack

Antoinette Jones

Introduction

Outpatient oncology care is delivered in a variety of settings. In this chapter, infusion centers (ICs) are introduced as a setting where comprehensive outpatient oncology care is provided. The history of ICs, considerations when planning such a center, nursing roles and practice models, types of services that may be offered, and other administrative considerations are reviewed.

Overview of Outpatient Cancer Care

Until the 1990s most cancer care was delivered in an acute-care inpatient setting. In the 1990s there was an unprecedented growth and shift to outpatient services for all types of care, including oncology (Lamkin, 1994; Summers & Chisholm, 1997). Today, outpatient care is recognized as an appropriate and less costly alternative to acute inpatient care, comprising 80% to 90% of all cancer care, with continued growth projected (Lamkin, 1994). The major driving forces behind this shift in cancer care delivery include diagnostic-related groupings, new technologies, the need for cost savings, and improved efficiencies (Ashley

& Cross-Skinner, 1992). In the past, outpatient cancer care was directed toward patients who were recovering from treatment but who were capable of self-care. Today, cancer outpatients receive highly complex and technical procedures and treatments. The current emphasis on increasing efficiency while maintaining desirable clinical outcomes has resulted in efforts that rely on shifting the site of delivery from inpatient to outpatient care. In many cases, the patient requirement for care remains unchanged.

A variety of cancer services are offered in the outpatient setting and can be broadly categorized under three headings: prevention, screening and detection, and treatment. Prevention services include patient education regarding modifications in diet, exercise, stress management, and chemoprevention. Screening and detection services include providing regular physical examinations, mammography, a clinical breast exam, a pelvic exam , pap smears, a colonoscopy, a sigmoidoscopy, a digital rectal exam, and a testicular examination (National Cancer Institute, 2003). Treatment modalities include surgery, radiation therapy, chemotherapy, biotherapy, and supportive therapies, such as intravenous hydration, electrolyte replacement, blood/cellular product infusions, antibiotics, and immunoglobulins. These modalities can be delivered in a variety of settings, including hospitals, ICs, 23/24-hour day hospitals, outpatient clinics, physician's offices, hotels, and patient homes (Lamkin 1994, 1993; Lamkin & Rice, 1993). Here the role of the IC in ambulatory care is discussed.

"Day hospital" and "IC" are often used interchangeably. The difference between the two is typically dependent on their location, the scope of services provided, and the hours of operation. Both provide traditional services at nontraditional times that make them more convenient for patients who are often balancing the demands of work, family, and therapy (Sands, Galassi, Chisholm, Dimond, Caubo, & Jenkins, 1993). Day hospitals are frequently hospital based and provide a range of services, including outpatient surgery (Clark, 1986). Hours and days of operation can be extended to 23/24 hours, seven days a week. ICs can be hospital or office based and typically concern themselves with the delivery of chemotherapy and supportive therapies. Similar to day hospitals, ICs can operate seven days a week, although hours of operation may be limited to 12 to 16 hours per day (Lamkin, 1994).

ICs

ICs are often associated with chemotherapy and supportive therapies. First established as hospital-based, these facilities provided limited chemotherapy services during the traditional Monday through Friday business hours. Today, complex chemotherapy regimens and supportive therapies such as blood product infusions, antibiotic therapy, hydration, peripheral blood stem cell transplantation (PBSCT), and symptom management along with education and counseling are given in freestanding or hospital-linked outpatient ICs. In many settings, extended hours and seven day a week services have been instituted to enable the administration of dose-intensive regimens in the ambulatory care setting (Gurlach & Macklis, 1995). The development of many chemotherapy

regimens has occurred with ICs in mind, resulting in tremendous increases in the volume of patients treated in the outpatient setting. Patients are likely to be hospitalized only when their complications are too severe to be managed on an outpatient basis (Richter & Felix, 1999; Schim, Thornburg, & Kravutske, 2001).

Hospital-based programs continue to be the most common. They are preferable because of the proximity of specialized diagnostic equipment, continuity of care, and highly trained medical and nursing staffs that can provide specialized services. Consults with nutrition, psychiatry, social work, and pharmacy departments are easier to obtain. Hospital-based programs offer the convenience of extended hours and weekend visits. Freestanding clinics have clear separation from the traditional hospital environment, and some patients prefer treatments delivered in a freestanding facility and find them less intimidating when compared with those that are administered in the hospital setting; however, support services are limited. Sophisticated treatments such as blood product administration and transplant services typically cannot be offered in an office because of time and space limitations. Although hospital-based programs often have more resources that are readily available to patients and their families, a well-designed, office-based IC program can meet many patient and family needs.

The concept of an IC is more attractive than a traditional outpatient treatment setting because of its ability to deliver complex treatments over an extended period without the financial and emotional burden of an inpatient stay. ICs allow patients flexibility in meeting cancer care needs while maintaining a sense of control and normalcy within their lives by remaining as much as possible in their home environment (Lamkin, 1994; Sands et al., 1993; Summers & Chisholm, 1997).

Planning an IC

The initial step in planning an IC consists of

completing a thorough analysis of the healthcare environment, organization, and identified customer needs (Lamkin, 1993). The organization should answer several assessment questions before developing an IC (**Table 6.1**).

Customer Needs

Patients are asking for comprehensive, compassionate, and quality care. Other important considerations include convenience, availability of services, continuity of care, and relationship with staff (Lamkin, 1994). Can this type of care be achieved along with the important goals of healthcare organizations, namely providing cost-effective and efficient care? The answer is yes, although careful consideration and planning must be given to the services provided. A program that is cost effective alone in the absence of therapy that is comprehensive and caring will not remain competitive if consumer satisfaction decreases.

Table 6.1 ORGANIZATIONAL CONSIDERATIONS WHEN PLANNING AN IC

What fits with the organizational vision and philosophy?

What scopes of services will be provided?

Is the center for-profit or non-profit?

What are competitors offering?

What types of services are needed?

How many patients/visits are anticipated?

How many providers will be involved in the delivery of care?

What types of providers are needed to provide care?

What ongoing training and education are available for providers?

What types of reimbursement are available?

Will there be multiple referral sources?

What does the organization already do well?

How can the center improve organizational and patient outcomes?

Alternatively, the provision of comprehensive care without attention to opportunities to manage costs and maximize efficiencies will result in program failure.

Organizational Needs

The design of outpatient ICs includes planning the facility, anticipating the scope of services, and determining workload and staffing requirements (Lamkin, 1993). Too often, regardless of the setting, ICs are physically located in a space that is shared with the delivery of other services. Careful design and planning will result in the creation of an IC that has adequate space for waiting areas, treatment rooms, supplies, and equipment, as well as other support services, such as a satellite pharmacy or laboratory.

Building an IC requires a team who is prepared to meet with architects and engineers to assure that the design is not only aesthetic but also properly constructed and equipped to accommodate the patients' care needs. Reading blueprints and learning safety codes and standards that affect accreditation are necessary skills that must be acquired. The nurse manager should be familiar with the American Institute of Architects Academy of Architecture for Health's Guidelines for Design and Construction of Hospital and Health Care Facilities, Joint Commission of Accreditation of Healthcare Organizations (JCAHO), and the health department requirements.

Environmental Needs

ICs must create a healing environment that provides individuals with a sense of caring and well-being. The design of the center can be accomplished by providing an environment in which individuals have a sense of control over their surroundings. To promote a sense of caring, attention should be paid to physical convenience and comfort, ease of navigation, physical comfort, relaxation, diversion, and the opportunity for social interaction (Reed, 1995; Summers & Chisholm, 1997; Walker, 1994).

A sense of caring can be established before the patient enters the outpatient facility by providing convenient drop-off and pick-up areas, accessible parking, and clearly identified walkways and entrances that facilitate navigation through the facility. Valet parking can be made available where public parking is limited. Entry into and navigation through an unfamiliar environment heightens an individual's sense of anxiety; thus a well-placed reception desk and clearly marked hallways may ease apprehension. Wheelchair accessibility and transport service to and from various destinations in the facility should be considered for individuals who are not ambulatory or who are weak from disease or treatment.

Attention to the waiting area is important. The waiting area should be clearly marked and visible from the reception desk or treatment area so that patients who are concerned or anxious can be reassured that they are not being forgotten. Attention should be paid to temperature, lighting, color scheme, artwork, and comfortable seating. Ideally, waiting areas should provide social and personal space. A choice of seating arrangements allows the patient to choose a comfortable level of socialization. If the waiting area is enclosed, glass walls allow patients to feel a part of what is going on without feeling confined (Reed, 1995; Summers & Chisholm, 1997). The American Institute of Architects recommends that two spaces of waiting area per treatment area equipped with handicapped fixtures (2001).

Waiting areas should provide individuals with snacks and diversions that entertain, amuse, or distract, such as audio and videotapes, television, and computer access. A public toilet must be immediately accessible from the waiting area (AIA, 2001). The use of nature, either through natural lighting, indoor plants, windows overlooking gardens, or fish tanks, engages the senses and provides a calming diversion. A dedicated education and reading area offers a place to pass time and provides individual or classroom education.

Patients should be offered the choice of a bed, a recliner, or a comfortable chair to maximize their comfort. Space is often restricted, and many ICs have a limited number of beds that are typically reserved for those undergoing treatments that are more than two hours or for those who are unable to tolerate a recliner or chair. Considerations in selecting a treatment chair or recliner include comfort, durability, and the ability to place the patient in a variety of positions, including those conducive to emergency treatments and resuscitation (Lamkin, 1993, 1994; Summers & Chisholm, 1997).

The treatment areas should be designed to maximize efficiency while providing a private or semiprivate area for the patient to receive therapy. Often friends and family accompany the individual to his or her outpatient treatment. Areas should be designed to accommodate a visitor while providing adequate space for the staff to treat the patient. Adjacent toilet space is necessary (one for every two treatment areas). Each treatment area must be equipped with either portable or piped-in oxygen and suction (AIA, 2001).

Architectural considerations must interface with patient and staff needs to ensure successful operations (**Figures 6.1** and **6.2** are two examples of infusion centers). This can be accomplished by creating a breezeway between two treatment rooms. This design opens the room and allows the nurse to care for up to four patients without leaving the area, but patient privacy is still maintained. Each room should contain a supply cart and computer access so that the nurse has all of the necessary equipment to provide care in one convenient location.

Rooms for isolating patients with infectious processes are an important consideration, particularly given the immunocompromised status of the oncology patient. An infection-control risk assessment can determine the need for and number of airborne isolation rooms (AIA, 2001). Typically, centers will convert a single occupancy room to an isolation room when needed.

The type of supplies and equipment needed in the IC is dependent on the scope of services. A

Figure 6.1 Warren Grant Magnuson Clinical Center Outpatient Cancer Center

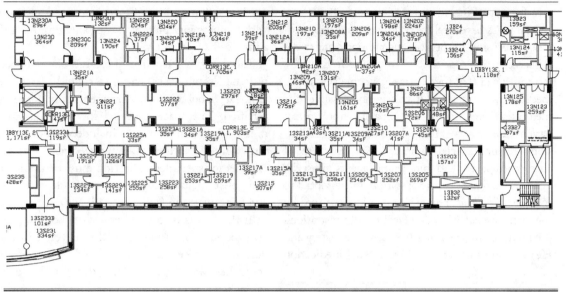

Figure 6.2 M. D. Anderson Cancer Center Ambulatory Treatment Center

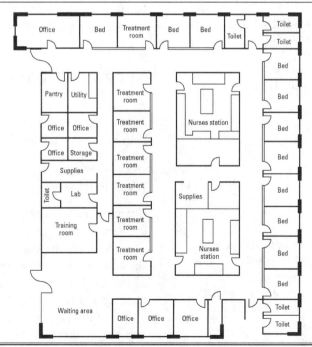

common list of supplies is provided in **Table 6.2**. Generally, one large supply room services the individual treatment rooms. Establishing a system for restocking the rooms is essential.

Many ICs have satellite pharmacies and laboratories. Dispensing of medications are done under the supervision of a registered pharmacist. It is highly recommended that the pharmacy assume the role of medication preparation. If this is not possible, the medication area should be separate from direct patient care activities. Individuals preparing medications require special training. The mixture of chemotherapeutic and biotherapy agents must be done in a laminar flow work station. It is essential to maintain the laminar air airflow work as outlined by the Occupational Safety and Health Administration's (OSHA) recommendations (Occupational Safety and Health Administration, 2003). The medication

preparation room must be well lit and ventilated and provide enough room for a drug storage and preparation area, a sink, and sufficient counter space (AIA, 2001). Staff must be fully educated and supplied with the necessary protective equipment to mix and administer agents safely.

Laboratories located in most ICs offer limited tests and services. Laboratories should ideally be Clinical Laboratory Improvement Amendments certified. The space allocated for the laboratory must be sufficient and must include work counters with a sink, a vacuum, gas, and electrical services. An area for specimen collection must be available and must include seating space, work counters, and hand-washing facilities (AIA, 2001).

If the IC plans to provide services to the pediatric population, this should be reflected in the design of the center. There should be a separate controlled waiting area (AIA, 2001). Other considerations include a playroom area and a pediatric-sized table, chairs, and treatment chairs. Hallway handrails should be positioned for the pediatric patient. Treatment rooms should be outfitted accordingly with appropriate pediatric-sized equipment. A list of space recommendations is provided in **Table 6.3**.

Table 6.2 COMMON SUPPLIES AND EQUIPMENT

Infusion pumps
Large needle buckets
Chemotherapy waste buckets
Automated blood pressure devices
Thermometers
Disposable gloves and gowns
Chemotherapy gowns and gloves
Scale
Pulse oximeter
Blanket warmer
Supply carts
Intravenous tubing
Butterflies
Intravenous catheters
Needleless syringes
Specimen collection tubes
Catheter-related dressing and equipment
Emergency/code cart: AED, portable oxygen,
    suction, backboard, ambu bag, air way
    maintenance equipment, defibrillator jackets,
    epinephrine, bicarbonate
Chemotherapy spill kit
Medication refrigerator
Specimen refrigerator

Services Provided

As noted previously, oncology ICs provide a wide array of services in a variety of settings, including hospitals, free-standing clinics, and physician's offices.

Chemotherapy

Chemotherapy services range from a brief encounter that is less than 30 minutes to those that are extending eight to ten hours. Nurses in the ambulatory care setting require certification in the handling and safe administration of cytotoxic agents (Oncology Nursing Society [ONS], 1996). Many ICs that conduct research are using complex research protocols through cooperative groups (e.g. Southwestern Oncology Group

Table 6.3   RECOMMENDED SPACE ALLOCATION

Type of Room	Square Feet
Patient treatment rooms	80–120
Procedure and exam rooms	120
Utility room (clean and soiled)	100
Pharmacy	150
Nurses' station	150
Waiting rooms	15 per person; 2 spaces for each treatment room
Offices	80
Conference rooms	25 per person
Bathrooms (each)	60

Note: From the American Institutes of Architects Academy of Architecture for Health Care: Guidelines for Design and Construction of Hospitals and Healthcare Facilities, 2001.

(SWOG), Eastern Cooperative Oncology Group (ECOG), National Cancer Institute (NCI)) for therapies administered in the outpatient setting. This further emphasizes the ongoing complexities of educational requirements (Summers & Chisholm, 1997). Cancer patients often have venous access devices (VAD) to ease the long-term impact of cancer treatment. Chemotherapy infused via VAD may be solely administered within the centers or via ambulatory pumps. In addition, the chemotherapy can be given via intraperitoneal or intrathecal routes based on treatment needs.

Supportive Therapies

Patients treated at ICs receive many complex supportive therapies, including intravenous hydration, electrolyte replacement, blood products, antibiotics, immunoglobulin, and total parenteral nutrition (TPN). Many therapies are administered by staff, whereas others require patient/family teaching so that therapies can be administered at home.

Procedures

Recoveries from procedures can be done in ICs. A bed/treatment chair design allows for a variety of procedures to be done. Blood work, bone marrow biopsies and aspirations, paracentesis, thoracente-

sis, lumbar puncture, and liver, renal, skin, and lymph node biopsies are done at the bedside for diagnosis and staging. In addition, patients receive postprocedure monitoring with or without sedation for bronchoscopy, colonoscopy, and VAD placement (implanted ports, Hickman and Groshong catheter). Procedures requiring sedation are ideal for ICs because of the cost-efficiency.

Education

Patient education rooms are essential for ICs. Providing a variety of reading materials helps the patient to understand his or her disease process and treatment options. A computer with Internet access provides patients with additional information and serves as a mode of distraction for those who are waiting for treatments to begin. Many classes can be provided in the patient education room based on patient need, staff expertise, and space. IC nurses who are skilled in working with patients who have VADs can conduct classes. PBSCT classes can be incorporated before and after transplant. Nurses also can collaborate with the ONS or other oncology organizations to provide education regarding such topics as "Fatigue Awareness" and "Lung Cancer Awareness" and to recognize special days such as "Cancer Survivors

Day" and "Race for the Cure." Nurses can collaborate with the American Cancer Society to provide "Look Good, Feel Better" classes for patients and family members. Some hospitals have designated areas for a "Boutique" to provide health-promotion materials and items such as wigs, turbans, and scarves. Providing education empowers patients/families as partners in their care.

Practice Models

Ongoing changes in healthcare have resulted in concurrent shifts in care delivery and nursing practice models. The goals of care delivery include production of high-quality care and achievement of improved patient outcomes and satisfaction levels. An increased emphasis on cost effectiveness and cost containment, evidenced-based practice, and practice standards contributes to the appropriate development, selection, and deployment of care delivery and practice models (Deutschendorf, 2003). Practice models determine the structure and method by which assignments are made and care is delivered.

Just as it is unreasonable to expect that one model of care delivery is applicable across inpatient settings, the same is true in outpatient settings (Deutschendorf, 2003). Issues to consider include the patient population, acuity and severity of illness, types of services offered, interventions required, and types of healthcare providers available to staff the center (Deutschendorf, 2003; Summers & Chisholm, 1997).

To meet the goals of high-quality care at the lowest cost, practice models must account for the variety of levels of skill and knowledge of healthcare providers (Richter & Felix, 1999; Schim, Thornburg, & Kravutske, 2001). Frequently, the role and the contributions of the professional nurse are misunderstood, misused, and underestimated (Richter & Felix, 1999; Schroder, Trehearne, & Ward, 2000a, 2000b). Practice models often focus on productivity, frequently

defined as a "task accomplishment." Unfortunately, this does not take into consideration the critical thinking that is required to analyze and assess complex situations and then apply appropriate clinical interventions (Deutschendorf, 2003). It also does not account for the "hidden work" of nurses, including working with and compensating for bureaucracy, coordinating the efforts of the healthcare team, troubleshooting, serving as a buffer for the physician, providing leadership, serving as the primary source of information, and acting as the patient's advocate (Schroder et al., 2000a, 2000b).

The process of selecting a care delivery model can proceed in an organized manner if structure is applied to the process. This should include a review of factors that affect care delivery (**Table 6.4**) (Walter, 1994). During these times of healthcare upheaval, it is imperative that the healthcare provider is assigned responsibilities appropriate to his or her skill level (see **Table 6.5**) (Deutschendorf, 2003).

Once this review is complete, the practice model of the IC can be determined. One common model is primary nursing. First proposed by Manthey (1980), primary nursing is a delivery model that is grounded in the individual nurse's responsibility and accountability for clinical decision making and quality of care, making assignments using the case method, and matching patient needs with nurse skills. The focus is on continuity of care and accountability for patient outcomes (Manthey, 1980, 1991).

Primary nursing requires that the center be staffed with a sufficient number of professional nurses. The primary nurse is responsible for developing the patient's plan of care, continually assessing progress and outcomes, and adjusting the plan accordingly. Although the primary nurse often provides care to the patient at each visit, this is not required. The primary nurse is responsible for directing the care and may delegate to other staff as appropriate. The benefit of primary

---

Table 6.4 FACTORS TO CONSIDER IN SELECTING A CARE DELIVERY MODEL

Infusion center
- Physical design
- Proximity to support services
- Operating hours and days
- Patient scheduling patterns

Patient
- Acuity
- Volume
- Age groups

Personnel
- Categories and roles of practitioners and support staff

Support services
- On-site versus off-site centralized services (rehabilitation, nutrition, and social work)

Services
- Scope of nurse-managed service

---

nursing includes enhanced continuity of care, increased patient and nurse satisfaction, and improved clinical outcomes.

Workload Analysis

Determining nursing workload and providing the right "mix" of staff to care for patients are not easy for nurse managers. A variety of tools are used in the inpatient setting to assist in the examination of patient acuity/intensity methods used to develop staffing patterns. The nursing care needs in ambulatory care have a different focus, and inpatient acuity/intensity tools cannot be easily applied. The development of such tools in the outpatient setting, although greatly needed, presents another challenge for the manager in ambulatory care.

Nursing workload in the outpatient setting has three major influences: patient volume/census, patient care demands, and the role of the nurse. Patient census is the volume of patients requiring care during a specific time period and can be quantified through the use of an appointment system. Patient care demands are factors that dictate the level of nursing care needed, including diagnosis, plan of care, and nursing acuity/intensity. The role of the nurse is a compilation of direct and indirect care required to deliver patient care, including telephone triage, coordination of care, and clerical and administrative duties. These influences help to determine workload, which can be defined as the required number of hours of staff time per workload interval (Hastings, 1987).

In the ambulatory setting, each patient interaction can be defined as an encounter. An encounter can be a direct contact between a patient and the nurse or an indirect contact between the nurse and any other person/department/system involving coordination of care around a specific patient. An encounter can be as brief as a 1-minute telephone call to an extensive 6- to 8-hour chemotherapy infusion. A nursing acuity/intensity system can be used to collate encounters and to determine workload.

Nursing acuity/intensity systems use one of two methods to sort patient encounters into levels to predict nursing care requirements (Haas, Hackbark, Kavanagh, & Vlasses, 1995). The prototype method is composed of four to five levels and sorts patients according to priority and care requirements, with each level containing a brief description. This method is subjective and relies on the nurses' judgments to reflect accurately the care needs from shift to shift. The factor method considers the most visible activities and correlates them with a time factor. The sum of the times designates the patient category.

The major issues associated with using acuity/intensity systems are assuring validity and reliability. Performance improvement indicators must be created, implemented, and reviewed frequently. It is important when developing an intensity tool that each descriptor be defined in a way that is meaningful for the staff. Staff should be in-serviced about the tool before use. Ongoing feedback must be given to the staff from implementation of the tool throughout its use to ensure consistency.

Nursing Roles

As outpatient care has evolved, so has the role of the outpatient nurse. Historically, the role of the nurse in ambulatory care had been to direct traffic, answer the telephone, complete paperwork, and order supplies. The work of the nurse in ambulatory care has become increasingly complex (Schim et al., 2001). As the demand for outpatient care services increased, nurses began to "assume more responsibility for health maintenance, treatment, and disease prevention" (Lamkin, 1994).

Managers and Administrators

Although the nurse manager and nurse administrator generally do not provide direct patient care in the outpatient setting, the roles remain important. The primary responsibility of the manager is to provide a dynamic environment for patients, families, and healthcare providers that is conducive to teamwork, efficiency, and quality care. Managerial responsibilities include defining the scope of practice, developing and assessing standards of care, determining appropriate staffing skill mix and patterns, planning the budget, developing and maintaining performance-improvement programs, and providing educational opportunities for clinical staff. Managers must have a good understanding of the patient

Table 6.5   ALLOCATION OF WORK AMONG IC STAFF

Role	Assignments
RN	Coordinates care, makes decisions independently, delegates and supervises assistive personnel, conducts patient education, acts as patient advocate, provides follow-up and ensures continuity of care, delivers complex care, administers chemotherapy and blood products, performs telephone triage, manages care in collaboration with a licensed independent practitioner
Unlicensed assistive personnel	Assists patient's with activities of daily living, performs simple intake (vital signs, height/weight) and other clinical duties as delegated and within competency set, stocks and sets up rooms, escorts patients and families, chaperones patients during exams
Administrative personnel	Makes appointments, ensures that patient medical records and other required documents are present for patient visit, validates demographic and insurance information, orders supplies, maintains administrative records, provides clerical support

(Deutschendorf, 2003).

population being served, the cancer treatments that are available, and the comprehensive needs of the oncology patient.

In this role, becoming knowledgeable of the national standards regarding ambulatory care of the cancer patient, intravenous therapy, and infection control will arm the manager with the necessary background to direct the staff in the various areas of patient care for which they will assume responsibility. The Intravenous Nursing Society, the American Academy of Ambulatory Care Nurses (AAACN), and the ONS are professional organizations that can be invaluable resources to the nurse manager of the IC as standards of practice, policies, and procedures are developed and implemented.

An effective appointment system must be developed. A variety of appointment types in an IC exist; these consist of cancer and other types of immunocompromised patients. A strategy to examine these appointment types and to develop a scheduling system to maximize the number of treatments that can be completed in a day is crucial if patient and staff satisfaction, as well as fiscal success, is to be achieved. Many outpatient areas struggle with patient scheduling, thus finding that they receive complaints about long waits and delays. Ongoing evaluation using a patient satisfaction survey provides information that can be used to adjust the system and improve the service provided.

A performance improvement program that has customer service and positive patient outcomes as its nucleus, along with commitment and involvement from the entire IC staff (manager, nurses, clerks, housekeepers), will have a significant influence on the success of the center. The nurse manager that understands the effect of a well-implemented and maintained performance improvement program on patient and unit outcomes will share its importance with the staff and lead them to incorporate performance improvement activities into their daily work in a meaningful and practical manner.

Clinical Nurse

The role of the clinical nurse in outpatient settings varies widely depending on the setting, the philosophy, and the practice model of the setting (Haas et al., 1995; Richter & Felix, 1999; Schim et al., 2001; Schroder et al., 2000; Summers & Chisholm, 1997). In ICs, this role is pivotal. The clinical nurse serves as the liaison between the hospital, physician, and home setting as well as provides the foundation for nursing care delivery. The clinical nurse assists patients in understanding the effects of their illness and treatments on their daily lives and translates diagnosis and treatment into practical plans that can be understood and controlled. Clinical nurses must possess a comprehensive understanding of oncology and immunology, be autonomous, and possess excellent skills in physical assessment, patient education, time management, organization, and communication. Comprehensive patient assessments address physical, psychosocial, and financial issues.

The ONS's standards for oncology practice are a framework for patient assessment, intervention, and education planning (Cooley, Lin, & Hunter, 1994; Oncology Nursing Society & American Nurses Association, 1996). Patient and family education should include providing information about the disease process, symptom management, self-care strategies, and when indicated, treatment options. Psychomotor skills, such as venipuncture and the management of VADs and other equipment, also are needed. The importance of time management and the ability to prioritize in the outpatient IC setting cannot be overstated. Treating multiple patients at one time and handling emergencies and unplanned visits, which are not uncommon, require the clinical nurse to triage and redirect nursing and patient care activities continually (Summers & Chisholm, 1997). Managing appointments must be done so that the maximum number of patients can be seen daily.

Telephone triage is a major component in the workload of the oncology nurse in the outpatient setting. The clinical nurse is frequently responsible for initiating and following patients who are not physically present. Nurses triage patients based on telephone triage etiquette and assessment skills and determine whether the patient should be seen emergently by a local physician or managed over the phone. These nurses must become adept in an environment that requires a strong sense of independence and excellent clinical judgment, as well as an increased scope of responsibility for positive patient outcomes (Wheeler, 1993).

Today many outpatient ICs provide care to patients receiving PBSCT. This may encompass patient and donor preparation, including stem cell harvest, the administration of the conditioning preparative regimens, patient and family education, reinfusion of cells, and immediate care after transplant follow-up. Therefore, nurses in the outpatient setting must possess the knowledge and abilities that were at one time limited to inpatient PBSCT nurses. This includes exceptional assessment skills and the ability to provide patients with direction on the management of anticipated complications during treatment and follow-up. In addition, excellent communication skills are essential when telephone assessments are conducted to triage patient problems. These practice requirements challenge many nurses in outpatient settings because they have not historically cared for such acutely ill patients undergoing such complex treatments. Nurses must ensure that they receive the appropriate education to care competently for patients on these complex regimens.

Unlicensed Assistive Personnel

The escalating cost of healthcare and the current nursing shortage have led to exploration and use of assistive personnel in providing nursing servic-es to patients (Barter, McLaughlin, & Thomas, 1994; Haas & Gold, 1997; Krapohl & Larson, 1996). These individuals have been trained to function as assistants to registered nurses in the provision of clinical nursing care (Barter et al.,1994; Haas & Gold, 1997; Johnson, 1995; Krapohl & Larson, 1996; Summers & Chisholm, 1997). The intended use of unlicensed assistive personnel (UAP) is to extend or complement care traditionally provided by the professional nurse. UAP includes nurses' aides, medical technicians, and patient care technicians as well as other position titles developed by individual institutions. UAP use has been addressed by professional organizations and the JCAHO, state boards of nursing, and state health departments. These agencies' regulations will vary from state to state.

Professional nursing organizations have issued statements related to the use of UAP. The American Nurses Association, the AAACN, and ONS have each developed position papers on the use of the UAP in healthcare settings. All three organizations share the belief that the professional nurse best accomplishes the overall accountability, coordination, and management of nursing care. All underscore the importance of validating the knowledge, skills, and competence of both professional nurses and UAP to provide care for individuals with clearly defined needs. The delivery of care by the UAP is performed as a delegated and supervised activity, with the professional nurse remaining responsible and accountable for the outcomes of care. UAPs need to be adequately trained for their work. Competency levels must be validated before allowing the UAP to function without direct supervision (Haas & Gold, 1997). The clinic nurse in the outpatient IC must maintain a role focus as the coordinator of care in its entirety. The decision to delegate care activities is accompanied by the obligation to supervise the delivery and outcomes of care and to integrate the clinical information gained about the specific patient as a result of that care (Haas & Gold, 1997; Medvec, Pelusi, Camp-Sorrell et al., 1996).

Recruitment and Retention

Two of the advantages of the nursing profession that have been touted for years are the abilities to practice in a variety of work settings and scheduling flexibility. Nurses work in hospitals, business and industry, schools, clinics, homes, and ICs. A nurse can find an array of work schedules that are compatible with his or her obligations to home and family. Despite this variety and flexibility, the nursing shortage is affecting the outpatient setting as well as the hospital bedside. Although national data are inadequate to describe the actual effect of the current shortage on the outpatient cancer areas, the U.S. General Accounting Office (GAO) reported that registered nurse employment has experienced a 2% overall decline from 1996–2000 (GAO, 2001). Job dissatisfaction, which is related to many factors (i.e., wages, workload, staffing, hours, overtime, lack of respect), is reportedly having a huge influence on the supply of nurses who provide direct patient care; therefore, focused recruitment and retention efforts are greatly needed (GAO, 2001; Aiken, Clarke, Sloane et al., 2002; Berliner & Ginzberg, 2002; Lamkin et al., 2001; Mee & Robinson, 2003).

As previously discussed, the role of the nurse in the ambulatory setting is expanding. With managed care and the movement of many patient treatments to the outpatient setting, what was considered complex patient care reserved for the inpatient has become normal for cancer patients in the outpatient setting (Richter & Felix, 1999). Long ago, the image of the nurse in the outpatient setting was someone who spent his or her day as an office manager using minimal nursing skills (Schim et al., 2001; Brenchley & Robinson, 2001). This misconception is disproved daily as the complex needs of cancer patients are met by high-caliber nursing care delivered in this setting. The IC provides an area of practice in which astute nursing assessment and intervention are constantly in demand. Nurses in the IC learn and use problem solving, critical thinking, communication, management, leadership, and advocacy skills. This setting attracts the best and the brightest because of the autonomy that it requires and the inherent potential for professional growth and development.

When recruiting for this area, the nurse manager or nurse recruiter should search for nurses who have experience in both oncology and ambulatory care. The experienced nurse desiring to work in the IC must demonstrate leadership skills that are developed through experiences such as charge nurse, team leaders on specific projects, and other career-enhancing opportunities. A candidate must demonstrate outstanding oral and written communication skills that are obtained through formal and informal presentations, precepting, serving in the charge nurse role, development of patient teaching tools, peer review activities, and annual evaluations. The uses of assertiveness, advocacy, and autonomy are traits that will ensure success for the nurse in this setting. The ability to multitask and to attend to detail is essential.

Recruitment to this area does not exclude the new graduate nurse, although their employment in the outpatient cancer setting remains controversial. Some advocate that the clinical nurse in the outpatient setting should be prepared at the baccalaureate level and have a minimum of 1 year of inpatient oncology experience. Advocates of these prerequisites believe that these practice experiences provide a foundation on which the nurse can build the additional knowledge and abilities required in the outpatient setting (Cooley, Lin, & Hunter, 1994). Conversely, this viewpoint is not universally accepted, and new graduates have been successfully integrated into select outpatient cancer centers. Successful transition from the new graduate to the competent clinician depends on a comprehensive orientation/ preceptor program and personal qualities of the individual nurse. Qualities that equip the new graduate for success include a willingness to take risks and practice in an area not traditionally viewed as "comfortable" for the novice practitioner, enthusiasm, professional maturity, and strong self-esteem.

Current Issues

Reimbursement

Reimbursement of services brings another set of issues to the cancer care arena. A current issue hotly debated in the press is concern of the "chemotherapy concession." Oncologists are being accused of purchasing chemotherapy and selling it to patients/payers at inflated prices, thus generating huge revenues. Drug companies are experiencing lawsuits related to accusations of physician inducement to purchase their drugs over competitors (Abelson, 2003; Abelson & Glater, 2003). Oncologists counter that the parameters through which chemotherapy is purchased, sold, and reimbursed is a complex structure (American Society of Clinical Oncology [ASCO] Statements, (2002); Grigsby, Bouda, Brown, & Sanchez, 1996). The "spread" between the price oncologists pay for the drug, the fee that they bill to Medicare, and the copayment that Medicare passes on to patients is used to offset the other expenses associated with chemotherapy administration and the basic costs of running an oncology practice (Benson, 2001; Dixon, 2003). Private health insurers pay doctors in a similar, although less rigid manner as the Medicare system (Dixon, 2003). Oncologists report that today's reimbursement levels for cancer drugs are used to help pay for highly trained oncology nurses to administer chemotherapy and to provide patient education and psychosocial support for patients and their families (Grigsby, Bouda, Brown, & Sanchez, 1996; ASCO, 2002; Abelson & Glater, 2003).

While the resolution of these issues is pending, the IC continues to prove to be a viable option for meeting the healthcare needs of the sick for less money. Benson reports that approximately 80% of cancer patients receive their chemotherapy treat-ments in the doctor's office or other freestanding facilities. Additionally, the government is continually reviewing the Medicare system as it relates to the payment of outpatient services (Arnold & Vastag, 2000). As long as patients are able to receive quality care in a setting that has the skill to provide high-level assessment and intervention at a reasonable cost, ICs will remain. Many centers have already expanded their scope of services and availability to 23/24 hours, allowing maximal flexibility without requiring an inpatient stay. Nurse-managed clinics with physician consultation are a cost-effective alternative. Collaborative programs (NP/MD partnerships) to expand the role of the nurse are being implemented (Richter & Felix, 1999).

Planning for the Future

What is the future of the IC in this new millennium? Experts estimate that by 2005, nonhospital care will capture 20% to 30% of the demand for acute hospital services (Richter & Felix, 1999). This supports the notion that ICs are here to stay.

How can we make the IC better? Creating a system of access to support services (social work, dietician, radiology) would make the freestanding IC an even greater success. Another approach is the implementation of educational programs that could decrease unnecessary visits. Building a wellness room to provide a place to meditate quietly and relax and having the use of complementary and alternative therapies such as massage therapy, relaxation, music therapy, visualization, therapeutic touch, and aromatherapy are ideas to explore. The possibilities are endless. Patients could conceivably receive their blood transfusion or chemotherapy after dinner or later in the evening and sleep through many side effects. Patients could have their blood drawn, work a full day, and come in after work for electrolyte replacement, antibiotic therapy, or intravenous hydration. These and other conveniences are possible through ICs, empowering patients and nurses toward favorable outcomes and overall satisfaction.

References

Abelson, R. (2003, January 26). Drug sales bring huge profits and scrutiny to cancer doctors. *The New York Times*.

Abelson, R. & Glater, J. D. (2003, February 13). New York will sue 2 big drug makers on doctor discount. *The New York Times*, pp. A1.

Aiken, L. H., Clarke, S. P., Sloane, D. M., Sochalski, J., & Silber, J. H. (2002). Hospital nurse staffing and patient mortality, nurse burnout and job dissatisfaction. *JAMA*, 288, 1987–1999.

American Institute of Architects Academy of Architecture for Health Care: Guidelines for Design and Construction of Hospitals and Healthcare Facilities. (2001). Washington, DC: AIA

American Society of Clinical Oncology: Statement on Reimbursement of Cancer Chemotherapy. Retrieved February 14, 2004 from *http://www.asco.org/ac*

American Society of Clinical Oncology: ASCO response to New York Times article entitled overpriced cancer drugs'. Retrieved February 14, 2004 from *http://www.asco.org/ac*

American Society of Clinical Oncology: ASCO policy watch weekly. Retrieved December 20, 2002 from *http://www.asco.org/ac*

Arnold, K. & Vastag, B. (2000). Medicare to cover routine care costs in clinical trials. *Journal of the National Cancer Institute*, 92, 1032.

Ashley, B.W. & Cross-Skinner, S. (1992). Oncology nursing care delivery issues in the ambulatory care setting. *Current Issues in Cancer Nursing Practice Updates, 1*, 1–10.

Barter, M., McLaughlin, F. E., & Thomas, S. A. (1994). Use of unlicensed assistive personnel by hospitals. *Nursing Economic$, 12*, 82–87.

Benson, L. R. (2001). Reimbursing cancer care: Medicare policies challenged. *Journal of the National Cancer Institute, 93*, 1595–1597.

Berliner, H. S. & Ginzberg, E. (2002). Why this hospital nursing shortage is different. *JAMA, 288*, 2742–2744.

Brenchley, T. & Robinson, S. (2001). Outpatient nurses: From handmaiden to autonomous practitioner. *British Journal of Nursing, 10*, 1067–1072.

Clark, M. (1986). A day hospital for cancer patients: Clinical and economic feasibility. *Oncology Nursing Forum, 13*, 41–45.

Cooley, M. E., Lin, E. M., & Hunter, S. W. (1994). The ambulatory oncology nurse's role. *Seminars in Oncology Nursing, 10*, 245–253.

Dixon, K. (2003, January 30). *Cancer Doctors Defend Chemotherapy Payments*. Science—Reuters.

Deutschendorf, A. L. (2003). From past paradigms to future frontiers: Unique care delivery models to facilitate nursing work and quality outcomes. *Journal of Nursing Administration, 33*, 52–59.

Grigsby, J., Bouda, D., Brown, E., & Sanchez, R. (1996). Panel discussion: Impact of guidelines on third party payors and hmos. *Oncology*, (Suppl.), 195–201.

Gurlach, R. W. & Macklis, R. (1995). Accomodating modern cancer treatment procedures in an outpatient facility. *Journal of Ambulatory Care Management, 18*, 8–15.

Haas, S. & Gold, C. (1997). Supervision of unlicensed assistive workers in ambulatory settings. *Nursing Economic$, 15*, 57–59.

Haas, S. A., Hackbark, D. P., Kavanagh, J. A., & Vlasses, F. (1995). Dimensions of the staff nurse role in ambulatory care: Part II—comparison of role dimensions in four ambulatory care settings. *Nursing Economic$, 13*, 152–165.

Hastings, C. E. (1987). Classification issues in ambulatory care nursing. *Journal of Ambulatory Care Management, 10*, 50–64.

Johnson, E. M. (1995). Assistive personnel in ambulatory care. *AAACN Viewpoint, 17*, 1, 4.

Krapohl, G. L. & Larson, E. (1996). The impact of unlicensed assistive personnel on nursing care delivery. *Nursing Economic$, 14*, 99–110, 122.

Lamkin, L. (1993). The new oncology ambulatory clinic. In P. C. Buchsel & C. H. Yarbro (Eds.), *Oncology Nursing in the Ambulatory Setting: Issues and Models of Care* (pp. 107–130). Sudbury, MA: Jones and Bartlett Publishers.

Lamkin, L. (1994). Outpatient oncology settings: A variety of services. *Seminars in Oncology Nursing, 10*, 229–236.

Lamkin, L. & Rice W. W. (1993). Cancer program development: Is your hospital ready? *Hospital Topics, 71*, 11–19.

Lamkin, L., Rosiack, J., Buerhaus, P., Mallory, G., & Williams, M. (2001). Oncology nursing workforce survey part I: Perceptions of the nursing workforce environment and adequacy of nurse staffing in outpatient and inpatient oncology settings. *Oncology Nursing Forum, 28*, 1545–1552.

Manthey, M. (1980). *The Practice of Primary Nursing*. Boston, Blackwell Scientific Publications.

Manthey, M. (1991). Delivery systems and practice models: A dynamic balance. *Nursing Management, 22*, 28–30.

Medvec, B. R., Pelusi, J. L., Camp-Sorrell, D., Klein-Schmidt, P., Krebs, L., & Mooney, K. (1996). Assistive personnel: Their use in cancer care—An Oncology Nursing Society Position Paper. *Oncology Nursing Forum, 23*, 647–651.

Mee, C. L. & Robinson, E. (2003). What's different about this nursing shortage? *Nursing, 33*, 51–55.

National Cancer Institute. (2003). Cancer Prevention and Screening. Retrieved February 14, 2004 from *http://www.cancer.gov/cancerinfo/screening*

Occupational Safety and Health Administration. (2003). Controlling Occupational Exposure to Hazardous Drugs. Section VI, Chapter 2. Retrieved February 14, 2004 from *http://www.osha.gov/SLTC/hazardous-drugs*

Oncology Nursing Society and American Nurses Association, Statement on the Scope and Standards of Oncology Nursing Practice. (1996).

Richter, P. & Felix, K. G. (1999). Adding value by expanding RN roles in ambulatory care. *Nursing Economic$, 17*, 225–228.

Reed, R. A. (1995). Creating a healing environment by design. *Journal of Ambulatory Care Management, 18*, 16–31.

Sands, D. A., Galassi, A., Chisholm, L., Dimond, E., Caubo, K., & Jenkins, J. (1993). A cancer day hospital: An alternative approach for patients in clinical trials. *Oncology Nursing Forum, 20*, 787–793.

Schim, S. M., Thornburg, P., & Kravutske, M. E. (2001). Time, tasks and talents in ambulatory care nursing. *Journal of Nursing Administration, 31*, 311–315.

Schroder, C. A., Trehearne, B., & Ward, D. (2000a). Expanded role of nursing in ambulatory managed care part I: Literature, role development and justification. *Nursing Economic$, 18*, 71–78.

Schroder, C. A., Trehearne, B., & Ward, D. (2000b). Expanded role of nursing in ambulatory managed care part II: Impact on outcomes of costs, quality, provider and patient satisfaction. *Nursing Economic$, 18*, 71–78.

Summers, B. L. Y. & Chisholm, L. M. (1997). Opportunities and challenges for oncology nursing in ambulatory cancer care. *Oncology Nursing Updates, 4*, 1–14.

U.S. General Accounting Office (2001). *Nursing Workforce: Emerging Nurse Shortages Due to Multiple Factors.* (General Accounting Office, Publication No.01–944). Washington, DC: Author.

Walker, J. K. (1994). Nurse managers making a difference: Creating a healing place. *Seminars in Nursing Management, 2*, 234–238.

Walter, J. M. & Robinson, S. H. (1994). Nursing care delivery models in ambulatory oncology. *Seminars in Oncology Nursing, 10*, 237–244.

Wheeler, S. (1993). *Telephone Triage: Theory, Practice and Protocol Development.* Albany, NY: Delmar Publishers.

Chapter 7

Outpatient Surgery in the Oncology Setting

Randi Z. Moskowitz

Introduction

Surgery as a potential cure for cancer is one of the oldest known methods of treatment for this illness. John Abernathy, an English surgeon, was one of the first physicians to consider that malignancies were local phenomena, and he proposed the possibility of surgical resection as a form of therapy. Today, surgery is still a major intervention in cancer treatment, and in 90% of patients with curable solid malignant tumors, surgical resection alone or in combination with other modalities is the treatment of choice (Fleming, 2001). According to the American Cancer Society, it is estimated that in the United States men have a little less than a one in two lifetime risk of developing cancer; for women, the risk is a little more than one in three (American Cancer Society, 2004). Thus, it is expected that a large number of patients may require surgical intervention.

Many advances in cancer diagnosis and treatment offer promise for less invasive procedures. The likelihood and length of hospital admissions are declining, and the proportion of care delivered in an inpatient setting is expected to represent less than 10% of total cancer patient care (Gerlach & Macklis, 1995). These factors have given rise to the number of ambulatory surgery centers dedicated to the diagnosis and treatment of cancer.

With the overwhelming mandate for hospitals to produce revenue while delivering quality care, many hospital administrative teams have instituted or enlarged alternative care sites. Outpatient surgical centers have grown at an unprecedented rate. It is imperative that clinical and administrative staff understand various clinical concerns and models and that nurses working in these areas can be called on to consult in the design, development, and renovation of these units.

Ambulatory surgery is a formal, organized program of elective surgery in which patients arrive at the facility, undergo their procedures, and are discharged on the same day (Lagoe & Milliren, 1990). These programs, which hospitals or independent providers sponsor, have become commonplace in the United States over the past 40 years. In this chapter, the important issues related to ambulatory surgery and its future trends in oncology care are addressed.

Historical Perspectives

The concept of ambulatory surgery is not new. Nicholl first documented the practice in 1909 at a meeting of the British Medical Association; he described 8,000 surgical procedures performed on outpatients at the Royal Glasgow Hospital for Children (Lyons & Petrucelli, 1978). In 1916, Waters opened the Down-Town Anesthesia Clinic in Sioux City, Iowa, for dental cases and minor surgery (Lyons & Petrucelli, 1978; Henderson, 1991). In 1937, Herzfeld reported more than 1,000 hernia repairs performed on children, many with general anesthesia on an ambulatory basis. In the late 1950s, a shortage of hospital beds in Canada provided the impetus for expanding outpatient surgery (Henderson, 1991).

In the United States, the modern era of ambulatory surgery began in the early 1960s. The first unit opened in 1961 in Butterworth Hospital in Grand Rapids, Michigan; the second opened a year later at the University of California at Los Angeles (Henderson, 1991). Other hospitals planned similar programs, and in 1970, the first successful freestanding ambulatory surgery facility was opened in Phoenix, Arizona. The unit was developed to provide quality care to the patient whose operation was too complicated to be performed in the physician's office, but not enough to require hospitalization. The most common procedures performed included hernia repairs, breast biopsies, interocular lens replacements, and minor orthopedic procedures (Burns & Ferber, 1984).

Trends in Ambulatory Surgery

The increase in ambulatory surgery is one of the most significant trends in healthcare. In 1995, more than 50% of the surgical procedures completed in the United States were done on an outpatient basis (Pandit, 1999). Based on an analysis that the SMG Marketing Group performed in January 2001, currently in the United States, 65% of operations performed in hospitals were done in the outpatient setting (Pandit, 1999; Burden & DeFazio Quinn, 2000; Burns, 2001; National Center for Health Statistics, 2004).

At cancer centers, many surgical procedures performed are diagnostic in nature, and most can be easily performed in ambulatory surgical centers. This shift presents a significant challenge to the ambulatory care nurses in preparing the patient and family for outpatient procedures that may be critical to prevention, early detection, and prompt treatment of cancer.

Major changes in healthcare in recent years have attempted to improve the quality of care, reduce duplication of services, and contain costs. The development of ambulatory surgery has become a significant factor in meeting these challenges. The growth in ambulatory surgery can be attributed to three factors (Highland, 1998):

- There has been an increase in the number of surgical procedures overall.
- Procedures previously performed on an inpatient basis are now performed on an outpatient basis, but in essentially the same way.
- New, less invasive surgical technologies (such as laparoscopic surgery) have been developed, enabling performance on an outpatient basis.

Technologic change accounts for each of these sources of growth in ambulatory surgery (Highland, 1998). First, new and better techniques with the potential to improve patients' lives can account for the overall growth of surgery. These techniques have caused the overall number of surgeries to increase as advances make significant improvements in quality of life. Second, the growth in medical and surgical technology, along with their costs, has led to an increasingly expensive inpatient setting, placing more emphasis on the potential savings of procedures performed in the ambulatory setting. This has accelerated the shift from inpatient to outpatient surgery. Finally, profit opportunities for techniques that can avoid the use of the inpatient setting have become greater. Outpatient surgery has allowed patients to undergo treatment with less time off from work and with less pain. This has encouraged even greater use of new technology by those who in the past would not have undergone treatment.

Other major factors in the development of ambulatory surgery are strong market forces, such as patients' demand for new and more convenient services, physicians' desire for greater participation, and hospitals' strategies for meeting competition (Burns & Ferber, 1984; Highland, 1998). Finally, the risks from anesthesia have decreased dramatically in the hospital setting over the past decade, leading to the growth of ambulatory surgery (Aker, 2001).

Advantages of Ambulatory Surgery

Advantages of ambulatory surgery include the following (Poole, 1999):

- Decreased cost because of decreased length of stay
- Decreased nosocomial infection rates because of decreased exposure to critically ill patients
- Decreased anxiety for the patient
- Convenience for the patient, necessitating minimal lifestyle changes.

Cost

Reduced cost is one of the most significant features of ambulatory oncologic surgery (Henderson, 1991). Fewer laboratory tests and medications are prescribed for outpatients because they are not a significant risk for surgical-related complications and are often well. Consequently, they are under medical supervision for a shorter period of time. In addition, the surgeon's time is used more efficiently with the decrease in prehospital and posthospital visits.

Outpatient oncologic surgery supports cost-effective hospital services in two ways: (1) Hospital beds, otherwise occupied for minor procedures now being done in outpatient areas, are available for acutely ill patients. (2) Safer use of

anesthesia and operating room services has significantly decreased intraoperative mortality; thus, more mortality-free procedures can be performed in a shorter period of time (Lagoe & Milliren, 1990; Aker, 2001).

Quality of Care

Ambulatory surgical patients receive more individualized attention because units are designed so that the focus of care remains on the outpatient in an atmosphere of wellness. Patients can return home to their families on the day of the procedure, avoiding hospital routines and restrictions. There is less risk of disability and hospital-acquired infection because there is less contact with other patients, staff, and equipment (Aker, 2001). Patients return to work earlier because they are discharged the same day, ambulate better, and return to normal activity almost immediately. Anxiety associated with hospitalization is reduced, especially for children who recover more easily at home.

Disadvantages of Ambulatory Surgery

Disadvantages to ambulatory surgery include the following (Poole, 1999):

- A lack of adherence to preoperative instructions by the patient
- A lack of transportation to and from the facility
- A lack of competent or affordable assistance at home
- A lack of immediately available supportive or resuscitative equipment at home
- An exclusion of uninsured or rural populations

Because the surgical oncologic patient is not onsite at the hospital the evening and morning before the procedure, he or she may not follow preoperative instructions. Mechanisms for preventing this situation include preprocedure telephone calls and written instructions for patients and their caregivers. In the past, the fear of pulmonary aspiration of gastric contents prompted anesthesiologists to forbid any ingestion of solid or liquid food after midnight before the day of the elective outpatient procedure. Current guidelines for preoperative oral intake adopted by the House of Delegates of the American Society of Anesthesiologists in 1988 allow solid food eight hours before, a light, low-fat and low-protein breakfast six hours before, human breast milk for infants four hours before, and clear liquids two hours before elective surgery (Pandit, 1999). These new guidelines may help decrease procedure cancellations due to noncompliance.

Most ambulatory surgery discharge criteria prohibit the patient from driving home after sedation. Certain groups of patients, particularly the older population and those of lower socioeconomic status, may not have easy access to and from the center. If this problem is identified early, social services may be able to arrange for transportation. Otherwise, an expensive and unnecessary overnight admission may be required. Patients living alone, especially older persons, may not have access to caregiver support of family or friends for immediate postoperative care and may also require an unnecessary overnight admission. Oncology nurses working in physicians' offices can provide this type of social information when scheduling outpatient surgical procedures and can arrange for an overnight volunteer or home care.

Types of Procedures Performed

Ideally, outpatient procedures should result in minimal bleeding and should not involve major intervention into the cranial vault or abdominal or thoracic cavities. In addition, they should be short to moderate in duration, should be associated with minimal to no complications or pain, and should not require extensive recovery time. The appropriateness of a procedure for ambulatory surgery depends on the patient's ability to recover from anesthesia and to be discharged to perform self-care at home (Ebbert, 1992).

Ambulatory surgical procedures that are specifically for patients with cancer can be found in **Table 7.1**.

Table 7.1 AMBULATORY SURGERY CANCER-RELATED PROCEDURES

Biopsy
Breast reconstruction, first and second stage
Bronchoscopy
Colonoscopy
Cystoscopy
Dental reconstruction
Endoscopic ultrasound
Esophagoscopy
Facial reconstruction
Gastrostomy
Insertion and removal of stent
Insertion and removal of vascular access devices
Laryngoscopy
Loop Electrosurgical Excision Procedure (LEEP)
Lumpectomy
Mastectomy with or without tissue expander
Parotidectomy
Prostate seed implants
Sentinal node biopsy
Sigmoidoscopy
Transurethral resection of the bladder
Thyroidectomy, total and subtotal

Types of Ambulatory Surgery Facilities

Ambulatory surgery is performed in a variety of settings, most often in hospitals, and is classified according to the governance of the facility. Forty-three states and the District of Columbia license ambulatory surgery centers (*http://www.fasa.org/ acsregulations.html*, August 1, 2002). These centers are some of the most highly regulated healthcare providers in the country.

In addition to state and federal inspections, many centers choose to go through voluntary accreditation processes that organizations such as the Joint Commission on Accreditation of Healthcare Organizations conduct. Medicare recognizes the Joint Commission on Accreditation of Healthcare Organizations for its rigorous adherence to the highest standards of quality care. All accredited ambulatory surgery centers must meet specific standards that are evaluated during onsite inspections. As a result, patients can be assured that the centers provide the highest quality of care.

There are three basic types of ambulatory surgery facilities: hospital-based units, hospital satellite units, and freestanding units (Marasco & Schirmer, 1998; DeFazio Quinn, 2000).

Hospital-Based Unit

The hospital manages the hospital-based unit, often by converting operating room and surrounding facilities used for inpatient surgery to an outpatient function. Scheduling and administration are usually intermixed with inpatient surgery, and scheduling conflicts and emergencies often adversely affect the efficiency of the outpatient unit. It also triggers a sequence of inconveniences for the patient and family. This model contributes to lower expenditures, allowing the institution to curb capital outlay, and consequently provides minimal financial risk to the hospital (Lyons & Petrucelli, 1978; Henderson, 1991). Equipment can be shared easily because supplies are kept in a central location. In addition, surgical staff can be cross-trained and work with minimal difficulty in several surgical units.

Facilities are available for the surgeon to perform more complex procedures, allowing for increased use of the program. For example, if unanticipated complications develop, the patient can be admitted to the hospital. The unit also offers readily available resources for resuscitation or emergency. A disadvantage of this type of facility includes scheduling delays because of emergencies in the inpatient setting. In addition, the "wellness" component of ambulatory oncology surgery centers is lost because of the integration of well outpatients with more acutely ill surgical patients. The fixed costs of inpatient operating rooms are generally higher than those of a dedicated ambulatory surgery facility. Furthermore, many states have requirements and standards applicable to all users of an inpatient facility, regardless of the magnitude of the operation that may be in excess of what is appropriate to the ambulatory case (Allo, 1998).

Hospital Satellite Units

The hospital manages and is attached to the hospital satellite unit, although the actual facility is separate from the inpatient unit (Marasco & Schirmer, 1998). This arrangement offers access to more sophisticated equipment and techniques because the equipment can be used in conjunction with the hospital. Immediate access to emergency services then is available (DeFazio Quinn, 2000). Physicians also like the idea that they can be in close proximity to their inpatients. This layout permits significant cost savings, and patients and staff tend to prefer this (Allo, 1998). Cost savings relate to having a dedicated staff dealing with one type of service and working in a dedicated space. In facilities that separate inpatients from outpatients, the outpatients receive appropriate and undivided attention.

Operating efficiency increases because the unit is designed for a specific service that is performed repeatedly. Scheduling becomes easier with no inpatient competition for operating rooms. The market share increases because of proven expertise in specific procedures, such as breast lumpectomy (Henderson, 1991). Physicians not presently on staff may be more likely to be recruited. Making the ambulatory care oncology patient the focus of care increases staff morale and patient satisfaction as well.

Although there are many advantages to this plan, disadvantages exist. The hospital administration may still base decisions on the inpatient operating room model. The overall mindset of employees is that of a hospital setting, where they must abide by the hospital bureaucracy in order to get things done. Cost is also a factor as the offering of duplicate services requires a high capital investment (DeFazio Quinn, 2000). Operating rooms, equipment, and skilled personnel are employed in both the inpatient and outpatient settings. Revenue-generating ambulatory surgery hospital satellite units usually carry the load for non–revenue-generating departments, such as medical records and finance. This dollar amount can be significant enough to have a negative impact on profit.

Finally, access to parking may be a problem if the unit is attached to the hospital and hospital parking is at a premium (Marasco & Schirmer, 1998). Supplemental valet parking and escort services help some hospitals solve this issue (DeFazio Quinn, 2000).

Freestanding Units

Freestanding units are not affiliated with any hospital, are autonomous, and operate as an entity. Physicians most often own these units (DeFazio Quinn, 2000). There is maximal flexibility in design, location, and scope of services (Allo, 1998). The "wellness" concept in architectural structure can be achieved more readily to promote a cheerful atmosphere for patients and staff. These units may serve single or multiple specialties. They employ, regulate, and control both the professional and business staffs of the facility. From the patient's perspective, the environment of a freestanding unit is more pleasing and less threatening than the hospital (DeFazio Quinn, 2000). Parking does not usually present itself as a problem.

Freestanding centers have mastered the process of cost containment. They do not incur the high overhead costs that are frequently associated with the hospital setting. When cases are finished for the day, they have the ability to shut down and save on electricity, labor, and other costs (DeFazio

Quinn, 2000). Where there is a high volume of certain specialty procedures, staff members become very proficient, providing the service in the most cost-efficient manner.

A disadvantage of the freestanding center includes the inability to keep the patient overnight in the event of slow recovery from anesthesia or if there is a major complication. In addition, construction and start-up require a considerable capital investment, and a profit may not be realized for years.

Other Ambulatory Surgery Models

OFFICE-BASED SURGICAL CARE

Office-based surgical care has increased exponentially during the past decade, basically because of the development of new technologies (Aker, 2001). An estimated 20% of all outpatient surgery is done in the office setting (Pandit, 1999). Other factors, including more personalized surgical care, single surgical specialty-based office practices, and third-party payers' exploration of less expensive options have also influenced this trend. Additionally, office-based surgery has not been subject to the same state and federal licensing and credentialing guidelines as the hospital-based center. This trend, however, is rapidly changing.

After reports of patient deaths in office-based facilities, California, Florida, Pennsylvania, Rhode Island, Texas, and New Jersey are leading the movement to regulate office-based surgery (Aker, 2001). These states are implementing regulatory mechanisms, which include reporting, certification, accreditation, and anesthesia standards; facility preparedness and emergency equipment and procedures; and staffing requirements.

According to Aker (2001), review and accreditation address several clinical issues that are important for quality patient care in the office-based surgical practice and include the following:

- Documentation is done of complete medical history, appropriate laboratory testing, and medical clearance before the procedure.
- Policy and procedure is available for preoperative and postoperative evaluation and care, especially in the event of an emergency.
- A licensed professional provides anesthesia.
- Procedure and anesthesia time is limited.
- Surgeons and all healthcare professionals are credentialed and licensed.
- All equipment should be current, maintained, and reflect current standards of care.
- All members of the surgical team are evaluated through a peer-reviewed morbidity and mortality conference.

ENDOSCOPIC AMBULATORY SURGERY CENTERS

Endoscopic ambulatory surgery centers that perform gastrointestinal procedures have also grown steadily in recent years (Deas & Durup, 1999). They must meet the expectations of patients, payers, specialist medical staffs, and primary care physicians. Skilled single specialty gastrointestinal staffs produce a higher quality, lower risk, and more stress-free environment for patient care. The survival of these centers depends on their ability to meet the demands of a rapidly changing healthcare marketplace. Endoscopic ambulatory surgery centers are particularly well adapted to thrive under the dominant forces that will drive the future of healthcare, consumer expectations, cost containment, quality of care, and consolidation.

FACILITIES FOR POSTOPERATIVE CARE

Facilities for postoperative care have allowed surgeons to perform more complicated outpatient procedures on sicker patients (Pandit, 1999). In the 23-hour admission or overnight stay unit, postoperative patients are observed overnight but are discharged early the next morning, within 23 hours of the surgery. This concept meets the criteria for reimbursement as an outpatient procedure.

Freestanding recovery units are newer concepts. They are privately run, entrepreneurial units for those patients who prefer not to go home after the procedure. Hospital hotels are facilities located near the hospital where the patient and family, especially those from out of town, can stay for a couple of days after the surgery, in case of a complication or emergency.

Patient Care Issues

Admission Criteria

Proper selection of the patient is the key to successful outpatient surgery. Selection depends on age, physical status, and complexity and duration of the operation (Pandit, 1999). Nonmedical contraindications for outpatient surgery include situations in which patients are unable or unwilling to cooperate and patients with significant communication or psychological problems. Many other areas of concern still exist and include morbid obesity, significant sleep apnea, fragile diabetes, severe chronic obstructive pulmonary disease or asthma, significant epilepsy, patients susceptible to malignant hyperthermia, premature infants, and patients with acute substance abuse (Pandit, 1999).

The final decision for eligibility should be made through surgeon, anesthesiologist, and nurse assessments. Family burden must be evaluated critically because all benefits of convenience and cost effectiveness of outpatient surgery may be lost if care burden outweighs the benefits of short stay surgery.

Physiological and Psychological Factors

Most ambulatory surgical centers use the American Society of Anesthesiology Physical Status Scale classification system to assess admission criteria (Dunn, 1998). Previously, only patients with American Society of Anesthesiology class 1 (no comorbid disease) status were accepted for ambulatory surgery (Pandit, 1999). Currently, even older patients with well-controlled and stable physical status (American Society of Anesthesiology class 3 or class 4 physical status are accepted for outpatient surgery). These are patients with severe systemic disease that may or may not be incapacitating. This is especially important for cancer centers, where many patients fall into this last category. As an example, patients currently undergoing active treatment may be at considerable risk for bleeding secondary to thrombocytopenia. Cancer patients with documented psychiatric problems that medication cannot control may require admission for surgery.

Age

The patient's age is an important criterion. Young children, including infants, can have successful and safe ambulatory surgical procedures if standard and emergency pediatric equipment are available. Pediatric oncology patients typically have underlying medical conditions, such as immunosuppression, and are at risk for infection, bleeding problems, and anemia. Appropriate blood component support should be available.

Currently, there is no upper age limit for outpatient surgery, as long as concurrent medical conditions are well-controlled (Pandit, 2000). The level of care required during the first 24 hours after surgery is very important. Many older patients live alone or have a spouse who is unable to provide care. Options for continuing care must be explored and arranged before the procedure. If needed, community or social service agencies should be contacted for assistance.

Social Factors

Travel distance to the ambulatory surgery center is an important consideration. It is not desirable for the patient to be more than an hour's distance from the center because of difficulty returning to the surgeon quickly enough in case of an emergency. Family support is another factor to consider. A postoperative patient who has had sedation or anesthesia is not allowed to travel home unsupervised. The patient's "care partner," a responsible adult, should be available to accompany the patient home, and assist the patient for the first 24 hours after the surgery.

The patient and caregiver are given written instructions during the presurgical testing visit and after the procedure before discharge. The instructions about postoperative care should include a telephone number to call for advice and a handout that specifies the care needed and the symptoms of complications (see **Figure** 7.1). The nurse should be available to answer any questions that the patient or caregiver may have.

Preprocedure and Postprocedure Telephone Calls

In most ambulatory surgery centers, a nurse telephones each patient within a few days of the procedure to confirm the appointment time, review patient learning needs, give final instructions, and answer questions. Nursing staff generally contact patients within 24 hours after discharge or on the next working day if the procedure took place on a Friday or on a day before a holiday. The purpose of the call is to check on the patient's progress and to answer questions. The time may also be used to discuss issues of satisfaction or dissatisfaction. Before discharge, certain information about the call should be clarified with the patient, including telephone number and preferred contact time. This will help to maintain patient privacy. From a public relations standpoint, both calls provide a positive statement about the center and its philosophy of care.

Figure 7.1 Ambulatory Surgery Post Operative Instructions

Saint Vincent
Catholic Medical
Centers

AMBULATORY SURGERY
POST OPERATIVE INSTRUCTIONS

DATE:_____ SURGEON: _____ SURGICAL PROCEDURE: _____

1. ANESTHESIA
For your surgery you had: ❑ General Anesthesia   ❑ Local anesthesia with IV sedation   ❑ Regional with sedation
IF YOU HAVE RECEIVED ANESTHESIA YOU MAY EXPERIENCE:

       *Dizziness   *Muscle Aches   *Nausea/Vomiting
       *Headaches   *Sore Throat   *Drowsiness
You must have a responsible person take you home.
You should not drive a motor vehicle, ride a bicycle, or engage in other activities that require coordination and the ability to respond quickly.
You should not operate machinery and power tools or handle dangerous items such as hot grease, boiling water, smoking, etc.
You should not consume alcoholic beverages.
You should not engage in sports, perform heavy work, or lift heavy objects.
❑ If you had general anesthesia, you may have a sore throat for the first 24 hours following surgery due to an airway placed inside your windpipe during your operation. Immediately telephone your doctor if you have difficulty with breathing, swallowing, or swelling of your throat.
2. DIETARY
❑ Return to Regular diet.
❑ Clear liquids advancing to normal diet as tolerated.
Begin with liquids and light foods such as crackers, Jell-O, soup, 7-UP, and bouillon.
Progress to your normal diet if you are not nauseated.
Report continued nausea and vomiting to your doctor.
3. BATHING
❑ No restriction   ❑ No tub bath   ❑ May shower after 24 hrs.
4. MEDICATION
GENERAL INFORMATION: Even minor surgery can cause swelling and injury to the tissue. Once you are at home, you may experience pain. This pain can affect the way you act and feel. It is important to keep your pain level low so that you are comfortable.
❑ Prescription sent with you. Use as directed.
❑ You may take a non-prescription type medication. Do not take aspirin or aspirin by-products.
❑ Resume your daily prescription medication schedule.
❑ Medication instruction sheet given.

INSTRUCTIONS:
   1. Be sure to take your pain medication as directed to stay comfortable
   2. **Do not drink alcohol or drive while you are taking narcotic pain medication.**
   3. Ask your doctor before taking other medications.
   4. Constipation is a common side effect with many narcotic pain medications, so increase the fluids and fiber in your diet. A fiber diet includes: wheat bread, graham crackers, cheese, brown rice, raw fruit and vegetables, and soups.
CALL YOUR DOCTOR IF:
   1. You have no relief from your pain medication.
   2. You have side effects such as nausea, vomiting, or a rash.
   Time and Dose last pain medication was given in hospital: _____
5. FOLLOW-UP
❑ Call and confirm follow-up appointment with surgeon on _____. Follow-up appt. _____
❑ OPD appt. _____
SPECIAL INSTRUCTIONS
❑ Observe the operative area for signs of <u>excessive bleeding</u> (slow, general oozing that saturates the dressing completely or frank red bleeding). In either case, apply pressure. Elevate if possible and call your physician at once.
❑ Observe operative site for signs of infection: redness, swelling, foul odor, drainage, or a <u>fever over 101 degrees</u>. Such signs and symptoms may become apparent only after 36-48 hours. Call your doctor at once if one or more symptoms are present.
IN CASE OF EMERGENCY:
   Attempt to reach your doctor. His phone number is _____. If you are unable to reach your doctor, call Ambulatory Surgery at (212) 604-7852, Mon-Fri 7 AM – 8 PM. Between the hours of 8 PM – 11PM, call (212) 604-7909.
   At any other time call our Emergency Department at (212) 604-8000 or go to your local Emergency Room.
   Patient/Escort _____ Telephone # (_____) _____
   Nurse's Signature _____ Date _____ Time _____

Presurgical Testing

The need for a proper anesthesia evaluation before outpatient surgery has prompted many institutions to develop onsite preadmission testing centers (Pandit, 1999). In these settings, the anesthesiologist has a chance to identify patients at risk and can prescribe an optimal preoperative preparation regimen, including ordering of laboratory tests. The physician can also plan appropriate care, provide patient education, and develop a rapport with the patient. Significant reductions in laboratory testing, consultation charges, and cancellation of procedures offset the costs of running a preadmission testing center (Pandit, 1999). These centers also fulfill regulatory requirements.

With changes in reimbursement and patient convenience and satisfaction issues, fewer patients may be able to make an extra visit to the hospital for their preoperative evaluation. Other means of evaluating the patient's physical status, such as health evaluation questionnaires, telephone interviews, and evaluation on the day of surgery have been developed (Pandit, 2000) (see **Figure 7.2**). A major responsibility for screening may fall on the surgeon, who must decide whether a consultation from an internist is indicated and which diagnostic tests must be ordered.

Intraoperative Care

A high proportion of patients undergoing surgery in the ambulatory setting are healthier and have lower risks from surgery; however, the risks from anesthesia remain. The same high quality equipment used in the inpatient facility is required in the outpatient setting. All equipment must meet appropriate regulatory standards and guidelines.

Intraoperative care of the surgical patient begins when the patient enters the operating room and ends when the patient is taken to the postanesthesia care unit (PACU) (Geuder, 2000). Care of the ambulatory surgery oncology patient

is similar to that of traditional hospitalized patients. The nursing staff must understand the needs of the patient, which include education, identification, safety, consents, site identification and preparation, positioning, equipment operation, emotional support, and documentation. In addition, the nurse must assess and plan for the entire continuum of care because the patient will be discharged the same day. The nurse's goal is to implement each procedure as safely, efficiently, and compassionately as possible.

PACU and Recovery

Postoperative patients are required to recover in a PACU where, according to Ferrara-Love (2000), the focus of care is on the following:

- To observe the patient's physiologic status and to intervene appropriately in a way that encourages uneventful recovery from anesthesia and surgery
- To provide a safe environment for the patient experiencing limitations in physical, mental, and emotional function
- To avoid or immediately treat complications in the immediate postoperative period
- To uphold the patient's right to dignity, privacy, and confidentiality
- To encourage a sense of wellness and self-confidence needed for early discharge

The hospital's inpatient PACU can be used; however, most ambulatory surgery centers have a designated section for PACU recovery for the day surgery patient.

The phase II or "step-down" recovery area provides a different form of care for the ambulatory surgery patient. It is usually a separate unit that is used for the care of awake patients who are nearing discharge. Because the unit provides care for patients and families who have experienced a period of significant stress related to surgery,

Figure 7.2 PREOPERATIVE HEALTH SURVEY

Saint Vincent
Catholic Medical
Centers

PREOPERATIVE HEALTH SURVEY
(TO BE FILLED OUT BY PATIENT)

PATIENT'S
NAME_____ SURGEON_____

DATE OF
SURGERY:_____ AGE:_____ SURGICAL PROCEDURE: _____

CHECK THE "YES" OR "NO" BOX FOR EACH OF THE FOLLOWING QUESTIONS:
1. **Have you ever had any problems with your heart?** . . . .   YES ❑   NO ❑

    If yes, please respond to the following:
        Have you ever had a heart attack or a cardiac arrest? . . . . YES ❑   NO ❑
        Within the last 3 months? . . . . YES ❑   NO ❑
        Do you have a history of chest pain or angina . . . . YES ❑   NO ❑
        If so, have your symptoms increased recently? . . . . YES ❑   NO ❑
        Do you have a history of congestive heart failure? . . . . YES ❑   NO ❑
        If so, have your symptoms increased recently? . . . . YES ❑   NO ❑
        Do you have a cardiac arrhythmia (irregular heart beat)? . . . . YES ❑   NO ❑
        If so, do you take medication for treatment? . . . . YES ❑   NO ❑
        Do you have any problems with your heart valves? . . . . YES ❑   NO v
        If so, does this problem limit your physical activity? . . . . . YES ❑   NO ❑

2. **Do you have high blood pressure?** . . . .   YES ❑   NO ❑
        If yes, do you take medication for treatment? . . . . YES ❑   NO ❑
3. **Are you diabetic?** . . . .   YES ❑   NO ❑
        If yes, do you use insulin? . . . . YES ❑   NO ❑

4. **Have you had a stroke or TIA (mini-stroke) or seizure?** . . . .   YES ❑   NO ❑
    If yes, please describe: _____

5. **Have you had problems with your lungs or breathing?** . . . .   YES ❑   NO ❑
    If yes, check one:
    ❑ Asthma,   ❑ Emphysema (COPD),   ❑ Bronchitis,   ❑ Other _____
    Have you been hospitalized for this problem? . . . . YES ❑   NO ❑
    Does this problem limit your physical activity? . . . . YES ❑   NO ❑
    Date and location of your last Chest X-Ray: _____

6. **Have you ever had liver problems or hepatitis?** . . . .   YES ❑   NO ❑
    If yes, check one:
  ❑ Hepatitis A,   ❑ Hepatitis B,   ❑Hepatitis C,   ❑Do not know type
    Describe other liver problems: _____
    Date and location of last liver function test _____

7. **Have you ever had problems with kidney function?** . . . .   YES ❑   NO ❑
    If yes, describe problem _____
    Do you have renal failure? . . . . YES ❑   NO ❑

8. **Have you ever been treated for cancer?** . . . .   YES ❑   NO ❑
    If yes, please list type of cancer _____
    Did you receive radiation therapy? . . . . YES ❑   NO ❑

9. **Do you have a bleeding disorder, bruise easily, or take blood thinner like coumadin?** . . . .   YES ❑   NO ❑
    If yes, please describe: _____

10. **Is there any chance you could be pregnant?** . . . .   YES ❑   NO ❑

11. **Do you take a diuretic (water pill), digoxin (Lanoxin), or a steroid?** . . . .   YES ❑   NO ❑

(continues)

Figure 7.2   PREOPERATIVE HEALTH SURVEY (CONT'D)

Patient's Name: _____

12. Have you been treated for TB? . . . .   YES ❑   NO ❑
     List dates of treatment. _____

13. Do you smoke cigarettes? . . . .   YES ❑   NO ❑
     Approximate number of packs per day _____
     When did you last smoke? _____

14. Do you drink alcohol? . . . .   YES ❑   NO ❑
     Approximate number of drinks per day _____, per week: _____.

15. Have you or any family members had major problems with anesthesia? . . . .   YES ❑   NO ❑
     If yes, please describe: _____

16. Do you have hiatal hernia, frequent heartburn, or food regurgitation? . . . .   YES ❑   NO ❑

17. Have you seen a medical physician (internist, cardiologist, etc.) within the last six months? . . . .   YES ❑   NO ❑

     Physician's Name: _____ Phone # : _____
     If so, has your health worsened in any way since that visit? . . . .   YES ❑   NO ❑

18. Please list any other medical problems not discussed above:
_____

ACTIVITY LEVEL
In the past month, have you experienced difficulty:

YES ❑	NO ❑	Walking indoors around your home?
YES ❑	NO ❑	Walking a block or two on level ground?
YES ❑	NO ❑	Doing light work, such as washing dishes?
YES ❑	NO ❑	Climbing a flight of stairs or walking up a hill?
YES ❑	NO ❑	Participating in moderate exercise such as golf, dancing etc.?
YES ❑	NO ❑	Doing heavy work around your home, like scrubbing floors or yard work?
YES ❑	NO ❑	Participating in strenuous activities like running or tennis?

If you have answered yes, is there a specific medical condition that limits your level of activity (for example: arthritis, angina)?

_____

Specifically, are you limited by shortness of breath? . . . .   YES ❑   NO ❑

PLEASE LIST :

MEDICATIONS	ALLERGIES	PREVIOUS SURGERIES
NONE ❑	To Medications: NONE ❑	NONE ❑
	To Foods:	
	To Latex:	

HEIGHT _____

WEIGHT _____

Home Phone: _____ Work Phone: _____ Best Time to Call: _____

Form filled out by Patient: _____   _____
                            SIGNATURE   DATE

Filed out by person other than patient: _____   _____
     Via: interview   telephone   SIGNATURE   DATE

INTERVIEWING ASU RN: _____   _____
                            SIGNATURE   DATE

anesthesia, and the diagnosis, the following goals should be the focus (Smith, 2000):

- To provide close assessment of and close attention to the patient's physical, emotional, and educational needs in the postoperative period
- To provide an environment and personnel who are prepared for emergency interventions at all times
- To provide family-oriented care that stresses the concept of wellness and acknowledges the intimate relationship of the patient, family, or other supporting adult
- To encourage the patient toward as much self-sufficiency as possible, given the type of surgery and anesthesia performed, and the patient's health status
- To respect the patient's right to confidentiality, privacy, and respectful, compassionate nursing care
- To maintain accurate records of patient-related care and environmental preparedness
- To interact with physicians and other healthcare providers in a professional manner that results in high-quality patient care
- To provide patients and families with a resource for questions, comments, and nursing information during their stay and the immediate period after discharge.

During this phase, the patient ambulates, is given nourishment, voids, visits with family, given postoperative instructions, and is discharged.

PACU bypass or "fast tracking" is a relatively new concept in ambulatory anesthesia. With the introduction of modern anesthetics and in-depth monitoring, many patients may actually meet the clinical criteria for phase II recovery in the operating room and will be able to go directly to phase II, bypassing the PACU. An awake, alert patient with no airway difficulty, stable cardio-vascular and respiratory functions, and appropriate oxygen saturation is considered to have acceptable clinical criteria (Pandit, 1999).

Advantages of PACU bypass include significant cost savings, reduced administrative paperwork, rapid turnover of cases reducing PACU overcrowding, and rapid discharge. It is estimated that 80% of patients receiving monitored sedation could be eligible for PACU bypass (Pandit, 1999).

Discharge

Evaluation of the patient for discharge is conducted with the aid of a scoring system. In 1970 Aldrete and Kroulik developed the universally acceptable system for discharge from the PACU. It focused on activity, respiration, circulation, and consciousness. It was updated to include the ability to monitor oxygenation in 1994 (Aldrete, 1970). Aldrete also introduced a criteria-based scoring system that is specific to the ambulatory setting. It includes five additional criteria, including dressing, pain, ambulation, fasting-feeding, and urinary output (**Figure 7.3**).

The anesthesiologist and surgeon make the discharge decisions based on the status of the patient. The nurse plays an important role in making the initial assessment and communicating readiness for discharge to the physician.

A responsible adult who can remain with the patient for the first 24 hours after the procedure should escort adult and pediatric ambulatory surgery patients home. In most settings, this policy is a requirement for patient eligibility. The caregiver must be responsible enough to know when, how, and where to seek emergency care if complications arise.

Complications and Emergencies

In 1981, the Freestanding Ambulatory Surgery Association established the definition of a complication as an abnormal condition resulting from care associated with ambulatory surgery (Natof, Gold, & Kitz, 1991). A major complication (e.g.,

Figure 7.3   POSTANETHESIA RECOVERY SCORE FORM

Criteria	Score	On Arrival	30 Minutes	1 Hour	1.5 Hours	2 Hours	3 Hours	At Discharge
Can move 4 extremities	2							
Can move 2 extremities	1							
Can move 0 extremities	0							
Able to deep breathe and cough	2							
Dyspnea/limited breathing	1							
Apnea	0							
Baseline B/P____								
B/P± 20% of baseline	2							
B/P± 21–49%of baseline	1							
B/P± 50% of baseline	0							
Fully awake	2							
Arousable	1							
Not responding	0							
$SpO_2 > 92\%$	2							
Requires O_2 to maintain $SpO_2 > 90\%$	1							
$SpO_2 < 90\%$ with O_2	0							
Dressing clean and dry	2							
Wet but stationery	1							
Increasing wetness	0							
No pain	2							
Mild pain relieved by oral medication	1							
Severe pain requiring intravenous or intra-muscular medication	0							
Can stand and walk	2							
Vertigo when standing	1							
Dizziness when lying	0							
Able to drink	2							
Nauseated	1							
Vomiting	0							
Voided	2							
Unable to void with no discomfort	1							
Unable to void with discomfort	0							
Totals								

* *Discharge criteria: Patient must have a total score of 18 or more in order to go home.*

hemorrhaging, infection, serious sequelae from the administration of anesthesia, or other medical problems requiring hospitalization) has the potential for serious harm. A minor complication (e.g., transient nausea and vomiting, weakness, headache, myalgias, sore throat, or dizziness) has minimal or no potential for serious harm. Certain major complications are more likely to occur during specific procedures, regardless of whether the patient is an inpatient or an outpatient. For example, immunosuppressed patients who require general surgery are at higher risk for septic shock, excessive bleeding, and anemia. Conversely, the incidence of nosocomial infection is substantially lower in the ambulatory surgery population because the patients are not exposed to hospital routines for long periods of time. Medication, patient identification, and laboratory errors are less frequent, possibly because of the simplicity of admission and preparation.

Ambulatory surgery patients who develop major complications are usually admitted to the hospital in order to receive medical care, skilled observation, or further treatment. All phases of ambulatory surgery require a medical and nursing staff that is alert, is knowledgeable about potential complications, and has superior communication skills (Mamaril, 2000). It is imperative that patients and their caregivers receive clear discharge instructions, specifically about the possibility of complications and their treatment.

Planning and Developing an Ambulatory Surgery Center

Successful strategic planning is the key to establishing a sound ambulatory surgery facility. Important aspects of the process include a needs assessment, development of a business plan for program functions, and a marketing strategy analysis. A team effort is essential and should include representatives from surgery, oncology, pediatrics, anesthesia, nursing, radiology, laboratory, and administration.

Basic Requirements

The development of any new facility begins with a planning and programming phase. Space and cost are the primary issues that determine feasibility for an oncology day surgery center. In terms of space, the functional objectives of the facility must be defined; in terms of cost, it is necessary to formulate a budget for design, construction, capital equipment, and interior furnishings (Allo, 1998).

The most elementary and sensible approach is to establish a task force. The planning staff must be aware of the current community surgery capabilities and the limitations of the institution, as well as, for example, the number of surgery suites available. The cost relative to time and availability of expert staff in planning the unit is a major concern. The chair of the task force might consider and benefit from an objective, independent consultant regarding patient traffic flow, staff education, and materials management. Budgeting considerations are paramount and will play an even larger role after the original brainstorming is completed. Recognition of potential changes of the institution's mix of surgical inpatients should not be underestimated. Community trends require analysis to identify shifts in practice and referral patterns. The planning staff must be committed to the development of such a unit so that it will truly benefit the institution, the patients, the medical and surgical staff, and the community.

Program Analysis

The needs assessment begins with a conservative estimate of the volume of operations likely to be done. The service area is analyzed in order to ascertain its size and scope. Once this area is defined, the character of the patient population needs to be identified. A profile of surgeons in the community also needs to be developed in order to identify specialty, practice patterns, and recruit ment needs. Other factors to analyze include surgical procedures, volume trends, comparisons to other institutions, and relationships with competitors (Marasco & Schirmer, 1998).

Functional Design

As the process of financial feasibility is conducted, the aim and purpose of the facility should be kept in mind. Financial issues constrain choices made for exterior and interior design. Functional design takes into account all of the major areas of ambulatory surgery: lobby and reception area, waiting area, business and administrative area, consultation and diagnostic area, patient dressing area, admitting and preoperative unit, the operating room, PACU, phase II recovery area, storage and utility areas, staff dressing area, hallways, and circulation space (Marasco & Schirmer, 1998; Burden & DeFazio Quinn, 2000).

The certificate of need process governs the establishment and construction of healthcare facilities. The application process is required for all healthcare facilities in most states that propose construction, acquisition of major medical equipment, changes of ownership, and the addition of services (*http://www.health.state.ny.us/nysdoh/cons/about.htm*). The certificate of need must include long-range plans, schematic drawings, and a financial feasibility study. After approval, detailed drawings, which include mechanical systems, major equipment, and specifications, are sent to contractors for bids.

Accountability

Administrative accountability—channels of communication and reporting responsibilities—must be determined. Questions include the following: Will this unit be autonomous and self-contained? Will it be offsite or an extension of the inpatient operating room? Will it be under the jurisdiction of ambulatory services? The unit should have an administrator who is responsible for the quality of care, finances, proper staffing, and maintenance of

the physical plant. The medical director should be responsible for managing the clinical components of the unit. The nurse manager should be responsible for overseeing and evaluating the nursing care.

Clinical, administrative, and nursing decisions cannot be made in isolation. The task force can assist in the development of policies for preadmission testing, procedures to be performed, and admitting and discharge criteria. Performance improvement and risk management issues also need to be addressed.

Day-to-Day Operations

The days and hours of operation, staffing patterns, and training issues need to be established. Policies for admission to the hospital, if required, also need to be developed. A subcommittee of the task force can identify patient flow systems and accountability. A performance improvement committee, with input from patients and consumers, can perform an ongoing evaluation of the day surgery program.

Space

Space needs are largely interdependent, with goals and concepts developed during the planning phase. The minimum space required for an ambulatory surgery center is based on anticipated workload requirements. Space needs depend on the number of surgical procedures to be performed, the time required for each procedure, and the efficiency of turnover between cases (Allo, 1998). Once the necessary space has been designated, adjacent areas and traffic patterns are considered because other space needs may be identified that were not previously allocated.

Ambulatory surgery centers, whether they are part of a hospital system or are freestanding, must be designed to accommodate changing needs over a 20- to 30-year span (Allo, 1998). They must be versatile enough to adapt to technological advances. Open meetings with the architectural and surgical staffs can avert costly mistakes in both function and form.

Equipment

There are legal equipment requirements that vary by locality, and it is imperative that the planning task force is aware of these mandates. The mandates include emergency generator power supply, firewalls, and provisions for gas and suction lines (Marasco & Schirmer, 1998). The same high quality equipment required for the inpatient operating rooms should be used in the ambulatory setting and must meet appropriate safety standards and guidelines.

Table 7.2 identifies the nine major steps in equipment planning (Dean, 1991). Equipment planning is necessary to ensure that proper supplies and equipment are available for the new facility. Efficient inventory will keep costs consistent with usage. The first step in the equipment planning process is programming, which is the assessment and documentation of equipment needs for the new facility. The next step is the evaluation and inventory of existing equipment. Lists should consider usable inventory and equipment that needs to be purchased. Cost estimates for new equipment and installation as well as repairs of existing equipment are to be obtained. It is advantageous to have the architectural staff lay out equipment on drawings on which room function, workflow, and equipment use are considered.

Once these initial steps are completed, the purchasing department becomes involved in the planning process. Equipment is categorized by supplier and installer. Purchases should be made through requests for proposals (bids). Coordination and scheduling of equipment delivery and installation help to avoid chaos as the unit nears completion and opening.

Equipment is categorized as fixed, movable, and small (Dean, 1991). Fixed equipment is permanently affixed to the structure and has a life of 10 years or more. Sterilizers, surgical lights, and X-ray machines are examples. Movable equipment has a life expectancy of 5 years and includes stretchers, wheelchairs, operating tables, and refrigerators. Small, durable items, such as surgical instruments and chart holders, are easily transported and have a life expectancy of 3 years or more. An active materials management and inventory program should be established (Dean, 1991; Knauer, 2000). Two to four weeks before the opening of the unit, staff should be trained for special technical needs. The staff, along with the biomedical engineering department, needs to develop a schedule for preventive maintenance of equipment.

Personnel and Staffing Issues

ADMINISTRATION

Decision-making authority and accountability should be given to the individuals responsible for the successful implementation and operation of the program. The medical director, administrator, and nurse manager should be designated to manage the ambulatory surgery program. The medical director is usually an anesthesiologist or surgeon who can navigate institutional politics and is available to assist in problem solving. The administrator is traditionally responsible for planning, marketing, operations, human resources,

---

Table 7.2   STEPS IN PLANNING FOR EQUIPMENT

1. Programming
2. Inventory and evaluation
3. Budget estimation
4. Architectural planning and design
5. Purchase specifications
6. Bid evaluation and purchasing
7. Equipment delivery
8. Staff orientation and training
9. Preventive maintenance programming

Dean, 1991.

and financial decisions related to day-to-day management. A clear understanding of insurance controls and negotiations, and reimbursement is imperative to success (DeFazio Quinn, 2000).

NURSING STAFF

Leaders in nursing administration require proactive and insightful outlooks to affect positively the hospital administration and community at large. Nurse managers and their staffs can develop a philosophy of patient- and family-centered care dedicated to the patient with cancer. Successful nursing in the ambulatory surgery unit involves motivation, initiative, enthusiasm, and teamwork.

Marketing

As the opening of a new center nears, marketing should be targeted to specific groups, including hospital- and community-based physicians and surgeons, hospital personnel, community organizations and leaders, and prospective patients (DeFazio Quinn, 2000). A staff that possesses exceptional public relations and marketing skills will assist in developing a center that has a positive reputation. This can be accomplished through proper training. When patients and their families are satisfied, they are certain to pass on positive experiences, as patient satisfaction is an indicator of good quality care (Yellen & Davis, 2001).

Performance Improvement

A setting committed to efficient, service-oriented, clinically excellent care will determine the ultimate success of an ambulatory surgery center (Allo, 1998). According to Schick (2000), performance improvement activities should do the following:

- Identify problems and concerns in the care of patients
- Evaluate the frequency, severity, and source of suspected problems and concerns

- Resolve identified concerns and problems
- Re-evaluate (after studies are completed, there is a restudy process to ensure that corrective measures instituted have achieved the desired results)
- Report performance improvement activities to the proper personnel and governing body
- Take suggestions and directives from the governing body to the staff for review and implementation

Measurement instruments in the areas of utilization management and review, outcome measurement, and practice standards are important as both internal indicators of the quality of care delivered and marketing tools (Allo, 1998). To perform these functions successfully, a well-designed information system is essential.

The program stresses these outcome measures: patient satisfaction, preoperative delays and incidents, preoperative cancellations, readmission to the hospital after discharge, occurrences in all areas of PACU and recovery, turnover times, discharge delays, unexpected admissions directly from the unit, infection control, incident reports, equipment repairs and failures, employee and physician surveys, and environmental safety (Schick, 2000).

A performance improvement committee with representation from surgery, anesthesia, nursing, and administration can be successful in identifying potential problem areas and policies and procedures to prevent their occurrence.

Legal Issues

STAFF SELECTION

Hiring the appropriate staff ensures a quality ambulatory surgery center. The hiring process must comply with applicable state, federal, and collective bargaining agreement guidelines (Cittan, 2000). Ideally, oncologic ambulatory surgery centers recruit personnel who have experience in the care of patients with cancer.

Professional licensing and credentials are to be verified. If the center has a human resources department, they can assist in this endeavor.

PROCEDURE SELECTION

The final approval of the types of surgical procedures to be performed in the ambulatory setting should be contingent on the type of unit developed (i.e., hospital based vs. freestanding). The primary consideration in this determination is the availability and proximity of emergency care.

PATIENT SELECTION

Patient selection begins with the surgeon and anesthesiologist, who evaluate the patient's physical condition and needs against the capabilities of the facility (Burden, 2000). Patient education can minimize the liability for patient care (Sabia, 1992). Patients who understand what is to be expected are less likely to bring legal action against staff members of the unit. Because contact with the patient and family is more limited in this setting, the staff needs to provide proper, easy-to-understand information so that the experience will be more positive.

The limited interaction with the patient also has an affect on proper documentation (Sabia, 1992). The short-term stay places the nurse at a disadvantage for evaluating care, and thus, nurses are required to be more diligent in their documentation.

Financial Considerations

REIMBURSEMENT

Financing and reimbursement are of paramount importance to the success of the ambulatory surgery center. Over the past 20 years, third-party payers have realized that there is a cost savings for performing surgery on an ambulatory basis and has had an influence on increasing the popularity of ambulatory surgery (Schirmer & Detmer, 1998). Although ambulatory surgery saves money for insurance companies on a per-case basis, the increase in the number of procedures has negated savings by becoming a cost-cutting target for the third-party payers. This presents a challenge to the ambulatory surgery center to provide cost-effective care while maintaining quality and attractiveness of services to the surgeon and patient.

On August 1, 2000, the Health Care Financing Administration (renamed the Centers for Medicare and Medicaid Services on June 14, 2001) initiated a new prospective payment fee structure for Medicare reimbursement for outpatient services, including ambulatory surgery (*http://www.chpsconsulting.com/ai/faq.htm*). Called Ambulatory Payment Classifications, it is expected that other third-party payers will adopt this payment method, which will certainly have an impact on the revenue flow of these centers.

Example of an Oncology Ambulatory Surgery Center

Ambulatory surgery centers specific to the patient with cancer are an innovative approach to continuity of care. Economically, this approach has the potential for new business development in cancer centers. The following description of a successful ambulatory surgery center located in a cancer center of a major metropolitan area can serve as a model to plan for an oncology ambulatory surgery center (**Figure 7.4**).

In 1999, the Ambulatory Surgery Unit of the St. Vincent's Comprehensive Cancer Center opened. This facility is part of a 100,000 square foot outpatient cancer center located in New York City. The Cancer Center was formed in 1996 as an alliance between St. Vincent's Hospital-Manhattan (a campus of Saint Vincent Catholic Medical Centers of New York) and Salick Health Care (*http://www.svccc.com/about/index.html*). Salick Health Care, a wholly owned subsidiary of AstraZeneca, provides consulting services and manages the operation of numerous comprehensive cancer centers throughout the United States. These centers are

Figure 7.4   PHOTOGRAPH OF OPERATING ROOM, AMBULATORY SURGERY UNIT, ST. VINCENT'S COMPREHENSIVE CANCER CENTER

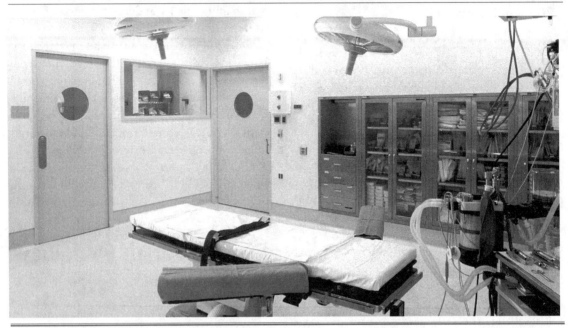

Used with permission: St. Vincent's Catholic Medical Centers, N.Y.

affiliated with many of the nation's leading medical institutions (*http://www.salick.com/company/relation ships.html*).

The ambulatory surgery facility provides state-of-the-art care for outpatients with cancer who require diagnostic and surgical procedures that enable the patient to return home the same day. The unit consists of a reception area and a waiting space for families, two patient changing rooms with lockers, two operating rooms, a dedicated pathology and cytopathology laboratory, a 4-bed PACU, a step-down PACU consisting of four lounge chairs, staff locker rooms and lounge, an office for the nurse manager, clean and dirty utility rooms, a sterile instrument room, a supply room, an anesthesia workroom, and an operating room control desk. Staff members include a nurse manager, who reports directly to the vice president/executive director of the Cancer Center, six registered nurses who rotate through the operat-

ing room and PACUs, one operating room technician, one housekeeper, one receptionist, and two aides who stock rooms and rotate between anesthesia and transport.

Approximately 1,100 procedures are performed a year. Procedures generally take three hours or less. Even though 85% of the cases are referred from the Breast Center, other types of procedures are also done in the center. They include prostate seed implantation, skin biopsies, insertion and removal of venous access devices, LEEP procedures for cervical cancer, and nasopharyngeal endoscopies (P. Garcia, personal communication, September 13, 2002).

The patient population in the cancer center presents unique problems for the ambulatory surgical staff. Many cancer patients present with multiple medical problems requiring diverse diagnostic and treatment procedures. Patients are evaluated during the presurgical testing phase (either onsite or through their referring physician), and if they do not meet the eligibility criteria for admission to ambulatory surgery, they are referred for inpatient surgery. This system is successful, and only 1.44% of all patients treated in this center were admitted to the hospital after the surgery in 2001 (P. Garcia, personal communication, September 13, 2002).

Future Trends

Recent developments in the ambulatory surgery industry will affect the delivery and financial performance of future models of day surgery programs. Because there are a large number of services for which inpatient care is the only option, the movement of services from inpatient to outpatient may be reaching its natural limit. Home care growth may be able to shift a small number of additional services out of the inpatient setting, but this will be limited by the degree to which patients and families are willing to tolerate this approach. The increased aging population will contribute to more required surgery, most of it performed in the ambulatory setting. Less invasive technology may improve the health status of older patients. As "baby boomers" age, this area of surgery will experience significant growth (Highland, 1998).

One critical area of development is the growth of payment systems for surgeons that place them at financial risk for the services they provide to patients. Capitated and "fixed-price" bundles of services present surgeons with different incentives that they have traditionally faced in the past (Highland, 1998). At this point, there is no documented evidence of the impact on ambulatory surgery. These payment incentives may encourage surgeons to avoid services that are of marginal value, which may, in turn, decrease the use of ambulatory surgical services. Conversely, when ambulatory surgery can be a cost-effective substitute for more expensive forms of care, incentive payment systems will encourage growth. An important issue for future research is the importance of the counteracting forces on the growth of ambulatory surgery.

References

About certificate of need (CON). (n.d.). Retrieved September 29, 2002 from *http://www.health.state.ny.us/nys-doh/cons/about.htm*

Aker, J. (2001). Safety of ambulatory surgery. *Journal of Perianesthesia Nursing, 16*, 353–358.

Aldrete, J. A. (1994). Discharge criteria. In D. Thompson & E. Frost (Eds.), *Bailliere's Clinical Anesthesiology: Postanesthesia Care* (pp. 763–773). London: Bailliere Tindall.

Aldrete, J. A. & Kroulik, D. (1970). A postanesthetic recovery score. *Anesthesia and Analgesia, 49*, 924–933.

Allo, M. D. (1998). Integration of ambulatory surgery into the healthcare system. In B. D. Schirmer & D. W. Rattner (Eds.), *Ambulatory Surgery* (pp. 41–47). Philadelphia: W.B. Saunders Company.

American Cancer Society. (2004). *Cancer Facts and Figures*. Atlanta, GA: Author.

APC frequently asked questions. (n.d.). Retrieved September 27, 2002 from *http://www.chpsconsulting.com/ai/faq.htm*

Burden, N. (2000). The specialty of ambulatory surgery. In N. Burden, D. M. DeFazio Quinn, D. O'Brien, & B. S. Gregory Dawes (Eds.), *Ambulatory Surgical Nursing* (pp. 3–22). Philadelphia: W.B. Saunders Company.

Burden, N. & DeFazio Quinn, D. M. (2000). The environment of care. In N. Burden, D. M. DeFazio Quinn, D. O'Brien, & B. S. Gregory Dawes (Eds.), *Ambulatory Surgical Nursing* (pp. 83–119). Philadelphia: W.B. Saunders Company.

Burns, L. & Ferber, M. (1984). Ambulatory surgery in the United States: Trends and developments. In L. Burns (Ed.), *Ambulatory Surgery, Developing and Managing Successful Programs* (pp. 1–18). Rockville, MD: Aspen Publications.

Burns, S. (2001). The state of ambulatory surgery and perianesthesia nursing. *Journal of Perianesthesia Nursing, 16*, 347–352.

Cittan, P. A. (2000). Personnel management selection and development. In N. Burden, D. M. DeFazio Quinn, D. O'Brien, & B. S. Gregory Dawes (Eds.), *Ambulatory Surgical Nursing* (pp. 136–147). Philadelphia: W.B. Saunders Company.

Dean, A. (1991). Fundamentals for success. In B. Wetchler (Ed.), *Anesthesia for Ambulatory Surgery* (pp. 574–592). Philadelphia: J.B. Lippincott.

Deas, T. M., Jr. & Durup, D. M. (1999). Endoscopic ambulatory surgery centers: Demise, survive, or thrive? *Journal of Clinical Gastroenterology, 29*, 253–256.

DeFazio Quinn, D. M. (2000). Business aspects, program development, and marketing. In N. Burden, D. M. DeFazio Quinn, D. O'Brien, & B. S. Gregory Dawes (Eds.), *Ambulatory Surgical Nursing* (pp. 23–55). Philadelphia: W.B. Saunders Company.

Dunn, D. (1998). Preoperative assessment criteria and patient teaching for ambulatory surgery patients. *Journal of Perianesthesia Nursing, 13*, 274–291.

Ebbert, D. W. (1992). Ambulatory surgical nursing. In S. Summers & D. W. Ebbert (Eds.), *Ambulatory Surgical Nursing, A Nursing Diagnosis Approach* (pp. 3–11). Philadelphia: J.B. Lippincott.

Ferrara-Love, R. (2000). Immediate postanesthesia care. In N. Burden, D. M. DeFazio Quinn, D. O'Brien, & B. S. Gregory Dawes (Eds.), *Ambulatory Surgical Nursing* (pp. 409–476). Philadelphia: W.B. Saunders Company.

Fleming, I. D. (2001). Surgical therapy. In R. E. Lenhard, R. T. Osteen, & T. Gansler (Eds.), *The American Cancer Society's Clinical Oncology* (pp. 160–165). Atlanta, GA: The American Cancer Society, Inc.

Gerlach, R. W. & Macklis, R. (1995). Accommodating modern cancer treatment procedures in an outpatient facility. *Journal of Ambulatory Care Management, 18*, 8–15.

Geuder, D. L. (2000). Introperative care. In N. Burden, D. M. DeFazio Quinn, D. O'Brien, & B. S. Gregory Dawes (Eds.), *Ambulatory Surgical Nursing* (pp. 381–408). Philadelphia: W.B. Saunders Company.

Henderson, J. (1991). Ambulatory surgery: Past, present and future. In B. Wetchler (Ed.), *Anesthesia for Ambulatory Surgery* (pp. 574–592). Philadelphia: J.B. Lippincott.

Highland, J. P. (1998). Economic incentives and cost effectiveness. In B. D. Schirmer & D. W. Rattner (Eds.), *Ambulatory Surgery* (pp. 11–20). Philadelphia: W.B. Saunders Company.

Knauer, J. (2000). Materials and equipment management. In N. Burden, D. M. DeFazio Quinn, D. O'Brien, & B. S. Gregory Dawes (Eds.), *Ambulatory Surgical Nursing* (pp. 120–127). Philadelphia: W.B. Saunders Company.

Lagoe, R. & Milliren, J. (1990). Changes in ambulatory surgery utilization 1983–1988: A community-based analysis. *American Journal of Public Health, 80*, 869–871.

Lyons, A. & Petrucelli, J. R. (1978). *Medicine: An Illustrated History*. New York: H.S. Abrams.

Mamaril, M. E. (2000). Clinical emergencies and preparedness. In N. Burden, D. M. DeFazio Quinn, D. O'Brien, & B. S. Gregory Dawes (Eds.), *Ambulatory Surgical Nursing* (pp. 205–239). Philadelphia: W.B. Saunders Company.

Marasco, R. & Schirmer, B. D. (1998). Determining the feasibility of an ambulatory surgery center. In N. Burden, D. M. DeFazio Quinn, D. O'Brien, & B. S. Gregory Dawes (Eds.), *Ambulatory Surgical Nursing* (pp. 21–36). Philadelphia: W.B. Saunders Company.

National Center for Health Statistics. Retrieved December 29, 2003 from *http://www.cdc-gov/nchs/fastats/outsurg.htm*

Natof, H., Gold, B., & Kitz, D. (1991). Complications. In B. Wetchler (Ed.), *Anesthesia for Ambulatory Surgery* (pp. 437–474). Philadelphia: J.B. Lippincott.

Pandit, S. K. (1999). Ambulatory anesthesia and surgery in America: A historical background and recent immovations. *Journal of Perianesthesia Nursing, 14,* 270–274.

Pandit, S. K. (2000). Anesthesia management. In N. Burden, D. M. DeFazio Quinn, D. O'Brien, & B. S. Gregory Dawes (Eds.), *Ambulatory Surgical Nursing* (pp. 243–253). Philadelphia: W.B. Saunders Company.

Poole, E. (1999). Ambulatory surgery: The growth of an industry. *Journal of Perianesthesia Nursing, 14,* 201–206.

Sabia, D. (1992). Issues in nurse/patient management. In S. Summers & D. W. Ebbert (Eds.), *Ambulatory Surgical Nursing, A Nursing Diagnosis Approach* (pp. 249–256). Philadelphia: J.B. Lippincott.

Salick Health Care. Company overview. (n.d.). Retrieved September 30, 2002 from *http://www.salick.com/company/relationships.html*

Schick, L. (2000). Quality improvement. In N. Burden, D. M. DeFazio Quinn, D. O'Brien, & B. S. Gregory Dawes (Eds.), *Ambulatory Surgical Nursing* (pp. 149–164). Philadelphia: W.B. Saunders Company.

Schirmer, B. D. & Detmer, D. E. (1998). Reimbursement issues. In B. D. Schirmer & D. W. Rattner (Eds.), *Ambulatory Surgery* (pp. 37–42). Philadelphia: W.B. Saunders Company.

Smith, S. (2000). Progressive postanesthesia care. In N. Burden, D. M. DeFazio Quinn, D. O'Brien, & B. S. Gregory Dawes (Eds.), *Ambulatory Surgical Nursing* (pp. 477–503). Philadelphia: W.B. Saunders Company.

St. Vincent's CCC. About us. (n.d.). Retrieved September 9, 2002 from *http://www.svccc.com/about/index.html*

The regulation of ambulatory surgery centers. (n.d.). Retrieved August 1, 2002 from *http://www.fasa.org/acsregulations.html*

Yellen, E. & Davis, G. C. (2001). Patient satisfaction in ambulatory surgery. *AORN Journal, 74,* 483–498.

Chapter 8

Radiotherapy Treatment Centers/ Ambulatory Dimensions

Susan Weiss Behrend

Introduction

Evolution of Radiotherapy Treatment Settings

Radiotherapy treatment centers have historically represented a conceptual framework for the development of ambulatory oncology healthcare. The clinical requirement for the administration of multidisciplinary-based radiation treatment regimens to individuals requires a flawless system that administers complicated protocols within an ambulatory environment. It is this distinction that has differentiated radiation treatment centers from other oncology-related specialties as the forerunner of ambulatory oncology systems. Evolutionary changes in radiotherapy treatment settings have led to the key integration of radiation departments in a variety of cancer care settings. Radiation treatment sites are commonly considered central to contemporary ambulatory oncology practice.

Radiation oncology is a primary treatment modality for cancer. The development and refinement of high-voltage equipment coupled with improved diagnostic procedures have enhanced the planning and administration of therapeutic radiation. Dosage and fractionation schedules have become more precise and tailored to specific tissue types. Improved treatment planning, equipment, and techniques have enabled the most effective use of radiation by targeting the tumor volume with the highest therapeutic dose while sparing surrounding vital tissues and organs. Research supporting the development of radiosensitizers has led to the definition of tumor radiosensitivity and has the potential to improve clinical outcomes. Radiotherapy serves as a critical intervention to cure, control, and palliate tumors. Research has substantiated the use of radiation alone or in combination with chemotherapy, immunotherapy, and/or surgery.

The previously mentioned advances in cancer care and specifically in the delivery of radiation for cancer treatment require that facilities offering radiation treatment be dynamic, flexible, and responsive to both general and specific patient care issues. The majority of radiation treatment is given to ambulatory populations that are discharged after treatment to home environments. It is, therefore, important that facilities offering radiation therapy provide patients in diverse areas equal access to this vital treatment technology.

Because rural, urban, freestanding, academic, and institutionally based settings all have unique administrative structures, it is necessary for these settings to ensure valid quality-assurance monitors in these highly technical and clinically complex ambulatory environments. The advancements in radiotherapy have enabled this specialty to flourish as an ambulatory treatment modality. These nuances have provided patients with the opportunity to receive complex antitumor therapy while avoiding confinement and ultimately maintaining their lives within their own surroundings.

Overview/History

Radiation therapy is a local–regional therapeutic method that uses high-energy X-rays to target tumors located in a variety of anatomic areas. The aim of radiation therapy is to deliver a precisely measured dose of radiation to a defined tumor volume, with minimal damage to surrounding healthy tissue. Radiation therapy will eradicate the tumor, prolong survival, maintain quality of life, and effectively palliate or prevent symptoms of cancer, including pain, restoration of luminal patency, skeletal integrity, and organ function (Chao, Perez, & Brady, 1999). This treatment may be used solely or commonly in combination with other treatment modalities such as chemotherapy, surgery, and immunotherapy.

Historical roots of therapeutic radiation are founded on the principles of diagnostic radiology and began at the end of the 19th century. At this time, X-rays with the unique ability of penetrating a few feet from the source were discovered. Subsequently, the discovery of radium, which provided the forerunner for interstitial radiotherapy, was a landmark pinnacle for therapeutic radiation (McCarty & Million, 1994). At the beginning of the 20th century, radiotherapy was used to treat external tumors of both benign and malignant origins. The differentiation between therapeutic and diagnostic radiology was evolving at this time. The limitations during these early years centered on the inability to quantify radia-

tion doses, which led to few responses, as these early techniques were unsuccessful at penetrating deep-seated tumor beds.

The development of dose fractionation highlighted post World War I discoveries. This is the radiobiologic principle that governs the clinical application of therapeutic radiation. Fractionation is the division of the total treatment course into equal doses over a prescribed course of time, which allows healthy cells time to repair and repopulate. The development of radiotherapy continued after World War II with the advent of megavoltage and supervoltage equipment, as well as radioactive Cobalt-60, a synthetic substitute for radium. At that time, the original unit of radiation measurement, the roentgen, was replaced by the RAD (radiation absorbed dose), which represents the amount of radiation that the tissues absorbed.

The decades from 1970 to the present have brought the development of high-powered, electrically charged machines known as linear accelerators, betatrons, and electron-beam treatment units. These advances were the result of the collaboration of biomedical engineering, medical physics, and medical and radiation oncology. The machines have the capability of penetrating deeply imbedded tumors while sparing surface skin effect and adjacent organs.

Presently, computerized axial tomography (CT) (1972), magnetic resonance imaging (MRI) (1977), single photo-emission tomogrpahy (SPECT) and positron emission tomography (PET) (tomography using gamma radiation and positron-irradiated nuclides), and ultrasound diagnostics have led to dramatic improvements in the anatomic basis of individual dose planning. Radiation doses are now planned and administered with the precise visual capabilities of three dimensions using advanced computer programs. Technical safety has matured with improved methods for in vivo dosimetry as well as computer-controlled verification of all parameters for every treatment. Research is now focused on the impact of different fractionation schedules on the effects of radiation, minimizing treatment-related side-effect profiles, and the most effective uses of combining radiotherapy with other antitumor modalities.

Radiation Treatment Centers: Ambulatory Oncology Models

Ambulatory care has been defined as personal healthcare provided to individuals or a population of individuals who are not occupying a bed in a healthcare institution or at home (Mezey, 2002). Ambulatory care is characterized as a vast array of health services offered to an aggregate of the American public. This model of care is broad based and includes all health services on a continuum from community-based issues to primary care to emergency services. Oncology care, specifically radiation oncology care, is further differentiated as a subset of ambulatory care within this large model (Mezey, 2002). Subspecialty care is characterized as care given by members of a healthcare team who are not generalists and are therefore dedicated to a specific facet of a population's healthcare requirements. Typically, ambulatory care is provided in a variety of settings: freestanding clinics, hospital-based clinics, community based institutions, and academically affiliated institutions. Both external and internal forces determine patient referral sources to ambulatory oncology subspecialty practices. Primary care practitioners, subspecialists representing both oncology and other medical specialties, multidisciplinary healthcare team members, and/or self-referral are common ways that patients are referred to ambulatory oncology settings. The latter route is not as prevalent because of healthcare insurance constraints that may impose financial costs that are associated with bypassing the required primary care referral system.

Current trends in healthcare require that ambulatory settings provide a full range of economically feasible services. The recent significant decline in both hospital admissions and length of stay as well as increases in the use of both emergency and nonemergent ambulatory facilities has dramatically increased access of ambulatory health services (U.S. Department of Health and Human Services, 2000). The trajectory of cancer care exemplifies a disease entity that encompasses both acute and chronic components. It is a prime example of a major disease that contemporary multidisciplinary health teams are willing and trained to treat in ambulatory environments. Hence, the volume of cancer care and all of its concomitant specialties has increased significantly within the domain of outpatient healthcare venues.

This chapter is a comprehensive review of ambulatory radiation oncology. Both historical and contemporary discussions focus on operational/administrative structures of radiation treatment centers, including a review of past and present practice settings, as well as a glimpse of the future. Commentary on the avant-garde distinction of radiation therapy as a premier ambulatory oncology care model provides new comparative knowledge for professionals working in radiation oncology. Personnel highlights focus on the multidisciplinary team, with emphasis on the unique challenges and opportunities posed when working as a member of this group of specialists. Every dimension of the professional radiation oncology nursing role is studied. These highlights include the nurse manager, advanced practice roles, staff nurses, research nurses, data managers, consultants, and educators.

Specific dimensions of ambulatory radiation oncology care are discussed. Patient care trajectory, including assessment dimensions, patient education, treatment and side-effect management, emergency care, follow-up care, multimodality treatment regimens, and clinical trial management, is emphasized. Special topics of importance provide an overview of both external and internal environmental forces that impact ambulatory radiation oncology. These issues include operational/administrative/economics, international practice issues, legal/ethical/quality-assurance programs, the impact of new treatment modalities, integrating complementary/alternative modalities into practice, and creation of patient support networks. The completion of this work touches on the "grace notes" of practice, in this stimulating environment in which the union of oncology clinical practice and research, academic medicine, and the ultimate in oncology nursing expertise meet.

Past Present Future Settings

What Did They Look Like: 1950–1970?

Radiation oncology centers have historically been institutionally based. The physical plants of these early radiation oncology settings were frequently situated near diagnostic radiology departments where equipment and even personnel may have been shared. The delivery of radiation treatment was a brief encounter and concluded with patients discharged to home. The details of these initial settings focused on the technologic delivery of treatment (Loescher, 2000). The presence of the diverse multidisciplinary team was absent in these early settings, and thus, this required some nurses to develop a thorough foundation in the science of radiation treatment planning. Many nurses were trained on the job to operate treatment technology and to administer treatment. This subsequently evolved into the formal licensure of registered nurses (in the mid-1960s) as radiation therapy technologists (Sitton, 1992). This combination of technical expertise and clinical management was advantageous for patient care, as the same professional treating the patient on a daily basis was also able to educate, assess, and manage individuals experiencing treatment-related side effects. This combined role lasted

until the late 1980s when the increase in dedicated radiation therapy technology programs coupled with federal and state regulations forced the need to separate these specialties (Shepard & Kelvin, 1999). Radiation therapy centers of the 1950s to late 1970s were dedicated to the technologic aspects of care and were maintained by a few radiation oncology professionals to support the patient experience.

What Do They Look Like: 1980 to the Present?

Contemporary radiation treatment centers exemplify the ultimate blend of technology and clinical oncology. Settings are no longer confined to the proximity of large urban tertiary healthcare institutions. Radiation oncology facilities are now commonly found in a variety of demographic regions. These may include urban, suburban, and rural communities. Additionally, today's radiation oncology departments are characterized as either independent, freestanding, private-practice settings, or those affiliated with institutions. The affiliated centers may be located either on the campus of a healthcare facility or off site and considered a satellite center. Technology and clinical oncology have impacted the environmental architecture of radiation oncology departments as both patient comfort and equipment space requirements need to be accommodated. Organizational planning for radiation oncology sites includes the collaborative effort of a multidisciplinary team of professionals such as architects, construction managers, interior designers, and space planners. These project teams work together with radiation oncology professionals to identify strategic goals that will ultimately define the environmental design (Arneill & Nuelsen, 1999). Planning today's radiation oncology departments requires consideration of a variety of clientele and organizational system needs to create an integrative project. Including both administrative and staff personnel in this process ensures an outcome that provides a functional and desirable work environment as well as safe, comfortable, and efficient patient care surroundings. Developing and honoring staff evaluations and wish lists when planning a department will ensure full participation in the design and may also provide previously unidentified and critical information (Arneill & Nuelsen, 1999; Bell, 1999). Radiation oncology departments today contain precision-based treatment equipment as well as dedicated patient care support systems.

Some contemporary radiation oncology departments are created in response to needs assessments that indicate inadequate access to services in a particular demographic area. These departments are formed when community hospitals partner to develop regional radiation sites to serve a community that had not had accessible radiation therapy care. Services like this are developed to provide equitable distribution of the complete spectrum of oncology services to populations and to establish and maintain patient focused standards of practice (Salner, Edwards, Kuzmicas, McIntyre, & Rice, 1999).

The presence of enhanced equipment such as telegamma devices and accelerators for external radiotherapy and new radionuclides for remote-controlled local application is evidence of the recent progress in current radiation oncology practice settings. With the use of CT, MRI, SPECT, PET, and ultrasound diagnostics as simulation devices, the anatomic basis for individual dose planning has improved dramatically. In many settings, CT on rails systems, working in concert with MRI simulator units, may now be seen. Additionally, the use of radiosurgery and stereotactic instrumentation to treat central nervous system malignancies is not limited to tertiary radiation oncology settings. Another advance includes instillation of multileaf collimators, which have replaced the need for creating hand-molded custom lead blocks for many treatment fields.

In summary, present-day radiation oncology departments are burgeoning sites of technologic advancement and clinical practice. The rapid pace of radiobiologic developments is quickly translated to clinical practice, and professional staffs are required to keep pace with these cutting-edge therapeutic modalities. Patients are the beneficiaries of well-equipped, well-maintained, and expertly staffed radiation oncology practices. Most of these treatment advances are available to ambulatory cancer patients. This provides individuals with the invaluable opportunity of receiving advanced treatment modalities while maintaining the rhythm of their personal lives.

What Will They Look Like and What Will The Future Bring?

Technologic advancements will continue to shape radiation oncology departments of the future. Healthcare trends will have an impact on every aspect of this oncology specialty from departmental design to treatment capabilities to clinical care. It is probable that the existing multidisciplinary team will expand to include professionals with specialty training in supportive care services. These may include the addition of psychotherapists and practitioners of complementary and alternative modality therapy. An initial assessment that includes a broadened team of specialists to facilitate the treatment journey will be beneficial to patients. Departments will have patient education resource centers featuring interactive libraries. New technologic realities will shape actual treatment requirements and will include remote reading of port and simulation films via the Internet, enhanced treatment planning/simulation using conformal radiation therapy, intensity-modulated radiation therapy, ultrasound-based positioning, (BAT) CT on rails systems, and MRI units to maximize tumor location, minimize side effects, and perfect reproducibility of treatment fields.

Enhanced linkage of professional staff with technology is predicted for the future (Lowenstein, 2002). This will be accomplished by creating proactive/alternative staffing systems with linkages that enable the seamless integration of radiobiologic principles of treatment with clinical patient management. Radiation oncology nurses have exemplified the union of technology and patient care and have been identified as technologic optimists (Loescher, 2000). Radiation oncology nurses have and will continue to function as interpreters of technology and as a link for the patient and the treatment trajectory. The future presence of the radiation oncology–nursing role will focus on the integration of clinical case management systems and the coordination of a broadened radiation oncology professional team (Shepard & Kelvin, 1999). The future of clinical radiation oncology is limitless. Continued research focusing on high-voltage treatment equipment coupled with high-resolution diagnostic methods for defining tumor boundaries will lead to more effective clinical responses and minimal side effects. Optimization of treatment fields and refined quality-improvement plans will increase curative intent profiles.

Operational Structures of Radiation Oncology Centers

Provision/Coordination of Clinical and Administrative Services

Radiation oncology facilities are either institutionally affiliated or independent and freestanding. The former are hospital sponsored either by tertiary care centers, comprehensive cancer centers, community-based individual medical centers, or a consortium of community-based sites. Independent sites are typically privately owned (often by groups of medical professionals) and sometimes by groups of business associates.

Institutionally affiliated sites may be located either on the campus of an institution or at a distance and considered a satellite division. Personnel and/or sharing of equipment and services link satellite sites to the main facility.

Independent radiation oncology centers are clinically, administratively, and financially internally governed and negotiate with clinical affiliates (to establish referral bases and expanded services) of their designation. Both types of centers present benefits and challenges for offering coordination of clinical radiation oncology patient treatment and administrative management. In some demographic regions, patients have a choice about the type of center that they will access; in many areas, however, though this option does not exist, and thus, it is necessary that both types of operational structures provide similar therapeutic options.

Institutionally Affiliated Radiation Oncology Centers

Hospital-sponsored radiation oncology centers serve as the most common setting for the integration and delivery of radiation oncology treatment regimens. The approximation of these departments to hospitals provides readily accessible resources to facilitate the trajectory of cancer care. The support services historically available in these departments include social service consultation, nutritional support, advanced practice nursing specialists, and health insurance counselors (Iwamoto & Gough, 1993). Social service may include individual and group psychotherapy, as well as focused support-group discussions. Additionally, social workers assist with daily transportation requirements as well as arrangements for nearby temporary housing for individuals and families. Nutritional support services are integral to symptom management of patients at risk. Nutritionists provide patient education material regarding specific dietary suggestions, nutritional supplementation, and assistive interventions (parenteral feedings).

Professional nursing services abound in hospital-based radiation oncology departments. If the center is affiliated with a comprehensive cancer center, nurses are dedicated oncology specialists, many are distinguished as an oncology certified nurse or as an advanced oncology certified nurse. A variety of nursing specialists are key to successful patient management (Wengstrom & Forsberg, 1999). Tertiary-care centers employ advanced practice nurses (APNs) representing diverse nursing specialties that provide clinical and consultative services for ambulatory cancer patients and families. Nurse specialists representing medical oncology, radiation oncology, pain management, infectious disease, neurology, and cardiology are available to interact with the multidisciplinary team for the enhancement of patient care.

Hospital-based radiation oncology nurses are able to access an array of professional opportunities that multispecialty institutions provided. Some of these venues are available: journal clubs, nursing grand rounds, continuing education courses, nursing research, study/discussion groups, and multidisciplinary educational offerings. In turn, radiation oncology nurses are considered professional resources and are often invited to share knowledge with colleagues representing other disciplines.

The department of nursing or interdepartmental structures may sanction administrative direction of radiation oncology nurses in institutional environments. Nurses practicing in these settings have an advantage because practice standards, clinical policies and procedures, and human resource guidelines are pre-established, uniform, and adapted by all disciplines.

Many patients and families carry the burden of fiduciary responsibility for ambulatory cancer treatment. Dedicated financial counselors are available in hospital-based centers to provide information regarding health insurance coverage and departmental charges. In these times of fiscal constraint and economic hardship, many patients and families consider financial services equally as important as those that focus on clinical issues.

Patients treated in hospital-based departments have many clinical services that are conveniently available to support their experience. The proximity of pharmacy, laboratory, diagnostic radiology, other oncology and healthcare professionals, supportive/palliative care, and emergency services is easily accessed. A prime example of the effective blending of administrative and clinical dynamics within institutionally based departments occurred at a Regional Cancer Center in Canada. This clinical ambulatory cancer center identified the need for a dedicated system for palliative radiation services and formed a palliative radiation therapy rapid response clinic. This clinic provided immediate appointments, the services of a skilled interdisciplinary team, and prompt administration of radiation to relieve symptoms and complications of advanced disease (Andersson & Sousa, 1998).

The opportunity for ambulatory radiation oncology patients to partake in clinical trials is an integral component of contemporary cancer care. Hospital-based departments are members of clinical trial cooperative groups and also may participate in pharmaceutical and institutional-sponsored trials. Radiation therapy trials compare radiation delivery methods, schedules, or different combinations of therapeutic modalities. Additionally, these trials measure both actual tumor response and local regional control (Works, 2000). Quality-of-life dimensions of radiation clinical trials have been added to a majority of radiation therapy oncology group (RTOG) trials.

Transportation options to hospital sites are convenient, economical, and scheduled to meet required appointment times. A combination of private and public funding provides patients and families with a broad range of ancillary resources that are invaluable to those seeking both general and specific information. Additionally, many institutions have begun to fund opportunities for the provision of complementary therapies as adjunct modalities to standard treatment regimens.

Hospital-based radiation oncology departments provide holistic care for patients and families. However, there are some administrative issues that can impede this process. Hospital systems, whether community or academically based, are notoriously complicated and difficult for patients to navigate. From the patient perspective, this environment is potentially unfamiliar, frightening, and alienating. To ease patient adjustment, some institutions conduct orientation sessions to familiarize those new to treatment. These programs may involve presimulation departmental tours to ameliorate fear of the unknown. Additionally, written material describing clinical and administrative services, commonly asked questions and responses, and key contact telephone numbers is given to all patients on both active and follow-up schedules.

From a professional perspective, hospital-sponsored radiation departments require a great deal of time to implement new or revised practice standards, documentation forms, and clinical protocols. Organizational committee structures require that changes in clinical practice be approved before implementation. This mechanism can be delayed and can become a source of frustration for professionals. To fast track prioritized needs, steps can be taken to educate colleagues who are external to the practice about unique dimensions of radiation oncology practice.

Freestanding/Independent Radiation Oncology Facilities

Freestanding ambulatory radiation centers have evolved in all demographic regions of the United States. These sites were originally established to fill the need of rural communities and those without tertiary settings in close proximity. These facilities provide invaluable access for patients and families who heretofore may not have the treatment modality of radiation oncology available. The Joint Commission on Accreditation of Healthcare Organizations does not administer accreditation criteria for these centers. Standards and accrediting are administered by the American College of Radiology and the Association for the Accreditation of Ambulatory Health Care. Accreditation for ambulatory centers is optional, whereas the federal government requires institutionally affiliated centers to be credentialed. Ambulatory care facilities require review by the state department of public health for conformance with the public health code or the Guidelines for Design and Construction of Hospital and Healthcare Facilities (published by the American Institute of Architects), depending on the regulation in the state in which the project is to be constructed. When planning an ambulatory center, a preliminary review of regulatory requirements and a schematic design of the project should be incorporated into the design (Bell, 1999).

Freestanding/ambulatory radiation facilities have demonstrated an amazing capacity to keep pace with hospital-based departments. Technologic advances in the field have provided these settings with the capabilities to provide similar protocols and advances as their counterparts. Expert teams of professionals administer advanced treatment techniques in much the same way as in hospital centers. Linear accelerators with multiple energies (photon and electron), simulators, brachytherapy capabilities, three-dimensional planning computer systems, and staffing with radiation oncologists, radiation oncology nurses, medical physicists, dosimetrists, engineers, and technologists all exist within freestanding centers.

Designs of ambulatory care centers involve collaborative teams of architects, administrators, consultants, builders, facility managers, governing boards, and staff (Arneill & Nuelsen, 1999). These professionals consider both external and internal requirements to plan an ambulatory environment that is conducive to safe and effective patient care. Issues to be considered at the beginning of the project include patient, personnel, and equipment needs; life safety/building codes and classifications; employee/patient safety and accessibility; and regulatory/accreditation requirements. Design teams often tour comparable facilities; develop treatment, examination, and waiting room mock-ups; consider staff evaluation/wish list requests; and consult vendors to assess equipment purchases (Bell, 1999).

Freestanding centers often combine oncology-related services such as medical oncology, an infusion center, surgical oncology, and patient support services on site. This provides patients with a full array of oncologic management (Salner et al., 1999). Freestanding centers have become vital components of ambulatory radiation care and are located in rural, urban, and suburban regions. The tremendous costs involved in building a freestanding site require a prospective multifactorial needs assessment. These needs may begin with qualitative studies done by regional cancer centers that may indicate underusage of radiation oncology services in urban and rural areas (Salner et al., 1999).

A lack of access to ambulatory healthcare is a major national crisis. An estimated 40-million Americans lack health insurance coverage, and for millions of others, access to care may be limited because of demographics, language, and educational differences (Mezey, 2002). Freestanding specialty healthcare has evolved to meet these needs. In order to do this effectively, some centers partner with tertiary settings. An example of this was the development of a regional radiation oncology network in a northeastern region of the United States. Through a detailed needs assessment, it was determined that many cancer patients in that area were not receiving adequate oncology care. The unique evolution of this process was that the region's community hospitals, which had been competitors, partnered to develop two regional radiation sites. The partnering of these sites with a tertiary care center completed the plan for augmenting services. The following are essential components of this model: integration with community-based cancer-related organizations; simulation, treatment planning,

and electron and high-energy photon treatment to be done at the tertiary center; installation of a 6 megavoltage computer-controlled linear accelerator at each freestanding site with a computerized record and verification system; simulation and upgrade ability with shielding and base frame for higher energy photons and electrons; tertiary center radiation staff at freestanding site; dedicated professional nursing staff with clerical support staff at each site; contractual agreement for nutritional support; social services with tertiary center; and dedicated patient resource center. This model was instituted to enhance patient access for radiation treatment in a cost-effective way while maintaining high standards of clinical practice parameters (Salner et al., 1999).

Freestanding radiation oncology centers present a blend of opportunity and challenge for nurses. Demands on nurses include the development of practice parameters, including patient assessment, informed consent, and symptom management. Nurses may be required to generate practice-related forms, including documentation tools and patient education material; and be prepared to establish policy and procedure guidelines applicable to both routine and emergent clinical care. Another integral component of care in radiation oncology is the establishment of quality-assurance parameters that produce measurable outcome criteria as a basis for the evaluation and improvement of care. Nurses in this environment exhibit flexibility and willingness to perform independently. The dimensions of the radiation oncology nursing position in a freestanding, privately owned center have been described as a multifaceted role that requires flexibility and independence (Anderson & Bruce, 2002). The myriad of questions can be overwhelming to even an experienced oncology nurse. Questions may relate to a variety of care dimensions including symptom management, transportation needs, nutritional concerns, and palliative care. Often, a nurse manager is not budgeted for the clinical support team (Anderson & Bruce, 2002). Nurses in this setting resort to creative practice plans that include job sharing with other colleagues and the development of position descriptions and standards of practice (Anderson & Bruce, 2002).

The organizational structure of freestanding centers may be less complex than hospital-based sites, thereby simplifying administrative and clinical decision-making processes (Iwamoto & Gough, 1993). Radiation oncology nurses can use professional affiliations such as the Oncology Nursing Society (ONS), the Radiation Oncology Special Interest Group of the ONS, and the American Society of Therapeutic Radiology Oncology (ASTRO) Nursing Committee as resources for assistance with the establishment of the previously mentioned aspects of clinical care.

An additional advantage of freestanding sites is the potential for greater net income because of direct control of expenditures. This structure can be beneficial to the nursing staff, as increased resources may be available to fund professional development. Nurses should be aware of the financial structure of the department in order to seek opportunities proactively to supplement nursing endeavors. Examples of some of these opportunities include national and international conference participation; professional dues, text book, and journal subscription reimbursement; grant money; and nursing research funding.

In the past, the primary limitation of freestanding sites was the lack of a seamless system for comprehensive patient support services, i.e., social service, nutrition counseling, pain management, hospice care, laboratory, diagnostic and radiology, and pharmacy services. If these vital services were not on site, patients were required to travel to other facilities to access them. Many freestanding radiation centers today are approximated near multidisciplinary and specialty ambulatory settings that may include some or all of the services described. Additionally, these affiliations also provide patients with equal access to clinical and cooperative group trials that on-site clinical research teams administer. The provision of care

at independent centers has evolved into comprehensive programs that are characterized by efficiency and the provision of a full array of oncology management.

Ambulatory Radiation Operations/Identifying Therapeutic Options/Treatment Process

Please refer to the series of photographs in the appendix that provide a pictorial sequence of pivotal equipment and procedures that are used to administer a variety of radiation therapy treatment modalities to individuals. This equipment is used to provide treatment to both ambulatory and hospitalized patients; the unique engineering of this equipment allows for the majority of radiation therapy procedures to be given to an ambulatory population. These photos depict simulation machinery, a selection of treatment machinery and equipment, and immobilization devices that are essential for precise and effective radiation treatment delivery.

Therapeutic options offered in a radiation oncology setting are numerous. It is important for nurses to be familiar with both the technical and clinical aspects of treatment choices in order to coordinate patient care. It is well established that radiation therapy is a treatment option used either alone or concomitantly with other modalities. Individuals with a cancer diagnosis may receive radiation as an initial or subsequent treatment intervention. It is important that flawless coordination of services occurs to assure continuity of complex regimens.

Radiation therapy is a multifaceted process. A thorough consultation occurs initially, in which the patient and family meet the radiation oncologist and oncology nurse. This consultation includes a thorough review of the patient's history, a physical and psychosocial assessment, a histologic reconfirmation of the cancer diagnosis, discussion of treatment options, and obtaining informed consent. Treatment recommendations are based on the potential for disease response and the risk of acute and long-term toxicity.

Many types of radiation treatment modalities may be offered, including external beam alone or a combined regimen with internal radiation. The type and length of treatment vary according to diagnosis, radiation sensitivity of the tumor, and patient performance status. Once these parameters are considered, the patient is offered a therapeutic plan. The radiation oncologist in conjunction with medical physicists develops the radiation prescription. Treatment planning is a precise process that requires a series of radiographic studies to identify tumor type, size, and location. Simulation involves a series of fluoroscopic films that when combined with a computerized planning program circumscribe the tumor and vital organs and tissues in the local regional area. This information is used to determine the exact dose that is required for the target volume and surrounding normal tissues (Behrend, 2000).

The initial appointment in the treatment area is for simulation that may require from 1 to 2 hours. Patients and families should be prepared for a lengthy visit. During this session, the treatment field is identified and measured, and small tattoos are injected on the patient's skin to mark the treatment area and enable daily replication of the target treatment field. Patients are told that they would be partially disrobed during the simulation and daily treatments. The patient may be required to drink radio-opaque contrast or to have intravenous contrast injected to enhance visualization of the tumor and treatment field. Additionally, mold room technicians may take measurements and readings to create immobilization devices and custom lead blocks to shield vital organs from scatter radiation and to secure the patient safely during the procedure. At this time, the physician obtains the final informed consent. Depending on the facility policy, the patient may be required to return before the initial radiation

procedure to confirm radiation parameters of the plan before actual administration. These collective series of events are unfamiliar and frightening for patients and families. It is therefore vital that professional radiation oncology nurses provide environments where patients feel physically comfortable and psychosocially supported (Behrend, 2000).

During the initial consultation, the patient and family learn about the treatment process. The patient is required to maintain the same position throughout the treatment session. The machinery (linear accelerator) rotates around the patient, and the average treatment time varies between 10 to 15 minutes. Radiation beams are odorless, colorless, and painless. The patient is comfortably situated alone in the treatment vault and is monitored at the therapist's control station with audiovisual cameras. Patients may require pretreatment medication with antiemetics, cortocosteroids, or analgesics. Pediatric patients may need sedation or anesthesia to diminish the risk of movement during the treatment session (Ruble & Kelly, 1999). The typical treatment course is daily for 5 days and varies in the total number of weeks. The radiation oncologist checks weekly planning films to monitor beam placement. Weekly appointments are scheduled so that the patient can be assessed for the development of acute toxicities and overall status (Behrend, 2000).

The planning and simulation processes depend on highly accurate measurements of patient characteristics to provide for differences in dose distribution. Dosimetric planning requires expert medical physicists, dosimetrists, and equipment. The data that the physicists require in order to plan treatment include body contour, outline and depth of internal structures, and location and size of the target. Mechanical, optical, ultrasonic, and CT equipment can determine patient contours. Internal structure identification provides vital information about the size and location of critical organs. These quantitative data complement qualitative diagnostic radiographic findings that are essential for the identification of actual contours. Transverse tomography, CT, ultrasound, treatment simulators, and port film techniques and devices are used for localizing internal structures to facilitate treatment planning.

Patients who are receiving radiation therapy must have coordinated service so that the treatment course is uninterrupted and so that side effects are minimized. Ambulatory radiation patients may require hospitalization to ameliorate the side effects of toxic concomitant regimens. It is vital that radiation nurses establish clear and consistent interdepartmental communication systems so that transitions for patients from ambulatory to acute-care settings are well coordinated.

Patients receiving radioactive implant therapy and intraoperative radiation require the coordination of many services within both the department and the medical center. Interdepartmental communication procedures need to be established with the admissions department: preoperative clinic, anesthesia, operating room, laboratories, the nursing department, physician's schedules, and the radiation department. Nursing protocols can be invaluable for standardizing interdepartmental responsibilities to provide a continuity of care to meet complex needs (Hendrix & deLeon, 2002). A group of oncology nurses at a comprehensive outpatient cancer treatment clinic developed and coordinated therapeutic options when an outpatient radioimmunotherapy treatment model was proposed (Hendrix & deLeon, 2002). The coordination of this treatment team involved the medical director, a clinical trials nurse, the nuclear medicine director, a radiation safety officer, a pharmacist, and an outpatient clinical manager. These nurses provided staff and patient education, planned treatment schedules, and maintained principles and policies of radiation safety.

Radiation nurses must also be available to communicate with an external contingency of healthcare team members such as medical oncology specialists, hospital-based nurses, home care/hospice agencies, social workers, and pharmaceutical and equipment representatives. The trajectory of cancer care is far reaching, and it is vital that every phase of the patient's course (home, community, and hospital) be considered.

The Multidisciplinary Team

Radiation oncology centers exemplify the essence of collaborative teamwork. A core group of expertly trained multidisciplinary professionals supports this work ethic. It is important that each team member know the function and role of the other to achieve a collegial effort. Patients and families should be introduced to team members and their functions. This will help individuals to understand the vital need for collaboration of technologic and clinical aspects of care. The effective blending of professionals and support staff can predict department vitality and patient satisfaction. When the entire multidisciplinary team is located at the same site, communication and consultation can occur expeditiously. In many centers, part of the team may intervene on a consultative basis and may not be working at the same site daily. This structure presents greater challenges for achieving continuity of care. Team members must prioritize the development of a collaborative multidisciplinary team through the establishment of consistent and concise communication channels.

The radiation oncologist is responsible for planning and prescribing appropriate treatment, assessing patients' physical and psychosocial needs before treatment, monitoring the patients' medical status and side-effect profile throughout the course, and planning short- and long-term follow-up care. The radiation oncology nursing role components include patient assessment, education, support, and counseling. Physical care, continuity of care, research, administrative, leadership, and mentorship are all part of this multifaceted nursing role. Radiation oncology nurses work collaboratively with radiation oncologists and the entire multidisciplinary team to provide a full spectrum of patient management. Variations in staffing patterns and role implementation exist throughout the specialty. Recently, there has been increasing interest in the development of APNs and physician assistants in radiation oncology centers (Shepard & Kelvin, 1999).

Registered radiation therapists (RTTs) are technically and academically cross-trained to assist in treatment planning during simulation. They are also responsible for operating machinery related to all aspects of radiation oncology treatment. RTTs are key team members in daily contact with patients throughout the treatment course. RTTs escort the patients to the treatment machines and verify that they are positioned safely during the treatment session. The RTTs interface with all other team members regarding patient care issues and assess patients for subtle changes in status that may require clinical consultation.

Medical physicists and dosimetrists determine the actual tumor target volume to be treated and create specific plans to accomplish this goal. These team members collaborate with the radiation oncologists to establish the most suitable direction and size of the radiation beam. This team is responsible for dosimetric planning and distribution. Medical physicists are responsible for maintaining local regional protection of vital organs and structures.

The radiation safety officers monitor Nuclear Regulatory Commission (NRC) regulations and safety guidelines, incorporate these guidelines into policy and procedure, and document facility compliance for insuring the safe discharge of patients treated with radioactive material. The radiation safety officer maintains personnel exposure records and submits monitoring badges to the NRC.

Mold and cast technicians are trained to create custom assistive devices and lead blocks. Patient positioning and immobilization are critical components of radiation delivery. To achieve the goals of tumor kill and preservation of normal organs and tissues, it is mandatory that the daily treatment be reproducible and accurate. If patient positioning is not exact and if immobilization, positioning devices, and lead blocks are inadequate, lethal consequences could occur.

Medical engineers are employed in some centers with many linear accelerators, advanced simulation equipment, and dedicated high-dose rate and implant programs. High-voltage machinery and concomitant accessories are technologically sensitive and often need multiple daily fine adjustments and calibrations. On occasion, treatment machines may not be operating, and the presence of an on-site engineer is an advantage for immediate problem solving and repairs. In smaller centers, engineers work as consultants and may be shared among sites.

Administrators are part of the multidisciplinary radiation oncology team. They are dedicated to the business/fiduciary functioning of the center. They focus on the overall delivery of services, associated charges, and reimbursement structures. Additionally, they oversee the accountability and cost effectiveness of departmental services and are involved in negotiations with both internal and external vendors and third-party payers. Administrators have oversight of staffing issues and plan strategies for recruitment and retention of both clinical and support personnel. Administrators may have educational training and professional training that include both healthcare administration and advanced clinical training.

Social workers play an integral role in the successful clinical management of patients and families. Some centers have dedicated professional social workers, while others contract for social services from external sources, or share services with other sites or departments. It is important that patients, families, and the staff know the types of services that are offered and the availability of this important dimension of patient care. Dedicated social service support should have a broad-based consultation system to access this assistance. Patient needs can be uncovered at all levels of staff interaction, and thus, social workers should encourage consultations from patients, families, and the entire radiation oncology staff.

Contemporary ambulatory radiation centers may employ individuals who provide complementary services to patients and families throughout active treatment. These services may include massage therapy, hypnotherapy, art therapy, and yoga. These services usually are not reimbursed by third-party payers and typically are offered at either subsidized rates or with no associated charge.

Ancillary support staff includes secretarial, file clerks, messengers, transport, and volunteers. This staff often serves as the unofficial ambassadors of the radiation oncology department. It is important to train staff in proper telephone etiquette, in basic personnel skills, and in privacy issues. These functions can enhance the quality of care for patients facing a difficult experience.

Dimensions of Professional Radiation Oncology Nursing Role

In 1990, the American College of Radiology appointed a task force of radiation oncology nurse experts to create the first official definition of the role of radiation oncology nursing. The definition is as follows: "The nurse will assess and provide appropriate nursing intervention for the actual or potential problems that the patient and family may experience related to the disease process, treatment course, and follow-up period. This role includes the teaching, counseling, and supportive functions needed to assist the patient and family to cope with and adjust to the diagnosis and treat-

ment of cancer. It is recommended that minimal qualifications for the radiation oncology nurse include a baccalaureate degree in nursing, two years of general medical-surgical nursing experience, and one year of oncology nursing" (Bruner, 1990). In 1991, the American College of Radiology first published the minimum nursing staffing requirements, which focused on development of quality-assurance parameters in radiation oncology (American College of Radiology, 1991). In 1992, the ONS published the first edition of the *Manual for Radiation Oncology Nursing Practice and Education*, which provided initial guidelines and practice standards for radiation oncology nursing. In 1998, the ONS published a second edition of the manual. This publication further expanded and defined the scope of practice for radiation oncology nurses as follows:

"The radiation oncology nurse is, at minimal preparation, a bachelor's-prepared, registered professional nurse who specializes in the care of individuals receiving radiation therapy to treat cancer. Radiation oncology nursing practice is based on the philosophic tenets identified in ONS's Statement on the Scope and Standards of Oncology Nursing Practice" (Oncology Nursing Society, 1996).

These standards and the Statement on the Scope and Standards of Advanced Practice in Oncology Nursing (Oncology Nursing Society, 1997) provide the framework that delineates these roles.

The radiation oncology nurse is an integral member of the healthcare team and collaborates with the radiation oncologist, radiation therapist, and other radiotherapy staff to coordinate services, ensure quality patient care, and provide continuity of care. The nurse is responsible for interdependently assessing, planning, implementing, and evaluating the care delivered to the patient who is receiving radiation therapy. During the treatment course and follow-up period, the nurse will assess and provide appropriate nursing intervention for actual or potential problems that the patient and family may experience related to the disease process and treatment (Bruner, Dunn-Bucholtz, Iwamoto, & Strohl, 1998).

The radiation oncology nurse must also demonstrate the following professional capabilities:

- Ability to provide holistic, individualized care for patients and families
- Ability to understand physiologic and psychosocial human responses as they relate to a cancer diagnosis and to radiation therapy as a specific treatment modality
- Ability to incorporate quality-of-life parameters in all domains of clinical care
- Ability to focus on long-term goals such as rehabilitation and reintegration to home and work environments

The practice of the staff radiation oncology nurse involves direct patient care and includes patient and family education, symptom management, and counseling. This nurse is an advocate for patients and assesses referral needs for ancillary healthcare services.

The APN is master's degree or doctoral degree prepared and functions as a direct care provider, coordinator, educator, researcher, and administrator. This nurse combines theoretical knowledge with clinical oncology expertise. The APN is considered a clinical nurse specialist (CNS) and also may be a certified nurse practitioner (NP) (Bruner et al., 1998).

The effort at defining the role of radiation oncology was vital for the perpetuation of this specialty. Nurses need to articulate their position to fellow colleagues, to members of the multidisciplinary team, to administrators, and to representatives of other clinical specialties. If nurses are able to describe, actualize, and document key role components, the security of the specialty will be enhanced. Presently, with healthcare focused on cost containment and multitasking, there is an on-going threat of eliminating professional nursing presence in radiation centers. Unfortunately,

degradation of the radiation–nursing role has begun to occur by replacing the professional practice model with ancillary nursing personnel having minimal oncology experience. In some instances, radiation therapists have identified the nursing shortage as an opportunity for their specialty to broaden the scope of practice to include patient caregiving skills in order to ensure expanded employment opportunities. This is an additional threat to the survival of radiation oncology nursing (Hinrichs, 1997).

Before 1980, radiation oncology departments had not had a strong nursing presence. Oncology nurses practiced in acute-care settings and in medical and surgical oncology. Nurses began to seek positions in radiation oncology as patient care evolved with the use of multidisciplinary treatment regimens, and symptom management became paramount. The definitions of radiation oncology nursing should serve to set the standards of professional requirements for those nurses seeking positions within the specialty. Radiation oncologists, oncology nurses, administrators, and affiliated professional organizations need to endorse the requirements established for radiation oncology nursing practice and be committed to invoking these parameters in staffing guidelines.

The following Recommendations for Practice have been developed as a framework for professional radiation oncology nursing services:

1. Radiation oncology nursing care services are provided to address the physical psychological, social, and educational needs of patients with cancer and their families.
2. Policies and procedures exist to ensure effective patient care management, radiation safety, effective communication, and quality assurance for the radiation oncology nursing services provided.
3. Documentation of nursing assessment, nursing interventions, and evaluation of patient outcomes are included in the patient's treatment record.
4. The quality and appropriateness of nursing care services must be monitored, eval-

uated, and identified; problem resolution must be addressed.

5. Radiation oncology nurses provide consultation to nurses and healthcare providers regarding healthcare needs and nursing care of the patient with cancer undergoing radiation treatment.

Radiation oncology nursing has evolved over the past 25 years as a multifaceted, collaborative specialty that is integral to the broad spectrum of cancer care. Scholars and clinicians have described dimensions of the role that include patient care, rehabilitative, administrative, research, and consultation (Bucholtz, 1987; Downing, 1998, 2001; Hilderley, 1980; Rosenal, 1985; Strohl, 1988).

Specific clinical and academic responsibilities have differentiated and guided the radiation oncology–nursing role. A comprehensive framework has been conceptualized as a structure for identifying key components of the radiation oncology role. These are as follows: patient assessment, patient education, support and counseling, physical care, and continuity of care (Shepard & Kelvin, 1999). Additionally, radiation nurses are challenged to understand the radiobiologic principles that determine treatment regimens as well as the equipment used to plan and deliver radiation therapy. The need to know the technologic basis for treatment to predict and manage patient care and associated side effects presents a great challenge for nurses because actual treatment administration is not a nursing function (Behrend, 2000).

Nursing functions vary according to the radiation oncology practice setting. It is advisable to evaluate initially the particular needs of the setting. Such information ultimately determines professional nursing staff requirements. Factors that influence the implementation of the radiation oncology nursing functions are geographic location, type of setting (hospital or freestanding), physical layout, hours of operation, patient volume and type, physician practice, types of treatments administered, nursing practice, and strength and function of clinical and support staff (Kelvin et al., 1999). Less staff support is associated with more nonnursing functions that are delegated to nurses and limits direct patient care interventions (Iwamoto & Gough, 1993).

A written position description for the radiation oncology nurse can describe the nurse's role to the entire multidisciplinary team as well as to healthcare professionals external to the center. This information can avoid conflicts related to staff functions and overlap of responsibilities. **Figures 8.1** through **8.6** provide examples of nursing position descriptions at a comprehensive cancer center department of radiation therapy. **Figure 8.1** describes the clinical nurse coordinator role. **Figure 8.2** is a general position description for the registered nurse practicing in radiation oncology. **Figures 8.3** through **8.5** are position descriptions illustrating a clinical ladder system for nursing skill levels ranging from competent and proficient to expert. **Figure 8.6** is an example of the role of the on-treatment visit registered nurse (RN) triage and special procedure functions. These position descriptions can be used as a foundation for practice in a multitude of settings.

Radiation oncology nurses serve as professional resources for other colleagues. Radiation is a unique discipline that is unfamiliar to many healthcare professionals. The radiation oncology nurse serves as a resource throughout the trajectory of treatment for patients and families. As patients evolve through the ambulatory treatment phase, they may require concomitant therapy, need an acute care stay, develop a side effect that requires immediate intervention, or require home care support. It is incumbent on the radiation oncology nurse to support patients through the care continuum and to provide nurses outside of the specialty with patient-management skills. This effort can facilitate complex patient care and assist with the accomplishment of long-term follow-up goals.

Figure 8.1 JOB DESCRIPTION FOR CLINICAL NURSE COORDINATOR

FOX CHASE CANCER CENTER
JOB DESCRIPTION

Job Title: Clinical Nurse Coordinator   **Department:** Radiation Oncology

Name: **Date:** October 2002

PRIMARY FUNCTION:

Under the direct supervision of the clinical director and/or chairman of radiation oncology and the general supervision of staff physicians, the clinical nurse coordinator is responsible for directing nursing staff and assessing departmental nursing needs. The clinical nurse coordinator is responsible for initiating appropriate interventions for patients in the department according to the departmental philosophy, goals, policies, and procedures and coordinating with the nursing department. The clinical nurse coordinator coordinates and conducts educational programs for staff, develops and conducts QA studies, and attends monthly departmental faculty meetings. The clinical nurse coordinator serves as liaison with nursing department and/or other FCCC departments, representing FCCC at other requested meetings. The clinical nurse coordinator prepares nursing staff and assists the department in preparing for JCAHO surveys and/or any other necessary licensure inspections. The clinical nurse coordinator is responsible for maintaining good communication with physicians, ensuring efficient patient flow and physician coverage, and making systems changes when necessary to ensure efficiencies and maximum use.

ACCOUNTABILITIES:		Essential Function
The following description of job responsibilities and standards is intended to reflect the major responsibilities and duties of the job but is not intended to describe minor duties or other responsibilities as may be assigned from time to time.	Percentage of time	(Yes or No)
A. Direct Caregiver	20%	Yes

    1. Provides for teaching needs of patient and/or family, as evidenced by chart documentation of patient/family understanding.
    2. Documents patient teaching on appropriate records.
    3. Collaborates with interdisciplinary members of the healthcare team to administer patient care and implement changes as needed, as evidenced by chart documentation.
    4. Documents nursing interventions and patient's response on the patient's record, in accordance to established standards.
    5. Provides nursing support for the clinical director and/or departmental physicians when necessary.
    6. Evaluates the outcome of patient care.
    7. Recognizes changes in patient status and informs physician. Charts documentation.
    8. Assures that all patients are treated with respect and consideration, that their right to treatment or service is respected, that confidentiality, privacy, and security are maintained; and that they are involved in all aspects of their care.
    9. Maintains confidentiality, security, and integrity of data and information.

(continues)

Figure 8.1 JOB DESCRIPTION FOR CLINICAL NURSE COORDINATOR (CONT'D)

10. Develops and maintains a unit base orientation program, including cultural competencies of the population served, in conjunction with staff development and unit preceptors.
11. Demonstrates an understanding of basic principles of physical and psychosocial assessment related to adult development.
12. Demonstrates ability to assess, interpret, and provide interventions based on age-specific data.
13. Demonstrates knowledge for geriatric and adult patients
    • of skills to provide appropriate patient care.
    • of principles of growth and development over the life span.
    • of mandated reporting laws.
    • of ethnic, religious, and cultural impact in the diagnosis and treatment of chronic illness.
14. Participates in hospital-wide quality-improvement program. Makes recommendations for appropriate revisions, as evidenced by patient care.
15. Evaluates patient's need for continuity of care and initiates appropriate requests for interaction with other hospital services.
16. Assures that patients are safely transported to and from the radiation oncology department. Initiates and reviews documented incidents of patient injury and/or complaints.
17. Promotes exceptional patient relationships, as evidenced by positive feedback questionnaires, gathered by guest relations.
18. Possesses good communication skills.
19. Is punctual with a good attendance record and sees that the nursing staff has same.
20. Has ability to maintain professional attitude at all times and maintain confidentiality.
21. Has continuous attention to details.
22. Has knowledge of the departmental computer system.
23. Is responsible for job descriptions, performance appraisals of nursing staff, and disciplines in conjunction with physicians.
24. Possesses the ability to work independently and as part of a team. Demonstrates leadership management skills required for optimum patient care.
25. Develops and maintains standards of practice for the department, as evidenced in written standards and evaluation of compliance.
26. Supervises and provides leadership to other nursing personnel and assists team members with patient care as needed in accordance with their scope of practice and hospital regulations.
27. Participates in staff development and section meetings, as indicated by meeting minutes.
28. Demonstrates the ability to use all channels of communication to address interdepartmental and intradepartmental concerns, solves problems, and addresses conflicts.
29. Demonstrates effective time management by completing commitments within negotiated time frames.
30. Able to take the initiative to facilitate necessary actions and changes recommended for the department.

Figure 8.2 JOB DESCRIPTION FOR REGISTERED NURSE

**FOX CHASE CANCER CENTER
JOB DESCRIPTION**

Job Title: Registered Nurse   Department: Radiation Oncology

Name: _____   Date: 3/31/99 (revised 8/1/01)

PRIMARY FUNCTION:

The radiation oncology nurse is responsible and accountable for the nursing care provided to an unassigned caseload of patients treated with radiation therapy. The registered nurse is accountable for coordinating services required during treatment for their caseload.

ACCOUNTABILITIES:	Percentage of Time	Essential Function
1. Direct Caregiver Carries out a systemic assessment process in determining the needs of the patient and family on all new patients by the third outpatient visit. Follows patients undergoing treatment and assesses them each visit for therapy and toxicity management. Plans for care are developed mutually with the patient. Implementation of the plan is evaluated in terms of patient outcomes.	50%	Yes
A. Nursing care is provided according to the Fox Chase Cancer Center Standards of Nursing Care.		
B. Symptom management is provided to the patient in collaboration with the radiation oncologist and surgical and/or medical oncologist. Symptoms commonly managed include anorexia, nausea or vomiting, diarrhea, constipation, stomatitis, dysphagia, dehydration, fatigue, pain, infection, impaired skin integrity, mobility, ventilation, weight loss/gain, menstrual irregularities, vaginal dryness, alopecia, decreased blood counts, impotence, or infertility.		
C. Assesses and intervenes as needed when patient requires assistance with his or her coping mechanisms, psychosocial interactions, or interpersonal relationships. Refers patients to appropriate resources when counseling is beyond the expertise of the nurse.		

(continues)

Figure 8.2 Job Description for Registered Nurse (cont'd)

D. Demonstrates an understanding of basic principles of physical and psychosocial assessment related to adult development.
E. Documents the four components of the nursing process—assessment, planning, intervention, and evaluation—in a timely, organized manner aimed at achieving the planned goals and outcomes.

2. Teacher
   Identifies areas in which the patient/family lack   15%   Y
   knowledge regarding the disease process and therapy
   and provides that information.
A. Provides general information and orientation to the radiation oncology department.
B. Provides specific information about cancer and the treatment of cancer, clarifying and expanding on the physician's explanation.
C. Teaches rationale and dosing schedule of medications ordered.
D. Provides preventive education in the areas of nutrition, elimination, mouth care, skin care, immunosuppression, and other self-care measures, including early detection.
E. Serves as a resource for other nurses in the institution caring for patients receiving radiotherapy.

3. Collaborator   10%   Y
   Coordinates services and communicates with other nurses, physicians, technologists, departments involved in care planning, and other health team members. Maintains confidentiality. Assures patient/family comfort and safety. Makes referrals as appropriate. Provides continuity of care by initiating telephone follow-up or being available to patients between outpatient visits to take patient questions for problems and direct them appropriately for resolution by triage of patient/family telephone calls.

Figure 8.2 Job Description for Registered Nurse (cont'd)

4. <u>Research</u>   5%   Y
    Supports nursing and departmental research activities.   (Except F)
A. Identifies current researchable problems in radiation   (Except G)
    oncology nursing.
B. Supports patients involved in clinical trials by
    clarifying information, assisting in patient education
    before informed consent, and identifying patients
    appropriate for protocols.
C. Evaluates research findings in the area of oncology
    nursing for use in practice.
D. Protects the rights of human subjects.
E. Collaborates with other health professionals in the
    development and use of research findings.
F. Develops research studies, particularly in the 11 ONS
    high-incidence problems areas and areas affecting the
    quality-of-life of patients treated with radiation
    therapy.
G. Presents and publishes research findings.

5. <u>Departmental Responsibilities</u>   10%   Y
    Supports the achievement of nursing and radiation
    oncology department goals in providing a positive,
    open, and creative environment.
A. Coordinates the flow of patients in the physician's
    practice.
B. Identifies learning needs on an ongoing basis and
    seeks to fulfill them.
C. Communicates plan of care with physicians.
D. Adheres to departmental policies and procedures.
E. Participates in the department question and answer
    program.
F. Attends radiation oncology conferences.
G. Attends nursing staff meetings and in-services.
H. Is concerned with the financial implications of
    ambulatory healthcare and assists where possible in
    keeping costs down.
I. Performs other duties as assigned.

(continues)

Figure 8.2 JOB DESCRIPTION FOR REGISTERED NURSE (CONT'D)

---

6. <u>Professional Responsibilities</u>   10%   Y
   Continuously strives to improve care and increase   (Except F)
   knowledge.
   A. Accountable for patient caseload.
   B. Identifies learning needs on an ongoing basis and
      seeks to fulfill them.
   C. Evaluates on an ongoing basis yearly objectives and
      assumes the responsibility for achieving these goals.
   D. Serves as a preceptor for new employees and
      graduate students in the department.
   E. Shares clinical expertise and seeks other expertise
      when needed.
   F. Assists in orienting technologists and volunteers in
      the radiation oncology department.
   G. Completes yearly skill credentialing and mandatory
      in-service training sessions.

Radiation Oncology Nursing Practice

A model of professional radiation oncology nursing practice is contingent on the type of nursing practice structure (team, primary, collaborative, case management, shared governance), size and academic preparation of the nursing staff, affiliation with a hospital nursing department, and the presence of policies, procedures, quality-assurance parameters, and standards of care.

Primary Nursing

Primary nursing is the most commonly used practice model for the delivery of patient care in radiation oncology centers. This model is most effective for providing consistent care along the trajectory of the patient's experience. Within this system, nurses provide patient assessment and education, treatment evaluation visits, as well as episodic intervention. Primary nursing involves a spectrum of basic assessment skills. In addition, nurses working within this model are required to perform psychomotor skills related to patient

care, such as dressing changes, assessment of medically related equipment, intravenous therapy, nutritional support devices, and assistance during invasive procedures (laryngoscopic, pelvic examinations). Staff nurses in radiation centers have broad educational backgrounds. Although the American College of Radiology guidelines describe the need for baccalaureate preparation with oncology and medical surgical experience, it is not always actualized in this model of care.

Four levels of nursing care have been described in this model:

Level I: the nurse focuses on clinic care, which includes supportive, operational actions that enable the radiation oncologist to see patients (answering telephones, scheduling, stocking rooms, cleaning instruments, retrieving diagnostic study results).

Level II: the focus remains on clinic care; expansion of scope of nursing practice to incorporate patient teaching (patient care by the nurse remains limited and physician directed).

Figure 8.3 JOB DESCRIPTION FOR RADIATION ONCOLOGY NURSE

FOX CHASE CANCER CENTER
JOB DESCRIPTION

Job Title: Radiation Oncology Nurse   **Department:** Radiation Oncology
             Level III (Competent Nurse)

Name:_____   **Date:** August 2000

PRIMARY FUNCTION:

The level III radiation oncology nurse is responsible and accountable for the nursing care provided to an unassigned caseload of patients treated with radiation therapy. The level III (competent) radiation oncology nurse assesses, plans, implements, and evaluates the following criteria on patients who have <u>intermediate care</u> needs and coordinates services required during treatment for their caseload.

ACCOUNTABILITIES:	Percentage of Time	Essential Function** (Yes or No)
A. Direct Caregiver	20%	Yes

    Carries out a systematic assessment process in determining the needs of the patient and family on all new patients by the third outpatient visit. Follows patients undergoing treatment and assesses them each visit for therapy and toxicity management. Demonstrates increased skill in assessment of biopsychosocial parameters. Provides the patient/family with quality care based on the assessment. Plans for care are developed mutually with the patient. Implementation of the plan is evaluated in terms of patient outcomes.

    1. Nursing care is provided according to the Fox Chase Cancer Center Standards of Nursing Practice.

    2. Symptom management is provided to the patient in collaboration with the radiation, surgical, and/or medical oncologist. Symptoms commonly managed include anorexia, nausea or vomiting, diarrhea, constipation, stomatitis, dysphagia, dehydration, fatigue, pain, infection, impaired skin integrity, mobility, ventilation, weight loss/gain, menstrual irregularities, vaginal dryness, alopecia, decreased blood counts, impotence, or infertility.

    3. Assesses and intervenes as needed when patient requires assistance with his or her coping mechanisms, psychosocial interactions, or interpersonal relationships. Refers patient to appropriate resource when counseling is beyond the expertise of the nurse.

    4. Demonstrates an understanding of basic principles of physical and psychosocial assessment related to adult development.

    5. Documents the four components of the nursing process—assessment, planning, intervention, and evaluation—in a timely, organized manner aimed at achieving the planned goals and outcomes.

    6. Answers all patient phone calls and communicates change in patient status in a timely manner to the physician.

    7. Organizes and establishes priorities for work load.

(continues)

Figure 8.3 JOB DESCRIPTION FOR RADIATION ONCOLOGY NURSE (CONT'D)

B. Teacher   20%   Yes
    Identifies areas in which the patient/family lack knowledge regarding the
    disease process and therapy and provides that information.
    1. Provides general information and orientation to the radiation oncology
        department.
    2. Provides specific information about cancer and the treatment of
        cancer, clarifying and expanding on the physician's explanation.
    3. Teaches rationale and dosing schedule of medications ordered.
    4. Provides preventive education in the areas of nutrition, elimination,
        mouth care, skin care, immunosuppression, and other self-care
        measures, including early detection.
    5. Serves as a resource for other nurses in the institution caring for
        patients receiving radiotherapy.
    6. Seeks guidance from resource personnel to determine alternate
        teaching strategies as needed.

C. Collaborator   25%   Yes
    Coordinates services and communicates with other nurses, physicians,
    technologists, departments involved in care planning, and other health
    team members. Maintains confidentiality. Assures patient/family comfort
    and safety. Makes referrals as appropriate. Provides continuity of care by
    initiating telephone follow-up or being available to patients between
    outpatient visits to take patient questions for problems and direct them
    appropriately for resolution by triage of patient/family telephone calls.
    1. Assists other individuals to select and use unfamiliar patient care
        resources and support services.
    2. Acts as a resource to licensed graduate practical nurse (LGPNs) and
        nursing assistants (Nas_ in the evaluation of identified patient
        needs/problems. Acts as a preceptor and serves as a positive role
        model.
    3. Displays positive verbal and nonverbal behavior when communicating
        with patients, families, physicians, and colleagues.
    4. Documents all nursing assessments in a timely organized manner
        aimed at achieving the planned goals and outcomes.
    5. Answers all patient phone calls and communicates change in patient
        status in a timely manner to the physician.

D. Research   10%   Yes
    Supports nursing and departmental research activities.
    1. Identifies current researchable problems in radiation oncology nursing.
    2. Supports patients involved in clinical trials by clarifying information,
        assisting in patient education before informed consent.
    3. Evaluates research findings in the area of oncology nursing for use in
        practice.
    4. Protects the rights of human subjects.

Figure 8.3 JOB DESCRIPTION FOR RADIATION ONCOLOGY NURSE (CONT'D)

E. Departmental Responsibilities   15%   Yes
    Supports the achievement of nursing and radiation oncology department
    goals in providing a positive, open, and creative environment.
    1. Coordinates the flow of patients in the physician's practice.
    2. Identifies learning needs on an ongoing basis and seeks to fulfill them.
    3. Communicates plan of care with physicians.
    4. Adheres to departmental policies and procedures and supports the
        achievement of the department and the department goals.
    5. Participates in department question and answer program with data
        collection.
    6. Attends radiation oncology conferences.
    7. Participates in radiation oncology conference.
    8. Attends nursing staff meetings and in-services.
    9. Is concerned with the financial implications of ambulatory healthcare
        and assists where possible in keeping costs down.
    10. Performs other duties as assigned.

F. Professional Responsibilities   10%   Yes
    Continuously strives to improve care and increase knowledge,
    1. Is accountable for patient caseload.
    2. Identifies learning needs on an ongoing basis and seeks to fulfill them.
    3. Evaluates on an ongoing basis yearly objectives and assumes the
        responsibility for achieving these goals.
    4. Serves as a preceptor for new employees and graduate students in the
        department.
    5. Shares clinical expertise and seeks other expertise when needed.
    6. Assists in orienting technologists and volunteers in the radiation
        oncology department.
    7. Completes yearly skill credentialing and mandatory in-service training
        sessions.
    8. Maintains confidentiality.
    9. Appreciates the legal implications of nursing.
    10. Maintains yearly credentialing skills.
    11. Complies with personnel policies.
        a) Follows dress code.
        b) Reports to duty as scheduled.
        c) Follows policy regarding notification of absence.
    12. Acts as preceptor to department if needed.

Figure 8.4 JOB DESCRIPTION FOR RADIATION ONCOLOGY NURSE LEVEL IV (PROFICIENT)

FOX CHASE CANCER CENTER
JOB DESCRIPTION

Job Title: Radiation Oncology Nurse Level IV (Proficient) **Department:** Radiation Oncology

Name:_____   **Date:**   August 2000

PRIMARY FUNCTION:
The level IV radiation oncology nurse is responsible and accountable for the nursing care provided to an unassigned caseload of patients treated with radiation therapy. The level IV (proficient) radiation oncology nurse assesses, plans, implements, and evaluates the following criteria on patients who have complex care needs and coordinates services required during treatment for their caseload.

ACCOUNTABILITIES:

	Percentage of Time	Essential Function** (Yes or No)
A. Direct Caregiver	20%	Yes

Carries out a systematic assessment process in determining the needs of the patient and family on all new patients by the third outpatient visit. Follows patients undergoing treatment and assesses them each visit for therapy and toxicity management. Demonstrates increased skill in assessment of biopsychosocial parameters. Provides the patient/family with quality care based on the assessment. Plans for care are developed mutually with the patient. Implementation of the plan is evaluated in terms of patient outcomes.

1.   Nursing care is provided according to the Fox Chase Cancer Center Standards of Nursing Practice.
2.   Symptom management is provided to the patient in collaboration with the radiation oncologist and surgical and/or medical oncologist. Symptoms commonly managed include anorexia, nausea or vomiting, diarrhea, constipation, stomatitis, dysphagia, dehydration, fatigue, pain, infection, impaired skin integrity, mobility, ventilation, weight loss/gain, menstrual irregularities, vaginal dryness, alopecia, decreased blood counts, impotence, or infertility.
3.   Assesses and intervenes as needed when patient requires assistance with his or her coping mechanisms, psychosocial interactions, or interpersonal relationships. Refers patient to appropriate resource when counseling is beyond the expertise of the nurse.
4.   Demonstrates an understanding of basic principles of physical and psychosocial assessment related to adult development.
5.   Documents the four components of the nursing process—assessment, planning, intervention, and evaluation—in a timely, organized manner aimed at achieving the planned goals and outcomes.
6.   Answers all patient phone calls and communicates change in patient status in a timely manner to the physician.
7.   Organizes and establishes priorities for work load.
8.   Assists level III nurses with the development of assessment skills.

Figure 8.4 JOB DESCRIPTION FOR RADIATION ONCOLOGY NURSE LEVEL IV (PROFICIENT) (CONT'D)

B. Teacher   20%   Yes
   Identifies areas in which the patient/family lack knowledge regarding the
   disease process and therapy and provides that information.
   1. Provides general information and orientation to the radiation
      oncology department.
   2. Provides specific information about cancer and the treatment of
      cancer, clarifying and expanding on the physician's explanation.
   3. Teaches rationale and dosing schedule of medications ordered.
   4. Provides preventive education in the areas of nutrition, elimination,
      mouth care, skin care, immunosuppression, and other self-care
      measures, including early detection.
   5. Serves as a resource for other nurses in the institution caring for
      patients receiving radiotherapy.
   6. Seeks guidance from resource personnel to determine alternate
      teaching strategies as needed.
   7. Independently provides feedback to peers related to readings and/or
      educational programs.

C. Collaborator   25%   Yes
   Coordinates services and communicates with other nurses, physicians,
   technologists, departments involved in care planning, and other health
   team members. Maintains confidentiality. Assures patient/family comfort
   and safety. Makes referrals as appropriate. Provides continuity of care by
   initiating telephone follow-up or being available to patients between
   outpatient visits to take patient questions for problems and direct them
   appropriately for resolution by triage of patient/family telephone calls.
   1. Assists other individuals to select and use unfamiliar patient care
      resources and support services.
   2. Acts as a resource to level III nurses in the evaluation of identified
      patient needs/problems. Acts as a preceptor and serves as a positive
      role model.
   3. Displays positive verbal and nonverbal behavior when
      communicating with patients, families, physicians, and colleagues.
   4. Documents all nursing assessments in a timely organized manner
      aimed at achieving the planned goals and outcomes.
   5. Answers all patient phone calls and communicates change in patient
      status in a timely manner to the physician.

D. Research   10%   Yes
   Supports nursing and departmental research activities.
   1. Identifies current researchable problems in radiation oncology
      nursing.
   2. Supports patients involved in clinical trials by clarifying information,
      assisting in patient education prior to informed consent, and
      identifying patients appropriate for protocols.
   3. Evaluates research findings in the area of oncology nursing for use in
      practice.
   4. Protects the rights of human subjects.
   5. Collaborates with other health professionals in the use of research
      findings.

(continues)

Figure 8.4 JOB DESCRIPTION FOR RADIATION ONCOLOGY NURSE LEVEL IV (PROFICIENT) (CONT'D)

E. Departmental Responsibilities	15%	Yes

    Supports the achievement of nursing and radiation oncology department goals in providing a positive, open, and creative environment.

    1.   Coordinates the flow of patients in the physician's practice.

    2.   Identifies learning needs on an ongoing basis and seeks to fulfill them.

    3.   Communicates plan of care with physicians.

    4.   Adheres to departmental policies and procedures and supports the achievement of the department and the department goals. Provides input for goal and objective development.

    5.   Participates in department question and answer program with data collection.

    6.   Attends radiation oncology conferences.

    7.   Participates in radiation oncology conference.

    8.   Attends nursing staff meetings and in-services.

    9.   Is concerned with the financial implications of ambulatory healthcare and assists where possible in keeping costs down.

   10. Other duties as assigned.

   11. Assists others to respond to unplanned events.

   12. Acts as a positive role model and resource person to level III staff registered nurses. Participates in the informal teaching and guidance of other staff.

F. Professional Responsibilities	10%	Yes

    Continuously strives to improve care and increase knowledge.

    1.   Is accountable for patient caseload.

    2.   Identifies learning needs on an ongoing basis and seeks to fulfill them.

    3.   Evaluates on an ongoing basis yearly objectives and assumes the responsibility for achieving these goals.

    4.   Serves as a preceptor for new employees and graduate students in the department.

    5.   Shares clinical expertise and seeks other expertise when needed.

    6.   Assists in orienting technologists and volunteers in the radiation oncology department.

    7.   Completes yearly skill credentialing and mandatory in-service training sessions.

    8.   Maintains confidentiality.

    9.   Appreciates the legal implications of nursing.

   10. Maintains yearly credentialing skills.

   11. Complies with personnel policies

       a. Follows dress code.

       b. Reports to duty as scheduled.

       c. Follows policy regarding notification of absence.

   12. Acts as preceptor to department if needed.

   13. Presents a positive unit and nursing image when communicating with other departments, nursing units, colleagues, and physicians.

   14. Assertively communicates concerns, issues, and information through appropriate channels. Displays appropriate degree of confidence in self. Communication and interpersonal skills enhance teamwork and the delivery of patient care.

   15. Participates in the development of nursing standards of practice as needed.

   16. Begins to participate in the development of alternative resources when dealing with changes on unit.

Level III: three basic role functions of the nurse are operationalized: patient care, teaching and counseling, and the coordination of services with other members of the multidisciplinary team (ancillary staff is necessary to perform nonnursing functions).

Level IV: the nurse functions at the advanced practice role and is usually prepared at the master's level. Activities are more comprehensive and include consultation, research, and administrative functions (Bruner, 1993).

In 1991, the American College of Radiology recommended that staffing include one nurse for direct patient care per 300 patients treated annually. The nurse was considered the key clinical staff member to evaluate the patient during treatment and in follow-up examinations with the radiation oncologist. Ancillary clinic activities (vital signs, weight, assistance with procedures, transport) were to be performed by licensed vocational nurses and nursing assistants (American College of Radiology, 1991).

The primary nursing model in radiation centers prevails today but is evolving due to both internal and external forces. Issues such as administrative and department restructuring, changes in practice and administrative philosophies, and diminished retention of established staff are examples of internal forces. The most profound external force is the nursing shortage. The diminished lack of qualified nursing professionals to assume positions within radiation oncology centers has led to the use of ancillary nursing personnel as primary care providers.

A collaborative practice model of care evolved from the primary model in radiation oncology centers. Collaborative practice models focus on the sharing of a specific patient practice by a nurse and a physician. These professionals have prescribed roles and responsibilities within the practice model, and patients are managed collaboratively throughout the treatment course

(Hilderley, 1991; Moore, 1996). Radiation practices lend themselves to collaborative work, as many radiation oncologists specialize in one or a few site-specific treatment areas. This kind of focused practice provides the foundation for the establishment of a collaborative clinical work. The following components of collaborative practice have been identified: mutual trust, understanding, open communication, flexibility, common goals, competence, independence, interdependence, and the desire for the collaboration to be successful (Hilderley, 1991). This model can evolve beyond the clinical arena and can extend to professional activities related to academic presentations, collaborative writing projects, and research and development of this clinical care model.

The Advanced Practice Role in Radiation Oncology

The APN is a registered nurse who is prepared with an advanced education such as a master of nursing science or a doctoral degree. APNs may also hold specialty certifications from professional organizations such as the American Academy of Nurse Practitioners or the ONS. APNs function as either CNSs or nurse practitioners (NPs).

The CNS role evolved during the mid-20th century with the purpose of developing an advanced practice nursing role dedicated to patient care. The major focus of the CNS is direct patient care in ambulatory and acute centers. The oncology CNS is expertly trained in all aspects of clinical oncology and typically subspecializes in a particular area such as medical oncology, surgical oncology, or radiation oncology. The CNS can also specialize in site-specific cancer diagnoses and management of patient populations with specific diagnoses. In addition to the clinical focus of the CNS, the role encompasses leadership, education, consultation, and research. The CNS functions to develop enhanced clinical programs, provide patient and staff education, consult on issues

Figure 8.5 JOB DESCRIPTION FOR RADIATION ONCOLOGY NURSE LEVEL V (EXPERT NURSE)

FOX CHASE CANCER CENTER
JOB DESCRIPTION

Job Title: Radiation Oncology Nurse Level V(Expert Nurse) **Department:** Radiation Oncology

Name:_____   **Date:** August 2000

PRIMARY FUNCTION:

The level V radiation oncology nurse is responsible and accountable for the nursing care provided to an unassigned caseload of patients treated with radiation therapy. The level V (expert) radiation oncology nurse assesses, plans, implements, and evaluates the following criteria on patients who have <u>complex care</u> needs and coordinates services required during treatment for their caseload.

ACCOUNTABILITIES:

	Percentage of Time	Essential Function (Yes or No)
A. Direct Caregiver	20%	Yes

   Carries out a systematic assessment process in determining the needs of the patient and family on all new patients by the third outpatient visit. Follows patients undergoing treatment and assesses them each visit for therapy and toxicity management. Demonstrates increased skill in assessment of biopsychosocial parameters. Provides the patient/family with quality care based on the assessment. Plans for care are developed mutually with the patient. Implementation of the plan is evaluated in terms of patient outcomes.

   1. Nursing care is provided according to the Fox Chase Cancer Center Standards of Nursing Practice.

   2. Symptom management is provided to the patient in collaboration with the radiation oncologist and the surgical and/or medical oncologist. Symptoms commonly managed include anorexia, nausea or vomiting, diarrhea, constipation, stomatitis, dysphagia, dehydration, fatigue, pain, infection, impaired skin integrity, mobility, ventilation, weight loss/gain, menstrual irregularities, vaginal dryness, alopecia, decreased blood counts, impotence, or infertility.

   3. Assesses and intervenes as needed when patient requires assistance with his or her coping mechanisms, phychosocial interactions, or interpersonal relationships. Refers patient to appropriate resource when counseling is beyond the expertise of the nurse.

   4. Demonstrates an understanding of basic principles of physical and psychosocial assessment related to adult development.

   5. Documents the four components of the nursing process—assessment, planning, intervention, and evaluation—in a timely, organized manner aimed at achieving the planned goals and outcomes.

   6. Answers all patient phone calls and communicates change in patient status in a timely manner to the physician.

   7. Organizes and establishes priorities for work load

   8. Assists level III and level IV nurses with the development of assessment skills.

Figure 8.5 Job Description for Radiation Oncology Nurse Level V (Expert Nurse) (cont'd)

   9. Augments initial assessment data with experiential knowledge.
  10. Integrates verbal and nonverbal behaviors exhibited by patient and/or significant others.
  11. Identifies underlying pathophysiological processes associated with abnormal findings.
  12. Provides direct care to the patient by performing nursing interventions with a high degree of mastery in accordance with standard of practice guidelines.
  13. Anticipates and responds to impending emergencies.

B. Teacher   20%   Yes
   Identifies areas in which the patient/family lacks knowledge regarding the disease process and therapy and provides that information.
   1. Provides general information and orientation to the radiation oncology department.
   2. Provides specific information about cancer and the treatment of cancer, clarifying and expanding on the physician's explanation.
   3. Teaches rationale and dosing schedule of medications ordered.
   4. Provides preventive education in the areas of nutrition, elimination, mouth care, skin care, immunosuppression, and other self-care measures, including early detection.
   5. Serves as a resource for other nurses in the institution caring for patients receiving radiotherapy.
   6. Develops alternate teaching strategies as needed.
   7. Independently provides feedback to peers related to readings and/or educational programs.
   8. Provides feedback to peers regarding strengths and developmental needs.

C. Collaborator   25%   Yes
   Coordinates services and communicates with other nurses, physicians, technologists, departments involved in care planning, and other health team members. Maintains confidentiality. Assures patient/family comfort and safety. Makes referrals as appropriate. Provides continuity of care by initiating telephone follow-up or being available to patients between outpatient visits to take patient questions for problems and direct them appropriately for resolution by triage of patient/family telephone calls.
   1. Assists other individuals to select and utilize unfamiliar patient care resources and support services.
   2. Acts as a resource to level III and level IV nurses in the evaluation of identified patient needs/problems. Acts as a preceptor and serves as a positive role model.
   3. Displays positive verbal and nonverbal behavior when communicating with patients, families, physicians, and colleagues.
   4. Documents all nursing assessments in a timely organized manner aimed at achieving the planned goals and outcomes.
   5. Answers all patient phone calls and communicates change in patient status in a timely manner to the physician.
   6. Arranges for active involvement of patient and family participation in planning nursing and/or self care activities.
   7. Uses "intuitive sense" in dealing with patient problems.

(continues)

Figure 8.5 Job Description for Radiation Oncology Nurse Level V (Expert Nurse) (cont'd)

D. Research Supports nursing and departmental research activities. 1. Identifies current researchable problems in radiation oncology nursing. 2. Supports patients involved in clinical trials by clarifying information, assisting in patient education prior to informed consent, and identifying patients appropriate for protocols. 3. Evaluates research findings in the area of oncology nursing for use in practice. 4. Protects the rights of human subjects. 5. Collaborates with other health professionals in the development and use of research findings.	10%	Yes
E. Departmental Responsibilities Supports the achievement of nursing and radiation oncology department goals in providing a positive, open, and creative environment. Participates in strategic planning for the unit. 1. Coordinates the flow of patients in the physician's practice. 2. Identifies learning needs on an ongoing basis and seeks to fulfill them. 3. Communicates plan of care with physicians 4. Adheres to departmental policies and procedures and supports the achievement of the department and the department goals. Provides input for goal and objective development. 5. Participates in department question and answer program with data collection. Develops monitoring tools. 6. Attends radiation oncology conferences. 7. Participates in radiation oncology conference. 8. Attends nursing staff meetings and in-services. 9. Is concerned with the financial implications of ambulatory healthcare and assists where possible in keeping costs down. 10. Other duties as assigned. 11. Assists others to respond to unplanned events. 12. Acts as a positive role model and resource person to level III and level IV staff RNs. Participates in the informal teaching and guidance of other staff. Uses principles of learning in the education of patients and colleagues. 13. Evaluates standards of care and identifies unsafe care practices, and initiates change. 14. Demonstrates self-motivation for professional and personal development.	15%	Yes
F. Professional Responsibilities Continuously strives to improve care and increase knowledge. 1. Accountable for patient caseload. 2. Identifies learning needs on an ongoing basis and seeks to fulfill them.	10%	Yes

Figure 8.5 JOB DESCRIPTION FOR RADIATION ONCOLOGY NURSE LEVEL V (EXPERT NURSE) (CONT'D)

3. Evaluates on an ongoing basis yearly objectives and assumes the responsibility for achieving these goals.
4. Serves as a preceptor for new employees and graduate students in the department.
5. Shares clinical expertise and seeks other expertise when needed.
6. Assists in orienting technologists and volunteers in the radiation oncology department.
7. Completes yearly skill credentialing and mandatory in-service training sessions.
8. Maintains confidentiality.
9. Appreciates the legal implications of nursing.
10. Maintains yearly credentialing skills.
11. Complies with personnel policies.
    a. Follows dress code.
    b. Reports to duty as scheduled.
    c. Follows policy regarding notification of absence.
12. Acts as preceptor to department if needed.
13. Presents a positive unit and nursing image when communicating with other departments, nursing units, colleagues, and physicians. Assertively communicates concerns, issues, and information through appropriate channels. Displays appropriate degree of confidence in self. Communication and interpersonal skills enhance teamwork and the delivery of patient care.
14. Able to incorporate alternative resources when dealing with changes on unit. Initiates referrals and uses available resources within and outside the institution.
15. Encourages mutual trust and respect among coworkers by maintaining open communication systems.
16. Formulates and evaluates nursing standards of practice to reflect trends in radiation oncology nursing.

related to symptom management and staff mentoring, coordinate research protocols, and apply research findings to clinical practice. The CNS functions to integrate organizational philosophy and healthcare services (Bigbee, 1996; Galassi & Wheeler, 1994; Shepard & Kelvin, 1999).

The CNS role in radiation oncology has developed in tandem with increased nursing presence. Many CNSs have an extensive background in clinical oncology and can serve as an invaluable patient, staff, and community resource. CNSs are integrated into the nursing component of the radiation department and work closely with all members of the multidisciplinary team to provide care for patients and families throughout the treatment and follow-up experience. CNS activi-

ties may also include developing standards of practice, writing staff policies and procedures, administering quality-assurance programs, and facilitating nursing-related research and writing activities.

The CNS functions in diverse types of radiation centers. Successful collaboration with a radiation oncologist in private practice has been documented and is considered the prototype for this model of healthcare (Hilderley, 1991). Collaborative nursing focuses on the expert delivery of patient care through the integration of medical and nursing functions; this concept is supported by the physicians' acceptance of advanced nursing practice. In order for the CNS in radiation oncology to function, it is necessary

Figure 8.6 Job Description for OTV RN: Triage/Special Procedures

FOX CHASE CANCER CENTER
JOB DESCRIPTION

Job Title: OTV RN: Triage/Special Procedures **Department:** Radiation Oncology

Duties to Include

1. Assure efficient/priority flow of patients in on treatment visit (OTV) area.
2. Assess/triage patients coming to the radiation clinic area.
   Document assessment/frequent monitoring on appropriate forms.
   Provide appropriate information for transfer to receiving area.
3. Provide direction for clinic licensed practical nurse (LPN)-delegate appropriate tasks, ensure adequate stock of clinic supplies, ensure necessary information is available (films, reports, etc.) when requested.
4. Monitor and provide care to patients in stretcher holding area.
5. Respond to request of technologists concerning patient's intravenous alarms, need for suctioning, pain management (administer medications as per physician orders), etc.
6. Obtain clinic data for department question and answering monitoring.
7. Provide complete patient care for special procedures (high dose rate (HDR), low dose rate (LDR), nasopharngolaryngoscopy, transrectal ultrasound (TRUS).
   Coordination of scheduling
   Preprocedure teaching
   Medication administration as ordered by physician
   Intraprocedure case/monitoring
   Postprocedure care/monitoring
   Postprocedure education
8. Assist OTV nurse
   Complete patient flow sheets in absence of OTV nurse.
   Provide coverage for OTV nurse for scheduled meetings, lunch, or mandatory inservices.
9. Other duties as assigned.

QUALIFICATIONS:

Licensure/Degree	Registered nurse with Bachelor Science Nursing (BSN) degree, licensed in Pennsylvania.
Certification Required	Oncology Certified Nurse (OCN) & Advanced Certification Life Support (ACLS), intravenous therapy.
Experience Required	Oncology experience necessary. Outpatient experience a plus, or experience necessary. Excellent time management skills required. Public speaking skills needed.

that the entire multidisciplinary team embrace this type of practice. Staff nurses and ancillary nursing support staff working with the CNS must support the role and appreciate the significant clinical and professional benefit.

When the NP role evolved in the 1960s the primary purpose was to increase access to primary healthcare in underserved areas. The NP is a registered nurse educated at the master's level in adult, child, or family health. The basis for NP training was primary healthcare; this has expanded into specialty areas. Based on the blending of the medical and nursing model, NPs function in all specialty areas of oncology. In radiation oncology, NPs provide primary care to patients, which includes obtaining medical histories and physical examinations; diagnosing acute and chronic physical and psychosocial issues; ordering and interpreting laboratory, radiologic, and other test results; and prescribing medical treatment, including certain classes of medications and counseling; and educating patients and families. Additionally, NPs monitor and manage symptoms of cancer and treatment and in some practices prescribe radiation treatment plans (Shepard & Kelvin, 1999).

The APN's role in healthcare has been evaluated and has demonstrated a high degree of acceptance by patients and medical colleagues over many years (Boyle, 1995; Girouard, 1996; Riportella-Muller, Libby, & Kindig, 1995). Additionally, APNs were found to perform specific tasks with equal proficiency as physicians and have a positive impact on patient outcomes. No research had been conducted on the role of nonphysician providers (NPPs) in radiation oncology. In response to this, the American Society for Therapeutic Radiology and Oncology (ASTRO) in 1997 established a joint committee of radiation oncology physicians, residents, and nurses working in both hospital based and private practice settings. The goal of this committee was to describe the roles of CNSs, NPs, and PAs in the practice of radiation oncology throughout the United States.

Changes in reimbursement and a decrease in the number of radiation oncology residents have led to new ways of providing high-quality patient care in radiation oncology. One way to achieve this goal was to invoke NPPs such as APNs and PAs. The definition by the ASTRO task force of each type of NPP includes educational background, clinical roles and responsibilities, regulatory issues, collaborative practice agreements, and philosophy of practice. The information provided can assist physicians, nurses, and administrators to decide whether an NPP is appropriate for their practice, what type of provider would be most effective, and plans for role implementation (Kelvin et al., 1999).

The task force further discussed the following issues regarding APN and PA roles in radiation oncology that includes role definition, regulatory mechanisms, prescriptive authority, reimbursement structures, and implementation of the role, educational requirements, and total impact on resident training programs. The role of the NPP is considered complementary to and not as a replacement for radiation residents and radiation oncologists. It was determined that the NPP can assist in the diagnostic evaluation of patients, manage symptoms, provide education to patients and families, and assist them in coping. This role can facilitate the radiation oncologists' ability to focus on the technical aspects of prescribing treatment (Babcock, 2000; Kelvin et al., 1999).

A survey of oncology APNs was conducted to identify critical issues impacting on the APN role. Oncology APNs demonstrated a lack of professional practice definition and standards, reimbursement, and billing discrepancies for services rendered, incomplete documentation and validation of practice outcomes, variance in educational preparation, credentialing, and prescriptive authority, and the merging of clinical roles. This survey demonstrated the intense need for the development of APN outcomes research to describe and validate the existence and perpetuation of APNs in oncology care (Lynch, Cope, & Murphy-Ende, 2001). The APN's role in radiation oncology must be developed and promoted. A clinical practice model based on comprehensive multidisciplinary cancer care can only be complete if the dimension of advanced nursing practice is supported and actualized (Lynch et al., 2001).

Role of the Research Nurse in Radiation Oncology

Radiation therapy centers participate in cooperative research studies through association with the RTOG, the Southwest Oncology Group, and Eastern Oncology Group. Clinical trials are also accessed through the National Cancer Institute (NCI), hospital protocols administered by institutional review boards, site-specific research consortiums such as the Gynecologic Oncology Group, as well as pharmaceutical trials. Access and participation in clinical trials provide patients in both hospital-based and freestanding facilities equal opportunity to benefit from current treatment advances, including multimodality regimens and innovative treatment methods.

The RTOG was organized in 1971 with the purpose of conducting clinical trials related to radiation oncology. The RTOG is a national cooperative research organization headquartered in Philadelphia, PA under the auspices of the American College of Radiology and funded by the NCI. Principal investigators are leaders of research teams and represent participating institutions. Nurses functioning as data managers for clinical trials are responsible for reinforcing informed consent, patient education, obtaining required trial data, and submission of written reports to study administrators. The RTOG is responsible for coordinating research efforts by randomizing and registering study patients, collecting and distributing study-related materials, and performing data analysis. Participating institutions are required to maintain adherence to study participation and are also responsible for specific accrual requirements to maintain active status.

The role of the nurse in radiation oncology has evolved from that of data manager to independent researcher. This has been due, in part, to the presence of APNs working in radiation oncology as well as the establishment of departments of nursing research within institutions and the success of the Radiation Special Interest Group of the ONS established in 1989. These structures have enabled radiation oncology nurses to identify specific clinical topics for investigation and to pursue scientific inquiry to substantiate these needs. Early descriptive radiation oncology nursing studies have evolved and now include clinical topics such as patient information and educational needs, treatment-related experience, symptom management, late effects, and survivorship issues (Dow, 1997).

Radiation centers can provide a climate for nursing research to be fostered by initiating different activities that promote critical thinking. Practice settings can be evaluated for their potential to support research by posing the following questions:

- Do nurses talk about research in this setting?
- Do they identify gaps in practice?
- Is there a nursing research committee to facilitate nursing inquiries?
- Do nurses have the same support mechanisms as other researchers?
- Does the setting hold formal continuing education programs related to nursing research?
- Does the setting conduct informal educational programs related to nursing research such as journal clubs?
- Are there graduate students or a nursing faculty conducting research in the setting?
- Are there any rewards related to conducting clinical research related activities? (Haberman, 2000)

Nursing research in radiation oncology continues to develop in the areas of symptom management, patient education, and research use.

Radiation nursing research provides an opportunity for expanded nursing functions, for provision of research-based patient care, and for the ability to study and test nursing interventions on the impact of patient responses to treatment. It is vital that nurses are supported in their effort to conduct research and that funding sources be available and used. Promising clinicians and graduate students must be encouraged to consider research as a career. The development of novel strategies for research dissemination and utilization must be developed and tested to ensure that oncology nursing practice becomes progressively evidence based (Haberman, 2000).

Role of the Nurse Administrator in Radiation Oncology

The scope of practice of the nurse administrator (also referred to as the nurse manager or clinical nurse coordinator) in radiation oncology depends on the type of facility in which the position exists. If the nurse administrator works in a comprehensive ambulatory oncology center, management may include other oncology-related specialties such as medical and surgical oncology. If the nurse administrator works in a freestanding radiation center, that setting may be the sole focus of responsibility. General responsibilities of the nurse administrator have been summarized as follows:

- Achieving departmental business and clinical goals
- Ensuring quality patient care; hiring/retention of skilled nursing personnel
- Participating in development of patient-related policy and decision making
- Participating in hospital, professional organizations, and community committees (Sporkin, 1997)

The nurse administrator's position description defines the scope of practice, and organizational structures define the nurse manager's authority. Size, complexity, and ownership of the radiation facility need to be considered when determining where nursing's place is within the organizational structure (Iwamoto & Gough, 1993). Nurse administrators reporting requirements vary depending on the facility. Institutionally affiliated radiation departments may require nurse administrators to report to the department of nursing governing the facility. Additionally, nurse managers may be required to serve on a hospital-wide nursing council. This type of organizational structure includes the radiation nurse manager in hospital nursing activities. In freestanding centers, nurses may report to a physician or to a chief therapist. In some settings, the nurse manager may report to a business administrator. Nurse administrators must understand both reporting mechanisms and the scope of authority when assuming a managerial role. Concerns related to these administrative parameters should be clarified before the nurse assumes an administrative position.

The role of the nurse manager has the potential to be multifaceted and requires an individual to have the broad capacity to coordinate complex clinical care as well as oversee both operational and personnel issues. Key aspects of the nurse manager's position have been identified as patient care management, operational management, and human resource management (Iwamoto & Gough, 1993). The patient care management role includes providing leadership in the development, implementation, and maintenance of patient care standards. Operational management includes leadership in areas of departmental planning, policymaking, staff assessment, and motivation. Additional operational skills include serving as a professional liaison within the medical center and with external agencies and managing clinically related budgetary guidelines. The human resource management aspects of the nurse administrator role includes promoting staff educational opportunities, establishing guidelines for implementation of nursing research, and developing staff leadership and professional skills.

In some settings, the administrative responsibilities of the radiation oncology nurse manager are limited to the supervision of a clinical department and staff. In some instances, the title of nurse manager is not conferred; therefore, staff nurses and APNs may assume administrative tasks in the absence of a formal title. In a recent survey of licensed nursing personnel employed in radiation oncology in North America, of 255 respondents, the majority (88%) reported having the responsibility for supervising staff, with 59% of APNs and 34% of staff nurses reporting responsibility for the task. Nurse managers reported responsibility for writing nursing policies and procedures (80%), and 47% reported writing nonnursing policies and procedures. Nurse managers reported participating in a variety of clinically related quality-assurance activities (Moore-Higgs et al., 2003a).

Nurse administrators are required to ensure that patient care needs are met with adequate staffing. They are responsible for hiring, planning orientation, retention, and evaluation of qualified nursing staffs. Staffing requirements are dependent on the hours of the radiation oncology center, the type of services offered, and demographic locations. If the radiation center operates with extended and weekend hours, then the department will need to offer flexible working opportunities to accommodate these requirements. The nursing staff coordinates with radiation oncologists to ensure that routine and emergent clinical coverage is available. If the center offers specific treatment regimens requiring increased planning and treatment time, staffing will need to be reconfigured to accommodate these particular needs. Staffing requirements of suburban/rural centers may be more challenging then urban settings. It is imperative that staffs have access to reliable modes of transportation to accommodate both distance and varied hours of operation.

Recruiting and retaining quality radiation oncology nursing personnel are currently the greatest challenges that are facing nurse managers. A profound decline in nursing school enrollment and the attraction of competing career paths are only two of the contributing factors to this national crises. The ONS developed a study to examine issues concerning the nursing shortage, a decline in dedicated oncology nursing units, and the potential impact on quality cancer care (Lamkin, Rosiak, Buerhaus, Mallory, & Williams, 2001). One finding indicated that oncology care reflects the direction of healthcare in general and that oncology nurses are in a prime position to become leaders in contributing to enhancing quality care in ambulatory settings. A survey of licensed nursing personnel (self-identified as ONS members and Radiation Therapy Special Interest Group [RT SIG] members) currently practicing in the specialty of radiation oncology in the United States and Canada revealed the following demographic information: Of 281 respondents, the majority (94%) were female, between 40 and 49 years of age (46%) with a bachelor's degree as the highest level of education (40%). Sixty-eight percent were oncology-certified nurses. The majority of respondents had spent more than 5 years in radiation oncology (64%), with 31% having more than 10 years of experience (Moore-Higgs et al., 2003a). Seventy-six respondents were 41 to 60 years old, reflecting the aging of the nursing workforce in North America and the resulting impact on the specialty of radiation oncology. The group held advanced educational preparation, with 58% having a bachelor's degree or master's degree. The respondents had a significant amount of experience in radiation oncology, with 64% reporting more than five years of employment in the field. Many of the nurses (36%) were within 10 years of retirement, which implies a significant future shortage of experienced nurses (Moore-Higgs et al., 2003a). These data exemplify the need for nurse administrators to develop proactive measures for renewal of the nursing profession.

The entire multidisciplinary radiation oncology team has been affected by personnel shortages

(Backus, 2001; Mazurowski, 2001). Although team members may differ in their professional contributions to the functioning of the radiation oncology setting, similarities exist that contribute to the shrinking pool of qualified personnel. Administrators should assess why people do not choose the profession, then why people leave, and what measures can be done to halt this cycle. The following are reasons for team members leaving the field of radiation oncology: uncompetitive salaries, a desire to seek specialty areas in competing institutions, stressful working conditions, private sector competition and expansion, rural/town life a disadvantage, undesirable locations in urban settings, contract agency opportunities at higher per diem rates (Backus, 2001; Luckett, 2000).

The following recommendations for enhancing recruitment and retention efforts have been suggested for both nurse and radiology administrators (Backus, 2001; Luckett, 2000; Mazurowski, 2001):

- Focus on the potential of future radiation oncology nurses.
- Create opportunities to present clinical topics in local universities with nursing curricula.
- Sponsor a career day for high school students and community participants.
- Highlight innovative technologic advances in radiation oncology, and explain the unique coupling of radiobiology with clinical practice.
- Although controversial, incentives can be effective. Sign-on bonuses coupled with a required length of service commitment, and referral bonuses can be attractive recruitment tactics. Loan scholarship programs can be provided as tuition reimbursement for existing staff and for those enrolled in healthcare programs that would be required to commit to future employment at the sponsoring facility. Implement and capitalize on the quality of life for employees (i.e., regular daytime hours; no shift rotation; attractive weekend only work packages; or 36 hours worked but 40 hours paid programs).
- Do not stress the negativity of the "shortage talk." Negative staff morale during difficult times can be damaging. Nurse administrators must remain optimistic and can ensure that other colleagues and staff project the same attitude. Resist the temptation to employ unqualified staff. Although the need to hire may be urgent, quick irrational decisions that lower quality personnel standards can be a disincentive to established and committed staff members.
- Serve as a clinical preceptor site for a nursing program. This opportunity could form an invaluable partnership to bring students into the facility. This environment motivates staff to maintain current clinical knowledge and provide a competitive environment for students seeking employment.
- Development of a clinical ladder system offers positions of greater responsibility at higher salaries, and provides an opportunity for staff to strive to develop professionally. Establishing criteria and job descriptions for competent, proficient, and expert nurses is another way to begin a clinical ladder system.
- Focus on teambuilding among all staff members. Recognition and praise should be immediate, intermittent, unexpected, and sincere. Mark budget dollars for continuing education help to build a competent and valued team. Provide reimbursement for conference attendance, professional association dues, journal subscriptions and textbooks, and certification examinations. Form a professional journal club. Offer incentives for conference participation and for writing for publications.

Arrange educational staff meetings that are meaningful and conducive to learning and to enhancing staff relationships.

- Encourage staff nurses to participate in the development of standards of care and quality-assurance programs. Promoting staff participation in shaping the nursing practice within the facility leads to autonomy, professional worth, and improvement of overall job satisfaction. Ensuring the most competitive wages and benefits for radiation oncology nurses enhances both recruitment and retention strategies. Comprehensive packages that include long-term retirement security plans are ideal. A recent survey of ONS members who practice in radiation oncology centers in North America reported a salary range of $41,000–$60,000 per year (Moore-Higgs et al., 2003a).

- Ensure that new staff members are welcomed and guided professionally with a comprehensive orientation program. An orientation manual with clinical resource information can include a refresher review of medical physics, radiobiology, an overview of radiation therapy, and patient care and symptom management across the continuum of radiation care. New nurses can be provided with an experienced radiation oncology nurse preceptor during their clinical practicum; the evaluation is to be based on a written evaluation protocol founded on current practice standards (Watkins Bruner, Bucholtz, Iwamoto, & Strohl, 1998). At one comprehensive cancer center, an annual radiation oncology nursing course is offered nationally and provides basic content that serves as a didactic overview for nurses new to radiation oncology (Fox Chase Cancer Center (FCCC) annual radiation oncology nursing course).

During this entire process, nurse administrators should strive to maintain high personal and staff performance goals consistently. Challenges of staff recruitment and retention are not insurmountable if creatively approached by nurse managers, addressed in a collegial forum to seek concrete solutions, and to ensure the future delivery of clinical radiation oncology care.

An understanding of the economics of the healthcare environment is essential for nurse managers. This fiduciary knowledge must also be imparted to staff nurses so that the entire clinical nursing team is educated and committed to delivering comprehensive oncology care that is economically feasible. Cost controlling is a central element of the nurse manager's role. The budget process varies among clinical facilities. Commonly, the total annual budget preparation and projection are under the auspices of a business administrator and accounting departments. Radiation oncology nurses need to be aware of financial concepts that govern healthcare services and to apply these tenets to the development of practice standards and decision pathways (Moore-Higgs et al., 2003b).

Budget processes usually occur annually and submitted prospectively for the forthcoming fiscal term. Radiation oncology nursing budgets may be funded by a variety of sources depending on the type of practice. In institutional settings, the hospital nursing budget or radiation department budget may fund the nursing component. In a freestanding facility, patient revenues may fund staffing needs. Potential changes in staffing requirements are also considered when prospectively planning budgets. Other considerations are increases in services and patient volume, nursing budgets to support clinical trial research, and competitive alignment of wages and benefit packages with the regional marketplace. The budget process is on a continuum and contingent planning for any possible needs is necessary to ensure an economically sound practice.

Fiscal planning considers the importance of providing third-party payers and government agencies with accurate documentation to substantiate billing to reduce losses, to improve patient access and satisfaction, and to ensure that the entire care continuum is approved for reimbursement. This process ultimately provides lower costs, higher quality of care, and few impediments to accessing approved services (Noa & D'Angelo, 2001; Sporkin, 1997). It is imperative that nurse managers impart this knowledge to staff so that the entire team is aware of the required documentation formats and the rationale for professionally supporting a fiscally responsible clinical environment. Depending on the practice site, radiation oncology nurse administrators are in pivotal positions to participate in the planning, developing, execution, and negotiation of facility budgets, resource management, capital budgets, operating budgets, third-party payer limitations, and key performance indicators (Moore-Higgs et al., 2003b).

Ambulatory Radiation Oncology/Trajectory of Patient Care

The ambulatory radiation oncology nurse is in a unique position to manage a patient population with evolving clinical needs. The trajectory of patient care in radiation oncology begins with expert nursing assessment, including physical, psychosocial, cultural, spiritual, and environmental dimensions, and evolves through the process of patient education and symptom management. The combination of these aspects of care requires that radiation oncology nurses have a thorough understanding of radiobiology, technical aspects of treatment delivery, physiologic indications for prescribing radiation as a cancer treatment modality, management of treatment-related side effects, and psychosocial issues that were extant and evolve during the trajectory of care.

Patient assessment and management occur over a course of time that includes pretreatment assessment, during treatment assessment/management, and follow-up care.

The relationship between the nurse and patients receiving radiation therapy has the potential to span a long time period. During this process, nurses are in pivotal positions to assess, intervene, and manage key clinical parameters that can ensure a safe and complete treatment course. During the pretreatment assessment, it is imperative that the nurse assesses the patients knowledge regarding the rationale for treatment and the expectations of the outcomes. Including patient family/support systems in the educational pretreatment phase will provide detailed information for the clinical team about the patient's level of understanding and anticipation of outcomes (Kelly, 1999). During the pretreatment phase, identification of individualized patient needs shoulc occur. These needs can be operational, administrative, or clinical. Some patients may need a specific treatment time scheduled. Some may need daily transportation, and others may require living arrangements closer to the facility (for hyperfractionated protocols or for those living at a distance). Insurance requirements must be prospectively arranged so that patients and families are aware of covered costs as well as out-of-pocket expectations. Included in these expenses are ancillary costs for attenuated salaries (disability income), extended childcare, and pharmaceutical and durable medical supplies. Specific clinical requirements such as fertility issues, dental/nutritional assessments, pain medication, oxygen therapy, assistive mobility devices all need to be assessed during the pretreatment phase (Kelly, 1999). If this information is provided before the course of treatment begins, then the likelihood of completing the entire prescribed course will be enhanced.

Consultation is the initial meeting of the patient and family with the radiation oncologist and radiation oncology nurse. At this visit, a review of the patient's presenting diagnosis, past medical history, operative procedure, and pathology and radiology findings occurs. A complete physical examination is performed, which may include a pelvic or rectal examination or an endoscopic examination of the head and neck region. The patient may be surprised at the need for these often-repeated examinations. It is necessary for the nurse to provide a rationale to validate and educate the patient about the necessity of the pretreatment assessment. After completion of a thorough review of the data, the radiation oncologist together with the multidisciplinary team develops a plan of care and presents it for discussion with the patient and family. Often the use of radiation therapy as a treatment modality is part of a multidisciplinary effort and must be carefully coordinated with other oncology-related disciplines. The physician obtains informed consent during the pretreatment phase of the initial consultation. The informed consent includes the goals of treatment, the number of days or weeks of therapy, and a discussion of short- and long-term side effects. The radiation oncology nurse participates and reinforces the process of informed consent. Nurses are able to evaluate patient understanding of the informed consent process and assess for potential barriers such as a compromised mental competency, sensory impairment, advanced age, and an inability to read and comprehend English. If limitations are identified, then the radiation oncology nurse can seek consultation with ancillary support services (translators, legal services, social services, government agencies) to ensure that an ethical informed consent process has occurred (Moore-Higgs et al., 2003b; Watkins Bruner et al., 1998).

Before obtaining signed informed consent, the following information is given to the patient: the purpose of treatment, the availability of pertinent clinical trials, the risk and benefit of treatment, the side-effect profile, the details of the treatment planning phase and the actual treatment experience, the follow-up schedule, and a discussion of other treatment modalities. The nurse assumes the role of patient advocate and assesses the individual's understanding of the consent information presented. Additionally, the nurse ensures ample

time for discussion of all viable treatment options and encourages patient's questions and provides complete answers to assist with decision making (Watkins Bruner et al., 1998). Providing thorough informed consent in ambulatory radiation oncology facilities is a pivotal aspect of the pretreatment assessment phase of patient care. During this time, the clinical team must devote a significant amount of effort to provide information, impart confidence, and encourage patients and families to become educated about the technologic and clinical dimensions of the complicated details of a radiation course. The pace and activities of ambulatory radiation facilities are busy, and prioritizing the informed consent aspect of the pretreatment phase of care can provide assurance of a comprehensive and effective clinical course.

Physical Assessment

During the initial consultation, the radiation oncology nurse completes a comprehensive nursing assessment, including a past and current medical history, a system review, a cancer history (patient and family), an emphasis on the present cancer diagnosis, previous and current cancer treatment, symptom distress, intercurrent disease involving the proposed treatment field, relevant laboratory data (hematology, chemistry, tumor marker assays), diagnostic data (radiology, CT, MRI, PET, endoscopic exams, pathology, staging studies), and assessment of functional, cognitive, and sensory domains (Catlin-Huth, Haas, & Pollock, 2002).

In addition to an initial physical assessment, it is vital that radiation oncology nurses assess patients during the course of active treatment. Patients receiving radiation may present with complex and yet subtle treatment related toxicity, which the radiation oncology nurse must carefully assess. If a patient is being assessed for dehydration, then orthostatic blood pressure changes are obtained. If positive, an infusion facility is consulted to consider if intravenous fluid support is required. Patients at risk for nutritional compromise are weighed routinely, and have a detailed assessment to evaluate nutritional status and plans for appropriate intervention (laboratory values, nutritional supplementation, and parenteral nutritional support). Laboratory studies are obtained routinely if the treatment field involves a large portion of proliferating bone marrow (such as the pelvis). It is essential that patients have routine hematology and chemistry values documented during treatment, especially if chemotherapy or biotherapy is being given concomitantly. Radiographic studies are also used to evaluate physiologic changes that may require additional clinical interventions. Site-specific regions of treatment fields require evaluation during the active treatment phase. For example, patients receiving head and neck irradiation, the oral cavity, external surface of the skin, and nodal region are assessed. Patients receiving chest irradiation require routine assessment of lung sounds. Throughout the course of radiation therapy, pain is assessed, especially for the patient receiving palliative treatment for bone metastasis. Pain assessment includes evaluation of medication regimens and treatment interventions.

Assessment and triage have been identified as two of the pivotal role dimensions of the specialty of ambulatory nursing (Haas, 1998). Combined modality therapy has broadened assessment profiles. When evaluating patients receiving combined modality therapy, it is essential to consider each treatment component and potential side effect before offering an intervention. It is vital that nurses are able to differentiate subtle changes in patient status, such as the development of a headache, nausea, vomiting, incontinence, and musculoskeletal weakness/pain. Also, radiation therapy patients may develop physical symptoms unrelated to the cancer diagnosis and treatment. Pathologic fractures, sepsis, and thrombophlebitis can occur independently and can require immediate intervention.

Psychosocial Assessment

A cancer diagnosis causes a profound psychosocial burden for individuals and their families. Cancer poses a threat to individual security and life patterns. The current cancer treatment continuum provides hope that many cancers are curable; however, profound fears of pain, suffering, and the ultimate outcome exist. These fears create anxiety that contributes to an individual's response to a cancer diagnosis and concomitant treatment course (Gorman, 1998).

It is vital that the psychosocial domain of cancer is assessed and interventions integrated into the total clinical care of patients and families. The psychosocial assessment and intervention process is dynamic and responds to continual change in patient status, disease course, and level of adaptation (LaRue, 2002). Radiation therapy can produce fear and anxiety. Most individuals do not have experience with this mode of treatment and have received lay information regarding the dangers of radiation exposure. It is challenging for the multidisciplinary team to explain the therapeutic rationale for delivery of radiation when preconceived notions are already in place. The process of receiving radiation therapy may create fear of the unknown, the need to establish trust with an new treatment team of professionals, and new scheduling requirements that create personal hardship (maintaining jobs, caring for families) (Gorman, 1998).

Patients may have preconceived ideas of the actual treatment experience, that need to be dispelled. Some individuals fear being burned; while others may balk at permanent skin tattoos (an indelible external reminder of a cancer diagnosis). The fears of being alone in the treatment room with dim lights, laser beams glowing, and the hum of the equipment may be profound. In addition, patient adjustment to the radiation process can vary from weeks to months. Patients who experience more severe side-effects tend to have more profound negative reactions than patients with fewer side effects (Holland, 1989; Walker, Nail, Larsen, Magill, & Schwartz, 1996). A thorough psychosocial assessment and appropriate interventions can reduce these fears.

A biopsychosocial model of assessing potential risk factors has been suggested as a most effective way of assessing and intervening in oncology settings. The biopsychosocial model in cancer care suggests that personal, social, and medical domains are integrated, and that each of these areas be assessed by the nursing staff in to create a relevant information source with critical information for intervention planning (LaRue, 2002).

The initial component of the assessment is a review of the patients' personal history. It is vital to understand the patients' prior experience with medical, personal, or family crisis. This part of the assessment elicits information about preconceived knowledge of the cancer experience, the patients' degree of realistic hopefulness regarding their diagnosis, the patients' ability to adapt to past life-losses, and the ability to identify appropriate support systems and to access them. This assessment phase then looks at current implications of the cancer diagnosis and poses the following questions:

- What are the patient's expectations about the diagnosis and response to treatment?
- What is current activity level and lifestyle and how will treatment change this?
- What developmental stage is the individual in, and how might this illness affect the ability to move through life tasks (parenting, wage earner, college attendance, and retirement)?

The last component of the personal history focuses on existential concerns. This is an assessment that helps the patient find meaning in the cancer experience. The following questions may be posed:

- What is the meaning of illness, life, and death for the patient?
- What are the spiritual concerns or connections that might affect the patient's adaptation to the diagnosis?

- Does the patient feel responsible for the cancer diagnosis? How will this affect the patient's adaptation and ability to access support?
- What expectations did the patient have before the illness about length and quality of life (LaRue, 2002)?

The second area of assessment focuses on the social context of the lives of patients. The social world in which individuals reside will affect response to cancer diagnosis. The following questions can be posed:

- What is the patient's perceived and actual support network?
- How will the cancer diagnosis affect the members of the network?
- What is the patient's role in family and community, and what is the influence of the cancer diagnosis on this role?
- What are the resources of the support network that may influence the patient's cancer experience?

The final phase includes the cancer status assessment. This refers to the impact of the diagnosis and prognosis on coping over time. For some patients, the effect of the diagnosis may be initially profound, while for others, the impact of the diagnosis and concomitant realities occurs over time. The following questions can be asked:

- What is the cancer diagnosis, stage, and prognosis?
- What is the potential significance/meaning of the side effects?
- What is the effect on physical functioning?
- What is the potential for rehabilitation?

A complete biopsychosocial assessment summary provides information about a patient's personal history, social context, and medical factors. These guidelines can be used in a radiation oncology setting to develop a biopsychosocial assessment of patients experiencing the trajectory of cancer care. This assessment can be shared among other members of the professional healthcare team thus, as patients experience different aspects of care and specialties, the information can serve as a guide for creating individual interventions in order to enhance adaptation (LaRue, 2002).

Psychosocial interventions incorporate the ability of each patient to adapt and to develop coping skills within their personal and social context. Once the patients primary concerns are identified, then interventions can be planned for the individual, for couples, and for families. Individual interventions may include psychotherapy, relaxation, and the development of stress-management skills, which can provide relief from anxiety or treatment-related symptoms. If a combined modality intervention is offered, then psychotropic medication may be indicated, along with psychotherapy. Psychotherapy with cancer patients typically focuses on illness-related concerns. It can also include exploration of past experiences and adjustment to the present situation as well (Holland, 1989). Patients experiencing treatment-related side effects require a combined interventional approach of medical care and complementary modalities such as guided imagery, music therapy, and massage therapy. The influences of the cancer experience for couples have indicated the following needs (Carlson, Bultz, Speca, & St. Pierre, 2000): find meaning in the cancer experience; the importance of communication, spousal supports, and marital satisfaction. Interventions for couples should focus on developing clear, consistent communication about the entire trajectory of the cancer diagnosis, treatment, and follow-up. Couples can be taught to prioritize their relationship and to seek external support services such as family, friends, healthcare professionals, and clergy to facilitate adaptation. The relationships of couples are multifaceted in today's contemporary world. It is important that professional radiation oncology nurses recognize the diversity of these relationships and focus on the couple's individuality, and the potential to apply interventions to enhance adaptation to a new and challenging life experience (Gritz, Wellisch, Siau, & Wang, 1990).

Family responses to cancer present complicated dynamics that require astute nursing intervention. Patients have the right to sanction the inclusion of families during medical team meetings. Family interventions focus on providing consistent information to designated family members, and ways to mobilize the family resources to assume the role of collective caregivers. Family therapy assists members in understanding the patient's physical and emotional response to the diagnosis and treatment. The overall goals of family therapy are to enhance the family members' ability to support each other and to evolve as a cohesive unit throughout the process (LaRue, 2002).

Providing comprehensive psychosocial assessments and interventions in ambulatory oncology facilities can be challenging for the healthcare team. Time and resources may not allow a full complement of services; however, it is imperative that radiation nurses prioritize this aspect of patient care and articulate the need for administrators in order to ensure access for patients and families. The following steps should be taken to ensure this process: Weekly interdisciplinary case conference meetings need to be held with a psychologist, clinical social worker, or psychiatrist as part of the team. All psychosocial services should be easily accessible and available to the patients. The healthcare team can attempt to normalize feelings associated with a stigma of seeking psychosocial services. Written information regarding available counseling services and appropriate contact information is essential. Psychosocial care is fundamental for a patient to achieve a more complete adjustment to the rigors imposed by the cancer diagnosis, treatment course, and follow-up. **Table 8.1** provides a comprehensive outline with examples of the psychosocial implications of the radiation treatment experience. This information can be used to assess patients and families before the onset of treatment, during the course of treatment, and in follow-up.

Table 8.1 THE RADIATION EXPERIENCE: CAPTURING THE PSYCHOSOCIAL PATIENT PERSPECTIVE

I. Factors that influence distress
  A. Medical
    1. Site of disease
    2. Clinical course
    3. Type of treatment
    4. Symptoms experienced
  B. Psychological
    1. Disruption of life goals
    2. Ability to modify life's plans
    3. Coping style/emotional maturity
  C. Social
    1. Available support network (family, community, belief system)
II. Dialogue with cancer experience
  A. Facing the fear
  B. Coming to terms
  C. Looking to the future
  D. Finding meaning
    1. Dialogue promptly
    2. Be resourceful
    3. Search for meaning
    4. Transcend the present (story telling)
    5. Total experience
    6. Need to talk
    7. Comfort in sharing
    8. Bibliotherapy (use of words in place of actions)
III. Trajectory of the experience
  A. Sample 1
    1. Diagnosis
    2. Pretreatment care
    3. During treatment care/experience
    4. Posttreatment follow-up
    5. Termination of active treatment/ rehabilitation
    6. Survival
  B. Sample 2
    1. Discovery/diagnosis
    2. Treatment
    3. Remission/Recurrence/Dissemination
    4. Terminal
  C. Sample 3
    1. Interpreting diagnosis

2. Confronting mortality
3. Reprioritizing
4. Coming to terms
5. Moving on
6. Flashing back
  D. Sample 4
    1. Revelation (diagnosis)
    2. Rupture (treatment)
    3. Re-entry (therapy completion)
    4. Regeneration (recovery)
IV. Cancer impact on the individual, family, and society
    1. Awareness
    2. Receiving the diagnosis
    3. Patient's response to the news
    4. Family reactions
    5. Life-span considerations
  A. Family defined
    1. Stages
      Transitional
      Beginning
      Young
      Middle
      Mature
      Old Age
    2. Contemporary variations
  B. Multicultural considerations
  C. General implications
    1. Awareness
    2. Receiving the diagnosis
    3. Patient's response to diagnosis
    4. Family response to diagnosis
    5. Life-span considerations
V. Psychological response to treatment
  A. Assessment parameters for the healthcare team
    1. Active treatment phase
    2. Recurrence
    3. Palliative care
    4. Terminal illness
    5. Survivorship
  B. Gender and age differences
    1. Stereotype

Table 8.1 THE RADIATION EXPERIENCE: CAPTURING THE PSYCHOSOCIAL
PATIENT PERSPECTIVE (CONT'D)

2. Coping
3. Developmental concerns
4. Age-based influences
5. Culture and gender
C. Spiritual response
   1. Definition
   2. Spiritual manifestation
   3. Spiritual assessment
   4. Interventions (prayer)
D. Body image
   1. Self-perception
   2. Predicting/defining physical changes
E. Sexuality
   1. Assessment
   2. Intervention
   3. Patient/partner comfort
F. Survivorship
   1. Definition
   2. Continuum/stages of survival
G. Complementary/alternative treatment
   1. Define
   2. Be knowledgeable
   3. Support without bias
   4. Urge integrative approach
H. Influence of fatigue
   1. Incidence
   2. Etiology and classification
   3. Identifying patterns
I. Death/dying/grief/end-of-life care
   1. Meaning
   2. Signs of grief
   3. Coping
   4. Communication
   5. Providing time
   6. Difficult responses

VI. Tips for communicating with patients
A. Prompt open-ended questions
   1. Listen
   2. Cue responses
   3. Avoid closed communication
   4. Role playing

VII. Tips for communicating with family
A. Determine power structure (hierarchy)
   1. How do members communicate?
   2. How do members share information?
   3. Compromise during conflict
   4. Avoid intruding
   5. Identify a "point" person
   6. Stress the positive
VII. Assessment of issues during the
cancer experience
A. How do patients respond to the diagnosis of cancer?
B. What is coping?
C. How do you assess patient coping?
D. When do you make appropriate referrals?
E. Therapeutic use of self-establishing a transpersonal relationship.
F. Going beyond hearing: developing effective listening skills.
G. What does hope mean to individuals with cancer?
H. How to respond to difficult questions.
I. Demystifying fears in a nonjudgmental way.
J. Coping with anxiety.
K. Use of support groups.
L. Unhelpful comments.
M. Helpful comments.
VIII. Practical questions
A. What types of losses have you experienced in the past?
B. How did you react or cope with that loss?
C. What or who helped you get through that difficult situation?
D. What have you been told about your illness and treatment?
E. How do you think your illness most affects you and your family?
F. How does the illness affect your feelings about God, faith, or self? What has bothered you most? How do you make sense of the illness?

Cultural Assessment

Cultural background needs to be considered when caring for patients and families. Due to the nature of this country, nearly every region has an ethnically diverse demographic profile, and each ethnicity has its own cultural aspects. Cultural values and beliefs in such areas as health and illness, family and community, diet, religion, and spirituality, can have a direct impact on patients' expectations and ultimate acceptance of a medical treatment regimen. Beliefs about illness are particularly important as some cultures have their own health professionals such as "shamans" or "curanderos" who could be helpful in the treatment process. It is obviously impossible to fully understand the myriad of cultures and subcultures a nurse may encounter, but it is important to avoid common stereotypes, as one cannot assume that all people of a particular culture are the same. Thus, it is imperative that the patient's own beliefs and values are assessed (Barhamand, 1998; Nishimoto, 1996). If language is a barrier, it is best to use a family member or friend as a translator, if possible; institutionally provided translators often may not be familiar with subtle difference in dialects, and may not be trusted by the patient. It is important that nurses understand potential cultural influences on oncology practice, and remain flexible when caring for these individuals. Development of a set of practice guidelines for assessing cultural values and beliefs can help overcome potential cultural barriers. **Table 8.2** provides an example of cultural assessment criteria for patients and families.

Spiritual Assessment

Spiritual care is an important aspect of the cancer trajectory. Cancer simultaneously challenges the physical, psychological, and spiritual dimensions of an individual (Taylor, 1998). Attention to the spiritual needs of patients and families is critical because a cancer diagnosis can cause spiritual distress that may be countered only by use of spiritual coping strategies to adjust to the illness. The Joint Commission on the Accreditation of Healthcare Organizations (JCAHO) has identified that for many patients, pastoral counseling and spiritual services are an integral part of healthcare. This has resulted in a Joint Commission on the Accreditation of Healthcare Organizations requirement to ensure that healthcare institutions provide pastoral and spiritual services (Taylor, 1998; The Joint Commission on Accreditation of Healthcare Organizations (JCAHO), 1996).

Asking well-phrased questions is key to conducting a comprehensive assessment. Questions should be carefully phrased to avoid the overt use of the words "religion" and "spiritual" (see **Table 8.3**).

The spiritual assessment is a continuous process that encourages patients to participate in information sharing. The rationale for obtaining a spiritual assessment begins after rapport has been established (Taylor, 1998). Because the patient trajectory can span over a significant block of time, nurses can develop a trusting patient/professional relationship. Although radiation facilities are primarily technical, insightful care that demonstrates the healthcare team has individualized interest is important.

Spiritual care is a reciprocal experience in which both patient and nurse exchange vital information that fortifies the patient's journey and enables the nurses role. The following interventions/actions are recommended for the completion of a spiritual nursing assessment:

- Provide the opportunity for patients to talk about spiritual and/or religious concerns.
- Listen and share personal spirituality with patients.
- Pray with patients.
- Be with the patient, especially during difficult moments.
- Provide/suggest religious materials (written material, audiovisual).
- Maintain a respectful, compassionate attitude.
- Arrange appropriate referrals. (Taylor, 1998)

Patient Education

The provision of comprehensive patient education regarding the complexity of radiation treatment will lessen patient and family anxiety, allay fears and misconceptions, and pave the way for the completion of the therapeutic plan. Patient and family education is a pivotal dimension of the clinical radiation oncology nursing. Every aspect of the trajectory of radiation therapy involves an educational domain. Patients require specific education as they experience informed consent, active treatment, radiation-related side effects, and completion of therapy. Family education encompasses an understanding of the current diagnosis, treatment options, and consequences. Patients and families are encouraged to be proactive decision makers so as to ensure treatment completion and commitment to long-term follow up (Haas, 2001; Moore-Higgs et al., 2003a).

A recent survey of staff nurses, nurse managers, and APNs described the activities associated with the patient education role: these activities included 1) providing patients and families with educational materials regarding radiation procedures and side effects, and 2) counseling for social service needs. A majority of staff nurses, nurse managers, and APNs reported spending time with new patients and families to provide education about RT (92%, 80%, and 93%), and many respondents provided symptom management education (98%, 92%, and 93%). In this study, respondents reported conducting patient education that included symptom management during the treatment period and during long-term surveillance (Moore-Higgs et al., 2003a). Radiation oncology nurses are in a pivotal position to provide clinical care based on a model of patient education that will enable the patients and families to understand the diagnosis and the rationale for treatment, recognize reportable consequences, and enhance self-care and family-care skills. A broad educational approach will ultimately facilitate continued care and maintenance (Moore-Higgs et al., 2003a).

Most patients and families welcome educational information; however, the material provided may vary from patient to patient depending on the potential for creating anxiety or negative reactions detrimental to treatment. Educational approaches are individually tailored to the patient's desires. Informing patients of the organizational expectations of the treatment trajectory can avoid unanticipated problems with schedules, such as changes in transportation and outside commitments (professional/personal). Alert patients to the time required for daily treatments and the weekly, routine clinical evaluation with the radiation oncologist and the nurse for the assessment of treatment-related side effects and the development of management interventions. Patients are encouraged to contact the team more frequently if needed and be assured that a clinical professional is available on a 24-hour basis for assistance. Reassure the patient that at the completion of radiation treatments, follow-up appointments will be scheduled and appropriate diagnostic studies and consultations arranged for evaluation of treatment regimen success. Self-evaluation forms are provided during follow-up visits to assess the patient's functional status, reintegration into personal lifestyle, and satisfaction with the overall clinical experience.

Educational material may be presented in a variety of formats to accommodate individualized learning styles of patients and families, including written material, audiovisual material, and/or computer generated educational modules (DVD format, Internet based). The patient's format preference, and ability to comprehend the information need to be assessed. Successful learning requires ample time and an appropriate environment that is quiet and private. Many ambulatory radiation facilities have resource areas specifically designed for patient and family education.

Table 8.2 CULTURAL ASSESSMENT GUIDELINES FOR THE FAMILY WITH CANCER

Assessment Criteria	Sample Questions
Ethnic/racial identity	• From what cultural group does your family originate? • Are both of your parents from the same cultural background? • Does your primary circle of friends and support system have a similar ethnic background?
Language spoken	• What language is spoken at home? • What language are you comfortable using with others away from home?
Place of birth	• Where were you born? Your parents? Your children?
Geographic mobility	• Where have you lived? How long have you been in the United States?
Family religion	• What is your family religion? Is it the same for your spouse? Your parents? • Do you attend religious services regularly? • Do you receive emotional support during times of crisis from clergy or members of your religious organization?
Dietary habits	• Do you follow a special diet? Are there religious or cultural restrictions to your diet?
Access to medical care	• Are there religious or cultural beliefs that affect the kind of medical treatment you can receive? • Does your culture commonly use folk medicine or alternative therapies?
Cultural beliefs about cancer	• Does a cancer diagnosis carry special meaning to people of your cultural background? To your family? • Do you feel comfortable revealing your diagnosis to others?

Note: From Family Nursing Research Therapy and Practice, 4th ed., p. 185, by M. M. Friedman, 1997, Stamford, CT: Appleton & Lange. Copyright 1997. Adapted with permission.

Active Clinical Treatment/Special Considerations in Radiation Oncology

General Clinical Management of Treatment-Related Side Effects

Refinements of radiotherapeutic techniques affect the frequency and degree of side effects that patients may experience. The goal of therapeutic radiation delivery is to maximize the dose of radiation to the target volume while minimizing the dose distribution to surrounding organs and tissue. Although clinically severe and debilitating side effects have lessened, they are not completely eliminated. With the use of dose-escalation techniques to achieve local control and improve survival, the potential for side effects may, in fact, increase. Radiation oncology nurses are expected to provide patients with skilled assessment, preventive management, and expert interventions if side effects are anticipated (Kelly, 1999). The provision of quality side effect management for the ambulatory population of patients receiving highly intense and complex treatment challenges the nurses' skills and abilities. Patients and families can play an important role in side effect management, and need to be encouraged and supported to develop the self-care/caregiver techniques required to do so. (**Table 8.4** details acute and delayed side effects.)

Radiation oncology side effects are categorized as either universal or site specific. Universal side effects are general and manifest independently of the treatment site. These side effects include fatigue and skin effect.

Fatigue

Fatigue is a common side effect of patients with cancer. It is difficult to manage and may be attributed to treatment, the physiologic process of cancer, and/or individual lifestyle. General feelings that patients describe include malaise, decreased energy, inability to perform activities of daily living, and exhaustion (Haylock & Hart, 1979; Mock, Dow, Mears et al., 1997; Piper, Dibble, Dodd et al., 1998). Mechanisms that cause radiation-related fatigue are not well identified. The increase in metabolism that occurs during radia-

---

Table 8.3 SUGGESTED QUESTIONS FOR THE ASSESSMENT OF PATIENTS' SPIRITUALITY

Without religious language

- How would you describe your philosophy of life? Of illness?
- How satisfactory is this philosophy to you now?
- How do you express your spirituality?
- What kinds of practices enhance your spirituality?
- How do you understand hope? For what do you hope?
- What helps you the most when you feel afraid or need special help?
- What is especially meaningful to you now?
- For what do you live? What is most important to you now?
- Has being sick made any difference for you in what or how you believe?
- What does (death, being sick, suffering, pain, etc.) mean to you?
- How do you handle feelings like (anger, doubt, resentment, guilt, bitterness, depression, etc.)? How does your spirituality influence how you respond to such feelings? Do you want spiritual support to deal with such feelings?
- Where do you get the (love, courage, strength, hope, peace, etc.) that you need?

With semireligious language

- How is your faith helping (or not helping) you with your illness?
- How do you experience God or whatever spiritual being(s) to which you relate? For example, is God loving? If so, in what ways?
- Where is God for you now? Where is God for you in this experience?
- How do your spiritual beliefs (or beliefs about the world) impact/influence how you respond to your illness? How does your illness influence your spiritual beliefs (or beliefs about the world)?

Note: Based on information from Dudley, Smith, & Millison, 1995, as well as the author's personal experience.

Table 8.4 ACUTE AND DELAYED SIDE EFFECTS

System/Site	Acute	Delayed/Late	Interventions
Central nervous system	Edema, alopecia, somnolence, radiation myelopathy, fatigue, skin reactions	Necrosis, cerebral atrophy, cranial neuropathies, endocrinopathies (in pituitary tumor), radiation myelopathies	Symptom management and education: steroid taper; teach safe parameters for activities of daily living; coping with loss of independence, understanding potential side effects/signs of recurrence. Identify sources of support: other patients/family and friend caregivers.
Head and neck	Skin reaction, fatigue, stomatitis, mucositis, xerostomia, monoliasis, pharyngitis, laryngitis, esophagitis, anorexia, taste alterations	Dental caries, xerostomia (permanent with > 30 Gy), osteoradionecrosis (with > 70 Gy), trismus	Nutritional assessment: nutritional supplementation, weight and laboratory values (albumin, glucose, electrolytes). Surgical defects healed before radiation begins. Oral cavity assessment: dental consultation; assess/manage stomatitis/mucositis; use oral assessment guides; promote mouth care; sodium bicarbonate, soft toothbrush/gauze/ sponge for cleaning, topical anesthetics for pain, monitor for infection. Dietary modifications (bland, soft food and liquid). New approaches: antibiotic pastille for mucositis; transdermal opioid for xerostomia; artificial saliva; amifostine; avoid tobacco/alcohol; dental consultation, fluoride application; extraction of nonrestorable teeth. Coordinate multidisciplinary support.
Breast	Skin reactions: erythema, hyper-pigmentation, moist or dry desquamation, pruritis, pain, lymphedema, fatigue	Skin changes, hyperpigmentation, telangiectasis, atrophy, fatigue, fibrosis, brachial plexopathy, second malignancies, lymphedema	Interventions focus on skin care, fatigue, and enhanced coping. Promote exercises related to mobility of affected limb and region; teach lymphedema/pneumonitis management if lungs/esophagus in field.

Table 8.4 ACUTE AND DELAYED SIDE EFFECTS (CONT'D)

System/Site	Acute	Delayed/Late	Interventions
Chest/lung (including esophagus)	Fatigue, pharyngitis, esophagitis, dysphagia, "heartburn," anorexia	Pneumonitis, esophageal stricture, fibrosis, cardiac (congestive heart failure, myocardial infarction)	Dyspnea management: repositioning; energy conservation; oxygen and humidification. Pharmacologic management: inhalers; opioids; expectorants; benzodiazepines; corticosteroids. Avoidance of environmental stimulants; monitor hgb/hct levels to assess anemia. Assessment/management of superior vena cava syndrome: emergency radiation/steroids. Manage pharyngitis and esophagitis: dietary modifications (soft, room temperature foods, dietary supplements, bland diets, clear liquids, small frequent meals.) Avoid tobacco, caffeine/alcohol. Special mouthwash: local anesthetic, antacid, antihistamine, and nystatin suspension equal parts prior to meals. Prevention/management of anorexia/cachexia. Manage radiation pneumonitis and fibrosis: teach signs and symptoms of radiation pneumonitis; manage corticosteroids. Ensure advanced treatment planning techniques to avoid pulmonary fibrosis.
Gastrointestinal	Gastritis, ulceration, anorexia, nausea and vomiting; proctitis; stool frequency, urgency, incontinence, tenesmus, pain, bleeding; enteritis; cramping, diarrhea	Fibrosis and vascular insufficiency (chronic ischemia), fistula, perforation ulcer, hemorrhage, obstruction, adhesions, diarrhea	Interventions focus on management of radiosensitivity of mucosa of the GI and GU tracts. Gastritis management: antacids, metoclopramide, sucralfate, and H2 receptor antagonists. Modify diet: small meals, bland food, proper positioning. Manage nausea and vomiting: metoclopramide, phenothiazines, $5HT^3$ serotonin antagonists.
Genitourinary	Cystitis, nocturia, hematuria, incontinence	Hematuria, persistent irritation, hemorrhagic cystitis, fistulas, impotence (prostate)	Radiation induced enteritis and colitis: antidiarrhea diet; low fiber, lactose-free, anticholinergics for diarrhea; bulk laxatives for constipation. Weekly electrolyte panels to assess hydration. Proctitis: assess perianeal skin integrity; sitz baths, skin care, pain medication and perineal pads. Cystitis: anesthetics, antispasmodics, and alpha-blockers.

(continues)

Table 8.4 ACUTE AND DELAYED SIDE EFFECTS (CONT'D)

System/Site	Acute	Delayed/Late	Interventions
Gynecologic	Decreased libido (in ovarian or testicular), hot flashes, dyspareunia, vaginal dryness, irritation, pruritis, skin reactions, diarrhea, cystitis, infections	Vaginal stenosis, dryness, decreased ovarian hormone production leading to early-onset menopause, fistulas	Late effect management: intestinal ulceration; stenosis; hemorrhage; bowel adhesion or obstruction. Focus interventions on surgical management; chronic diarrhea; bowel impairment. Sexual effect: symptomatic treatment; comfort and psychosocial support. Avoid intercourse until symptoms subside; vaginal stenosis; teaching; use of dilators. Fertility issues: impotence erectile dysfunction; access to research-based studies.
Hodgkin's and non-Hodgkin's lymphoma	Mild mucositis, xerostomia, taste alterations, alopecia (occipital area), penumonitis, esophagitis, diarrhea, nausea, vomiting, fatigue, thrombocytopenia, leukopenia	Dental caries, xerostomia, hypothyroidism, penumonitis, pulmonary fibrosis, pericarditis, myocardial infarction, increased risk of sepsis (in splenic radiation therapy or splenectomy), immunologic impairments and second primary cancers, ovarian failure, azoospermia	

tion treatment to eliminate toxic tumor by-products is one possible mechanism. In such cases, more energy is required to repair damaged tissue and cells (Sitton, 1997). The patient's energy reserves are often weakened from other physical and psychological needs. In addition, a relationship appears to exist between radiation dose, field size, and degree of fatigue. A patient who receives treatment of a large anatomic field at a high dose is more susceptible to fatigue than a patient who receives smaller doses to a narrow field. Other factors include underlying medical conditions such as cardiac/pulmonary compromise and depression, chemotherapy, surgery, medications such as antiemetics and narcotics, pain, anemia, respiratory compromise, distance from home, duration of the treatments, and pressure to maintain a normal lifestyle.

The experience of fatigue for the patient receiving radiation therapy can adversely affect the patient's quality of life during and after treatment. Assess the patient for the duration and intensity of fatigue, factors that increase or decrease fatigue, nutritional status, emotional status, the effect of fatigue on daily activities, usual rest and sleep patterns, and undertake appropriate laboratory studies (Beach, Siebeneck, Buderer, & Ferner, 2001). Management of treatment-related fatigue is based on individual needs, and focuses on encouraging self-management. Patients are informed that radiation-induced fatigue is an expected side effect and not necessarily an indication of tumor progression. Suggest that the patient maintain high-calorie and high-protein diet with adequate fluid intake and report signs and symptoms of infection. Monitoring of pertinent laboratory values also needs to be undertaken. Treatment times should be scheduled to accommodate the patients most energized times. Structuring an individualized program, which balances rest with exercise is helpful. Identification of a support network can also lessen treatment-induced fatigue (Sarna & Conde, 2001).

Skin Changes

Most patients receiving radiation will experience skin-related side effects. Skin cells originate from rapidly reproducing differentiated stem cells that are exquisitely radiosensitive. Radiation treatment has a cellular effect, which causes a localized tissue response on the protective mechanisms of the skin (Moore-Higgs & Amdur, 2001). Radiation treatment can affect the two layers of the skin, the dermis and the epidermis. Ionizing radiation affects the highly mitotic cells of the epidermis, hair follicles, and sebaceous glands. The three most common types of skin reaction are erythema and dry or moist desquamation. Erythema is a generalized reddening of the skin in the treatment field. This may occur after 5 to 10 treatments and is characterized by itchy, red, raised vesicles. Erythema occurs because of an increase in capillary blood flow that progresses from opening of the vessels to congestion. Dry desquamation appears as scaly, flaky skin, which causes itching, peeling, and shedding. This occurs in response to radiation damage to the basal cells of the epidermis. Moist desquamation is characterized by reddened, weeping skin that is warm and tight to the touch with a shiny appearance. Skin with moist desquamation produces a clear to cloudy drainage, with random areas of crust or scab formation. This occurs in response to complete destruction of the epidermis. Often erythema occurs before moist desquamation, looks like a second-degree burn; it is painful, and can develop a secondary infection such as Candida, cytomegalovirus, and aspergillus.

Skin assessment is undertaken before treatment begins to identify predisposing factors that may enhance skin reaction. A complete visual examination of the skin within the treatment field (including beam exit points) is conducted during treatment and at follow-up appointments. The following grading systems have been developed for early and late skin effects to radiation: the (NCI) Common Toxicity Criteria, Version 2.0. and The Radiation Therapy Oncology Group (RTOG), Toxicity Criteria, Version 2.0 or the RTOG SOMA Scales. Additionally, the ONS Radiation Therapy Patient Care Record for Skin is designed to assist nursing professionals with monitoring patients and accurately documenting care (Catlin-Huth, Haas, & Pollock, 2002).

Outcome management related to skin effect focuses on reducing identified risk factors for skin reaction, complying with practice guidelines for recommended skin products, minimizing trauma and irritation, preventing infection, and maintaining patient dignity and quality of life (Olsen et al., 2001).

Site-Specific Side Effects

Radiation-induced site-specific side effects occur in the local/regional area of the treatment field and are usually predictable. Site-specific side effect management focuses on the assessment and development of interventions related to a specific anatomical area of radiation treatment. This requires skilled assessment, expert teaching skills, anticipatory guidance abilities, provision of preventive measures, and understanding of techniques required for in-home care on the part of the radiation oncology nurse (Kelly, 1999). The knowledge fundamental to these skills is a solid grounding in the anatomy and physiology of specific treatment regions.

Side effect management, universal and site-specific, in a busy ambulatory setting poses a significant challenge and opportunity for radiation oncology nurses. Ambulatory oncology practice necessitates individualized patient and family management under conditions that often require rapid clinical response related to the entire trajectory of cancer care. The development and implementation of a practice model that is comprehensive, founded on a philosophy of quick and safe response, and able to provide effective care for acute or chronic, universal or site-specific problems is a priority need.

Special Clinical Considerations

The clinical practice of radiation oncology nursing has expanded from general professional functions to specific and intricate clinical capacities. The advancement of patient care requirements in radiation oncology has demanded that nurses manage the complex intricacies of every dimension of patient care. The radiation oncology–nursing role includes dimensions of assessment, triage, interdisciplinary collaboration, education, intervention, documentation, and evaluation (Moore-Higgs et al., 2003b). Contemporary radiation oncology nurses have extended these clinical dimensions and embraced the challenge of innovative practice. Nurses have assumed a proactive role by identifying the need for, and developing practice standards, with appropriate clinical guidelines, which ensure the safe delivery of highly technical care. One example is the development of clinical standards for the use of intensity-modulated radiotherapy, three-dimensional conformal radiotherapy, and dose-escalation studies for patients with implanted cardiac pacemakers in the treatment field (Hogle, 2001). Cardiac pacemaker malfunction can occur at radiation doses ranging from 1,500 cGy to 3,960 cGy. Policies regarding nursing care of patients with implanted cardiac pacemakers vary among facilities. Standardized recommendations for caring for implanted cardiac pacemakers patients receiving external beam radiotherapy were developed to facilitate patient assessment and to differentiate between pacemaker irregularities and treatment-related side effects (Hogle, 2001).

A second example of a proactive role involves radioimmunotherapy, which is now a viable ambulatory treatment option. Ambulatory oncology nurses facilitated the development of an outpatient radioimmunotherapy treatment model for patients with non-Hodgkin's lymphoma. This model addresses coordinated collaborative patient care, safe delivery of radioimmunotherapy in an outpatient setting, and the establishment of an education program for the interdisciplinary medical team, patient, and family. The goal of this model was to conserve inpatient resources, to enhance patient and caregiver morale and satisfaction by providing support in the home environment, and to improve patient compliance. This effort provided the framework for a classic acute level of care model for the ambulatory environment (Hendrix & deLeon, 2002). The development of a thorough educational template for professionals and for patients was a priority considered integral to the overall success.

Gamma knife stereotactic radiosurgery is a device often used during neurosurgical procedures. The gamma knife emits individual cobalt radiation beams that converge on a specific target to destroy it. The role of a radiosurgical subspecialty nurse is relatively new and evolving. This nursing professional serves as the liaison for the patient throughout the treatment process (DeLaune, Jawahar, & Nanda, 2002). Few formal orientation programs for this subspecialty exist; these nurses rely on professional colleague networking to delineate role dimensions, practice parameters, and standards of care. The role of the gamma knife nurse is a relatively independent one. Neurosurgical nurses have identified the special clinical considerations of this nursing role. Such nurses require a thorough understanding of neuroanatomy and principles of radiosurgery and technical patient care and management skills needed in this specialty practice. This exemplifies the need for nursing specialties to collaborate in determining educational and practice standards in response to technologic advances in the field.

Another special clinical consideration in radiation therapy focuses on the role of palliative services in managing the severe implications of advanced disease. An interdisciplinary team consisting of two radiation oncologists—one radiation oncology nurse and rotating radiation therapists—formed a palliative radiation therapy rapid response clinic to provide immediate radiotherapy relief for distressing symptoms of advanced disease (Andersson & Sousa, 1998). This innovation was in response to recognized delays, because of lack of personnel and technologic resources, for the treatment of terminally ill patients in Canada. Economic constraints also contributed to delays. Institutional, administrative, and government support was sought to support this effort, and marketing was initiated to encourage local and regional referrals. The success of this service was overwhelming, and the concept has been adopted at other distant facilities. This is a prime example of an interdisciplinary radiation team identifying a gap in cancer care, prioritizing the issue, gaining support, and promoting the service.

Quality-Assurance Parameters

Radiation therapy facilities are required to have an established quality-assurance program, with associated policies and procedures, to ensure the comprehensive administration, surveillance, and documentation of the quality of treatment regimens. Quality-assurance programs in radiation therapy vary depending on 1) whether standard treatment or a clinical trial is administered, and 2) whether the services are provided in a single or multiple institutional setting. For multiple institution programs, clear instructions and standardized parameters in dosimetry procedures, and treatment, planning, and administrative processes are required for all participants. Patterns of care studies have demonstrated a direct correlation between the quality of radiation therapy services and clinical outcomes (Behrend & Coia, 1999). The clinical director usually appoints a quality-

assurance committee that meets regularly to review the results of audits, physics quality-assurance reports, outcome studies, mortality and morbidity statistics, cases of "misadministration" or error where the delivery of greater than 10% of intended dose, and incident reports (Chao et al., 1999).

The administration of therapeutic radiation requires precise technology. Slight percentages of an increase or decrease in the intended dose level can represent the success or failure of the treatment course. Thus, precision of basic dosimetry for different types and qualities of radiation, applied dosimetry for dose planning, and in vivo dosimetry is an absolute requirement. External audits are employed to avoid systemic error and comparative dose measurements to establish variations within a department and between departments. Simulators and therapeutic equipment are to be checked regularly to assure that the direction of the radioactive beam and the field size complies with the plan. Margins that are too narrow can miss part of the target volume and increase the risk for relapse. If the margins are too wide, the potential for side effects involving nearby organs may present a clinical risk. Accessible field control images are to be integrated regularly, particularly when the margins between tumors and healthy organs are small (Behrend, 2000; Nicolaou, 1999).

The two primary dimensions of a quality-assurance program for radiation oncology facilities are a technical quality surveillance program for therapy services, and an organized quality improvement program to enhance organizational performance. The steps involved in the quality-assurance process include the identification of desired technical process and patient outcomes, with associated specific and measurable criteria for quality defined, for each service provided. The result of the process determines the level at which quality standards are achieved. If there are areas in which desired performance standards are not met, the quality improvement program identifies associated problems and the means for enhancing quality achievement.

An effective quality-assurance program involves all levels of staff in all components of the program. The processes or outcomes under review can be illustrated through the use of flow sheets and diagrams that clearly identify the desired clinical results and the measures for relevant data collection and statistical analysis (Bruner et al., 1998). If processes and outcomes do not meet expectations, the causes of variation are pinpointed and opportunities for improvement or correction are identified and developed. An example of the process of a quality improvement project in radiation oncology is shown in **Table 8.5**.

The blend of technology and clinical patient management in radiation oncology facilities creates a natural environment for the development and actualization of comprehensive quality improvement systems. With administrative support and full staff participation, a quality-assurance framework allows for improved facility function on a daily and future basis. Quality-assurance indicators provide data to support clinical, technical, and administrative outcome measures that serve to validate individual and collective professional practice standards. Radiation oncology nurses are in key positions to develop and administrate this vital aspect of professional accountability.

Documentation

Documentation of clinical care is an important component of professional nursing practice. In contemporary clinical environments, the medical record has tremendous value to patients, to the healthcare system, and to a variety of external systems that require institutional documentation of service delivery (Teytelman, 2002). Documentation systems validate what type of care is offered, how it is administered, what the outcomes are, and the patient response. Oncology nurses responsibilities include the completion of comprehensive documentation of patient care

(Stromborg, Christensen, & Elmhurst, 2001a). Emerging technology has created innovative ways to record, deliver, and receive patient records (facsimile, telephone, e-mail, computer charging) (Tuma, 2002). However, these emerging electronic venues for documentation carry a risk of compromising the privacy of patient records, and the institutional responsibilities and liability related to these records (Stromborg et al., 2001a). For instance, secured access to computerized patient records may be difficult to achieve, and is an ongoing concern. Nonetheless, a recent review of nursing documentation suggested that when nurses support institutional documentation requirements and guidelines, patient records are more accurately maintained and patient care is enhanced (Stromborg et al., 2001a).

Requirements for nursing documentation include written records of assessments and the specific interventions planned in response to assessments. Nurses are liable for improper or incomplete documentation of patient care; the law presumes that if the work is not documented it was not done (Stromborg, Christensen, & Elmhurst, 2001b). Oncology nurses are required to adhere to strict practice guidelines for documentation to avoid malpractice litigation, which occurs frequently and is very costly. Nurses are trained to avoid liability by keeping up to date on state-of-the-art practices, identifying risk factors associated with documentation, implementing risk-reduction practices, and adhering to these practices.

The specialty of oncology nursing has identified and responded to the need for improvement and standardization of documentation systems for oncology patients. In 1990, the ONS RT SIG created a work group to analyze existing documentation systems and to focus on improved documentation support of side-effect management and patient education encounters for individuals receiving radiation therapy. This work group together with ONS published the first edition of Radiation Therapy Patient Care Record.

Table 8.5 AN EXAMPLE OF THE PROCESS OF A QUALITY IMPROVEMENT PROJECT IN RADIATION ONCOLOGY

---

1. Select a process or outcome to improve.
   A. Functional care of patients
      1. Process: management of moist desquamation
      2. Outcome: treatment break for moist desquamation
   B. Rationale
      1. Primary treatment of breast cancer with radiation therapy involves a high volume of patients.
      2. Moist desquamation is a significant problem, resulting in pain, infection, or the need for treatment break.
2. Form team of knowledgeable staff to perform question and answer measures.
3. Clarify understanding of the process.
4. Measure the current level of performance.
5. Assess the data.
6. Improve the process.

This is now the standard radiation therapy documentation tool in many radiation facilities in the United States.

In 2002, the ONS and the RT SIG published a revised edition of the Radiation Therapy Patient Care Record (Catlin-Huth et al., 2002). This edition contains suggested modifications from RT SIG members for improved implementation of the tools. The revised edition provides nurses with general forms such as an initial nursing assessment/database (see **Figure 8.7**) and the patient medication form (see **Figure 8.8**). A series of radiotherapy site-specific assessment tools are provided using a flow sheet format with associated keys for assessment scales. A comprehensive teaching and instruction form accompanies each site-specific patient care record (see **Figure 8.9**).

Documentation of care in a busy ambulatory radiation oncology center can present a tremendous challenge for nurses with all of the concomitant responsibilities that arise during the course of a clinical day. It is imperative that time is allotted and used to document the care rendered and to validate the effort to institute interventions. Documentation is the essence of the patient nurse encounter. It validates the effort to assess, manage, and intervene. Documentation systems serve as invaluable means for interdisciplinary communication and collaboration. Radiation oncology settings need to be dedicated to ensuring that a documentation system tailored to the facilities specific needs is established, promoted, and used.

Ethical Dimension

Ambulatory oncology care is a complex component of healthcare that requires expert clinical skills of nursing professionals practicing in this specialty. The environment of ambulatory oncology blends highly technical application of cancer diagnosis, treatment, and symptom management with equally important functions of patient education, telephone triage, symptom management, and coordination of support networks (Christensen, 2002). A radiation oncology nurse's practice is characterized by many brief patient encounters. Potential ethical issues related to the brevity of the visit include the need to offer comprehensive patient education regarding technical aspects of treatment and symptom management, the use of telephone triage to manage patient needs, maintaining patient confidentiality, interfacing with multidisciplinary teams of professionals, and interrelating with the patient or the designated patient representative regarding personal and professional needs.

An effective patient/healthcare provider relationship is founded on ethical principles that define patient rights and directly influence quality of care. Mutual identification of patient expectations is vital for the establishment, of a lasting therapeutic relationship between the professional staff and patients and their families. Patient rights include:

- The right to be treated as a human being with respect and consideration, regardless of race, gender, creed, or national origin.
- The right to feel secure with the healthcare program. The patient has a right to obtain complete, current information concerning diagnosis, treatment, and prognosis in understandable terms.
- The right to privacy. Discussion of the patient's condition, examinations, or treatment records is confidential. Written permission is required for release of information
- The right to service. Requests for services are to be fulfilled, within reasonable limits.
- The right to understand the cost of treatment. A forum for discussion of financial arrangements is to be provided.
- The right to be advised of education or research activities. Patients need to know the identity and professional status of the multidisciplinary team. If the patient is treated in a teaching institution, student training programs (preceptorships/residencies/fellowships/internships) are to be explained. Patients are to be advised of opportunities to partake in clinical trials, with the associated right of refusal to participate. All trials must be institutional review board approved, and investigational consent forms must be signed.
- The right to counseling about consequences of refusal of treatment. Certified

letters, with return receipt required, are sent to individuals who refused to begin, to continue, or to follow-up with planned treatment course (Chao et al., 1999).

Conclusion

The nuances of radiation oncology practice are founded on the impressive evolution of this cancer treatment modality. The focus on the technologic aspects of radiobiology and medical physics coupled with clinical patient management has distinguished radiation practice as a unique entity. Radiation oncology facilities have embraced the ambulatory model of care long before other oncology subspecialties. The resiliency of this specialty in responding to external and internal forces that have influence on the environment of practice has been exemplary. The history of radiation oncology is a rich blend of basic science and clinical trials that enhance the effort to refine and improve this specialty. Scientists and clinicians routinely work together in multidisciplinary teams to translate the latest research findings into improved patient care in the clinical setting.

Operational and administrative structures of radiation facilities vary and are structured according to the type of setting, the demographic location, and available resources. The ambulatory model of radiation practice has provided this cancer treatment modality to individuals living in both rural and urban environments in the United States. Concomitant clinical and support services are available in regional areas, and provide a variety of therapeutic options and eliminate the stress of lack of access. The presence of a dedicated, progressive clinical team is a prerequisite for this complex cancer specialty area to function. Nurses are a pivotal component of the multidisciplinary radiation oncology team. The professional role of radiation oncology nursing has evolved to include the full realm of every aspect of the specialty. Continued professional role development of radiation oncology nurses will ensure this vital pres-

Figure 8.7 INITIAL NURSING ASSESSMENT/DATABASE FORM

RADIATION THERAPY
INITIAL NURSING ASSESSMENT/DATABASE

Patient _____ MR#/RT# _____ Radiation Oncologist _____ Date _____

Diagnosis _____ Prefers Appointment in: AM _____ PM _____

VITAL SIGNS			
Temp:	Pulse:	Resp:	O₂ Sat:
BP:	Height:	Weight:	Pain (0–10) ____Site _____ Describe:_____

HISTORY OF PRESENT ILLNESS
Chief complaint:

Prior radiation therapy? ____No ____Yes, site treated _____ Facility _____
Prior chemotherapy? ____No ____Yes, last treatment _____ Facility _____
Prior hormonal therapy? ____No ____Yes, last treatment _____ Facility _____

CURRENT MEDICATION/ALLERGIES
See Patient Medication Record

PAST MEDICAL HISTORY	
Medical:	Surgical:
Transfusion hx:	Family cancer hx:

SOCIAL HISTORY/HABITS				
Lives with _____		Transportation _____		
Tobacco ____Yes, Pack-year history _____ ____No ____Quit _____		ETOH ____Yes, freq _____ ____Quit _____		
Sleep hx:	Insomnia ____Yes ____No None _____	Difficulty getting to sleep _____	Difficulty maintaining sleep _____	Early AM awakening _____

REVIEW OF SYSTEMS				
Constitutional	Fatigue level 0–4 ____	Fevers ___Yes ___No	Night sweats ____Yes ___No	Weight loss ____No ____Yes, ___lb / ___months
Eyes	Vision blurred ___Yes___No	Blind ____Yes ____No	Requires: ____Glasses ____Contacts	
Ears, Nose, Mouth, Throat	Hearing loss ____Yes ___No (Circle) R / L / Both sides	Difficulty swallowing ___Yes ___No	New lumps ____Yes ___No Location:	
	Hearing aid(s) ___Yes ___No	Dentures ____None ____Upper ____Lower	Dental condition ____Good _____Fair _____Requires consult	
Cardiovascular/ Respiratory	Heart attack ____Yes ___No	Cough ___Yes ___No	Orthopnea ___Yes___No # pillows req _____	
	Stroke ____Yes ___No	Dyspnea __Yes __ No		
	Angina ___Yes ___No	O₂ @ ____L/min	Hemoptysis ___Yes ___No	
	Pacer ___Yes ___No		Other:	

Figure 8.8 PATIENT MEDICATION RECORD FORM

PATIENT _____ MR#/RT# _____ DATE _____

PATIENT MEDICATION RECORD

Allergies_____

Pharmacy_____ Telephone_____

CHEMOTHERAPY

NEOADJUVANT (N) CONCURRENT (C)		DRUGS	LAST COURSE	FUTURE COURSE(S)	MEDICAL ONCOLOGIST
N	C				
N	C				
N	C				
N	C				

MEDICATIONS

DATE (PTA = prior to admission)	MEDICATION	DOSE	ROUTE	FREQ	DC'D	SAMPLES	REFILLS Amt Dispensed/ # of Refills/ Date Refilled/Initials

_____ ( )   _____ ( )   _____ ( )
Signature   Initials   Signature   Initials   Signature   Initials

Figure 8.9 Radiation Therapy Patient Care Record—Skin Form

PATIENT _____ MR #/RT# _____ DATE _____

RADIATION THERAPY PATIENT CARE RECORD—SKIN

Site		Surgical Procedure	
Histology		**Keloid (Y / N)**	
Grade/Stage		**Protocol**	
Recurrence (Y / N) Location		**Other**	

ASSESSMENTS									
Dates									
(cGy or Gy) / Fx									
Comfort Alteration KPS									
Fatigue									
Pain Location									
Pain Intensity									
Pain Intervention									
Effectiveness of Pain Intervention									
Nutrition Alteration Weight									
Skin Alteration Skin Sensation									
Radiation Dermatitis									
Mucous Membrane Alteration									
Drainage									
Drainage Odor									
Emotional Alteration									
Coping									
Injury, Potential Bleeding/Infection Date									
WBC									
Hemoglobin/Hematocrit									
Platelets									
Vital Signs									
TPR									
BP									
Other									
INITIALS									

(continues)

Figure 8.9 RADIATION THERAPY PATIENT CARE RECORD—SKIN FORM (CONT'D)

PATIENT _____ MR#/RT# _____ DATE _____

TEACHING AND INSTRUCTIONS—SKIN

	DATES/ INITIALS	METHOD	EVALUATION	PLAN	COMMENTS
General Care Nutrition					
Social Service					
Discharge Care					
Referrals					
Site-Specific Simulation					
Initial Treatment					
Side Effects					
Fatigue Management					
Pain Intervention					
Skin Care					
Prevention/Other Skin Self-Exam					
Ultraviolet Protection					
Smoking Cessation					

Method Codes
A = Personal session
B = Family conference
C = Booklet (specify)
D = Demonstration
E = Audio/video resource

Evaluation Codes
UE = Unable to evaluate (explain)
V = Verbalizes concept accurately
D = Demonstrates skill accurately
R = Needs review
NR = Not receptive to learning at this time (explain)

Plan Codes
RC = Reinforce concept
RD = Return demonstration
LOM = Learning objective met
RF = Referral to other health care givers (specify)

SOCIAL INFORMATION
Lives With (specify relationships)
Agency in Home
Durable Medical Equipment in Home
Transportation
Prescription Coverage
Other

( )   ( )   ( )
_____ _____   _____ _____   _____ _____
Signature   Initials   Signature   Initials   Signature   Initials

ence. Nurses are infused in every aspect of radiation oncology care and have been integrated in the entire trajectory of patient care management, support services, clinical research, administration, and consultation. It is through the perpetuation of a strong radiation oncology nursing subspecialty that the success of facilities will depend.

Patients receiving radiation treatment require intense preparation, expert monitoring during treatment, and a methodical plan for continued surveillance once treatment is completed. The interdisciplinary team provides these aspects of care and focuses on the concomitant challenges of addressing complex needs while remaining dedicated to the tenets of an ambulatory care model. Interwoven in this ambulatory model are legal and ethical issues, regulatory and quality assurance requirements, fiduciary constraints, and competition for services. Radiation oncology continues to evolve by responding to challenging environmental cues. With a dedicated, well-educated, creative, and flexible professional team approach, it is possible for this specialty to continue to provide the progressive template for oncology ambulatory care models.

Appendix A

The following series of photographs provide an overview of the trajectory of requirements for the delivery of radiation therapy. Radiation Oncology is an integral specialty in the arena of cancer treatment. Refinements in treatment planning commonly referred to as simulation; coupled with precise tools to localize tumors and to protect surrounding vital anatomic structures provides patients with effective local-regional radiotherapy.

Photo 1 (Cat Scan Simulator) and **Photo 2** (MRI Simulator) are used to identify exact anatomic region of tumor target. These treatment-planning machines provide key information for medical physicists and dosimetrists to develop precise plans for radiotherapy beam placement. These plans include target volumes as well as identification of vital tissues and organs to be spared. The MRI Simulator (Photo 2) is useful for identification and localization of deeply seated tumors (such as genitourinary malignancies).

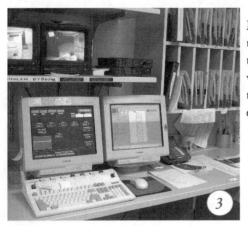
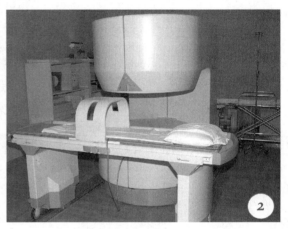

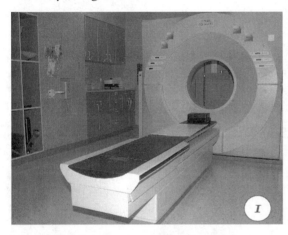

Photo 3 (Radiotherapist Control Center/Patient Monitoring Station) depicts computer terminals used by the radiotherapists for machine calibration according to the radiation oncologist's prescription. Additionally, the video screens provide both visual and audio monitoring of the interior of the treatment room, which is necessary to ensure patient safety and equipment function.

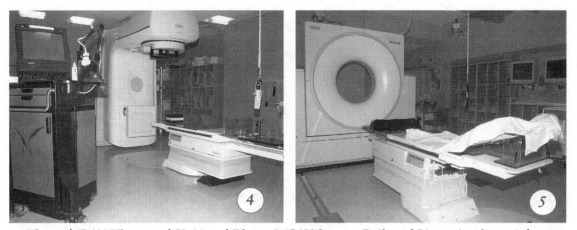

Photo 4 (BAT Ultrasound Unit) and **Photo 5** (CAT Scan on Rails and Linear Accelerator) demonstrate equipment used to deliver external beam (teletherapy) radiation. In Photo 4 the BAT Ultrasound Unit is used to localize the contours of deeply seated tumors such as the prostate gland and then to deliver simultaneous radiation treatment using the adjacent Linear Accelerator. Photo 5 demonstrates a CAT scan unit on a rail system (located on the floor of the treatment room). Prior to receiving treatment, the patient lies stationary on the Linear Accelerator treatment table and the mobile CAT scan unit moves along the rails and provides additional treatment field details such as tumor localization and precise anatomic region for tumor targeting.

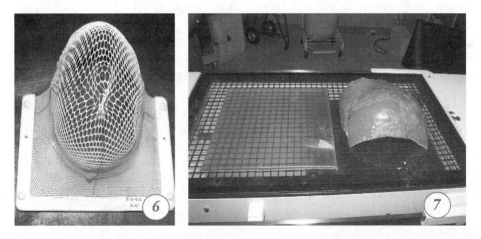

A course of radiation treatment depends upon successful replication of exact laser guided beam placement during each successive treatment. **Photo 6 (Aquaplast Head and Neck Immobilizer)** depicts immobilization equipment for the head and neck region, which is used to safely and comfortably position patients during treatment to avoid unnecessary movement that could alter the prescribed treatment beams. **Photo 7 (Bolus Material)** illustrates a selection of two types of bolus material; one of a firm gel substance and one of a wax mold that are used to increase the skin effect of the radiation beam.

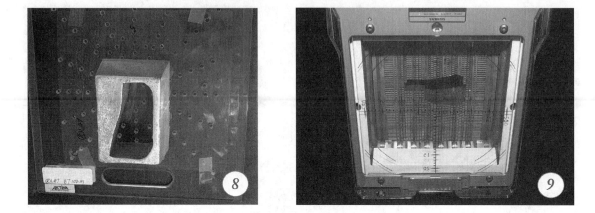

The essence of radiation treatment is the ability of the multi-disciplinary team to target the tumor and surrounding anatomic margins while sparing approximating tissues and vital organs. These photos provide visuals of two mechanisms used to accomplish this. **Photo 8 (Custom Lead Block)** depicts a custom lead block mounted on a plexi-glass shield that inserts into the gantry of the linear accelerator and is contoured to protect surrounding tissues and organs from radiation beams. **Photo 9 (Multi-Leaf Collimator)** shows a multi-leaf collimator unit, which is comprised of small lead leaves that are custom, adjusted by computerized programming to shield vital tissues and organs adjacent to the tumor target.

Photo 10 and **Photo 11** Illustrate a dedicated high dose rate treatment room and High Dose Rate (HDR) equipment respectively. This treatment area and equipment are used to administer and monitor the delivery of Brachytherapy and implanted radiation therapy sources. These are treatment regimens that are given safely and effectively to ambulatory populations utilizing implanted radioactive sources of high dose and short duration.

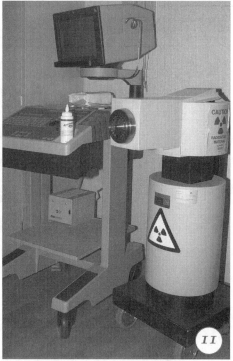

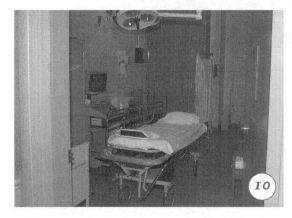

References

American College of Radiology. (1991). Radiation oncology in integrated cancer management: Report of the Inter-Society Council for radiation oncology. Reston, VA: Author.

Anderson, K. L. & Bruce, S. D. (2002). Putting your best foot forward in a challenging role: Finding the resources needed to work in a freestanding radiation oncology clinic. *Clinical Journal of Oncology Nursing, 6*, 225–227.

Andersson, L. & Sousa, P. (1998). In Profile - An innovative way of caring: Palliative radiation therapy rapid response clinic. *Canadian Oncology Nursing Journal, 8*, 146–147.

Arneill, B. P. & Nuelsen, P. H. (1999). Organize for success: Seven steps to a successful building project. *Journal of Ambulatory Care Management, 22*, 58–66.

Babcock, J. M. (2000). ARTICLE REVIEW of Non-physician practitioners in radiation oncology: Advanced practice nurses and physician assistants. *Clinical Excellence for Nurse Practitioners, 4*, 254–255.

Backus, A. (2001). R.T. Shortage: One college's search for answers. *Radiology Management, May/June*, 36–39.

Barhamand, B. A. (1998). *Coping with Cancer: Family Issues. In Psychosocial Dimensions of Oncology Nursing Care* (pp. 27–52). Pittsburgh, PA: Oncology Nursing Press.

Beach, P., Siebeneck, B., Buderer, N. F., & Ferner, T. (2001). Relationship between fatigue and nutritional status in patients receiving radiation therapy to treat lung cancer. *Oncology Nursing Forum, 28*, 1027–1031.

Behrend, S. W. (2000). Radiotherapy administration techniques. In C. H. Yarbro, M. H. Frogge, M. Goodman, & S. L. Groenwald (Eds.), *Cancer Nursing Principles and Practice* (pp. 300–322). Sudbury, MA: Jones and Bartlett Publishers.

Behrend, S. W. & Coia, L. R. (1999). Patterns of care in radiation oncology. *Seminars in Oncology Nursing, 15*, 303–312.

Bell, K. L. (1999). Planning ahead: Practical hints for designing ambulatory care facilities. *Journal of Ambulatory Care Management, 22*, 74–88.

Bigbee, J. L. (1996). History and evolution of advanced nursing practice. In A. B. Hamric, J. A. Spross, & C. H. Hanson (Eds.), *Advanced Nursing Practice: An Integrative Approach* (pp. 3–24). Philadelphia: W.B. Saunders Company.

Boyle, D. M. (1995). Documentation and outcomes of advanced nursing practice. *Oncology Nursing Forum, 22*(suppl), 11–17.

Bruner, D. W. (1990). Report on the radiation oncology nursing subcommittee of the American College of Radiology Task Force on Standards Development. *Oncology, 4*, 80–81.

Bruner, D. W. (1993). Radiation oncology nurses: Staffing patterns and role development. *Oncology Nursing, 20*, 651–655.

Bruner, D. W., Dunn-Bucholtz, J., Iwamoto, R., & Strohl, R. (1998). *Manual for Radiation Oncology Nursing Practice and Education*. Pittsburgh, PA: Oncology Nursing Press.

Bucholtz, J. D. (1987). Radiation therapy. In C. Ziegfield (Ed.), *Core Curriculum for Oncology Nursing* (pp. 207–224). Philadelphia: W.B. Saunders Company.

Carlson, L. E., Bultz, B. D., Speca, M., & St. Pierre, M. (2000). Partners of cancer patients: Part I. Impact, adjustment, and coping across the illness trajectory. *Journal of Psychosocial Oncology, 18*, 39–63.

Catlin-Huth, C., Haas, M., & Pollock, V. (2002). *Radiation Therapy Patient Care Record: A Tool for Documenting Nursing Care*. Pittsburgh, PA: Oncology Nursing Society.

Chao, K. S. C., Perez, C. A., & Brady, L. W. (1999). *Radiation Oncology: Management Decisions*. Philadelphia: Lippincott-Raven.

Christensen, A. (2002). Legal and ethical issues confronting oncology nursing. *Seminars in Oncology Nursing, 18*, 86–98.

DeLaune, A., Jawahar, A., & Nanda, A. (2002). The Gamma knife nurses: Defining roles and responsibilities. *Journal of Neuroscience Nursing, 34*, 25–29.

Dow, K. H. (1997). Nursing research in radiation oncology. In K. H. Dow, J. Dunn-Bucholtz, R. Iwamoto, V. Fieler, & L. J. Hilderley (Eds.), *Nursing Care in Radiation Oncology* (2nd ed., pp. 421–431). Philadelphia: W.B. Saunders Company.

Downing, J. (1998). Radiotherapy nursing: Understanding the nurse's role. *Nursing Standard, 12*, 42–43.

Downing, J. (2001). Oncology out-patients nursing: A challenge within the changing fact of cancer care. *European Journal of Oncology Nursing, 5*, 49–59.

Galassi, A. & Wheeler, V. (1994). Advanced practice nursing: History and future trends. *Oncology Nursing, 1*, 1–10.

Girouard, S. A. (1996). Evaluating advanced nursing practice. In A. B. Hamric, J. A. Spross, & C. M. Hanson (Eds.), *Advanced Nursing Practice: An Integrative Approach* (pp. 569–600). Philadelphia: W.B. Saunders Company.

Gorman, L. M. (1998). The psychosocial impact of cancer on the individual, family, and society. In R. M. Carroll-Johnson, L. M. Gorman, & N. J. Bush (Eds.), *Psychosocial Nursing Care: Along the Cancer Continuum* (pp. 3–25). Pittsburgh, PA: Oncology Nursing Press.

Gritz, E. R., Wellisch, D. K., Siau, J., & Wang, H. (1990). Long-term effects of testicular cancer on marital relationships. *Psychosomatics, 31*, 301–312.

Haas, S. (1998). Ambulatory care nursing conceptual framework. *AAACN Viewpoint, 20,* 16–17.

Haas, S. A. (2001). Ambulatory care nursing specialty practice. In J. Robinson (Ed.), *Core Curriculum for Ambulatory Care Nursing* (pp. 3–15). Philadelphia: W.B. Saunders Company.

Haberman, M. (2000). Advancing cancer nursing through nursing research. In C. H. Yarbro, M. H. Frogge, M. Goodman, & S. L. Groenwald (Eds.), *Cancer Nursing Principles and Practice* (pp. 1728–1740). Sudbury, MA: Jones and Bartlett Publishers.

Haylock, P. & Hart, L. (1979). Fatigue in patients receiving localized radiation. *Cancer Nursing, 2,* 461–467.

Hendrix, C. & deLeon, C. (2002). Establishing a radioimmunotherapy outpatient care clinical for non-Hodgkin's lymphoma. *Seminars in Oncology Nursing, 18* (Supplement-February), 22–29.

Hilderley, L. J. (1980). The role of the nurse in radiation oncology. *Seminars in Oncology, 7,* 39–47.

Hilderley, L. J. (1991). Nurse-physician collaborative practice: The clinical nurse specialist in radiation oncology private practice. *Oncology Nursing Forum, 18,* 585–591.

Hinrichs, M. (1997). Advanced radiation therapy practitioners: A specialty of the future? *Radiation Therapist: The Journal of the Radiation Oncology Sciences, 6,* 57–62.

Hogle, W. P. (2001). Pacing the standard of nursing practice in radiation oncology. *Clinical Journal of Oncology Nursing, 5,* 253–256.

Holland, J. C. (1989). Clinical course of cancer. In J. C. Holland & J. H. Rowland (Eds.), *Handbook of Psychooncology: Psychological Care of the Patient with Cancer* (pp. 75–100). New York: Oxford University Press.

Iwamoto, R. & Gough, S. (1993). Radiotherapy: Ambulatory care models. In P. Buchsel & C. H. Yarbro (Eds.), *Oncology Nursing in the Ambulatory Setting.* Sudbury, MA: Jones and Bartlett Publishers.

Kelly, L. D. (1999). Nursing assessment and patient management. *Seminars in Oncology Nursing, 15,* 282–291.

Kelvin, J. F., Moore-Higgs, G. J., Maher, K. E., Dubey, A. K., Austin-Seymour, M. M., Daly, N. R. et al. (1999). Non-physician practitioners in radiation oncology: Advanced practice nurses and physician assistants. *International Journal of Radiation Oncology Biology Physics, 45,* 255–263.

Lamkin, L., Rosiak, J., Buerhaus, P., Mallory, G., & Williams, M. (2001). Oncology Nursing Society workforce survey Part I: Perceptions of the nursing workforce environment and adequacy of nurse staffing in outpatient and inpatient oncology settings. *Oncology Nursing Forum, 28,* 1545–1552.

LaRue, L. J. (2002). Integrated psychosocial care of patients with cancer in the ambulatory setting. *Oncology Supportive Care, 1,* 7–18.

Loescher, L. J. (2000). The influence of technology on cancer nursing. *Seminars in Oncology Nursing, 16,* 3–11.

Lowenstein, G. (2002). New realities shape future radiology delivery models. *Radiology Management, 24,* 22–25.

Luckett, D. R. (2000). Recruitment and retention topics for a changing environment in medical imaging. *Radiology Management, September/October, 32–37.*

Lynch, M. P., Cope, D. G., & Murphy-Ende, K. (2001). Advanced practice issues: Results of the ONS Advanced Practice Nursing Survey. *Oncology Nursing Forum, 28,* 1521–1530.

Mazurowski, J. (2001). Recruitment & retention in seven easy steps. *Radiology Management, May/June,* 42–43.

McCarty, P. J. & Million, R. R. (1994). History of diagnosis and treatment of cancer in the head and neck. In R. R. Million & N. J. Cassisi (Eds.), *Management of Head and Neck Cancer: A Multidisciplinary Approach* (2nd ed., pp. 17–26). Philadelphia: J.B. Lippincott.

Mezey, A. P. (2002). Ambulatory care. In A. R. Kovner & S. Jonas (Eds.), *Health Care Delivery in the United States* (7th ed., pp. 173–198). New York: Springer.

Mock, V., Dow, K. H., Mears, C. J. Grimm, P. M., Dienemann, J. A., Haisfield-Wolfe, M. E. et al. (1997). Effects of exercise on fatigue, physical functioning, and emotional distress during radiation therapy for breast cancer. *Oncology Nursing Forum, 24,* 991–1000.

Moore, G. J. (1996). Issues in collaborative practice: Collaborative role of a nurse practitioner in a unversity radiation oncology department. *Cancer Practitioner, 4,* 285–287.

Moore-Higgs, G. J. & Amdur, R. J. (2001). Sustained integrity of protective mechanisms (skin, oral, immune system). In D. Watkins Bruner, G. J. Moore-Higgs, & M. Haas (Eds.), *Outcomes in Radiation Therapy: Multisciplinary Management* (pp. 493–518). Sudbury, MA: Jones and Bartlett Publishers.

Moore-Higgs, G. J., Watkins Bruner, D., Balmer, L., Johnson-Doneski, J., Komarny, P., Mautner, B. et al. (2003a). The role of licensed nursing personnel in radiation oncology Part A: Results of a descriptive study. *Oncology Nursing Forum, 30,* 51–58.

Moore-Higgs, G. J., Watkins Bruner, D., Balmer, L., Johnson-Doneski, J., Komarny, P., Mautner, B. et al. (2003b). The role of licensed nursing personnel in radiation oncology Part B: Integrating the ambulatory care nursing conceptual framework. *Oncology Nursing Forum, 30,* 59–64.

National Cancer Institute. (1999). National Cancer Institute's Common Toxicity Criteria, Version 2.0, with Radiation Therapy Oncology Group (RTOG) and European Organization for Research and Treatment of Cancer (EORTC) Acute Effects Criteria. Bethesda, MD: National Cancer Institute.

Nicolaou, N. (1999). Radiation therapy treatment planning and delivery. *Seminars in Oncology Nursing, 15,* 260–269.

Nishimoto, P. (1996). Venturing into the unknown: Cultural beliefs about death and dying. *Oncology Nursing Forum, 23,* 889–894.

Noa, C. & D'Angelo, L. (2001). Health care fiscal management. In J. Robinson (Ed.), *Core Curriculum for Ambulatory Care Nursing* (pp. 84–95). Philadelphia: W.B. Saunders Company.

Olsen, D. L., Raub Jr., W., Bradley, C., Johnson, M., Macias, J. L., Love, V. et al. (2001). The effect of aloe vera gel/mild soap versus mild soap alone in preventing skin reactions in patients undergoing radiation therapy. *Oncology Nursing Forum, 28,* 543–550.

Oncology Nursing Society. (1996). *Oncology Nursing Society Statement on the Scope and Standards of Oncology Nursing Practice.* Pittsburgh, PA: Author.

Oncology Nursing Society. (1997). *Oncology Nursing Society Statement on the Scope and Standards for Advanced Practice in Oncology Nursing.* Pittsburgh, PA: Author.

Piper, B. F., Dibble, S., Dodd, M. J., Slaugher, R. E., & Paul, S. M. (1998). The Piper Fatigue Scale: Psychometric evaluations in women with breast cancer. *Oncology Nursing Forum, 25,* 677–684.

Riportella-Muller, R., Libby, D., & Kindig, D. (1995). The substitution of physician assistants and nurse practitioners for physician residents in teaching hospitals. *Health Affairs (Millwood), 14,* 181–191.

Rosenal, L. (1985). Radiotherapy nurse: Develping a new role. *Canadian Nurse, 10,* 21–23.

Ruble, K. & Kelly, K. P. (1999). Radiation therapy in childhood cancer. *Seminars in Oncology Nursing, 15,* 294–302.

Salner, A., Edwards, A., Kuzmicas, P., McIntyre, P., & Rice, R. (1999). A regional radiation oncology network is developed to meet community needs. *Managed Care & Cancer, 1,* 10–13.

Sarna, L. & Conde, F. (2001). Physical activity and fatigue during radiation therapy: A pilot study using actigraph monitors. *Oncology Nursing Forum, 28,* 1043–1046.

Shepard, N. & Kelvin, J. F. (1999). The nursing role in radiation oncology. *Seminars in Oncology Nursing, 15,* 237–249.

Sitton, E. T. (1992). Clinical practice. In K. H. Dow & L. J. Hilderley (Eds.), *Nursing Care in Radiation Oncology* (pp. 361–369). Philadelphia: W.B. Saunders Company.

Sitton, E. T. (1997). Managing side effects of skin changes and fatigue. In K. H. Dow, J. D. Bucholtz, R. Iwamoto, V. Fieler, & L. Hilderley (Eds.), *Nursing Care in Radiation Oncology* (2nd ed., pp. 79–100). Philadelphia: W.B. Saunders Company.

Sporkin, E. (1997). Administrative issues in today's managed care environments. In K. H. Dow, J. Dunn-Bucholtz, R. Iwamoto, V. Fieler, & L. Hilderley (Eds.), *Nursing Care in Radiation Oncology* (2nd ed., pp. 386–391). Philadelphia: W.B. Saunders Company.

Strohl, R. (1988). The nursing role in radiation oncology: Symptom management of acute and chronic reactions. *Oncology Nursing Forum, 15,* 429–434.

Stromborg, M. F., Christensen, A., & Elmhurst, D. (2001a). Nurse documentation: Not done or worse, done the wrong way—Part I. *Oncology Nursing Forum, 28,* 697–702.

Stromborg, M. F., Christensen, A., & Elmhurst, D. (2001b). Nurse documentation: Not done or worse, done the wrong way—Part II. *Oncology Nursing Forum, 28,* 841–846.

Taylor, E. J. (1998). Caring for the spirit. In C. C. Burke (Ed.), *Psychosocial Dimensions of Oncology Nursing Care* (pp. 53–75). Pittsburgh, PA: Oncology Nursing Press.

Teytelman, Y. (2002). Effective nursing documentation and communication. *Seminars in Oncology Nursing, 18,* 121–127.

The Joint Commission on Accreditation of Healthcare Organizations (JCAHO). (1996). *Nursing Care Standards: Accreditation Manual for Hospitals.* Oakbrook Terrace, IL: Author.

Tuma, R. S. (2002). Communicating with patients via E-Mail: Help or hindrance? *Oncology Times, November,* 53.

U.S. Department of Health and Human Services. (2000). Health United States, 2000 (DHHS Publication No. PHS 01-1232). Washington, DC: U.S. Government Printing Office.

Walker, B. L., Nail, L. M., Larsen, L., Magill, J., & Schwartz, A. (1996). Concerns, affect, and cognitive disruption following completion of radiation therapy for localized breast or prostate cancer. *Oncology Nursing Forum, 23,* 1181–1187.

Watkins Bruner, D., Bucholtz, J. D., Iwamoto, R., & Strohl, R. (1998). *Manual for Radiation Oncology Nursing Practice and Education.* Pittsburgh, PA: Oncology Nursing Press.

Wengstrom, Y. & Forsberg, C. (1999). Justifying radiation oncology nursing practice—A literature review. *Oncology Nursing Forum, 26,* 741–750.

Works, C. (2000). Principles of treatment planning and clinical research. In C. H. Yarbro, M. H. Frogge, M. Goodman, & S. L. Groenwald (Eds.), *Cancer Nursing Principles and Practice* (5th ed., pp. 259–271). Sudbury, MA: Jones and Bartlett Publishers.

Chapter 9

Hematopoietic Stem Cell Transplant Outpatient Models

Kim Schmit-Pokorny

Introduction

High-dose therapy (radiation and/or chemotherapy) followed by autologous or allogeneic hematopoietic stem cell transplantation (HSCT) has become a frequently used treatment modality for many malignant and nonmalignant diseases. Historically, the high-dose therapy, infusion of hematopoietic stem cells, and hematopoietic recovery have taken place in an inpatient special care unit. In 1983, Stream first described outpatient care before and after transplant. Since that time, numerous articles have described ambulatory care of the transplant patient (Chielens & Herrick, 1990; Buchsel, 1991; Buchsel, 1993; Hurley, 1997; Buchsel & Kapustay, 1997). Since the early 1990s, many centers have shifted much of the care to outpatient clinics.

The demand to decrease healthcare costs has prompted transplant programs to develop innovative strategies to care for patients. The development of novel technology and new medications has also prompted the move of HSCT to the outpatient setting. Many investigators have reported the cost for an autologous or allogeneic transplant, and it varies widely (Bennett et al., 1995; Yee, 1998; Freeman et al., 1999). The costs of a hospital room, nursing, and supportive care are the most expensive components in the transplant process. Performing some or all of the transplant procedure in the outpatient clinic can significantly reduce the overall cost. Although inpatient transplantation provides some environmental control relative to infection, inpatients may experience more nosocomial infections or increased use of laboratory and diagnostic tests (McGuire, Tarantolo, & Reed, 1998).

The development and use of hematopoietic growth factors, including granulocyte colony-stimulating factor and granulocyte macrophage colony-stimulating factor, have markedly decreased the hematopoietic recovery time for transplant patients. Innovative technology, most significantly, the almost exclusive use of peripheral blood stem cells (PBSCs), has also allowed patients to engraft more rapidly. A shorter engraftment interval results in decreased infection rates, reduced hospital stays, and overall safer transplants. Improved antiemetic regimens, including the use of prophylactic antibiotics, have also helped patients to tolerate the transplant process better. Overall, transplant teams have gained experience and knowledge about the transplant process. All of these strategies have made it possible to move some, if not all, of the transplant to the outpatient setting and to address the need to decrease cost.

Models of Outpatient Transplantation

Early Discharge

In 1994, Peters and colleagues first described outpatient transplantation. This report described transplants occurring at the Duke University Medical Center between 1991 and 1993 for 110 patients with stages II, III, or IV breast cancer. All patients received cyclophosphamide, cisplatin, and carmustine followed by PBSCs. Initially, all patients received the chemotherapy and infusion of PBSCs as inpatients and were discharged approximately two days after transplant. As the study progressed and safety was established, patients were discharged after the final dose of chemotherapy. The median length of stay for patients was nine days (range, 7–12); however, the inpatient length of stay decreased to seven days (range, 5–11) once familiarity with the program was established.

After this study, many centers reported outpatient transplantations (**Table 9.1**) and various methods of conducting outpatient transplants were described (**Table 9.2**). Total outpatient, early discharge or subtotal outpatient, and modified outpatient are three modes of outpatient transplantation. In the total outpatient model, the patient may receive the high-dose therapy, transplant, and recover totally as an outpatient. In the early discharge or subtotal outpatient model, high-dose therapy may be administered in the inpatient setting. Then the patient is discharged, receives the transplant outpatient, and recovers as an outpatient. In the modified outpatient model, the patient may receive the conditioning therapy as an outpatient and then is admitted to the hospital. Another model of care that decreases the overall cost of transplant is the Cooperative Care model at the University of Nebraska Medical Center/Nebraska Health System (Schmit-Pokorny & Nuss, 2000; Wardian & Franco,

2001). In this model of care, the patient is admitted to an inpatient hotel-like setting. A care partner provides much of the basic care, and an outpatient staff is used instead of the traditional hospital setting. This model is discussed in greater detail later in this chapter.

The early-discharge model of outpatient care was also described by Burns, Tierney, Long, Lambert, & Carr (1995); and Meisinger, Sasse, & Schmit-Pokorny, (1996). Burns et al. (1995) described a protocol in which patients were discharged immediately after chemotherapy and received the PBSCs as outpatients. Patients are managed in the outpatient setting with prophylactic antibiotics and growth factors. This high-dose chemotherapy regimen was repeated every four weeks for four cycles. Meisinger et al. (1996) discharged 64 patients to the outpatient cancer center initially after the infusion of PBSCs, and then as experience and knowledge increased, discharge occurred before transplant.

Total Outpatient

The first description of total outpatient transplantation by Meisenberg et al. (1997) was for patients with various malignant diseases using disease-specific chemotherapy regimens. Initially, patients were offered to have their transplant performed in the subtotal outpatient transplant program (STOT). Patients received the high-dose therapy inpatient and were discharged the day after chemotherapy was completed. Once the STOT program was established, a total outpatient transplant program was developed. Patients were given the option of receiving their transplant in the traditional transplant unit, the STOT, or the total outpatient program. One hundred thirty-five patients were transplanted using STOT or the total outpatient option, and 70% were never readmitted. The authors concluded that a majority of transplants can be safely performed without the patient needing to be hospitalized.

In another early study, Jagannath et al. (1997) reported 251 patients with multiple myeloma who received autologous, planned tandem transplants between 1992 and 1994. Ninety-one patients were transplanted as total outpatients and compared with 160 patients receiving transplants as inpatients; however, for logistical reasons, only two total outpatient transplants were preformed per week. Consequently, some inpatient transplant recipients were eligible for outpatient transplants. Twenty-one percent of the outpatients needed to be admitted after transplant, with a median hospital stay of nine days. Jagannath et al. concluded that there was significant financial savings in the areas of pharmacy, hospitalization, and pathology/laboratory charges and that outpatient transplantation would be more accessible to patients in the future.

Outpatient Allogeneic Transplants

Rizzo et al. (1999) reported on the first outpatient allogeneic bone marrow transplants (BMTs). At Johns Hopkins University in Baltimore, MD the inpatient–outpatient (IPOP) program was started in 1995. The main objective of the study was to determine whether shifting the care of a transplant patient from the inpatient unit to an outpatient unit decreased charges to payers without increasing out-of-pocket costs or adverse complications to patients. All patients who planned to receive an autologous or allogeneic BMT were encouraged to participate in the IPOP program. Of the 132 patients who underwent transplant, 17 were eligible and chose to participate in the program. The researchers indicated that even though most patients were eligible, insurers' refusal to approve the outpatient procedure was the limitation to enrollment. Eight outpatients underwent an allogeneic BMT and were compared with 60 inpatients. The outpatient group of patients had a mean of 22 days as inpatients as compared with the inpatient group with a 47-day mean inpatient stay. Overall, the total number of days either group received care at the transplant center was not significantly different. Results from this study indicate that IPOP reduces the inpatient length of stay by 47% without increasing adverse complications. However, total hospital (inpatient and outpatient) charges were only 7% lower in the IPOP group. The investigators concluded that outpatient autologous and allogeneic transplants are feasible and safe.

Foreign Countries

Lowering the cost of transplantation is not unique to the United States. In developing countries, decreasing the cost allows individuals who may not be able to afford the treatment greater access to transplantation. Ruiz-Argüelles et al. (2001) reported on nonmyeloablative allogeneic transplants preformed on 21 patients in the outpatient setting. Patients received either fludarabine, busulfan, and cyclophosphamide or fludarabine and melphalan as a preparative regimen. One patient was admitted 15 days after the transplant because of graft-versus-host disease symptoms of jaundice and diarrhea. The median cost of the transplant in these patients was $18,000 (U.S. dollars).

Community Cancer Centers

Transplantation in community cancer centers has been described by several authors (Weaver, Schwartzberg, Hainsworth et al., 1997; Weaver, Schwartzberg, Zhen et al., 1997; and Schwartzberg et al., 1998). In the report by Weaver et al. (1997) patients were initially admitted to the hospital to receive the chemotherapy and transplant. After the transplant team acquired experience, the patients were maintained in an outpatient setting. However, of the 83 inpatient and outpatient cases reported, 96% (80 patients) needed to be hospitalized for a median of 14 days (range, 6–37). Only three patients remained as having total outpatient care. Weaver et al. (1997) concluded that transplant in the community setting is feasible and allows patients to have access to transplant therapy that may have been excluded because of geographic barriers, high cost, or perception that transplants must be carried out in a tertiary center.

Table 9.1   OUTPATIENT TRANSPLANTATION PROGRAMS (CHRONOLOGICAL BY YEAR OF ARTICLE PUBLISHED)

Name of Transplant Center	Date Study Published	First Author	Method of Outpatient Transplant	Diagnosis	Conditioning Regimen	Autologous or Allogeneic	Prophylactic Antibiotic Regimen
Duke University Medical Center	1994	Peters	Early discharge	Breast cancer	Cyclophosphamide, cisplatin, and carmustine	Autologous BM or PBSC granulocyte colony-stimulating factor or granulocyte-macrophage colony stimulating factor	Ciprofloxacin and rifampin
Stanford University Hospital	1995	Burns	Early discharge and total outpatient	Breast cancer	Mitoxantrone, thiotepa, and cyclophosphamide +/- paclitaxel	Autologous PBSC granulocyte colony-stimulating factor	Vancomycin and ceftriaxone
University of Nebraska Medical Center	1996	Meisinger	Early discharge	Non-Hodgkin's lymphoma and Hodgkin's disease	Disease specific	Autologous BM or PBSC Not noted	Not noted
Scripps Clinic and Research Foundation	1997	Meisenberg	First subtotal then total outpatient	Hematologic and non-hematologic diseases	Disease specific	Autologous PBSC granulocyte colony-stimulating factor	Ciprofloxacin and rifampin, acyclovir if HSV (+)
University of Arkansas	1997	Jagannath	Total outpatient	Multiple myeloma	Melphalan	Autologous (Tandem) PBSC + BM granulocyte-macrophage colony stimulating factor or granulocyte colony-stimulating factor	Ciprofloxacin, penicillin, V potassium, and mycelex

Table 9.1 OUTPATIENT TRANSPLANTATION PROGRAMS (CONT'D)

Response Oncology, Inc	1997	Weaver	Community cancer center	Non-Hodgkin's lymphoma	Carmustine, etoposide, cytarabine, and cyclophosphamide	Autologous PBSC	granulocyte colony-stimulating factor or granulocyte-macrophage colony stimulating factor	Fluconazole, acyclovir if HSV (+), antiviral agent if CMV (+)
Scripps Clinic and Research Foundation	1998	Meisenberg	Subtotal and total outpatient	Breast, ovarian cancer, or non-Hodgkin's lymphoma	Cyclophosphamide, thiotepa or etoposide, and carboplatin	Autologous PBSC granulocyte colony-stimulating factor	Ciprofloxacin and rifampin
University of Nebraska Medical Center	1998	McGuire	Total outpatient	Breast cancer	Cyclophosphamide, cisplatin, and etoposide	Autologous PBSC granulocyte colony-stimulating factor	Ceftazidime, acyclovir if HSV (+)
Mexico	1998	Ruiz-Argüelles	Total outpatient	Hematologic malignancies	Melphalan	Autologous PBSC granulocyte colony-stimulating factor	Ciprofloxacin and itraconazole
Johns Hopkins University	1999	Rizzo	Total outpatient	Hematologic malignancies	Busulfan and cyclophosphamide and other regimen(s) not noted	Autologous and Allogeneic BM Growth factors not routinely used	Not reported
Yale Cancer Center	1999	Seropian	Total outpatient	Non-Hodgkin's lymphoma and Hodgkin's disease	Carmustine, etoposide, cytarabine, and melphalan (BEAM)	Autologous PBSC granulocyte colony-stimulating factor	Ciprofloxacin and fluconazole acyclovir if HSV (+)
Mexico	2001	Ruiz-Argüelles	Total outpatient	Hematologic malignancies	Fludarabine, cyclophosphamide, and busulfan or fludarabine and melphalan	Allogeneic - Nonmyeloablative PBSC Growth factor usage not noted	Ciprofloxacin, itraconazole and ganciclovir if CMV (+)

Abbreviations: BM = bone marrow; PBSC = peripheral blood stem cell; CMV = cytomegalovirus; HSV = herpes simplex virus

Table 9.2 CARE SETTINGS FOR TRANSPLANT

Traditional	Inpatient admission for high-dose therapy, transplant, supportive care, and hematopoietic recovery
Outpatient	
Total outpatient	Outpatient high-dose therapy, transplant, supportive care, and hematopoietic recovery
Early discharge or subtotal outpatient	Inpatient high-dose therapy; inpatient or outpatient transplant; outpatient supportive care and hematopoietic recovery
Modified outpatient	Outpatient high-dose therapy; inpatient or outpatient transplant; inpatient supportive care and hematopoietic recovery
Cooperative care	Inpatient high-dose therapy, transplant, supportive care, and hematopoietic recovery in a hotel-like inpatient setting with a care partner providing basic care

Adapted from Buchsel & Kapustay, 1995.

Pediatric Outpatient Transplants

Children may also receive transplants in the outpatient setting. Schmit-Pokorny and Nuss (2000) noted that children, unlike adults, can never be left alone. Therefore, an additional caregiver other than the main caregiver was needed to give mutual respite care. They described a situation in which a nurse with intensive care and pediatric oncology experience became overwhelmed with the continual care for her child. However, with rotation of caregivers, educational resources, and psychological support, children may participate in outpatient transplant programs.

Advantages and Disadvantages of Outpatient Transplantation

Currently, many autologous transplants and frequently allogeneic transplants take place in an outpatient setting. What began in the early 1990s as a method to decrease cost has turned into the accepted manner of performing transplants. Clinical transplant staff, patients, and families are challenged to weigh the advantages and disadvantages associated with providing care in the outpatient setting [**Table 9.3**] (Cavanaugh, 1994; Schmit-Pokorny, Hruska, & Ursick, 1998). Outpatient transplantation may decrease cost while increasing patient satisfaction, independence, and control over daily routines. As an outpatient, the patient may be more active, because of the requirements of traveling to and from the outpatient clinic and his or her accommodations. Outpatient transplantation may also enhance the development of close, supportive relationships between family and friends, resulting in a decrease in the separation anxiety that may occur in a traditional hospital setting.

Disadvantages to be considered are the potential for increased out-of-pocket expenses, consisting of living expenses (housing and food) that are usually part of the inpatient room charges. Transportation to and from the transplant center may be costly and inconvenient. The burden of responsibility on the family care partner is also a major consideration. Care partners are required to perform much of the care that nurses traditionally give in the hospital setting. Young families often have other children besides the transplant patient to whom the caregiver is responsible; thus, young families may also need to consider additional expenses to pay for child care. Care partners must be able to identify potential complications and report them to the transplant team. It is possible that a delay in identification or reporting could affect the outcome of the transplant.

Patient Eligibility

Patients considered for outpatient transplantation are required to meet the protocol-specific eligibility criteria for the transplant. Their performance status is monitored closely for comorbid conditions that may compromise the success of the transplantation. Some centers require patients to speak English and have normal hearing capacity to facilitate communication (Rizzo et al., 1999). Ruiz-Argüelles et al. also selected patients with fair educational levels (1998). The patient's third-party insurance is assessed to determine whether there is outpatient coverage for housing and med-

---

Table 9.3 ADVANTAGES AND DISADVANTAGES OF OUTPATIENT TRANSPLANTATION

Advantages
> Decreased cost
> Increased patient satisfaction
> Increased independence
> Increased control over daily routines
> More active routine
> Development of close supportive
> relationships
> Increased self-care activities
> Less separation anxiety

Disadvantages
> Increased out-of-pocket costs
> Transportation
> Living expenses
> Care partner's lost wages because of
> missed work
> Child care
> Delayed treatment of complications

Used with permission, Meniscus, Incorporated. Schmit-Pokorny, Hjruska, & Ursick, 1998.
Data from Cavanaugh, C.A., 1994; Schmit-Pokorny, Hjruska, Ursick, 1998.

ications. Often considerable time is spent on education and negotiation with payers to explain the cost benefits and patient satisfaction derived from transplants performed in the outpatient clinics.

Care Partner Selection

A dedicated care partner is a key requirement for a patient undergoing an outpatient transplant. Early in the transplant process, the transplant coordinator should discuss the role and responsibilities of the care partner with the patient. The care partner needs to be a responsible adult and available to the patient 24 hours a day and may be a spouse, relative, or friend. Often, care partners rotate throughout the transplant process. Responsibilities of the care partner may range from assisting the patient with daily activities to administering intravenous medications (**Table 9.4**). As Meisenberg et al. (1997) discussed, not all patients are be able to identify care partners, and they suggested the possibility of hiring caregivers. Meisenberg et al. (1998) found that patients and their care partners like the outpatient transplant programs.

Patient and Care Partner Education

One of the most significant components in supporting and maintaining a patient and care partner in the outpatient setting is the presence of a strong and diverse education program. (Schmit-Pokorny, Hruska, & Ursick, 1998). A variety of methods, including one-to-one, classroom, handouts, and videos, can be used to instruct the patient and care partner. Each stage of the transplant should be described in detail. In a basic skills class, the patient and care partner are taught to use an incentive spirometer, to manage catheter care (dressing changes and flushing techniques), to administer medications (oral and intravenous), and to follow safety guidelines and emergency procedures. The care partner is taught how to take

Table 9.4   RESPONSIBILITIES OF THE CARE PARTNER

Assist the patient with activities of daily living
Keep a diary (including oral medication usage, input and output, and temperature graph)
Administer oral medications
Administer intravenous medications
Assess the patient for symptoms
Draw blood from the central venous catheter
Monitor oral intake
Monitor urine output
Assess temperature
Provide transportation
Contact the transplant team to report symptoms

Adapted from Schmit-Pokorny, Hjruska, & Ursick, 1998.

an accurate temperature, to measure the patient's input and output, to document procedures performed in a diary, and to manage basic side effects. Self-care for the patient includes oral care, rectal care, diet and nutrition, basic infection control strategies, coping strategies, and relaxation techniques.

Wardian and Franco (2001) suggested that one of the fundamental techniques in reducing anxiety in patients and care partners is to build on their current knowledge. Recalling past experiences and building on those may help patients to understand the complex transplant process. Wardian and Franco (2001) also proposed that the most demanding challenge is teaching the partnership—patient and caregiver—to work together. Control versus independence and support versus smothering are two areas in which patients and care partners struggle. Caregiver empowerment is essential because often times the care partner must make a decision sometimes against the patient's wishes.

Schmit-Pokorny and Sasse (1994) reported that opinions and commonly held beliefs instead of the actual guidelines were often conveyed to patients by the transplant staff (nurses, physician assistants, and physicians). To combat this phenomenon, all staff members were required to review education materials. Also, standardized classes and printed patient material were created to provide accurate and consistent information to patients and care partners.

Confirming that caregivers understand and can perform taught material is difficult to evaluate. Heerman et al. (2001) developed objective structured clinical examinations to teach and evaluate care partners' mastery of the information and skills. In their study, caregivers were provided with immediate feedback during the learning sessions. Response from caregivers was positive, and objective structured clinical examinations were found to increase comfort with the caregiving role.

The Outpatient Program

Transplant Team

Critical to establishing an outpatient program is a diverse multidisciplinary team. Crucial team members include transplant physicians, physician assistants, nurses, pharmacists, social workers, dietitians, home care nurses, and insurance coordinators. As with inpatient transplant programs, a wide variety of support services is needed. Buchsel and Kapustay (1997) described in detail the administrative, medical staff or consultants, nursing staff, support, and ancillary services that are necessary for outpatient transplant models.

Many reports indicated that nurses are key components to accomplishing an outpatient program (Peters et al., 1994; Burns et al., 1995; Jagannath et al., 1997; McGuire et al., 1998; Blume & Thomas, 2000). McGuire et al. (1998) underscored the importance of recruiting and retaining nursing staff who had inpatient BMT experience.

A transplant nurse case manager is essential for the coordination of clinical care for the transplant patient. A transplant nurse case manager is usually assigned to the patient before the consultation and then follows the patient throughout the entire transplant process. Coordination of care and services, education, and acting as a liaison among all transplant team members are the major roles of the nurse case manager. Burns et al. (1995) asserted that the transplant nurse case manager is integral to an outpatient transplant program.

Physical Resources

A dedicated outpatient clinic is required to support immunosuppressed patients. Red blood cell and platelet transfusions and administration of intravenous medications, including chemotherapy and antibiotics, are common procedures in the outpatient clinic. Large transplant units are usually open seven days a week, 24 hours a day and are staffed with physician, nursing, and pharmacy support. If this model is not available, patients are clinically evaluated for ongoing problems by the inpatient transplant team. Several transplant centers have developed outpatient programs in which the clinic is not open 24 hours a day, 7 days a week. Jagannath et al. (1997) maintained patients in the outpatient setting with a clinic that was open seven days a week from 8:00 a.m. to 5:00 p.m. Patients were able to contact a transplant physician for medical emergencies after hours. Outpatient transplant nurses also were available to assist the patient with malfunctioning infusion pumps. Stanford University Hospital (Burns, Tierney, Long, Lambert, & Carr, 1995) developed a four-bed day hospital to accommodate the outpatient transplant patients. This area, which included a treatment center and dedicated staff, was adjacent to the inpatient BMT unit and was open Monday through Friday from 7:30 a.m. to 5:00 p.m.

Housing close to the transplant center is imperative for an outpatient program to succeed. A hotel-like facility is ideal; however, third-party payers may not reimburse patients for these accommodations. Those patients who reside near the transplant center are allowed to remain in their own homes. Burns et al. (1995) required patients to live within 30 minutes of the transplant center, providing that a reliable support person was available at all times. Other BMT units will have variations of these policies. For example, Meisenberg et al. (1997) allowed patients to remain in their home if the residence was located less than 45 minutes from the clinic by car.

Homecare Management

Most transplant centers have policies that allow patients to receive medications and hydration in their housing accommodations. Usually ambulatory infusion pumps are used to deliver intravenous medications and hydration under the supervision of home care nurses. Before committing to a homecare agency, critical assessments are required to evaluate the skill level and knowledge of the nursing and pharmacy staff, in particular safe handling and mixing procedures of intravenous solutions. In Seropian et al.'s (1999) study, visiting nurses safely administered chemotherapy in the patients' home. Burns et al. (1995) also reported that home healthcare nurses administered chemotherapy, hydration, and platelets via infusion pumps. However, recipients requiring red blood cells transfusions were required to have them infused in the outpatient treatment center. Kelley et al. (2000) described the role of the transplant homecare nurse during the different phases of transplant. They stated that home care provides patients with easy access to services in their own environment. Homecare nurses are invaluable in the early identification of side effects associated with transplant.

Critical Pathways

Burns et al. (1995) developed an outpatient transplantation critical path to improve communication among team members and to provide a more standardized process. Flow sheets for documentation can be developed specifically for outpatient transplant patients. Burns and Tierney (1996) developed one example shown to decrease charting time, decrease time giving verbal reports, and daily assessments were more easily evaluated.

Outpatient Transplant Process

PBSC Collection

The collection of PBSCs for patients transplanted in the outpatient setting is similar to patients in the inpatient setting. Usually patients and allogeneic donors receive hematopoietic growth factors (patients may also receive chemotherapy) to mobilize stem cells. The stem cells are then collected via apheresis procedures until an adequate number of cells are harvested (Buchsel & Kapustay, 1995; O'Connell & Schmit-Pokorny, 1997). In most circumstances, the stem cells are cryopreserved by previously reported methods (Letheby, Jackson, & Warkentin, 2000).

In Ruiz-Argüelles et al.'s report (1998), noncryopreserved PBSC autotransplants in six patients with hematologic malignancies were performed entirely outpatient. PBSCs were collected on days −4, −3, and −2 before transplant and were stored in a conventional blood bank refrigerator at 4°C. High-dose melphalan was given to the patients on day −1. The patients received the stem cell products on days 0, +1, and +2, respectively. All patients achieved engraftment. The median time to reach more than 500 ml/mm³ granulocytes was 21 days (range, 16–40 days), and the median time to reach more than 20,000 mm³ platelets was 38 days (range, 21–48). All patients

remained outpatient for the entire procedure. The median cost for the total transplant procedure was $6,500.

High-Dose Therapy

Transplant preparatory regimens have been adapted to accommodate outpatient transplants. The two major evaluations that need to be considered are the toxicities associated with the high-dose therapy and the length of infusion time for the chemotherapy and hydration. Meisenberg et al. (1997) administered chemotherapy by a 4-hour infusion rather than by a continuous infusion to facilitate total outpatient transplant. To prevent the common adverse effect of hemorrhagic cystitis, hydration used to diminish this effect was changed from hyperhydration and bladder irrigation to using mesna and lesser hydration.

Peters et al. (1994) implemented the chemotherapy regimen of cyclophosphamide, cisplatin, and carmustine to minimize mucositis, a typical but painful adverse effect. When this protocol was instituted, the overall treatment-related mortality was approximately 3%. Peters et al. (1994) suggested that because of the reduction in toxicities is associated with high-dose therapies and peripheral stem cell transplants, the efficacy and/or cost-effectiveness of the chemotherapy agents should determine which agents are used in transplant.

McGuire et al. (1998) administered cyclophosphamide, cisplatin, and etoposide in conditioning regimens because of the low risk of mucositis and the overall low toxicity profile. An aggressive antiemetic regimen (ondansetron, dexamethasone, lorazepam, prochlorperazine, and diphenhydramine) was also initiated to prevent severe nausea and vomiting. The authors noted that this antiemetic regimen is extremely sedating, requiring that the care partner be exceptionally attentive to the needs of the patient during administration.

Another chemotherapy regimen that is reported to be associated with a low mucositis profile and is used in outpatient recipients with non-

Hodgkin's lymphoma or Hodgkin's disease is high-dose carmustine, etoposide, cytarabine, and melphalan (BEAM) (Seropian et al., 1999). Many transplant centers have identified chemotherapy protocols with decreased toxicities and ease in administration that are used in outpatient programs. A number of outpatient transplant programs used are listed in **Table 9.1**.

Transplant (Infusion of Hematopoietic Stem Cells)

The infusion of outpatient PBSCs remains essentially the same as for inpatient transplants. Intravenous hydration may be administered for several hours before, during, and after the infusion of cells. The use of chemotherapy and/or hematopoietic growth factors to mobilize PBSCs has decreased the overall volume of the cells infused. A lesser volume of cells results in a lesser volume of the cryoprotectant dimethylsulfoxide, thereby resulting in decreased side effects from the transplant (Kessinger, Schmit-Pokorny, Smith, & Armitage, 1990). Patients are usually premedicated to alleviate the side effects associated with the transplant. Common premedications may include a combination of lorazepam, diphenhydramine hydrochloride, meperidine hydrochloride, hydrocortisone, acetaminophen, or methylprednisolone. Common side effects (listed in **Table 9.5**) that the patient may experience during the transplant may be caused by the dimethylsulfoxide, volume of cells infused, or lysis of red blood cells contained in the product (Kessinger, 1990). Outpatients are encouraged to drink plenty of fluids, to continue to take antiemetics, and to rest. Care partners may be asked to measure urine output and to report red urine.

Transplant Complications, Engraftment, and Recovery

Patients transplanted in the outpatient setting may experience toxicities that are comparable to inpatient transplants. Complications or toxicities may include hematologic (neutropenia, anemia, thrombocytopenia), renal, hepatic, pulmonary, gastrointestinal, neurological, cardiac, hemorrhagic cystitis, graft-versus-host disease, skin, fatigue, and psychological effects from the transplant. This chapter addresses several complications that are common and significant to transplant patients in the outpatient setting. Detailed descriptions for other complications may be found in a number of other transplant publications. Several include Buchsel and Kapustay, (2000), Whedon and Wujcik, (1997), and Buchsel et al. (1997). As noted earlier, the use of chemotherapy protocols specifically chosen to result in fewer toxicities has also helped to decrease overall complications.

A transplant physician and nurse examine outpatient transplant recipients daily. Daily blood counts and serum chemistries are also assessed to determine possible toxicities. The administration of red blood cell and platelet transfusions, intravenous antibiotics, and fluid and/or electrolyte supplementation may be accomplished in either the outpatient clinic or via ambulatory infusion pumps.

NEUTROPENIA

One of the largest concerns with conducting transplants in the outpatient setting is the possibility of developing a serious infection during the neutropenic phase. Most outpatient transplant programs use a prophylactic antibiotic regimen. Usually no special cleaning procedures in the hotel room or home are required; however, good hand washing is strongly encouraged. McGuire et al. (1998) reported the use of intravenous ceftazidime every eight hours as an empiric antibiotic because of the potential severity of gram-negative infections. The morning and afternoon doses are administered in the clinic, and the night dose is given by a home healthcare nurse in the patient's hotel room. Vancomycin and occa-

Table 9.5   SIDE EFFECTS OF PBSC INFUSION (TRANSPLANT)

Potential Side Effect	Etiology	Assessment	Intervention
Nausea Vomiting	Dimethylsulfoxide	Evaluate amount and frequency	Give antiemetics lorazepam, diphenhydramine hydrochloride, ondansetron, prochlorperazine
Hemoglobinuria Elevated serum creatinine Elevated serum bilirubin	Lysis of red blood cells Dimethylsulfoxide	Baseline creatinine and bilirubin Hematest urine	Hydration
Chest tightness Cough Dyspnea Increased weight Hypertension Tachycardia Tachypnea	Volume of infusate	Vital signs every 15–30 minutes I/O hourly	Decrease rate of infusion Administer furosemide or mannitol Give oxygen
Chills, fever	Coldness of product	Temperature every 15–30 minutes	Provide warmth Give meperidine hydrochloride Give acetaminophen PRN
Garlic taste or smell	Dimethylsulfoxide	Ask patient if taste or smell noticed	Provide mints or gum
Anaphylactic reaction	Dimethylsulfoxide	Notify physician for care of itching, wheezing, skin rash, or erythema	Stop infusion Administer epinephrine
Miscellaneous Diarrhea Headache Flushing Abdominal cramping Malaise	Dimethylsulfoxide	Evaluate frequency and duration	Treat symptoms Decrease rate of infusions

Reprinted with permission from O'Connell & Schmit-Pokorny, 1997.

sionally empiric amphotericin may be added if a patient develops a fever while receiving ceftazidime. Patients who show symptoms consistent with the onset of gram-negative sepsis are admitted to the hospital (McGuire et al., 1998).

Jagannath et al. (1997) obtained daily blood cultures from outpatients while they were neutropenic. If a patient's temperature spiked to 38.3°C or more after clinic hours, the physician was contacted, and the patient or care partner infused vancomycin 1 grams and ceftazidime 2 grams. The antibiotics were provided to the patient before any report of fever and were stable for seven days. Patients continued to self-administer the antibiotics every 12 hours. Prophylactic antibiotics used by other transplant centers for outpatients are listed in **Table 9.1.**

NAUSEA AND VOMITING

Significant nausea and vomiting may require an outpatient to be admitted to the hospital. A study reported by Lawrence et al. (1996) found that nausea and vomiting caused significant distress in transplant patients. Uncontrolled nausea and vomiting in patients transplanted in the outpatient setting can result in not only readmission to the hospital but also inadequate nutrition and dehydration. They concluded that further research is necessary to decrease or prevent nausea and vomiting, especially in the outpatient setting.

A variety of oral and intravenous antiemetic regimens have been reported by outpatient transplant teams. Peters et al. (1994) used an antiemetic regimen consisting of intravenous ondansetron, oral prochlorperazine, and lorazepam. Dix et al. (1999) described an antiemetic regimen using an ambulatory infusion pump that the patient controlled. Three antiemetics were evaluated: diphenhydramine, lorazepam, dexamethasone (BAD). Starting with a continuous basal rate, patients were able to administer a bolus of medication themselves if necessary. Sedation or somnolence that patients experienced were managed by teaching the caregiver to adjust the dose titration. The patient was continued on this regimen until he or she was able to tolerate oral medications. Dix et al. (1999) found that the BAD infusion pump was safe and effective and facilitated outpatient transplantation.

Schmit-Pokorny et al. (1998) reported that supplies of medications, including lorazepam, prochlorperazine, and diphenhydramine, were given to outpatients. Patients and care partners were instructed on the use of these medications for administration at home. No problems occured. Additional intravenous medications used to prevent or control nausea and vomiting are ondansetron, dexamethasone, prochlorperazine, and diphenhydramine.

MUCOSITIS AND PAIN

Outpatient chemotherapy protocols, chosen specifically to decrease mucositis and esophagitis, have minimized swelling, ulcerations, and pain in the mouth; however, patients may still develop severe mucositis and esophagitis, resulting in intense pain and the potential for infection. Although pain management may be provided with oral, dermal, or intravenous narcotics, some patients may require hospitalization for larger amounts of opioids (Jagannath et al., 1997). Chapter 13 offers a complete discussion on dental care in ambulatory care settings.

Criteria for Admission to the Inpatient Unit

Patients who become febrile (or for other clinical indications) may need to be admitted or readmitted to the hospital. Often a hospital bed may be reserved for the outpatient population to ensure availability (Peters et al., 1994; Jagannat et al., 1997). Severe nausea, vomiting, or diarrhea may also require the patient to be admitted so that parenteral nutrition and intravenous antiemetics may be administered. Severe mucositis requiring intravenous narcotic analgesics may also necessitate readmission. Also, patients may request to be hospitalized, or the care partner may not be able to manage complicated toxicities. Peters et al. (1994) reported that the most common reason for readmission to the hospital was culture-negative febrile neutropenia. Other causes for readmission that Peters et al. reported were viral pneumonia, dehydration, suspected veno-occlusive disease, and thrombocytopenia. Jagannath et al. (1997) reported the need to hospitalize patients for capillary leak syndrome, hemodynamic instability, cardiac or respiratory distress, and pneumonia. Blume and Thomas (2000) stated that over 1,000 patients since 1993 have been treated in a day hospital at Stanford University. The readmission rate, mostly for fever, ranged from 20% to 40%.

Meisenberg et al. (1997) did not routinely admit patients to the hospital for febrile neutropenia unless complicated by other conditions. Thirty percent of the patients in the STOT program were readmitted for a mean of 8.7 days (range, 1–19) and 29% in the total outpatient program for a median of seven days (range, 1–34). The reasons for readmission were fever and mucositis, fever with rigors, refractory thrombocytopenia, renal failure, syncope, a lack of compliance, and a lack of a caregiver.

In a follow–up study by Meisenberg et al. (1998), specific criteria were used for readmission of a patient to the hospital. These criteria were patients with uncontrolled emesis, nausea, diarrhea, a rapidly rising creatinine, or unstable hemodynamics. Febrile neutropenia was not an indication for immediate readmission unless complicated by other organ toxicities such as hypotension and renal insufficiency (Meisenberg et al., 1998, p. 928).

McGuire et al. (1998, p. 21) readmitted 35% of their patients. Complications included cellulitis, *Clostridium difficile* infection, mucositis, vomiting and gastrointestinal bleeding, syncope, fluid and electrolyte requirements, and renal dysfunction. Patients who were readmitted were hospitalized for a median of five days. None of the complications were life threatening. Those patients who elected to receive their transplant in the outpatients department may verbalize disappointment and loss of control. However, transplant teams, patients, and caregivers understand that the patients may need to be admitted because of complications, caregiver burnout, or unforeseen circumstances.

Outcomes

Cost and Charges

Reviews of published studies indicate that outpatient transplantation does decrease cost; however, there is a wide range in reported savings. Peters et al. (1994) reported a 50% cost savings associated with outpatient transplantation. According to Burns et al. (1995), Stanford University Hospital reported that cost decreased, however, not by their targeted 40%, possibly because of all of the patients requiring a period of hospitalization. Rizzo et al. (1999) reported that even though IPOP reduces the inpatient length of stay by 47%, total hospital (inpatient and outpatient) charges were only 7% lower in the IPOP group. However, they suggest because patients with a standard risk of recurrent disease status incurred 34% lower hospital charges than patients in the traditional group and that selection of standard risk patients for outpatient programs may result in cost savings.

Also, insurer response to outpatient transplantation has not been consistent. Meisenberg et al. (1997) reported that the insurer response between their two methods of outpatient transplant, STOT, and total outpatient was not identical. They noted that some insurance companies supported a decreased length of stay, whereas others had no mechanism to cover outpatient housing. In many of the cases that Meisenberg et al. presented, a fixed global fee was paid to the transplant institution by the insurance company.

In a follow-up, prospective study, Meisenberg et al. (1998) reported that 94 patients received high-dose therapy followed by an autologous PBSC transplant in one of three settings: traditional inpatient, partial outpatient, or total outpatient. Determination of which type of treatment setting the patient was admitted to was based on the availability of a caregiver and patient preference. Beginning with the first day of chemotherapy and ending on day +30 post transplant, unless receiving treatment for transplant-related complications, all charges were assessed. Pretransplant evaluation charges were not included. Also, some charges (granulocyte colony-stimulating factor, central venous catheter insertion, and peripheral stem cell collection and preservation) were standardized to ensure an adequate comparison between settings. The cost of housing for the patients participating in the total outpatient program who stayed at a local hotel or apartment (64%) was applied to the outpatient bill. There were no statistically significant differences in toxicities, response rates, or disease-free survival noted between groups. Meisenberg et al. (1998) concluded that there was a substantial reduction in hospital charges and costs for outpatient transplants.

Charges for outpatient transplants that Jagannath et al. (1997) reported were adjusted for inflation. One hundred dollars was added for each outpatient day to cover room and board for the patient and care partner. One hundred dollars per day was added to estimate the care partner's time, and inpatient pharmacy charges were discounted to equal outpatient pharmacy charges. After reviewing many factors that might affect the overall charges, the only significant variable that was associated with financial savings was the outpatient setting.

Patient Out-of-Pocket Expenses

Patients transplanted in the outpatient setting may incur personal costs. Few studies have reviewed out-of-pocket costs. Rizzo et al. (1999) surveyed transplant patients who survived one year or longer. Patients were contacted one year after transplant and were asked to complete a questionnaire regarding out-of-pocket costs. Physicians, nurses, and social workers developed this survey, and it was piloted on a small group (n=17) of transplant patients. Transportation, lodging, meals, telephone, childcare, and household assistance costs were evaluated. Other indirect costs evaluated were employment status, changes in productivity, disability history, and lost income. Also included in the questionnaire were questions regarding unreimbursed medical costs and the perceived financial impact of transplant care. Results from the survey indicated that out-of-pocket costs

were no different between the groups. However, the authors noted that many patients wrote comments indicating that substantial nonfinancial assistance was provided by friends and community groups after transplant.

Patient Satisfaction/Quality of Life

Another area that must be evaluated when reviewing outpatient transplantation is patient satisfaction with the program and the patient's quality of life (QOL) in relationship to the outpatient program. Burns et al. (1995) reported on the QOL of five patients undergoing transplant as outpatients. The authors concluded that because patients felt they had more control over their care and schedule, their QOL was improved. The researchers also reported that patient independence increased, as patients have more responsibility over medication administration and symptom management. Blume & Thomas (2000) also identified a higher level of patient satisfaction in patients who were transplanted in the outpatient program.

Lawrence et al. (1996) reported on outpatient transplant patients perception of symptoms using the Symptom Distress Scale. They found that patients enjoy being out of the hospital, and medication compliance was greater than 90% in the outpatient setting. They further stated that medication noncompliance increases with additional doses of medication. They reported that the lowest compliance was in using clotrimazole troches five times daily (91%), whereas the highest compliance was with rifampin taken twice daily (98%). Overall, patient satisfaction with outpatient transplantation is good; however, more research in this area is needed.

Caregiver Burden

Care partners are essential for a patient to undergo an outpatient transplant. However, the transplant team needs to be aware that care partners may become overwhelmed and unable to care for the patient. Wardian et al. (1997) found that care partners were frustrated with patient coping patterns and management of symptoms. Support systems for the caregiver must be clearly addressed for outpatient transplant programs to succeed. Educational and psychological resources must be available for care partners. If care partners become overwhelmed while caring for the patient, the patient may need to be admitted to the hospital. McDonald et al. (1996) described the need for caregivers to become homecare managers. They describe the need for care partners to not only maintain the home environment but also to learn how to provide some of the basic medical care (assessing and reporting symptoms, providing emotional support, and dealing with emergencies). They stated that assuming the caregiver role requires a major shift in the caregiver's personal activities. Caregivers may take a leave from work, assume the patient work role, or temporarily make other adjustments to their responsibilities. The researchers suggested that the transplant team should provide educational opportunities, support groups, and counseling. Promotion of self-care strategies and active participation in the transplant process also help care partners cope with the challenges of the transplant.

Grimm et al. (2000) reported a study comparing inpatient transplant caregivers compared with the IPOP model of outpatient transplantation. Emotional responses and the needs of caregivers in terms of importance and satisfaction of informational, patient care, and psychological needs were studied. The authors found that IPOP caregivers had higher levels of satisfaction in these areas. They concluded that the IPOP model of outpatient transplantation is less emotionally distressing than the traditional inpatient transplant. Also, IPOP meets the needs of family caregivers more than inpatient transplantation. Overall, caregivers seem to have a positive experience in the outpatient setting, but continued research is necessary to evaluate the impact of outpatient transplantation on the caregiver.

Alternatives to Outpatient Transplantation: Cooperative Care

An alternative to outpatient transplantation is the Cooperative Care Center in the Lied Transplant Center at the Nebraska Health System/University of Nebraska Medical Center (Franco, 1998; Schmit-Pokorny & Nuss, 2000; Wardian & Franco, 2001). Cooperative Care, first introduced by Anthony Grieco, MD, at the University of New York Medical Center (Grieco, Garnett, Glassman, Valoon, & McClure, 1990) is a model of care in which the patient and caregiver actively participate in the treatment process. Patients and care partners assume responsibility for certain elements of inpatient care traditionally delivered by hospital staff. Patients who are admitted to the inpatient Cooperative Care Center must be ambulatory (may use a cane, walker, or wheelchair) and have a caregiver. The University of Nebraska Medical Center adapted the Cooperative Care model for transplant patients as an effort to help control transplant costs and to provide a supportive environment for patients and caregivers. The multidisciplinary transplant team is available 24 hours a day, seven days a week in the outpatient clinic and treatment center, one level below the inpatient Cooperative Care floor. Patients and their care partners stay in two room suites with hotel-like services and amenities. Other services available in the Lied Transplant Center for transplant patients are an exercise room, play rooms, laundry facilities, concierge, patient resource center, and outdoor garden area (Schmit-Pokorny & Nuss, 2000). Overall, the cost of the transplant process is less. Also, the patient and caregiver receive support that may not be available in the outpatient setting. Chwalow et al. (1990) reported on the use of the Cooperative Care model for medical and surgical patients. They found that not only did cost decrease, but patient satisfaction increased and patients' knowledge of their disease process, care, and treatment increased (Schmit-Pokorny, Franco, Frappier, & Vyhlidal, 2003).

Conclusion

Outpatient high-dose therapy followed by autologous HSCT and frequently allogeneic HSCT is becoming routine. Reports since 1994 confirm that outpatient transplantation is safe and feasible. Often outpatient transplantation costs less than inpatient transplantation. Patients and care partners seem to prefer this approach; however, more research is necessary to confirm this choice. Outpatient transplantation allows patients and care partners more freedom, control over daily care, and independence. However, not all patients are eligible for this approach, and not all patients will choose to be transplanted in an outpatient setting. Continued follow-up is needed to assess and compare QOL, complications, survival time, and cost issues between different models of outpatient and inpatient transplantation.

References

Bennett, C., Armitage, J., Armitage, G., Vose, J., Bierman, P., Armitage, J. et al. (1995). Costs of care and outcomes for high-dose therapy and autologous transplantation for lymphoid malignancies: Results from the University of Nebraska 1987 through 1991. *Journal of Clinical Oncology, 13*, 969–973.

Blume, K. & Thomas, E. (2000). A review of autologous hematopoietic cell transplantation. *Biology of Blood and Marrow Transplantation, 6*, 1–12.

Buchsel, P. (1991). Ambulatory care: Before and after BMT. In M. B. Whedon (Ed.), *Bone Marrow Transplantation: Principles, Practice, and Nursing Insights* (pp. 295–311). Sudbury, MA: Jones and Bartlett Publishers.

Buchsel, P. (1993). Ambulatory care for the bone marrow transplant patient. In P. C. Buchsel & C. H. Yarbro (Eds.), *Oncology Nursing in the Ambulatory Setting: Issues and Models of Care* (pp. 185–216). Boston: Jones and Bartlett Publishers, Inc.

Buchsel, P. & Kapustay, P. (1995). Peripheral stem cell transplantation. *Oncology Nursing: Patient Treatment and Support, 2*, 1–14.

Buchsel, P. & Kapustay, P. (1997). Models of ambulatory care for blood cell and bone marrow transplantation. In M. Whedon & D. Wujcik (Eds.), *Blood and Marrow Stem Cell Transplantation: Principles, Practice, and Nursing Insights* (pp. 525–561). Sudbury, MA: Jones and Bartlett Publishers.

Buchsel, P. & Kapustay, P. (2000). *Stem Cell Transplantation: A Clinical Textbook*. Pittsburgh, PA: Oncology Nursing Society.

Buchsel, P., Leum, E., & Randolph, S. (1997). Nursing care of the blood cell transplant recipient. *Seminars in Oncology Nursing, 13*, 172–183.

Burns, J. & Tierney, D. (1996). A daily flowsheet for an outpatient bone marrow transplant treatment center. *Oncology Nursing Forum, 23*, 1313–1316.

Burns, J., Tierney, D., Long, G., Lambert, S., & Carr, B. (1995). Critical pathway for administering high-dose chemotherapy followed by peripheral blood stem cell rescue in the outpatient setting. *Oncology Nursing Forum, 22*, 1219–1224.

Cavanaugh, C. A. (1994). Outpatient autologous bone marrow transplantation: A new frontier. *Quality of Life: A Nursing Challenge, 3*, 25–29.

Chielens, D. & Herrick, E. (1990). Recipients of bone marrow transplants: Making a smooth transition to an ambulatory care setting. *Oncology Nursing Forum, 17*, 857–862.

Chwalow, A., Mamon, J., Crosby, E., Grieco, A., Salkever, D., Fahey, M. et al. (1990). Effectiveness of a hospital-based cooperative care model on patients' functional status and utilization. *Patient Education and Counseling, 15*, 17–28.

Dix, S., Cord, M., Howard, S., Coon, J., Belt, R., & Geller, R. (1999). Safety and efficacy of a continuous infusion, patient controlled antiemetic pump to facilitate outpatient administration of high–dose chemotherapy. *Bone Marrow Transplantation, 24*, 561–566.

Franco, T. (1998). Reshaping care delivery in oncology: The cooperative care delivery model. *Oncology Nursing Forum, 25*, 312, (Abstract #20).

Freeman, M., Vose, J., Bennett, C., Anderson, J., Kessinger, A., Turner, K. et al. (1999). Costs of care associated with high-dose therapy and autologous transplantation for non-Hodgkin's lymphoma: Results from the University of Nebraska Medical Center 1989 to 1995. *Bone Marrow Transplantation, 24*, 679–684.

Grieco, A. J., Garnett, S. A., Glassman, K. S., Valoon, P. L., & McClure, M. L. (1990). New York University Medical Center's Cooperative Care Unit: Patient education and family participation during hospitalization—The first ten years. *Patient Education and Counseling, 15*, 3–15.

Grimm, P., Zawacki, K., Mock, V., Krumm, S., & Frink, B. (2000). Care giver responses and needs. *Cancer Practice, 8*, 120–128.

Heerman, J., Eilers, J., & Carney, P. (2001). Use of modified OSCEs to verify technical and skill performance and competency of lay care givers. *Journal of Cancer Education, 16*, 93–98.

Hurley, C. (1997). Ambulatory care after bone marrow or peripheral blood stem cell transplantation. *Clinical Journal of Oncology Nursing, 1*, 19–21.

Jagannath, S., Vesole, D., Zhang, M., Desikan, K., Copeland, N., Jagannath, M. et al. (1997). Feasibility and cost-effectiveness of outpatient autotransplants in multiple myeloma. *Bone Marrow Transplantation, 20*, 445–450.

Kelley, C., Randolph, S., & Leum, E. (2000). Home care of peripheral stem cell transplantation recipients. In P. C. Buchsel & P. M. Kapustay (Eds.), *Stem Cell Transplantation: A Clinical Textbook* (pp. 13.1–13.16). Pittsburgh, PA: Oncology Nursing Society.

Kessinger, A., Schmit–Pokorny, K., Smith, D., & Armitage, J. (1990). Cryopreservation and infusion of autologous peripheral blood stem cells. *Bone Marrow Transplantation, 5* (Supp. 1), 25–27.

Lawrence, C., Gilbert, C., & Peters, W. (1996). Evaluation of symptom distress in a bone marrow transplant outpatient environment. *The Annals of Pharmacotherapy, 30*, 941–945.

Letheby, B. A., Jackson, J. D., & Warkentin, P. I. (2000). Processing, cryopreservation, and storage of peripheral blood progenitor cells. In P. C. Buchsel & P. M. Kapustay (Eds.), *Stem Cell Transplantation: A Clinical Textbook* (pp. 4.1–4.20). Pittsburgh, PA: Oncology Nursing Press.

McDonald, J., Stetz, K., & Compton, K. (1996). Educational interventions for family care givers during marrow transplantation. *Oncology Nursing Forum, 23*, 1432–1439.

McGuire, T., Tarantolo, S., & Reed, E. (1998). Peripheral blood progenitor cells: Enabling outpatient transplantation. *Pharmacotherapy, 18*, 17S–23S.

Meisenberg, B., Ferran, K., Hollenbach, K., Brehm, T., Jollon, J., & Piro, L. (1998). Reduced charges and costs associated with outpatient autologous stem cell transplantation. *Bone Marrow Transplantation, 21*, 927–932.

Meisenberg, B., Miller, W., McMillan, R., Callaghan, M., Sloan, C., Brehm, T. et al. (1997). Outpatient high-dose chemotherapy with autologous stem-cell rescue for hematologic and nonhematologic malignancies. *Journal of Clinical Oncology, 15*, 11–17.

Meisinger, D., Sasse, S., & Schmit-Pokorny, K. (1996). Early discharge-autologous bone marrow/peripheral stem cell transplant patients: Outcomes. *Oncology Nursing Forum, 23*, (Abstract #75), 328.

O'Connell, S. & Schmit-Pokorny, K. (1997). Blood and marrow stem cell transplantation: Indications, procedure, and process. In M. Whedon & D. Wujcik (Eds.), *Blood and Marrow Stem Cell Transplantation: Principles, Practice, and Nursing Insights* (pp. 66–99). Sudbury, MA: Jones and Bartlett Publishers.

Peters, W., Ross, M., Vredenbrugh, J., Hussein, A., Rubin, P., Dukelow, K. et al. (1994). The use of intensive clinic support to permit outpatient autologous bone marrow transplantation for breast cancer. *Seminars in Oncology, 21*, 25–31.

Rizzo, J. D., Vogelsang, G. B., Krumm, S., Frink, B., Mock, V., & Bass, E. B. (1999). Outpatient-based bone marrow transplantation for hematologic malignancies: Cost saving or cost shifting? *Journal of Clinical Oncology, 17*, 2811–2818.

Ruiz-Argüelles, G., Gómez-Almaguer, D., Ruiz-Argüelles, A., González-Llano, O., Cantú, O., & Jaime-Pérez, J. (2001). Results of an outpatient-based stem cell allo-transplant program using nonmyeloablative conditioning regimens. *American Journal of Hematology, 66*, 241–244.

Ruiz-Argüelles, G., Ruiz-Argüelles, A., Pérez-Romano, B., Marín-López, A., & Delgado-Lamas J. (1998). Non-cryopreserved peripheral blood stem cells autotransplants for hematological malignancies can be performed entirely on an outpatient basis. *American Journal of Hematology, 58*, 161–164.

Schmit-Pokorny, K., Franco, T., Frappier, B., & Vyhlidal, R. C. (2003). The cooperative approach to delivery blood and marrow stem cell transplant care. *Clinical Journal of Oncology Nursing, 5*, 509–556.

Schmit-Pokorny, K., Hruska, M., & Ursick, M. (1998). Peripheral blood stem cell transplantation: Outpatient strategies. *Innovations in Breast Cancer Care, 3*, 52–56.

Schmit-Pokorny, K. & Nuss, S. (2000). Pediatric peripheral stem cell transplantation. In P. C. Buchsel & P. M. Kapustay (Eds.), *Stem Cell Transplantation: A Clinical Textbook* (pp. 16.1–16.24). Pittsburgh, PA: Oncology Nursing.

Schmit-Pokorny, K. & Sasse, S. (1994). *Perceptions of the Health Care Team Toward Patient Education in the Bone Marrow Transplant Setting*. Research Project for Master of Science in Nursing, Omaha: University of Nebraska Medical Center.

Schwartzberg, L., Birch, R., West, W., Tauer, K., Wittlin, F., Leff, R. et al. (1998). Sequential treatment including high-dose chemotherapy with peripheral blood stem cell support in patients with high-risk stage II-III breast cancer. *American Journal of Clinical Oncology, 21*, 523–531.

Seropian, S., Nadkarni, R., Jillella, A., Salloum, E., Burtness, B., Hu, G. et al. (1999). Neutropenic infections in 100 patients with non-Hodgkin's lymphoma or Hodgkin's disease with high-dose BEAM chemotherapy and peripheral blood progenitor cell transplant: Out-patient treatment is a viable option. *Bone Marrow Transplantation, 23*, 599–605.

Stream, P. (1983). Functions of the outpatient clinic before and after transplantation. *Nursing Clinics of North America, 18*, 603–610.

Wardian, S. & Franco, T. (2001). Cooperative care presents unique challenges in education. *Blood and Marrow Stem Cell Transplant Special Interest Group Newsletter, 12*, 1.

Wardian, S., Warren, J., & Eilers, J. (1997). Care partners to persons undergoing outpatient autologous stem cell transplant: The lived experience. *Oncology Nursing Forum, 24*, (Abstract 205), 341.

Weaver, C. H., Schwartzberg, L. S., Hainsworth, J., Greco, F. A., Li, W., Buckern, C. D., & West, W. H. (1997). Treatment-related mortality in 1000 consecutive patients receiving high-dose chemotherapy and peripheral blood progenitor cell transplantation in community cancer centers. *Bone Marrow Transplant, 17*, 671–678.

Weaver, C., Schwartzberg, L., Zhen, B., Mangum, M., Leff, R., Tauer, K. et al. (1997). High-dose chemotherapy and peripheral blood stem cell infusion in patients with non-Hodgkin's lymphoma: Results of outpatient treatment in community centers. *Bone Marrow Transplantation, 20*, 753–760.

Chapter 10

The Breast Cancer Clinic: Yesterday, Today, and Tomorrow

Cathy Coleman

Introduction

Breast cancer patients often have no way to correct problems they encounter. We need a healthcare system that is accountable for giving good care. Meanwhile, as patients we can do our part to make the system more accountable. We need a health care system that provides the right treatment, at the right time, every time. (National Breast Cancer Coalition, 2002)

Overview

During the past five years, six landmark reports from the Institute of Medicine (IOM) have instilled a new sense of national urgency related to the safety, quality, delivery, integrity, and economy of healthcare in the United States (Institute of Medicine, 1999–2003). Concurrently, major constituents, including providers, payers, policy experts, patients, and professional societies, have responded with comprehensive and innovative strategic and business plans to address the gaps in care and the costs of correcting them. Not surprisingly, the focus is on research-driven, evidence-based, and patient-centered care. As a result of two lawsuits by consumer groups, Kaiser Permanente (the nation's largest nonprofit health maintenance organization) has published treatment guidelines on its Website for hundreds of diseases (Freudenheim, 2004). The Department of Veteran's Affairs is on the frontier of evolving standards and systems for electronic health records to optimize communication and minimize medical errors (Department of Veteran's Affairs, 2003). The federal government, which purchases healthcare for 100-million Americans, is leveraging its unique role as regulator, provider, and researcher to create an example of new leadership and partnership models to improve safety and quality (IOM, 2002). As shown in **Tables** **10.1** and **10.2**, public policy experts such as Paul Ellwood are prescribing a heroic "cure" for the common healthcare system, including outcomes accountability, whereas other prestigious groups have declared new rules for redesigning healthcare, resulting in a new and unprecedented definition of patient expectations, including such terms as "individualization" and "transparency" (Ellwood, 2002; IOM, 2001).

Professional oncology organizations and breast cancer advocacy groups have also mobilized to translate and integrate new research findings and emerging data regarding care deficiencies into their plans for the future. Recently, the Oncology Nursing Society (ONS) published a Patient's Bill

Table 10.1 A "HEROIC" CURE FOR THE COMMON HEALTHCARE SYSTEM

H	Health Organization: a new infrastructure for a new medical culture.
E	Evidence-based medicine: links quality improvement to cost containment and allows us to quantify the value to patients of new technologies.
R	Responsibility: shared by the patient, provider, and payer
O	Outcomes accountability: routine measurement and reporting of health outcomes by all providers evidence of openness and trustworthiness to patients.
I	Information technologies: all major reforms are tied to an electronic medical record, enhancing decision support, outcomes analysis, and patient communication.
C	Commitment: continuously available follow-up care and advice over a lifetime with constant health insurance coverage.

Ellwood (2002).

of Rights for Quality Cancer Care (Oncology Nursing Society, 2003a) and after a monumental "think tank," the National Breast Cancer Coalition disseminated its guide to quality and accountability for breast cancer care (National Breast Cancer Coalition, 2002). However, while unacceptable variations in quality and safety were being publicized, major strides continued to be made nationally and internationally in cancer survival rates as well as new breakthroughs in translational research. Based on progress in exciting areas such as molecular epidemiology and bioinformatics, the National Cancer Institute (NCI) announced an optimistic new goal of eliminating cancer-related suffering and deaths by the year 2015 (Oncology, 2003). Clearly, the new century has begun with major national efforts to transform healthcare and to inform patients better. A unique opportunity exists for cancer nurses to build on this momentum of change by creating new site-specific models of delivery and accountability such as the breast cancer clinic. The breast cancer clinic, program, or center of the future could serve to align patient, payer, researcher, and provider needs and priorities. This chapter describes the historical, clinical, and practical considerations for developing such a comprehensive clinic or program in the ambulatory care setting.

Yesterday: The Courage to Change

There is a better way for everything. Find it.

Thomas Edison

Over the years, there has been remarkable progress in both the diagnosis of breast disease

---

Table 10.2 FORMULATING 10 NEW RULES TO REDESIGN AND IMPROVE CARE

Healthcare: what people should expect

1.	Beyond patient visits:	new methods of communicating via e-mail, phone, Internet.
2.	Individualization:	clinicians who adapt to meet personal needs/preferences.
3.	Control:	patient as the source of control of the care system.
4.	Information:	medical record for the patient to keep, read, and understand.
5.	Science:	evidence-based knowledge; excellence as system standard.
6.	Safety:	accountable health systems that will prevent/reduce errors.
7.	Transparency:	entitled to know about clinician performance/costs of care.
8.	Anticipation:	proactive efforts to restore and maintain health.
9.	Value:	money and time to be valued, not wasted; new innovation.
10.	Cooperation:	interdisciplinary, seamless coordination of care.

IOM (2001).

and the delivery of breast care. The possibility of detecting small, preclinical, and noninvasive breast cancer through an X-ray was unthinkable in the early days of radical mastectomy. Between 1890 and 1960, most breast cancer was detected clinically and treated surgically, with large tumors often representing inoperable or incurable disease. Beginning in the 1960s, research in breast imaging evolved and became an established radiologic subspecialty. Mammography now represents the most common imaging procedure that directly impacts a reduction in mortality from disease (Sickles, 2000). Today, most early breast cancers identified through high-quality mammography are both curable and operable, but with less invasive, more cosmetic procedures. Furthermore, emerging biomarker and genetic research as well as new imaging technologies is yielding promising and revolutionary changes in the detection and diagnosis of microscopic, preclinical disease and there is real hope for primary prevention (IOM/National Research Council, 2001; Oncology News International, 2003a, 2003b). Multimodality therapy is now becoming more individualized with less morbidity, and quality of life is being measured along with clinical trials to evaluate new drugs and medical devices. Clearly, the complexity and specialty of diagnosing and treating breast disease have required more satisfying and efficient systems to deliver care and conduct research.

Changes in providing ambulatory breast care have evolved from public health clinics to private practice offices to interdisciplinary centers. As early as 1931, leading surgeons began to form breast "services" at their academic institutions, and in 1937, the National Cancer Act was passed, which authorized the surgeon general to "cooperate with state health agencies in the prevention, control and eradication of cancer" (Coleman, 2000; Coleman & Lebovic, 1996). Breast cancer clinics first came into existence during the 1940s when community-based "cancer detection clinics" were formed as public health demonstration projects to provide clinical breast examination and to teach breast self-examination. When a more modern version of the National Cancer Act had been passed in 1971, a new research-driven organizational model was embraced by Congress and the public by funding and designating NCI cancer centers to focus on the disease and its diagnosis, treatment, and rehabilitation. Between 1974 and 1980, the NCI also funded 12 breast cancer network demonstration projects in association with both community and tertiary hospitals (Kane et al., 1981). In the 1970s, a new consumerism, the birth of "feminism," and political activism also contributed to societal changes with demands for more targeted research, better treatment options, improved communication, and coordination regarding breast cancer. In the late 1970s, the first privately funded breast "center" was developed in Van Nuys, CA whereas community and academic centers nationwide began to create more specialized "clinics." Interestingly, the inspiration to start the first freestanding breast center in the country came about because the politics and logistics of developing a truly patient-oriented, multidisciplinary breast clinic at the University of California at Los Angeles (UCLA) proved impossible for the dedicated and politically courageous breast surgeon who dared to challenge the status quo of fragmented, inefficient care (Silverstein, 2000). By the mid 1980s, at least three national breast care organizations (the American Society of Breast Disease, the National Consortium of Breast Centers, the National Alliance of Breast Care Organizations) had been founded (**Table 10.3**), and breast care "clinics, programs, or centers" became an increasingly value-added service or business unit driven by hospitals with accredited cancer programs or interested physicians and administrative leaders in radiology, medical oncology, women's health, or surgery. In 2003, yet another progressive, interdisciplinary breast center model involving the military and civilian communities emerged to address the new paradigms and challenges associated with translational research

(Hymowitz, 2003; Oncology News International, 2003c).

Common to all of these historical breast cancer "clinic" organizational structures are four fundamental goals and challenges:

- To decrease the morbidity, anxiety, and mortality from breast cancer in communities served
- To increase the coordination and communication between patients, multiple professionals, departments, and healthcare facilities
- To foster participation in clinical, behavioral, or translational research
- To define, measure, and monitor quality determinants of clinical, operational, and financial success for the sponsoring organization(s).

Dr. Benjamin O. Anderson, a breast center leader and surgeon from University of Washington in Seattle summarized the challenges of building a breast cancer clinic:

> *Our mission is to provide a full spectrum of care from high-risk evaluation to initial breast cancer diagnosis and treatment to advanced therapy for metastatic disease, and at the same time support clinical and translational research. The coordination is very challenging, particularly when we are trying to at least maintain cost neutrality in our clinical work. There is always a series of options and barriers around geography, but with creativity, flexibility and good space planners, compromises and committed staff, solutions can always be found. (personal communication, accessed by email on September 2, 2003)*

It has been estimated that the lag time between the discovery of more effective forms of treatment and their incorporation into routine patient care averages 17 years (IOM, n.d.). Considering this fact and the increasing capacity of bioinformatics to expedite research processes, it has been predicted that yesterday's advances may arrive in the clinic sooner rather than later.

Commenting on new findings to predict prognosis in breast cancer, Marc Lippman, MD, from the University of Michigan stated, "There is a tsunami of data...genetic signatures represent a technology that is going to transform practice in the next handful of years" (Kolata, 2002). From the detection of palpable tumors in public health clinics of the early 20th century to the laser microdissection of tumor cells in research labs of the early 21st century, breast cancer clinics will continue to present a unique opportunity for oncology nurses to facilitate more individualized care of patients and to foster interdisciplinary practice for professionals.

Today: Getting Started, Staying Focused, and Achieving Growth

Getting Started

> *Nothing will ever be attempted if all possible objections must first be overcome.*
>
> *Samuel Johnson*

Despite many political, financial, geographic, and operational barriers, breast cancer clinics, mammography centers, and comprehensive breast centers have been evolving in Europe and the United States for three decades. Critical success factors for these diverse organizational models have been extensively detailed elsewhere (Coleman, 2000; European Society of Mastology, 2000; Katterhagen, Barofsky, & Berliner et al., 1998; Lee, 2000; Parikh & Coleman, 2002; Piccart et al., 2001; Silverstein, 2000; Tabar et al., 2000). Currently, in the United States, there are no nationally developed consensus standards for developing or evaluating breast cancer clinics or breast centers, but leading organizations in Europe (European Commission/ Eusoma) and the United States (American College of Surgeons, American Society

Table 10.3 BUILDING A BETTER BREAST CANCER CLINIC: RESOURCES FOR QUALITY IMPROVEMENT AND PROGRAM DEVELOPMENT

Organization	Telephone	Website
Advisory Board Company	(202) 672–5600	http://www.advisoryboardcompany.com
Agency for Health Care Research and Quality	(301) 594–1364	http://www.ahrq.gov/ http://www.talkingquality.gov
American Association of Cancer Research	(215) 440–9300	http://www.aacr.org
American Cancer Society	(800) ACS–2345	http://www.cancer.org
American College of Radiology (& Society of Breast Imaging)	(800) ACR–LINE	http://www.acr.org/ http://www.sbi–online.org
ACR Mammography Interpretive Skills Assessment	(800) ACR–LINE	http://www.acr.org
American College of Surgeons Commission on Cancer	(312) 202–5000	http://www.facs.org/
American Health Information Management Association, Quality Management Section	(800) 428–4112	http://www.ahima.org/qms/about/index.html
American Health Quality Association	(202) 331–5790	http://www.ahqa.org/pub/quality
American Society of Breast Disease	(214) 368–6836	http://www.asbd.org/
American Society of Breast Surgeons	(301) 362–1722	http://www.breastsurgeons.org
American Society of Clinical Oncology	(703) 299–0150	http://www.asco.org/
American Society of Preventative Oncology	(608) 263–9515	http://www.aspo.org
American Society of Radiologic Technologists	(800) 444–2778	http://www.asrt.org
AVON Breast Cancer Crusade	(212) 244–5368	http://www.avoncompany.com
Blue Cross Blue Shield Association Technology Evaluation Center	(312) 297–6000	http://www.bcbs.org
Breast Diagnostic Algorithms for Primary Care Clinicians	(619) 594–2087	http://qap.sdsu.edu
California HealthCare Foundation The Quality Initiative	(510) 238–1040	http://www.chcf.org
Centers for Disease Control and Prevention	(888) 232–5929	http://www.cdc.gov
Centers for Medicare & Medicaid Services	(410) 786–3000	http://www.cms.gov
Clinical Breast Care Project Department of Defense/Walter Reed Army Medical Center	(202) 782–0002	http://cbcp.info
CMS–Quality Improvement Organizations	(410) 786–3000	http://cms.gov/qio
College of American Pathologists	(800) 323–4040	http://www.cap.org/pathfocus

(continues)

Table 10.3 Building a Better Breast Cancer Clinic: Resources for Quality Improvement and Program Development (cont'd)

Organization	Telephone	Website
Department of Defense, General Services Administration		http://www.arnet.gov/Library/OFPP/BestPractices
Duke Rohe–Weekly Reader on Performance Improvement		http://www.mdanderson.org drohe@mdanderson.org
European Commission, European guidelines for quality assurance in mammography screening		http://europa.eu.int http://eusoma.org
Food and Drug Administration	(800) 495–3232	http://www.fda.gov/cdrh/mammography/
Foundation for Accountability	(503) 223–2228	http://www.facct.org
Guidelines Clearinghouse		http://www.guidelines.gov
Healthcare Information and Management Systems Society	(312) 915–9237	http://www.himss.org
HealthLeaders Journal		http://healthleaders.com
Healthy People 2010, DHHS	(800) 367–4725	http://www.health.gov/healthypeople/
Johns Hopkins Breast Center	(410) 955–4851	http://www.hopkinsmedicine.org/breastcenter/treatment/billofrights.html
Institute for Healthcare Improvement		http://www.ihi.org
Joint Commission on Accreditation of Healthcare Organizations	(630) 792–5000	http://www.jcaho.org/
Kaiser Permanente		http://www.kp.org
Leadership Development	(800) 590–0799	http://banffleadership.com
Lehigh Valley Health Systems	(610) 402–0689	http://www.lvh.org
Lumetra (formerly CMRI)	(415) 677–2000	http://www.lumetra.com
Mammatech Corporation (CBE)	(800) 626–2273	http://www.mammacare.com
Mammography Education, Inc.	(480) 419–0227	http://www.mammographyed.com
Medicare Preventive Services, (Mammography Campaign)	(410) 786–3000	http://www.cms.gov/preventive services
Memorial Care Health Services Quality Report Card	(562) 933–1800	http://www.memorialcare.org
National Academy Press, Institute of Medicine	(888) 624–8373	http://www.nap.edu http://www.iom.edu
National Alliance of Breast Cancer Organizations	(800) 719–9154	http://www.nabco.org
National Breast and Cervical Cancer Early Detection Program	(888) 232–5929	http://www.cdc.gov/cancer/nbccedp
National Breast Cancer Coalition, Guide to Quality Breast Care	(202) 296–7477	http://www.natlbcc.org
National Cancer Institute (Search– Quality of Cancer Care)	(800) 4–CANCER	http://www.cancer.gov
National Committee for Quality Assurance	(202) 955–3500	http://www.ncqa.org

Table 10.3 BUILDING A BETTER BREAST CANCER CLINIC: RESOURCES FOR
QUALITY IMPROVEMENT AND PROGRAM DEVELOPMENT (CONT'D)

Organization	Telephone	Website
National Comprehensive Cancer Network; NCCN Guidelines	(800) 777–0965	http://www.nccn.org
National Consortium of Breast Centers	(219) 267–8058	http://www.breastcare.org/
National Quality Forum	(202) 783–1300	http://www.qualityforum.org
Oncology Nursing Society	(412) 494–4599	http://www.ons.org
Physician Insurers Association of America	(301) 947–9000	http://www.thepiaa.org
Rand Corporation	(310) 393–0411	http://www.rand.org
Rewarding Results Program; Robert Wood Johnson Foundation	(888) 631–9989	http://www.rwjf.org
SNOMED International (Systematized Nomenclature of Medicine)	(800) 323–4040	http://www.snomed.org
Society for Ambulatory Care Professionals	(312) 422–3902	http://www.sacp–net.org/mission.html
Susan G. Komen Foundation	(800) 462–9273	http://www.komen.org
Team Approach–Breast Imaging	(617) 384–8600	http://cme.med.harvard.edu
UCSF Radiology/Breast Imaging Courses & Visiting Fellowships	(415) 476–9776 (415) 476–5731	http://postgrad.radiology.ucsf.edu

of Breast Disease, and the National Consortium of Breast Centers) (**Table 10.3**) are beginning to create quality standards and specialized curricula for interdisciplinary breast care professionals in both postgraduate and continuing-education settings. In 2000, the European Society of Mastology published an article with the first position paper in the world on the requirements of a "specialist breast unit." This paper also represented the first published standards for "a high quality specialist breast service" in Europe that were collaboratively developed with scientists, clinicians, and breast cancer survivors. This seminal article is a blueprint for action for all interested parties relative to developing a first-class breast cancer clinic or center.

Like the nursing process, getting started begins with a plan, including assessment. Depending on the ambulatory practice setting (i.e., physician office, outpatient department, tertiary academic setting, community hospital, free-standing surgery center, cancer center) and the sponsoring organization (i.e., profit, not for profit, managed care), there are numerous and diverse factors to consider for success. One easy and focused tool to assist in the initial, baseline program assessment is to conduct a brief SWOT (strengths, weaknesses, opportunities, and threats) analysis (**Table 10.4**). One mistake that many administrative planners make is to limit the number of participants who are interviewed in the SWOT analysis or business plan development. Often, clinicians represent the majority when the departments of human resources, quality/performance improvement, case management, contracting, as well as nonclinical, operational support staff should be included for input from all levels of the organization.

From day one, it is important to create a unified working team with relevant smaller subgroups to oversee the development process. In

Table 10.4 SWOT ANALYSIS

A "SWOT analysis" is the term often used by marketing and other business professionals to provide a summary of the strengths, weaknesses, opportunities, and threats in a given situation or organization. Analogous to the nursing process components of assessment, planning, implementation, and evaluation, the SWOT analysis represents a planning tool to expedite the initial and ongoing assessment of any opportunity such as breast care program development.

S = Strengths, W = Weaknesses, O = Opportunities, T = Threats

Coleman & Lebovic (1996).

this initial stage, effective, well-respected leadership, even on an interim basis, is critical for the purposes of clearly defining, discussing, and debating issues, roles, and resolving conflicts as they arise over time (Coleman,1998; Gunderman, 2003). In setting up a breast care clinic, four primary areas should be considered in the SWOT analysis and strategic plan: organizational development, business plan development, space planning/facility development, and most importantly, the clinical program development. **Table 10.5** provides a sample checklist with key components that may serve as a starting point for discussion in any setting.

Staying Focused

> *The difference between a successful person and others is not a lack of strength, not a lack of knowledge, but rather a lack of will.*
>
> *Vincent Lombardi*

Strategic planning, budgeting, and benchmarking are critical to quantify the process and ultimate success of the breast cancer clinic, which may include both direct (core) and indirect (complementary) services. Many institutions are introducing a service-line orientation to specialty programs such as cardiac, cancer, or women's health services, including breast care and breast cancer. This is a more focused, proactive approach that will assist oncology nurse administrators in formulating a realistic business case for develop-

ment and/or expansion of existing core services into a more holistic, integrated, functional, and profitable program. Often, the direct revenue-generating services of the "core" program (i.e., infusion services or breast imaging center) will provide valuable, additional spin-off revenue for the sponsoring organization; however, it may not be easily tracked or visible to financial decision makers or senior leaders in the institution. The creation of an inclusive charge master for all direct and indirect services is advisable to map the source of initial program entry for the patient and to detail the associated services (both revenue generating and not) as well as the referral services forwarded to other departments, physicians, etc. This task is time consuming and tedious, but the investment of human and financial resources to create a realistic budget and high-quality program will serve not only to "sell" administrators but also to motivate donors, employees, and affiliated physicians. **Tables 10.6** and **10.7** describe key questions for strategic planning efforts and key attributes of cancer data systems that will promote accountability and quality within a breast cancer clinic, regardless of clinical setting or funding sources (refer to **Table 10.3** for additional reference organizations).

Achieving Growth

> *I never notice what has been done. I only see what remains to be done.*
>
> *Madam Curie*

Table 10.5 DEVELOPING A BREAST CANCER CLINIC: SAMPLE CHECKLIST AND QUESTIONS

Organizational development

1. Collaborative, experienced administrative manager/partner
2. Respected, credible physician leader/champion/medical director
3. Oversight by interdisciplinary (clinical and administrative) team or professional advisory board (i.e., cancer committee, women's health, surgery, radiology)
4. Mechanism for formal community participation in planning/development (i.e., community advisory board and/or liaison to organizations' board of directors)
5. Creation of patient advisory group
6. Organizational focus, including vision statement for breast cancer clinic/center/program (regardless of sponsoring/funding department)
7. Stable funding and access to capital
8. Senior leader support in administration and governing board
9. Liaison to finance and contracting for business plan development
10. Liaison to quality improvement program
11. Liaison to institutional review board
12. Liaison to education/training department
13. Liaison to case management department
14. Liaison to risk management department
15. Liaison to foundation or fundraising department
16. Accreditation by American College of Surgeons, Commission on Cancer or other relevant quality organizations

Business plan development

1. Vision statement
2. SWOT analysis
3. Programmatic development and growth strategy (past, present, future)
4. Business case
   * Baseline data-procedure charge master, payer mix, reimbursement rates
   * Financial projections and timeframe (define direct and indirect spin-off revenue, staffing ratios for sample projections, etc.)
   * Analysis of self-referred patients and referring physician patterns
   * Identification of primary, secondary, and tertiary geographic service areas
5. Operating budget (1–3 years)
6. Equipment budget (including information technology/cancer data system)
7. Marketing budget (including community outreach, advertising, etc.)
8. Define measures of success with clinical, operational, and financial metrics
9. Development dollars needed (from operational revenue, philanthropy, grants/contracts, etc.)
10. Return on investment and timeframe

Space planning and facility development

1. How does the clinic or center currently fit into the strategic space plan for the campus of the organization?
2. Define core program services, staff, locations, and primary contact for each.
3. Define associated program services, staff, locations, and primary contact for each

(continues)

Table 10.5 DEVELOPING A BREAST CANCER CLINIC: SAMPLE CHECKLIST AND QUESTIONS (CONT'D)

4. Compose a master equipment and space needs list; include each program component and associated staff (from a telephone and desk/workstation all of the way to a comprehensive infusion or radiation therapy center/department).
5. Create operational flow chart starting with intake and triage for all potential entry points of contact by patient (walk-in, telephone, e-mail, fax, appointment, etc.).
6. Create operational flow chart of physician coverage by service line (independent and interdisciplinary).
7. Ascertain which clinical, educational, research, case-management services require adjacency for either necessity or convenience of patients, physicians, or staff.
8. What is the existing space allotment and for which services/staff?
9. What are proposed space needs for each independent program and the interdependent program functions?
10. Is there room for growth?
11. How important is the geographic fragmentation in terms of patient, physician, and employee satisfaction?
12. Will the identity of the facilities be related or "connected" by the program and marketing materials if not by location or proximity?
13. Which program(s) will take the leadership or "driver" role? Women's health, medical oncology, surgery, radiology, other?
14. Will donors be contributing to the funding, naming, and location decisions?
15. Will there be access to professional space planners and interior designers?

Clinical program development: core service options

Note that this list describes only core services. An efficient, multientry (i.e., phone, e-mail, fax, walk-in) intake process also needs to be in place to assess, triage, and refer patients to appropriate departments/physicians. For more details about this process and other associated breast program services, please refer to **Table 10.3** and contact breast centers affiliated with either the ASBD or NCBC. Ideally, psychosocial, spiritual, educational, and research services should be developed and integrated within each "core" patient service or disease management category in conjunction with relevant cancer/other data systems and bioinformatics (Coleman & Lebovic, 1996).

Risk assessment, risk reduction, and counseling

1. Cancer risk and/or genetic counseling team available
2. Access to clinical trials for prevention/risk reduction
3. Support and educational groups for patients/families
4. Formal relationship with regional or national reference laboratory

Disease detection and diagnosis

1. Clinical breast examination and breast self-examination performed regularly and proficiently with standardized policies/procedures for all licensed practitioners
2. Mammography technologists specially trained in patient communications, positioning, pain assessment, equipment quality control, patient history, and correlative clinical exam for symptomatic patients; cross-trained in ultrasound, magnetic resonance imaging, interventional biopsy procedures, and medical–legal issues

Table 10.5 DEVELOPING A BREAST CANCER CLINIC: SAMPLE CHECKLIST AND QUESTIONS (CONT'D)

3. Breast imaging radiologist/subspecialist interpreting mammography reads at least 2,500 exams per year
4. Double reading of screening mammograms by radiologists or with computer-aided detection technology
5. Fine needle aspiration readily available by well-trained practitioners and expert interpreting pathologists who also serve as second opinion consultants
6. Routine imaging–pathology correlation conferences for all breast biopsies
7. Access to emerging breast imaging technologies such as digital mammography, magnetic resonance imaging, ductal lavage, positiron emission tomography scanning, or associated molecular pathology-clinical trials involving regional or national tissue banks

Staging and treatment planning

1. Weekly/regular interdisciplinary breast cancer treatment planning conference
2. Subspecialized surgeon or surgical oncologist
3. Access to stage specific clinical trials
4. Sentinel lymph node biopsy offered to appropriate patients by all surgeons
5. Access to initial or delayed breast reconstruction
6. Tumor registry or other data collection/patient tracking systems in place
7. Access to second/third opinion/consultation service for each specialty

Multimodality treatment

1. Nurse case manager or patient navigator/care coordinator available for newly symptomatic or diagnosed patients
2. Oncology infusion and radiotherapy services staffed by specialized oncology certified and/or advanced practice nurses
3. Integration of complementary medicine services/options
4. Fast track anesthesia
5. Access to clinical, basic, and translational research trials
6. Access to state of art radiation oncology centers
7. Educational resource library

Recovery and rehabilitation

1. Individual and group education and support
2. Cancer rehabilitation program
3. Nutrition and lifestyle counseling services
4. Peer/partner visitation/education/counseling program
5. Boutique for prosthetics, wigs, and scarves

Continuing care

1. Identification of primary care coordinator/case manager (i.e., office nurse)
2. Designation of one treating physician as "captain" of follow-up team
3. Patient/family education and communication regarding standardized protocols for quality of life assessment and follow-up
4. Ongoing education and support services
5. Pain and symptom management services as indicated
6. Terminal care services if indicated

Table 10.6 ACHIEVING HEALTHCARE PROFITABILITY: STRATEGIC PLANNING AND BUDGETING

Assess each service line:

Quantifying profitability:

Who?	Who is accountable for accomplishing specific tasks?
What?	What are the specific steps or measures needed to accomplish each objective?
Where?	Where are changes to be implemented, including the impacts on interdependent departments?
When?	When are changes to be implemented, accomplished, and evaluated? (Milestones)
How?	How is success going to be measured and monitored?
Why?	Communicate the plan to relevant employees in all departments.

Rohloff & Phifer (2003).

Once the initial program has been defined, hopefully the leaders and team members will feel a sense of accomplishment and pride. Conducting patient, employee, and referring physician satisfaction surveys on an ongoing basis will help to guide short- and long-term goals, needs, and milestones. Many breast care clinics have been generously funded or expanded based on measuring and achieving the clinical, financial, and operational objectives. The simplest model of developing a breast cancer clinic is probably the formation of a convenient tumor board or similar multidisciplinary care planning conference for discussing the management of individual patients. Another example is the creation of a mammography–pathology correlation conference to assess the appropriateness and accuracy of each breast biopsy performed and by whom in the institution(s). Auditing this dimension of breast care will ensure the evaluation of all clinical findings, tissue specimens, and radiographic images that might represent numerous providers and facilities. The complexity related to breast cancer patient care depends on the initial pathology, prognosis, and stage of disease; any effort to improve communication, collaboration, and case management

Table 10.7 THE IDEAL CANCER CARE DATA SYSTEM: TOP 10 ATTRIBUTES

1. A set of well-established core quality measures to address the spectrum of care

2. Reliance on computer-based patient records—patient care and outcomes

3. Standard reporting of cancer stage, comorbidity, and processes of care

4. National population-based case selection to assure generalizability/quality

5. Repeated cross-sectional studies to monitor national trends and progress

6. Established benchmarks for quality improvement

7. Data systems for internal quality assurance

8. Public reporting of selected aggregate quality scores for consumers/purchasers

9. Adaptability and flexibility

10. Protections to ensure privacy of health information

IOM (2000b).

Table 10. 8 OBSERVING HEALTHCARE: NEW DIRECTIONS FOR 2004

1. From a youthful society with low health costs to an aging society obsessed with costs and looking younger
2. From inpatient care to outpatient care
3. From prescription drugs as an incidental expense to prescription drugs as an intolerable cost burden
4. From costs absorbed by employers to costs shifted to employees
5. From national to world concerns about infectious disease
6. From enough physicians and nurses to a shortage of both
7. From laissez faire medicine to activist programs to prevent and manage disease
8. From a la carte care to standardized care to improve quality, consistency, and outcomes

---

Reese (2003).

around the mammography–pathology procedures will ensure quality and accuracy. The most complex model of a breast cancer clinic is expressed through the development of a comprehensive breast center. Published results have proven that comprehensive breast centers or programs can enhance the quality and efficiency of care. Public reporting of outcomes has even become a centerpiece for marketing as well as a central component of internal quality-improvement programs that increase morale and pride. Several leading breast care programs have shared their outcomes and report cards in a recent article published in Imaging Economics (Parikh & Coleman, 2002). Achieving and sustaining growth will also need to reflect new directions in healthcare delivery and reimbursement. Eight new directions to help plan for growth have been outlined in an excellent commentary by Reese at *www.healthleaders.com*; these are listed in **Table 10.8**.

Tomorrow: The Courage to Lead

The measure of success is not whether you have a tough problem to deal with, but whether it's the same problem you had last year.

John Foster Dulles

Referring to Florence Nightingale in a remarkable biography (Florence Nightingale, page 48), Woodham-Smith said:

She too had thought that the qualities needed to relieve the misery of the sick were tenderness, sympathy, goodness, and patience. Now her short experience had already shown her that only knowledge and expert skill brought relief; and her destiny, which was to lighten the load of suffering, could be fulfilled only if she were armed with knowledge. She must learn how to nurse.

Thanks to this extraordinary leader, we have learned how "to nurse." It is now time for oncology nurses "to lead." More specifically... to lead the transformation of cancer care at local, state, national, and international levels (Oncology Nursing Society, 2003b). Breast cancer is a global public health problem. Creating a breast cancer clinic or program in your practice setting may be the first step to focus attention on the multifaceted problems and to generate the multidisciplinary solutions associated with the complexity, quality, and delivery of breast care in the future.

References

Anderson, B. O. Personal communication, accessed by email on September 2, 2003.

Coleman, C. (2000). Building quality into comprehensive breast care: A practical approach. *Surgical Oncology Clinics of North America, 9*, 319–338.

Coleman, C. M. & Lebovic, G. (1996). Organizing a comprehensive breast center. In J. Harris, M. E. Lippman, M. Morrow, & S. Hellman (Eds.), *Diseases of the Breast* (pp. 963–970). Philadelphia–New York: Lippincott-Raven Publishers.

Department of Veteran's Affairs. (2003). Veteran's affairs electronic health records system pushing national standards. Retrieved April 18, 2003 from *http://www.va.gov/opa/pressrel/docs/HHSCPRS.doc*

Ellwood, P. M. (2002). A cure for the common health care system. *Decisions in Imaging Economics, 15*, 6.

EUSOMA (European Society of Mastology). (2000). Position Paper: The requirements of a specialist breast unit. *European Journal of Cancer, 36*, 2288–2293.

Freudenheim, M. (2003). Large HMO to make treatment guidelines public. *The New York Times.* Retrieved January 24, 2003 from *http://www.nytimes.com*

Goleman, D. (1998). What makes a leader? *Harvard Business Review*, 93–102.

Gunderman, R. B. (2003). Leadership and psychological development. *Radiology, 228*, 617–619.

Hymowitz, C. (n.d.). In the lead. How innovative leadership cured ailing medical center. *Wall Street Journal.* Retrieved August 28, 2003 from *http://www.wsj.com*

Institute of Medicine. (1999). M. Hewitt & J. V. Simone (Eds.), *Ensuring Quality Cancer Care.* Washington, DC: National Academy Press.

Institute of Medicine. (2000a). M. Hewitt & J. V. Simone (Eds.), *Enhancing Data Systems to Improve the Quality of Cancer Care.* Washington, DC: National Academy Press.

Institute of Medicine. (2000b). L. T. Kohn, J. M. Corrigan, & M. S. Donaldson (Eds.), *To Err is Human: Building a Safer Health System.* Washington, DC: National Academy Press.

Institute of Medicine. (2001). *Crossing the Quality Chasm: A New Health System for the 21st Century.* Washington, DC: National Academy Press.

Institute of Medicine. (2002). *Leadership by Example: Coordinating Government Roles in Improving Health Care Quality.* Washington, DC: National Academy Press.

Institute of Medicine. (n.d.). The Chasm in Quality: Select Indicators from Recent Reports. Retrieved September 22, 2003 from *http://www.iom.edu/subpage.asp?id=14980*

Institute of Medicine. National Research Council. (2001). S. J. Nass, I. C. Henderson, & J. C. Lashof (Eds.), *Mammography and Beyond: Developing Technologies for the Early Detection of Breast Cancer.* Washington, DC: National Academy Press.

Kane, R. A., Kane, R. L., Williams, C. E., Hopwood, M. D., Lincoln, T. L., Rettig, R. A. et al. (1981). *The Breast Cancer Networks: Organizing to Improve Management of a Disease.* Santa Monica: Rand Publishing.

Katterhagen, G., Borofsky, H., & Berliner, K. (1998). The use of evidence based guidelines to improve outcomes and drive down costs in a community based breast center. *Cancer Management, 3*, 8–14.

Kolata, G. (2002). Breast cancer: Genes are tied to death rates. *The New York Times.* December 19, 2002.

Lee, C. Z. (2000). Oncopolitical issues: Obstacles and options for success in a comprehensive breast center. *Surgical Oncology Clinics of North America, 9*, 279–294.

National Breast Cancer Coalition. (2002). Guide to quality breast cancer care (2nd ed.). Retrieved September 21, 2002 from *http://www.natlbcc.org*

Oncology. (2003). NCI aiming to meet goal of eliminating suffering and death from cancer by 2015. *Oncology, 17*, 1019.

Oncology News International. (2003a). Are we closing in on a blood test for breast cancer? *Oncology News International, 13*(Suppl.), 19–20.

Oncology News International. (2003b). Concept of running a clinical trial without genetic profiling may soon be unthinkable. *Oncology News International, 13*(Suppl.), 19–20.

Oncology News International. (2003c). Military – Civilian endeavor makes breast cancer strides. *Oncology News International, 12*, 22–23.

Oncology Nursing Society. (2003a). Patient's bill of rights for quality cancer care. *Oncology Nursing Forum, 30*, 13–14.

Oncology Nursing Society. (2003b). Leadership Development Institute. Mission and Goal. Retrieved September 1, 2003 from *http://www.ldi.ons.wego.net/index.v3page?p=2895*

Parikh, J. R. & Coleman, C. M. (2002). Building a better breast program. *Decisions in Imaging Economics, 15*, 60.

Piccart, M., Cataliotti, L., Buchanan, M., Freilich, G., & Jassem, J. (2001). Brussels statement document. *European Journal of Cancer, 37*, 1335–1337.

Sickles, E. A. (2000). Breast imaging: From 1965 to the present. *Radiology, 215*, 1–16.

Silverstein, M. J. (2000). The Van Nuys Breast Center. *Surgical Oncology Clinics of North America, 9*, 159–175.

Tabar, L., Dean, P. B., Kaufman, C. S., Duffy, S. W., &
      Chen, H. H. (2000). A new era in the diagnosis of
      breast cancer. *Surgical Oncology Clinics of North Amer-
      ica, 9*, 233–277.
Woodham-Smith, C. (1951). *Florence Nightingale*. Great
      Britain: Penguin Books.

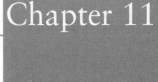

Chapter 11

Managing Pain in Ambulatory and Home Care

Carol P. Curtiss

Introduction

Unrelieved pain from cancer and other sources remains an important public health issue. Efforts to improve pain management continue in all healthcare settings, including ambulatory care. Since 2001, organizations are required to identify and treat pain in all patients as a basic part of clinical care in all settings. This chapter will review the principles for effective pain assessment and management in ambulatory care, describe strategies to develop and implement pain management initiatives, describe a variety of pain management services and offer recommendation for establishing and developing a pain management service.

The American Cancer Society estimates that approximately 1,368,030 people will be diagnosed with cancer in 2004 in the United States, and 536,700 will die from the disease. The overall 5-year survival rate for all cancers combined continues to increase and is now 62% (American Cancer Society [ACS], 2004). Approximately one-third of those people being treated for cancer have pain, more than two-thirds with advanced cancer experience pain (National Comprehensive Cancer Networks [NCCN], 2001). In the week before death, more than 50% of people experience severe unrelieved pain (SUPPORT Principle Investigators,

1995). Although the prevalence of pain in cancer survivors is unknown, many experience lasting pain from cancer, cancer therapies, or other causes that affect quality of life (Ferrell & Hassey Dow, 1997). Pain is one of the most common reasons that people seek healthcare, and ambulatory care services are a common site of entry into the healthcare system. Pain was one of the 10 most common reasons for calls to nurses for telephone advice in one large managed care plan, and inadequate pain relief was one of the most common reasons for member complaints (Donovan, Evers, Jacobs, & Mandleblatt, 1999). Simply stated, people with cancer at all stages of illness are at an increased risk for pain.

Cancer pain may be acute, chronic, chronic with acute episodes, constant, or intermittent. It may vary in intensity from minute to minute or day to day. Cancer, cancer therapy and treatment, or problems unrelated to either the illness or treatment can cause pain. Cancer pain is characterized as nociceptive (visceral or somatic), neuropathic, or mixed. Although cancer pain can be complex, relatively simple methods can relieve most cancer pain (American Pain Society [APS], 1999).

Attentive pain care is a patient right and a measure of quality care in all clinical settings.

The principles for assessing and managing cancer pain are well known (Jacox et al., 1994; APS, 1999) and are listed in **Table 11.1**. However, unrelieved cancer pain and poor clinical practices in managing pain are well documented and remain a major public health problem (National Institutes of Health [NIH], 2002; Bernabei et al., 1998; Cleeland et al., 1994; Jacox et al., 1994). A lack of knowledge on the part of healthcare professionals and the public, erroneous myths and misperceptions about pain and pain treatments, a lack of professional accountability for pain management, and healthcare systems that place a low priority on pain management are common barriers to adequate pain care (Oncology Nursing Society [ONS], 1998; Jacox et al., 1994).

In recent years, changes in reimbursement for cancer care and other healthcare systems changes have shifted the care of people with cancer from the inpatient setting to outpatient and home settings. It is estimated that approximately 90% of all cancer-related services occur in ambulatory settings, including hospital-based clinics and treatment centers, physician and nurse practitioner offices, and patient's homes (Haylock, 2001). Even the most complex procedures and therapies are currently performed as outpatient procedures. The responsibility for assessing and managing cancer pain has also shifted to these settings, placing ambulatory care staff, home care staff, and all oncology nurses in pivotal positions to provide effective leadership to improve pain and symptom management.

In 1999, the Joint Commission for Accreditation of Health Care Facilities (JCAHO) published new Pain Management Standards in all of its accreditation manuals, including its Comprehensive Accreditation Manual for Ambulatory Care (CAMAC) (JCAHO, 1999). JCAHO's new standards essentially require implementation of existing national standards and guidelines for managing all types of pain, including cancer pain. The standards require that pain is recognized, evaluated, and treated. An organization's response to pain should be based on the specific services provided in each clinical setting (JCAHO, 2001). All organizations accredited by the JCAHO are mandated to screen for pain routinely, assess those with pain, and address unrelieved pain (JCAHO, 1999; Dahl, 1999). An overview of the JCAHO pain standards is listed in **Table 11.2**. Regardless of the type of oncology services offered in an ambulatory setting, pain assessment and management are hallmarks of quality care.

Managing Pain in Ambulatory Care

Although the principles for managing pain in ambulatory care settings and the JCAHO requirements are similar to those in other care settings, ambulatory care presents several unique challenges to effective pain management. Patients' visits are short, and patients are often anxious and under stress. Pain may not be a priority for discussion with the nurse or physician, and patients may not realize that pain is not an inevitable consequence of cancer (Jacox et al., 1994). The time available for teaching may be limited, and depending on the ambulatory setting, nurses and doctors may or may not follow a caseload of

---

Table 11.1 PRINCIPLES FOR ASSESSING AND MANAGING PAIN

- Use, document, and display self-report whenever possible
- Screen for pain routinely
- Assess and reassess systematically
- Combine medications and nondrug strategies in a way that relieves each individual's pain
- Titrate medications to dose limits (nonopioids) or to individual response (opioids)
- Identify accountability
- Communicate the plan to those involved in care
- Identify and deal with barriers

Table 11.2 JCAHO PAIN MANAGEMENT STANDARDS

- Organizations must identify pain relief as a priority.
- All patients have the right to assessment, reassessment, and management of pain.
  - Pain is assessed routinely in all patients.
  - Assessment data are recorded in a way that facilitates reassessment and follow-up.
- Educate relevant clinical staff.
  - Include pain management education in orientation.
  - Assure competency of all relevant clinical staff.
- Educate the patient and family that pain control is an important part of care.
- Adopt policies that assure appropriate prescriptions/orders for the use of medicines and technology.
- Pain is monitored for pain intensity, quality, and response to treatment throughout the postprocedure period.
- Pain must not interfere with optimum level of function or rehabilitation.
- Include pain and symptom management in discharge planning.
- The organization collects data to monitor its performance.

Adapted from: Dahl, 1999; JCAHO, 1999.

patients over time. These and other challenges make it important for a healthcare facility to assess pain systematically and routinely and develop written, well-communicated plans to manage pain. Cancer pain management models and algorithms for ambulatory care are published (National Comprehensive Cancer Network [NCCN], 2000; Cleeland et al., 1986; Du Pen et al., 2000). Policies and practices must be in place to identify a basic standard of care for all patients within a healthcare system, including ambulatory care. **Table 11.3** describes components of a pain management standard for ambulatory care settings.

Another challenge for nurses providing care in ambulatory settings is that nursing assessment and management are often provided over the phone, with only verbal reports from the patient or family to guide assessment. Competent, systematic, well-honed assessment skills are essential for effective pain management while providing telephone nursing care. A sample telephone checklist for systematically assessing and managing pain is included in **Table 11.4**.

At discharge from ambulatory care areas or when an office or home visit is over, the patient and family are responsible for carrying out the pain management plan. Patient education and support are needed to anticipate and deal with common problems that patients experience at home. They include obtaining a prescribed medication, accessing information, tailoring prescribed regimens to meet individual needs, managing side effects, cognitively processing information, managing new or unusual pain, and managing multiple symptoms simultaneously (Schumacher et al., 2002). Educational materials should also include instructions for the safe storage of medications at home as well as other information to teach patients and families about the appropriate use of medications. **Table 11.5** lists key teaching points.

Integrating Pain Management into Clinical Care

Most people with pain can and should be treated by nonspecialty staff in all areas of healthcare as a routine part of competent basic clinical care. However, effective pain management requires updated knowledge and skills for all healthcare providers. However, knowledge and skills alone will not change practice or improve pain management (NIH, 2002). In order to improve pain assessment and management for all patients, organizations must make an institutional com-

Table 11.3   DEVELOPING A STANDARD FOR ASSESSING AND MANAGING PAIN

- All patients have a right to appropriate assessment and management of pain as a basic part of healthcare.
  - Include a commitment to pain management in mission statement, patient/family bill of rights, or service standards.
    Post a written statement on patient rights and responsibilities in examination rooms and other clearly accessible areas.
  - Identify groups and patients at high risk for pain and develop protocols to assess and manage high-risk patient's pain.
  - Distribute patient/family education brochures that teach that effective pain relief is an important part of care.
  - Integrate teaching about pain, pain assessment, and options for pain relief into presurgical teaching sessions, prenatal classes, public health fairs, and other educational efforts.
- Screen all patients for pain at first contact and routinely.
  - Select appropriate rating scales to meet the needs of patient populations and designate them as standard screening tools. These are examples:
    - 0–10 scale (with 0 being "no pain" and 10 being the "worst possible") for use for all adolescents and adults who are able to understand the scale
    - Faces scale for children and adults who cannot use the 0–10 scale
    - Premature Infant Pain Profile (PIPP) (Stevens, Johnston, Petryshen, & Taddio, 1996) for premature infants
    - Designate a specific alternative method to evaluate pain in those who are cognitively impaired, unconscious, or unable to verbalize pain
  - For specialty clinics, questions about pain may be targeted to the specific reason for the visit. For example, a patient being seen for breast cancer may be asked, "Do you have any pain from your breast cancer or your treatment?" A person who is being seen only for a procedure can be asked, "Do you have pain now?"
  - Postscreening tools should be in examination rooms where they are easily visible. For home care, use a "show and tell" approach with screening tools.
  - Identify a minimum required frequency for screening all patients and a level of pain intensity that requires intervention. This is an example:
    - Minimum required frequency—all patients are screened for pain at every visit and during follow-up phone calls.
    - On a scale of 0–10, pain greater than level 3 or any level unacceptable to the patient requires assessment and attention to the plan.
    - Include questions about pain in the routine questions asked all patients in the ambulatory setting (e.g., function, mobility, appetite, bowel management, comfort levels).
  - Record screening results in a way that facilitates reassessment and follow-up.
    - Integrate pain ratings into current documentation systems so that ratings are easy to find, easy to compare with one another over time, and easy to document.
    - Document pain ratings for easy access where other important clinical information is documented (e.g., flow sheets, graphic sheets).
  - Accept self-report as the single best indicator of pain and pain relief (Jacox et al., 1994; APS, 1999) in patient's who can report pain. Define pain as "whatever the person says it is, occurring whenever the person says it occurs." (McCaffery & Pasero, 1999)
  - Teach support staff to screen for pain and identify levels that must be reported to the nurse or physician for assessment.
  - In emergent settings, consider increasing the level of triage assigned to a person who reports pain.

Table 11.3   DEVELOPING A STANDARD FOR ASSESSING AND MANAGING PAIN (CONT'D)

- Systematically assess patients who report pain. Many published tools are available. (Jacox et al., 1994; Haylock & Curtiss, 1997; McCaffery & Pasero, 1999)
    - Include questions about the following:
        - Pain: onset, duration, location, quality, intensity, exacerbating and relieving factors, radiation, obtain pain rating
        - Pain relief: amount of relief, length of time for relief, pain relief rating, pain management history
        - Effects of pain on the person: function, sleep, appetite, mood, mobility, energy, ability to get around, work, play, socialize, etc.
        - Side effects: assessment for the presence of side effects and management of side effects
        - The plan: evaluate the plan for effectiveness, appropriateness, simplicity, and barriers to adherence
        - Patient's goal for relief (using the rating scale when possible; may also include functional goals)
        - A pain diary for the patient to record scores for pain, pain relief, function, activities, use of medications, and other strategies to relieve pain, side effects, and other concerns that is helpful for outpatient care providers to understand the pain experience
    - Initiate a telephone check list (**Table 11.4**) to evaluate pain when managing a patient's problems over the phone.
- Combine nondrug interventions and medications to meet individual needs for pain control.
- Screen for pain before, during, and after procedures. Assess those reporting pain.
    - Screen and document pain before procedures as a baseline.
    - Continue to evaluate the patient routinely during and after procedures.
    - Identify discharge criteria for pain relief. For example, "Patient may be discharged when pain is less than 3 on a scale of 0–10 or with any level acceptable to the patient."
    - Include questions about pain, response to pain treatment, and ability to rest or function in postprocedure follow-up phone calls.
- Maintain competency of all relevant clinical staff.
    - Include essentials of pain screening, assessment, and management in orientation of all clinical staff.
    - Include knowledge and skills in pain assessment and management as part of competency-based performance reviews within the scope of practice of the individual.
    - Make information about pain and pain therapy readily available to staff.
    - Hold staff accountable for effective assessment and management of pain.
- Teach patients and families that pain is an important part of care.
    - Teach rating scales and their purpose.
    - Make culturally and developmentally appropriate educational materials available to patients and families.
- Discharge plans include pain management plans.
    - Use written plans based on individual need.
    - Identify a contact person if pain is unrelieved or gets worse, new pain develops, or the person has questions about the plan.
- Collect data regarding pain assessment and management to monitor performance.
    - Evaluate current knowledge, skills, and attitudes of relevant clinical staff. Design educational and other programs to meet needs.
    - Investigate the care of patients with unrelieved pain.
    - Collaborate with pharmacists to evaluate appropriate use of medications for pain.
    - Identify problem areas and develop quality improvement plans to improve practices.
    - Identify high-risk patient populations and develop protocols to manage difficult types of pain common to particular settings.

Table 11.4 PAIN MANAGEMENT: TELEPHONE CHECKLIST

Assessment

- ❏ Pain history
  - ○ Pain onset, duration, location, severity
  - ○ Temporal pattern
    - • pain now versus old pain, continuous/intermittent, changes over time
  - ○ Quality
    - • sharp, dull, sore, throbbing, radiating, pressure, burning, shooting, etc.
  - ○ Exacerbating/relieving factors
    - • walking, sitting, coughing, lying flat, sleeping, eating, time of day, medicines, activity
  - ○ Intensity
    - • now, worst/best in last 24 hours, use a rating scale; record the ratings
  - ○ Current therapy for pain
    - • doses and frequency of medications actually used by person in last 24–48 hours; include opioid, nonopioid, adjuvant, and over-the-counter medications and nutritional/alternative supplements
  - ○ Analgesic side effects
    - • constipation: current bowel regimen, other side effects
  - ○ Pain relief
    - • how much relief: use the same rating scale; how long to achieve relief, how long does it last, what has worked in the past?
  - ○ Effects of pain on the person
    - • function, mood, energy, appetite, mobility, comfort, ability to work, socialize, play, etc.
- ❏ Psychosocial assessment
  - ○ For persistent pain, evaluate for depression
    - • time out of bed, activity level, changes in social interaction/communication, etc.
- ❏ Concurrent problems
  - • fatigue, anorexia, dyspnea, anxiety, delirium, etc.
- ❏ Treatment history
- ❏ Past history
- ❏ Diagnostic evaluation
- ❏ Compare ratings of pain and pain relief over time (as with other vital signs)

Possible interventions

- ❏ Increase/decrease scheduled and breakthrough opioid doses
- ❏ Increase aggressiveness of bowel management program to prevent constipation
- ❏ Change opioids (review equianalgesic conversion)
- ❏ Change routes (move from the oral route only for valid reasons (e.g., unable to take nutrition orally, unable to swallow, gut does not work, person is not conscious))
- ❏ Add tricyclic antidepressant (neuropathic pain; check cardiac history)
- ❏ Add anticonvulsant (neuropathic pain, after trial of tricyclics or as first line)
- ❏ Treat/manage side effects
- ❏ Add nondrug interventions (e.g., heat, cold, massage, transcutaneous electrical nerve stimulator, relaxation and imagery, etc.)
- ❏ Evaluate understanding and reinforce teaching (what to report, to whom, when; ask about actual use of medications, plan time for refills; look for barriers)
- ❏ Referrals as needed (social work, behavioral medicine, physical therapy, pain specialist, etc.)
- ❏ Does patient need to be seen for further assessment or teaching?
- ❏ Follow-up phone call to/from person/family within 24 hours to evaluate response to change

Sheidler, V. (1997, May) Telephone check list. Part of a handout for symposium held in conjunction with the annual meeting of the National Association of Orthopaedic Nurses. Philadelphia, PA. Adapted with permission by Curtiss, C. (1997). Pain management - telephone check list. Unpublished handout.

mitment to improving pain control. This commitment requires administrative support and leadership, along with a willingness to change polices, procedures, and practices throughout the healthcare system, with a goal of supporting and developing skills and accountability of all staff around pain-management issues. Steps to achieve this commitment include articulating a statement of administrative support and commitment; forming an interdisciplinary team with the authority and responsibility to improve pain assessment and management; analyzing current practices, attitudes, costs, and barriers; articulat-

ing a standard of care; establishing accountability for pain assessment and management; providing information about interventions to facilitate orders and implementation of orders; promising patients a quick response to pain; providing a program for ongoing education for staff and patients; establishing policies to ensure continuity and accountability across the care setting; and implementing a program for ongoing evaluation and quality improvement (Gordon, Dahl, & Stevenson, 2000; McCaffery & Pasero, 1999; Altilio, 1999).

Forming a Team to Improve Pain Management

Success in pain management occurs across settings when a team is inclusive and interdisciplinary and pain management is considered a standard practice for all clinicians (Ferrell, 1999). For a systems-wide team, select individuals from a variety of disciplines who are interested in pain management and who have the expertise or who are willing to learn about pain control. Choose those who are well respected among colleagues and who have a passion to champion the cause of effective pain management. Anticipate that the team will be a standing part of the organization rather than a temporary task force. Consider forming a "spin-off" interdisciplinary team to work on improving pain assessment and management in specific ambulatory care settings to complement and disseminate the work of an institution's pain management team. This "miniteam" will focus attention on issues specific to outpatient, home, or office care, as well as integrate systems-wide changes into ambulatory practice.

The Work of the Team

An initial plan should include strategies to examine current pain management practices in each particular setting. Surveys are published to evaluate knowledge and attitudes of staff members regarding pain and pain management (Gordon et

---

Table 11.5 SAFE USE OF MEDICATIONS: DO'S AND DON'TS FOR PATIENTS

DO

- Maintain a list of all medications and their dosage schedules; update the list when medications change.
- Keep medications in their original containers for accurate identification.
- Store medications in a safe, secure place away from children and pets.
- Read the label every time medicine is taken.
- Tell the nurse or physician about any side effects that you think the medication may be causing and about any allergies you have.

DON'T

- Share medication or take another person's medication.
- Chew, crush, or break tablets unless instructed to do so. Some pain medications are made to be slowly absorbed over many hours; crushing, chewing, or breaking releases too much medication at once.
- Store medications in direct sunlight or in humid places such as bathroom cabinets.
- Take more or less medication than prescribed. Call the physician if your pain is not relieved or if you are having side effects. Ask the physician to adjust the dose.

Institute for Safe Medication Practices (ISMP). Be an informed consumer/key questions. www.ismp.org/consumer/brochure.html. Accessed July 27, 2002.

al., 1999; McCaffery, Gordon, Pasero, & Ferrell, 1999). Results of these surveys can direct specific educational efforts. Improvement processes may include chart audits to determine whether pain screening is routinely performed and recorded by everyone, if patients who report pain are appropriately assessed and interventions are carried out to relieve pain, and most important whether pain was managed. If pain was unrelieved, chart audits may also reveal that assessment was absent or that the plan was ineffective or perhaps not appropriately changed. Evaluating these results in the aggregate can direct further efforts to target areas for improvement. In addition to examining current practice, a pain team must also articulate a standard of care, establish strategies to educate the public and professionals, and mentor and coach others to increase their skills and knowledge about pain control.

Ambulatory settings and home care agencies that are part of a wider healthcare system should adopt the organization's system-wide standard of care for assessing and managing pain, adapting it to ambulatory or home care as needed. Freestanding ambulatory centers and offices must adopt a standard of care based on national standards and guidelines. For freestanding services, collaborate with the facilities where patients are admitted to share standards and provide continuity of pain care across the trajectory of care.

Strategies to Improve Cancer Pain Management

Algorithms and pathways are published for managing pain in the outpatient setting (Georgesen, 1999; DuPen, Niles, Hansberry, & DuPen, 1997) and are consistent with the principles for assessing and managing pain elicited in national standards and guidelines. Using pathways and algorithms can help standardize options for care as well as educate staff about appropriate interventions for pain.

Many organizations have implemented some type of pain-management program to ensure that all patients receive competent pain assessment and management as a basic part of care. Many have instituted programs that are modeled after the Pain Resource Nurse (PRN) Program that Ferrell and colleagues developed (Ferrell, Grant, Richey, Ropchan, & Rivera, 1993) to provide advanced education and ongoing support to nurses who serve as decentralized and easily accessible resources to improve pain management. Nurses are selected for their interest, expertise, leadership abilities, and respect among colleagues. Some organizations see the role as a rung on a clinical ladder. In most models, participants attend an intensive educational session with information about pain, pain pathophysiology, barriers to effective pain management, assessment skills, management strategies, including medications and nondrug interventions, communication skills, and strategies to act as change agents. PRN nurses are then available to other staff for questions, consultation, and mentoring. Periodic educational and problem-solving updates and ongoing communication and support among PRN nurses are keys to successful programs. Members of interdisciplinary teams assigned to improve pain assessment and management in a facility may serve as resources for staff as well.

Pain Clinics, Centers, and Services

Most acute and cancer pain and some chronic pain can be treated by nonspecialty staff using the basic principles for managing pain shown in **Table 11.1**. In fact, as a core competency, any healthcare professional caring for people with cancer should be able to demonstrate the ability to screen for pain routinely, accurately assess and reassess patients with pain in order to evaluate pain and pain relief, and appropriately select and use medications and nondrug interventions to manage pain. Occasionally, the needs of individual patients may require consultation with or referral to pain-management specialists. These types of challenging pains may be extremely complex and require expert, interdisciplinary specialty consultation and care in order to evaluate patients and develop and carry out the most therapeutic strategies (Bonica, 1990). Although specialized pain services may result in improved care for some patients, by themselves, pain services, centers, and clinics do not solve the organization-wide problem of untreated pain (Pasero, Gordon, McCaffery, & Ferrell, 1999).

Pain clinics were first documented in the literature in the 1970s (Taricco, 1996) and continue to emerge in a variety of settings today. The primary goal for any pain-treatment facility or program is to provide effective, humane care for those who suffer from unrelieved pain (APS, 1996). The International Association for the Study of Pain [IASP] (1990) classified pain-management clinics as multidisciplinary pain centers, multidisciplinary pain clinics, pain clinics, and modality-oriented clinics, depending on a program's scope of care, services, and resources. A multidisciplinary pain center includes services for direct patient care, education, and research and often exists as a component of a medical school or teaching hospital. A wide array of healthcare specialists, including nurses, is required and will vary depending on the patient population and healthcare resources of the community. A multidisciplinary pain clinic differs in definition from a multidisciplinary pain center only because it does not include research and teaching activities as part of its regular programs. A pain clinic focuses on the diagnosis and management of patients with pain and may specialize in specific diagnoses such as cancer pain or other areas of specialization. However, this term should not be used to describe an isolated solo practitioner. A modality-oriented clinic offers a specific type of treatment and does not provide comprehensive assessment or management (IASP, 1990).

The American Society of Pain Management Nurses identifies eight care delivery models for pain management that include multidisciplinary and interdisciplinary models, case management models, pain resource nurse models, pain team models, hospital-based models, home healthcare models, outpatient clinics, and primary care models (Jerin, 2002). An interdisciplinary model of some type is usually established to treat complex pain problems through collaborative assessment and multimodel approaches to treatment. The Commission of Accreditation of Rehabilitation Facilities (CARF) requires an interdisciplinary model for accreditation. Examples include palliative care pain services, anesthesia services (Horlitz & Lucas, 1994), and cancer pain services (Williams et al., 1992). In a case management model (McMarburg, 1998), the goal of case managers is to follow the patient's progress, evaluate the overall plan in a systematic way, and optimize care in a cost/quality manner (Curtiss, 2001; Silverstein, 1998). PRN programs are briefly described previously here. Regardless of the model of care, most pain teams are comprised of at least the patient, nurse, and physician and may vary by clinical location and specialty focus (Jerin, 2002; Pasero et al., 1999).

The delivery of pain management services to people with cancer varies widely across healthcare settings, and many services are not organized like any of these models. Some services offer a restricted range of modalities, relying heavily on consultants for comprehensive treatments (Johnson, Abram, & Lynch, 2000). Others are organized as consultative and referral services and are often staffed by advanced practice nurses who provide patient consultation, staff education, and mentoring. Services may be available by staff request or written referral (Faucett, 1994; Williams et al., 1992). Some pain consultation services are organized as separate, interdisciplinary departments and provide cancer pain management using a team approach that is similar to that seen in hospice care. There is not a "right" structure to use when developing pain services. Each facility must determine its own specific needs and resources and design a service that is workable within the organization's structure and resources.

No matter what the structure or delivery system, every pain management program should offer comprehensive evaluation by competent staff before treatment is initiated, provide diagnostic resources as needed, maintain access to a variety of nondrug strategies and interventions, provide appropriately selected, scheduled, and accurately titrated medications, assure access to technology if necessary, and establish a method to follow patients over time to evaluate treatment outcomes.

Although many new and varied pain management programs are being developed across the country, making the decision to establish a pain management program, service, clinic, or center requires thoughtful introspection and analysis of existing as well as anticipated resources. Unless pain-related procedures are a part of the service (and most cancer patients do not require them), reimbursement for comprehensive pain assessment and treatment is often far less than the actual time required to assess a patient thoroughly, develop a treatment plan, and re-evaluate patient outcomes. Therefore, any pain service will require extensive administrative support, clinical support, and allocation of resources. Three elements common to successful programs are as follows: (1) team effort and coordination, (2) provision of education for professionals and patients, and (3) accountability and administrative support (Williams et al., 1992).

The first steps in deciding to develop a program include determining the need for the program, identifying the scope of the service, and identifying a patient population to use the services. In addition, identify currently available expertise, interest, and resources. Begin market research by surveying key groups to identify potential needs and ask what the ideal solution might be to meet the perceived needs related to effective pain management (Donovan et al., 1999). Determine whether other departments are already providing any of the proposed services, whether existing staff has the expertise to provide the service, and whether space and resources are available for the program.

Develop both a business and strategic plan to guide the process as it moves forward. Initial work should include plans to identify specific goals and strategies to develop the program; articulate the specific scope of services and the relationship of the program to other key services; acquire space, supplies, and equipment; recruit, hire, and educate staff; develop policies and procedures; establish job descriptions with clearly articulated time commitments, responsibilities, and lines of accountability; initiate plans for public, patient, and staff education and resources; develop the budget; identify initial quality-improvement and outcomes studies for the service; include marketing and advertising, coding and billing, and contracting with managed care organizations.

Develop specific goals and strategies to guide the process, and be sure to dream a little about new possibilities for services. Include proposed timelines for meeting specific goals and subgoals to develop and launch the program, and identify the person who will assume accountability for meeting each goal. Think ahead approximately two years to establish both long- and short-term goals and review the plans at predesignated intervals to measure progress.

The scope of service for a cancer pain program may encompass inpatients, outpatients, ambulatory patients, homecare, or all of these settings. It may accept patients by referral from healthcare providers or permit self-referral and may be structured as a separate service or integrated into routine clinical services. The scope of service may assign designated accountability to the department of nursing, medicine, or other organizational reporting structure and may have a dedicated staff, a core team, or staff that serve on a consultative basis. It may or may not include organization-wide resource nurses to serve as liaisons with other staff. It is vital to be clear about the organizational structure, the process for providing services, and the essential components of the service from the start.

Comprehensive programs for cancer pain management require staff with sophisticated knowledge and skills in pain, pain assessment, and pain management. Well-designed programs provide patients with a variety of opportunities for interdisciplinary specialty consultation, including, but not limited to the following team members: pain management and/or oncology nurses, oncologists, neurologists, anesthesiologists, pharmacists, social workers, counselors, physical therapists, occupational therapists, registered dieticians, clergy, and other team members appropriate to the needs of an individual with cancer. Interdisciplinary team members may be full-time staff or part-time staff, or they may be available as affiliates to the pain service.

Role of Team Members

The center of the team is the patient and his or her family or supporters in a partnership with other members of the interdisciplinary team. Identifying appropriate individual needs and goals of treatment with the person with pain is essential to effective care.

Nurses often provide the initial impetus to develop pain programs and are in a unique position to provide leadership to organize a new pain program. Identifying the roles and responsibilities of key team members early on is an important part of program development.

Ideally, once a decision is made to offer a comprehensive pain service, the medical director and key staff should be in place to participate in the initial strategic planning process. The medical director should possess medical and scientific knowledge about cancer pain and its management and also possess strong administrative skills, communication skills, and leadership. If the service is to be part of a pain center accredited by the Commission on Accreditation of Rehabilitation Facilities, the medical director must be American Board of Medical Specialties board certified in his or her specialty, have at least 2 years of experience in the interdisciplinary management of chronic pain, be a member of a regional or national pain society, participate in pain-related continuing medical education programs at least yearly, and be able to serve as team leader to provide direction to other staff (Johnson et al., 2000). Additional physician team members may include oncologists, neurologists, physiatrists, anesthesiologists, or physicians from other disciplines.

Nurses hold a variety of positions in pain management programs and are often key clinical leaders and/or coordinators. In smaller programs, a nurse may be the only individual dedicated to pain consultation. Donovan and colleagues (1999) identified these characteristics for successful coordinators: a strong clinical background, administrative experience, ability to be a team player, ability to mentor and coach others, excellent interpersonal and negotiating skills, self-motivation, skilled communication abilities, ability to be a champion for improving pain management, and creativity.

As in other settings, all nurses caring for people with pain use the nursing process to meet the needs of patients and their significant others to maintain optimum levels of wellness and effective pain control. In addition, national standards (American Society of Pain Management Nurses [ASPMN], 1998) also require that nurses who specialize in pain management facilitate the development, implementation, and ongoing evaluation of pain management practices to promote quality care and continuously evaluate personal professional performance. Furthermore, nurses must acquire and maintain current knowledge in the specialty of pain management nursing and promote professional growth and development of colleagues within the specialty. The standards also require integration of ethical principles into decisions about practice, collaboration with clients and team members to provide integrated care, contributions to the integration and advancement of scientific knowledge into clinical practice, and the use of available resources to promote safe, effective, and economical pain management (ASPMN, 1998).

In many pain programs, nurses are responsible for initial comprehensive assessment of patients, coordination of treatment plans, independent and dependent functions in providing interventions, patient education, reassessment, and evaluation of progress toward meeting designated goals. Depending on the program, advanced practice nurses may assume responsibility for a primary caseload of patients, coordinate a pain management program, assume the role of initial and ongoing consultant for the program, or work with other members of an interdisciplinary team to evaluate patients, develop treatment plans, and follow patients over time.

Common activities for nurses who practice in pain services and programs are as follows: participate in patient care rounds, screen for and assess pain, complete health histories and perform physicals, initiate and adjust medication doses and infusions using pre-established protocols, conduct phone triage and patient and family education, direct clinical care, direct participation in patient care conferences, assist with procedures, develop and lead support groups, and help with discharge planning and support at the end of life. Other roles include educator, manager, and researcher (Vanderveer, 2002). Most nurses also act as change agents to develop and implement broad-based services to meet the needs of patients with pain and to improve clinical practice for all patients in a healthcare setting.

Core competencies for caring for people with pain include knowledge of basic principles of pain management, including pain theory, physiology, and pathophysiology, common barriers that inhibit effective pain control, screening and assessment skills, appropriate use of analgesics

and other medications indicated for different types of pain, use of nondrug interventions, and side effect and risk management for medications (Gordon et al., 2000). Additional competencies such as initiating and maintaining patient controlled analgesia infusions (epidural, intravenous, or subcutaneous), assisting with nerve blocks and other procedures, and skills specific to the services that a particular program offered may also be required.

For other team members, each discipline's professional practice standards guides roles and responsibilities. For example, pharmacists bring knowledge and expertise about medications, assist to optimize medication therapy, monitor outcomes, collaborate for patient education and adherence, and serve as a resource to teach professionals appropriate selection and use of medications for pain. For most people, the crisis of cancer is like nothing else they have ever experienced (Loscalzo & Knight, 1999). Psychologists, social workers, and other counselors deal with the impact of pain on the person and his or her life and assist patients in identifying coping skills and other resources to deal with unrelieved pain and its consequences. Some also teach behavioral interventions such as relaxation and imagery, self-hypnosis, and other self-care strategies to decrease pain and pain perception. Ministers, rabbis, priests, chaplains, and other spiritual counselors provide support and assist patients and their families in their search for meaning from the experience and to place the illness experience within the context of spiritual beliefs and values. Physical and occupational therapists play key roles in increasing strength and endurance and other restorative activities. Other team members contribute their expertise based on individual patient's needs.

Conclusion

Effective pain assessment and pain management are a patient rights and a team responsibility in every clinical setting. Nevertheless, unrelieved cancer pain remains a major public health problem. Healthcare organizations must develop programs to assure that all people receive adequate pain assessment and management as a basic part of clinical care, including ambulatory care settings. In order to accomplish this, facilities must make an organizational commitment to improve pain practices, teach effective pain assessment and management, identify problem areas, and monitor progress via process improvement programs. All patients seen in ambulatory settings must be screened for pain routinely and assessed when pain is reported, and a plan must be devised to treat pain.

Resources are widely available to assist organizations to establish an organizational approach to effective pain care and to guide the management of pain in nearly any setting. When developing a pain service, center, or clinic, selecting a model that is appropriate to an organization's needs and resources is key. Successful pain services, centers, and clinics are organized to offer patients interdisciplinary, comprehensive assessment, reassessment, and follow-up with a sound plan of care based on national standards and guidelines. However, the bigger challenge is to integrate existing knowledge and skills about assessing and managing pain into clinical practice and to develop strategies to sustain clinical practice changes. People with cancer have a right to effective pain assessment and management. We have a responsibility to provide it—failing to treat pain brushes perilously close to inflicting it intentionally and violates the covenant of trust between our patients and ourselves (Morris, 1991). We must vigilantly continue efforts to improve pain management for people with cancer in all healthcare settings.

References

American Cancer Society. (2004). *Cancer Facts and Figures 2004*. Atlanta: Author.

American Pain Society. (1996). *1996 Pain Facilities Directory*. Glenview, IL: Author.

American Pain Society. (1999). *Principles of Analgesic Use in the Treatment of Acute Pain and Cancer Pain* (4th ed.). Glenview, IL: Author.

American Society of Pain Management Nurses. (1998). *Standards of Clinical Practice for the Specialty of Pain Management Nursing*. Pensacola, FL: Author.

Altilio, T. (1999). Building a pain management program: Background and basics. *Oncology Pain Management*. Rockville, MD: Association of Community Cancer Centers (ACCC).

Bernabei, R., Gambassi, G., Lapane, K., Landi, F., Gatsonis, C., Dunlop, R. et al. (1998). Management of pain in elderly patients with cancer. *JAMA, 279*, 1877–1882.

Bonica, J. J. (1990). Multidisciplinary/interdisciplinary pain programs. In J. J. Bonica (Ed.), *The Management of Pain* (2nd ed., pp. 197–207). Philadelphia: Lea & Febiger.

Cleeland, C. S., Gonin, R., Hatfield, A. K., Edmonson, J. H., Blum R. H., Stewart, J. A. et al. (1994). Pain and its treatment in outpatients with metastatic cancer: The Eastern Cooperative Oncology Group's Pain Study. *New England Journal of Medicine, 330*, 592–596.

Cleeland, C. S., Rotondi, A., Brechner, T., Levin, A., MacDonald, N., Portenoy, R. et al. (1986). A model for the treatment of cancer pain. *Journal of Pain and Symptom Management, 1*, 209–215.

Curtiss, C. P. (2001). Pain management: When the problem is the plan. *Disease Management Digest, 5*, 6–7, *In Care Management* 7(3).

Dahl, J. L. (1999). New JCAHO standards focus on pain management. *Oncology Issues, Sept/Oct*, 27–28.

Donovan, M. I., Evers, K., Jacobs, P., & Mandleblatt, S. (1999). When there is no benchmark: Designing a primary care based chronic pain management program from the scientific basis up. *Journal of Pain and Symptom Management 18*, 38–48.

Du Pen, A. R., Du Pen, S., Hansberry, J., Milleer-Kraybill, B., Millen, J., Everly, R. et al. (2000). An educational implementation of a cancer pain algorithm for ambulatory care. *Pain Management Nursing 1*, 116–128.

Faucett, J. (1994 April/May). *What is the Role of Nursing in the Multidisciplinary Pain Treatment Center?* APS Bulletin. Glenview, IL: American Pain Society.

Ferrell, B. R. (1999). Oncology pain management: A team approach. *Oncology Pain Management*. Rockville, MD: Association of Community Cancer Centers (ACCC).

Ferrell, B. R. & Hassey Dow, K. (1997). Quality of life among long-term cancer survivors. *Oncology, 11*, 565–575.

Ferrell, B. R., Grant, M., Richey, K. J., Ropchan, R., & Rivera, L. M. (1993). The pain resource nurse training program: A unique approach to pain management. *Journal of Pain and Symptom Management, 8*, 549–556.

Georgesen, J. (1999). A clinical pathway for outpatient cancer pain management. *Oncology Issues, Sept/Oct*, 23–26.

Gordon, D. B., Dahl, J. L., & Stevenson, K. K. (2000). *Building an Institutional Commitment to Pain Management* (2nd ed.). Madison, WI: U.W. Board of Regents.

Haylock, P. J. (2001). Advances in care – Cancer doesn't have to hurt. *AAACN Viewpoint, 23*, 1,12–14.

Haylock, P. J. & Curtiss, C. P. (1997). *Cancer Doesn't Have to Hurt*. Alameda, CA: Hunter House.

Horlitz, K. & Lucas, A. (1993). Implementation of an anesthesia pain management service program. *Cancer Practice, 1*, 129–136.

International Association for the Study of Pain (IASP) Task Force For Pain Treatment Facilities. (1990). *Desirable Characteristics for Pain Treatment Facilities*. Seattle: IASP Press.

Jacox, A., Carr, D. B., Payne, R., Berde, C. B., Brietbart, W., Cain, J. M. et al. (1994). *Management of Cancer Pain. Clinical Practice Guideline No. 9*. (AHCPR Publication No. 94-0592). Rockville, MD: Agency for Health Care Policy and Research, Public Health Service. U.S. Department of Health and Human Services.

JCAHO Department of Communications and Customer Service. (2001). Taking the ouch out of pain standards. *Ambulatory Care Advisor, Issue 2*. Retrieved September 5, 2002 from *http://www.jcaho.org/accredited+organizations/ambulatory+care/advisor/2001issue2/*

Jerin, L. (2002). Care delivery models for pain management. In B. St. Marie (Ed.), *American Society of Pain Management Nurses Core Curriculum for Pain Management Nursing* (pp. 491–497). Philadelphia: W.B. Saunders Company.

Johnson, J. L., Abram, S. E., & Lynch, N. T. (2000). Pain clinic organization and staffing. In S. E. Abram & J. D. Haddox (Eds.), *The Pain Clinic Manual* (2nd ed., pp. 3–11). Philadelphia: Lippincott Williams & Wilkins.

Joint Commission on Accreditation of Health Care Organizations. (1999). *1999-2000 Comprehensive Accreditation Manual for Ambulatory Care* (CAMAC). Oakbrook Terrace, IL: Author.

Loscalzo, M. J. & Knight, L. A. (1999). Using psychosocial resources effectively. *Oncology Pain Management: A Team Approach* (pp. 15–18). Rockville, MD: Association of Community Cancer Centers (ACCC).

McCaffery, M. & Pasero, C. (1999). Assessment. In M. McCaffery & C. Pasero (Eds.), *Pain: Clinical Manual* (2nd ed. pp. 35–102). St. Louis: Mosby.

McMarburg, B. (1998). Establishing a pain service within managed care. *APS Bulletin, 8*. Retrieved June 8, 1998 from *http://www.ampainsoc.org/bulletin/may98/clinic.htm*

Morris, D. B. (1991). *The Culture of Pain*. Berkeley, CA: University of California Press.

National Comprehensive Cancer Network (NCCN). (2000). *Practice Guidelines for Cancer Pain version 1.2000*. Rockledge, PA: Author.

National Comprehensive Cancer Network & American Cancer Society. (2001). *Cancer Pain: Treatment Guidelines for Patients*. (Version 1). Atlanta, GA: American Cancer Society.

National Institutes of Health. (2002 July 17). State of the Science Statement: Symptom Management in Cancer: Pain, Depression and Fatigue (draft statement). Retrieved October 1, 2002 from *http://www.nih.gov/ta/022/022_statement.htm*

Oncology Nursing Society. (1998). Oncology Nursing Society Position on cancer pain management. *Oncology Nursing Forum, 25*, 1–2.

Pasero, C., Gordon, D. B., McCaffery, M., & Ferrell, B. R. (1999). Building institutional commitment to improving pain management. In M. McCaffery & C. Pasero (Eds.), *Pain Clinical Manual* (2nd ed.). St. Louis, MO: C.V. Mosby Company.

Schumacher, K. L., Koresawa, S., West, C., Hawkins, C., Johnson, C., Wais, E. et al. (2002). Putting cancer pain management regimens into practice at home. *Journal of Pain and Symptom Management, 23*, 369–382.

Sheidler, V. (1997 May) Telephone check list. Part of a handout for symposium held in conjunction with the annual meeting of the National Association of Orthopaedic Nurses. Philadelphia, PA. Adapted with permission by Curtiss, C. (1997). Pain management – telephone check list. Unpublished handout.

Silverstein, W. (1998). Care management: The right balance of care and management? *Nursing Administration Quarterly, 22*, 66–75.

Stevens, B., Johnston, C., Petryshen, P., & Taddio, A. (1996). The Premature Infant Pain Profile: Development and initial validation. *Clinical Journal of Pain, 12*, 13–22.

SUPPORT Principle Investigators. (1995). A controlled trial to improve care for seriously ill hospitalized patients: The study to understand prognosis and preferences for outcomes and risks of treatments (SUPPORT). *JAMA, 274*, 1591–1598.

Taricco, A. (1996). Perils of payors: A pain center paradigm. In M. J. M. Cohen & J. N. Campbell (Eds.), Pain Treatment Centers at the Crossroads: A Practical and Conceptual Reappraisal. *Progress in Pain Research and Management, 7*, (pp. 109–116). Seattle, WA: IASP Press.

Vanderveer, B. L. (2002). The caregiver role. In B. St. Marie (Ed.), *American Society of Pain Management Nurses Core Curriculum for Pain Management Nursing* (pp. 499–505). Philadelphia: W.B. Saunders Company.

Williams, A., Kedziera, P., Osterlund, H., St. Marie, B., Gronbeck, W., Wenzl, C. et al. (1992). Models of healthcare delivery in cancer pain management. *Oncology Nursing Forum, 19* (Suppl.), 20–26.

Chapter 12

Palliative and Hospice Care Issues and Concepts in the Ambulatory Care Setting

Kim K. Kuebler

Introduction

The paradigm shift that is taking place in the evolving field of palliative care is remarkable. The genesis that initially spurred the hospice movement was in opposition to aggressive biomedical technology. This movement has also helped to promote the development and integration of palliative practices used in collaboration with acute care settings. This chapter discusses the evolution of change in the field and the emergence of palliative care by discussing the integration of palliative interventions throughout the patients' disease trajectory to promote quality of life for those living and dying from advanced illness.

How Americans Are Dying

It is predicted that by the year 2030, for the first time in history, the old will out number the young (USA Today, 2001). Americans are living longer, often with chronic illness. Currently, the leading causes of death in the United States include heart disease, cancer, stroke, chronic obstructive pulmonary disease, and dementia (von Gunten, Ferris, D'Antuono, & Emanuel, 2002).

Although most of these diseases have a relatively predictable course, most patients will live with chronic illness for many years before death. A vast majority of Americans, however, who die each year are older patients (a median age of 77 years) and typically experience a slow, progressive chronic disease trajectory before death (Brumley, 2002). It is predicted that women on average experience debilitating progressive illness for three years before death, whereas men often demonstrate two years of serious progressive disability before dying (Introcaso & Lynn, 2002). With this in mind, the traditional approach to end-of-life care is not meeting the current needs of the population nor does it address the burgeoning needs that will arise as a result of an aging society.

Most recently the World Health Organization (WHO) revised its definition to address this problem by broadening the approach to palliative interventions. The new definition indentifies that "Palliative care is an approach that improves the quality of life of patients and their families facing the problems associated with life-threatening illness, through the prevention and relief of suffering by means of early identification and impeccable assessment and treatment of pain and other problems, physical, psychosocial, and spiritual" (WHO, 2002).

The SUPPORT Study

Data generated from the infamous SUPPORT study (the Study to Understand Prognoses and Preferences for Outcomes and Risks of Treatments) have contributed to the paradigm shift that is currently underway in the United States. Study data about the manner in which Americans are dying shocked the investigators and funding agencies and have since stimulated change in the development and dissemination of palliative practice across the United States. Patients (more than 10,000) who enrolled in the SUPPORT study were dying in moderate to severe pain and died in acute care settings, often in the intensive care unit connected to mechanical ventilators despite their medical directives to die at home. These patients did not engage in communication with their physician regarding care options while facing the gravity of their illness (The SUPPORT Principal Investigators, 1995; Lo, 1995). This study has promoted many professional, legislative, and lay groups to initiate agendas to improve the care of the dying throughout the United States.

Current Research Agendas

The Institute of Medicine, the Veterans Administration, the Robert Wood Johnson Foundation, the National Institutes of Health, and State Legislative Initiatives among others have identified needed improvements in the areas of advance care planning, respecting patient and family preferences for the choice of death, and the use of aggressive interventions, pain and symptom management, and home healthcare and hospice care. These needs coupled with the interest in initiating major research initiatives to generate evidence-based solutions to improve care for those living with advanced illness are from the SUPPORT study which investigated characterizations of a "good" death (Tolle, Tilden, Rosenfield, & Hickman, 2000). The definition of a "good" death includes the following:

A good death is free from avoidable pain and suffering, in accord with the wishes of the patient and family, and reasonably consistent with clinical, cultural, and ethical standards. (Field & Cassel 1997; Council on Scientific Affairs, 1996; Scanlon, 1996; Emanuel & Emanuel, 1998; Singer, Martin, & Kelner, 1999).

In 1997, the Institute of Medicine called for social, behavioral, and health services research on dying because limited knowledge existed about where and how Americans were dying. This call was also in part to understand better what patients and families perceived as important about the care that they wished to receive during the dying experience (Field & Cassel, 1997). The current literature reflects a plethora of research that addresses advance directives, symptom management, and family support but was limited in the collection of family data (Tilden, Drach, Tolle, Rosenfield, & Hickman, 2002). The demands of caregiving for a loved one who is dying from advanced illness is overwhelming, and healthcare providers need to understand this area better to support the multiple needs of the patient.

Underuse of Hospice Care in the United States

After two decades, the hospice care model has provided the initial framework used to care for dying Americans. Despite this care model, most dying Americans are not enrolled in a hospice program. The steady rise in hospice access since 1985 went from 160,000 patients enrolled in Medicare hospice to 700,000 patients in 1999 (Ogle, Mavis, & Wyatt, 2002). Despite this rise, only 29% of all patients who died in the United States in 1999 were enrolled in a Medicare Hospice program (Ogle et al., 2002). Most Americans are dying in hospital or nursing home beds rather in their own home (Friedman, Harwood, & Shields, 2002). With less than one-third of the patients who are dying using hospice services, some leaders in the field believe that this underuse is a public health issue in the United States (Ogle et al., 2002). The limited use of hospice care in the United States is multifactorial and includes the following:

1. Western society is a "death-denying" culture in which many patients and healthcare professionals desire life-prolonging care.

2. Patients and their families often lack the knowledge regarding the availability of hospice services.

3. Physicians have difficulty in determining prognoses in terms of six months or less (Kuebler & Heidrich, 2001).

Last Acts Report

The most recent and comprehensive report since the SUPPORT study is the report by Last Acts also funded by The Robert Wood Johnson Foundation (Last Acts, 2002). The report rated each state and the District of Columbia on eight criteria as a basis for determining the state of end-of-life care in the United States (Last Acts, 2002). Despite what we have learned from the SUPPORT Study and the massive initiatives that have taken place in its wake Americans today can expect no more than a fair chance of finding adequate care for their loved ones or themselves when faced with advanced illness (Last Acts, 2002). To view these data and determine how your specific state looks in relationship to the rest of the United States go to www.lastacts.org.

Confusing Terms

Confusion exists between healthcare professionals and the public when describing various models of care for those living with a life-limited prognosis. The terms supportive care, hospice care, end-of-life care, and/or palliative care are frequently used to denote care when a cure is no longer offered. However, the European experience of integrating palliative care into the patient's plan of care sooner verses later serves as an exemplar for the American experience. In an editorial, respected

experts pointed out the distinction of palliative practices versus those that imply a "time-defined care model." End-of-life and hospice care, for example, are both quantitative rather than qualitative descriptors that exclude the purpose of care and fail to recognize the complex skills inherent to adequate palliative care (Davis, Walsh, LeGrand, & Lagman, 2003). They further describe that these terms wrongly advertise to both the public and professional colleagues that this care specialty is reserved for the imminently dying and contributes to the transitional "discontinuous" care model rather than a seamless "collaborative" care model with early referral (Davis et al., 2003).

Palliative care is not time defined but is rather goal oriented (WHO, 2002). The World Health Organization (2002) and the United Kingdom's Policy Framework for Commissioning Cancer Services (1994) described the use of palliative care early in the course of a patient's disease trajectory, including diagnosis until death. Both of these organizational definitions of palliative care are intended to be person directed versus time limited (Woodruff, 2002). Palliative care is not only applicable but relevant when a disease is no longer curable (patients may suffer for years before being considered "terminal") or when a cure is being attempted (Davis et al., 2003). Palliative care interventions, therefore, should not be reserved for the end of life when all other measures have been exhausted or when the patient's highly symptomatic and social supports are collapsing, but rather throughout the disease process until death (Davis et al., in press).

The Evolution of Palliative Care

Dr. Balfour Mount was the first to define palliative care when he opened the first hospital-based palliative care service at the Royal Victoria Hospital at McGill University in Montreal in 1975 (Doyle, Hanks, & MacDonald, 1998). The

McGill model followed the interdisciplinary framework of care that a team of experts provided to address the multiple needs of the dying patient and his or her family. The McGill model, however, was the first to include research and education in the area of pain and symptom management (Bennahum, 1996; Finn-Paradis, 1985). Innovative palliative care research continues to come from the McGill Model, which has influenced the development and evolution of palliative practices worldwide.

Palliative care recognizes that dying is a normal process that should be neither hastened nor postponed. The provision of symptom management that includes emotional and spiritual support for patients and their families is considered when developing a plan of care to promote an optimal dying experience followed by family bereavement (Doyle et al., 1998; McHale, 2002). Palliative philosophies that the Last Acts Palliative Task Force and the National Hospice and Palliative Care Organization (*www.NHPC0.org*) (Bednash & Ferrell, 2002) identify are as follows:

1. Palliative care provides support and care for persons facing a life-limited illness across all care settings.

2. Palliative care identifies death as normal and natural.

3. The dying process is profoundly individualized and occurs within the dynamics of the family.

4. Palliative care enhances the quality of life and integrates the physical, psychological, social, and spiritual aspects of care.

5. The interdisciplinary team addresses the multidimensional needs of the dying patient and his or her family.

6. Palliative interventions affirm life and neither hasten nor postpone death.

7. Appropriate palliative care and a supportive environment promote quality of life and healthy closure for the patient and family.

Integrating Palliative Care

A patient's position along the disease continuum largely determines the specific palliative interventions that would improve his or her quality of life. A comprehensive assessment is essential when determining the extent of disease and the effects of symptom burden. This assessment includes these considerations (Bruera & Lawlor, 1998):

1. Define the nature of the clinical finding and the effects of symptoms.

2. Perform a thorough history and physical examination, review current and tried medications, and evaluate a minimal set of diagnostics procedures to differentiate underlying pathophysiologic disorders from a reversible symptom.

3. Evaluate the problem within the context of the patient's situation and allow for prioritization. For example, the priority assigned an upper respiratory infection in a cognitively impaired, dehydrated, bedridden patient who is actively dying will be different from the treatment for the patient with an upper respiratory infection who remains alert, active, and ambulatory.

4. Define the "cost" of diagnostic and therapeutic interventions and the varying differences between patients. What may be considered appropriate therapy for one patient may be inappropriate for another; therefore, evaluating the risk versus the benefit of treatment options and the financial burden of unnecessary interventions is important.

5. Discuss the various care options with the patient and family and encourage informed decision making with a reality-oriented outcome. For example, it

would not be appropriate for the patient and family to expect to engage in a cross-country trip when the patient is unable to perform his or her activities of daily living, is bed bound to progressive weakness, and is severely dyspneic with accompanied anemia. However, this might be considered appropriate for a patient who remains ambulatory and active and has adequate symptom management.

Palliative interventions are individually based for the patient who is diagnosed with a noncurable illness but also for patients who are seeking a cure. An example is in the patient undergoing a bone marrow transplant with a diagnosis of acute myelogenous leukemia. Although the patient is seeking aggressive intervention, he or she may also experience pain, dyspnea, fatigue, and/or depression. All of these symptoms can interfere with the patient's perceived quality of life. Palliative interventions used to control these symptoms provide comfort and allow the patient to focus on important personal issues.

Ambulatory Palliative Care

The ambulatory nurse bridges the gap between the acute care setting and home (Farley, 1991). Nurses practicing in this area require a broad range of knowledge with a span from prevention and detection to symptom management and terminal care (Farley, 1991). The ambulatory care nurse who has knowledge and skills in pathophysiology, disease interventions, management of treatment and medication side effects, symptom control, and community resources is a key player in the provision of palliative care.

Integrating palliative interventions into the ambulatory care setting is not only necessary when attempting to reduce the burden of symptoms but also compliments the intended plan of care by promoting comfort and encouraging the patient and his or her family to live as long as pos-

sible with the best quality of life. Ambulatory care nurses who understand the importance of symptom management are able to identify palliative care needs and either provide these skills or identify skilled providers in the community who can address palliative needs in the home. Depending on the extent of illness, a skilled palliative care provider, such as a nurse practitioner, can provide interventions, or if the patient has a prognosis of six months or less, a referral to a hospice program may be sufficient. Integrating palliative care into the patient's plan of care to address unmanaged symptoms and to improve quality of life is the intended outcome. Here the main objective is to introduce the concept of palliative interventions and not to discuss individual symptom management.

Common symptoms that accompany advanced illness can include pain (neuropathic, somatic, and visceral syndromes), dyspnea, fatigue, depression, constipation, puritus, edema, anemia, anxiety, anorexia, and confusion among others. The key concept in palliative care is symptom management. Having a working knowledge of the underlying pathophysiology is also very important when considering specific interventions. Consider the following case example when exploring the integration of palliative interventions.

Case Example

T.B. is a 28-year-old man who is diagnosed with metastatic melanoma with positive cervical and mandibular lymphadenopathy the size of baseballs. He has liver metastasis, is jaundiced, and is experiencing severe lower extremity weeping pedal edema. Despite receiving over a gram of morphine, he continues to rate his pain intensity at an 8 on a scale of 1–10 and describes his pain as burning, sharp, shooting, and constant. Because of poor pain control, he has attempted to commit suicide by melting his previous sustained release oxycodone down and drawing it up into a syringe for self-injection. His bowels remain regular in spite of a high dose of opioids, and he has a good appetite. He has problems with insomnia as a result of poor pain control. He is agitated, myoclonic, and anxious about being in constant pain. The patient is married and has a 5-year-old daughter and says that he has many unfinished business issues that he needs to address before dying. T.B. is enrolled in a hospice program, but because of his age, he feels that his doctor has all but ignored him because of his imminent death.

It is clear that T.B.'s symptoms are multiple and that the interventions currently employed are inefficient. Understanding disease pathophysiology is very important when employing the appropriate interventions. No amount of opioid can manage neuropathic or somatic pain. The use of adjuvant analgesics such as baclofen would help reduce his neuropathic pain experience. T.B. has the potential of developing superior vena cava syndrome from the extensive lymphadenopathy. The use of a corticosteroid (i.e., dexamethasone) would help to prevent this oncologic emergency from occurring and is also useful for the treatment of somatic pain. His morphine dose requires adjustment. Whenever an opioid is used alone to control pain but is found to be inadequate, increasing the dose is not appropriate without considering the addition of an adjuvant analgesic. Evidence of myoclonus, agitation, and anxiety may indicate that the morphine dose is creating opioid toxicities by adding adjuvant analgesics. By decreasing the morphine dose, T.B.'s pain may be better controlled, which will help reduce many of his other symptoms and his attempts to commit suicide. His lymphedema in the lower extremities would benefit from the use of supportive stockings and elevation rather than a diuretic, as this edema is a result of a tumor and is not cardiovascular related. Another important consideration for this patient is the nurse's understanding of how medications are metabolized or the pharmacodynamics of specific medications. His previous pain medication was oxycodone, but because of his liver metastasis, oxycodone could not be adequately metabolized.

The use of baclofen requires ongoing assessment because it is metabolized in the liver. Weighing the benefit of specific interventions versus harm remains a constant balance of assessment and intervention in the palliative care setting.

Medication Selection

Medication selection in palliative care should be based on how many symptoms can be controlled by using the least amount of medication. The use of baclofen, for example, benefits neuropathic pain while alleviating anxiety because it is in the benzodiazepine drug group, which can also promote sleep. The use of dexamethasone is beneficial for the relief of both somatic and neuropathic pain, serves as an anti-inflammatory agent for lymph nodes, helps to reduce swelling in the liver, promotes a sense of well-being, improves appetite, and is a quick intervention to improve depression (Twycross, Wilcock, & Thorp, 1998). Because of T.B.'s lower extremity edema, the use of a corticosteroid will require titration and monitoring.

Nurses practicing in this challenging environment require extensive knowledge about medication interactions, which can be classified as being either pharmacodynamic or pharmacokinetic. Pharmacodynamics is what a specific medication does to the body. Pharmacodynamic medication interactions occur as a result of competition for the same drug receptor site, resulting in a synergistic or antagonistic drug action (Johnson, Newkirk, & White, 1999; Davis & Homsi, 2001). Using two different drug groups to control one symptom creates a synergistic or antagonistic reaction such as using both a monamine oxidase inhibitor along with a selective serotonin reuptake inhibitor to treat depression (Davis & Homsi, 2001).

Pharmacokinetic interactions are a result of adverse reactions caused by altered drug absorption, distribution, metabolism, and excretion (Bernard & Bruera, 2000; Davis & Homsi, 2001;

Johnson et al., 1999). Pharmacokinetic interactions contribute to the metabolism of one medication by adding a second medication (Bernard & Bruera, 2000; Davis & Homsi, 2001; Johnson et al.). Pharmacokinetic properties are the result of metabolism that occurs primarily in the liver through the process of the cytochrome p450-mediated enzyme system (Davis & Homsi, 2001). The predominant enzyme used in the metabolism of palliative medications (25%) is cleared by the CYP2D6 enzyme (Davis & Homsi, 2001). Another important consideration when choosing medications is how the CYP2D6 enzyme affects metabolism in different ethnic backgrounds. For example, Caucasians have adequate amounts of this enzyme, whereas Asians carry a limited amount, and African Americans are poor metabolizers (Davis & Homsi, 2001). Knowledge of this phenomena is important when considering optimal symptom control reduction of adverse effects and minimization of medication use at any given time.

Accessing the Interdisciplinary Team

Addressing T.B.'s depression should be considered and seeking interdisciplinary support to help articulate T.B.'s unfinished business issues and recent suicide attempt is an important consideration. The palliative care consultant or provider understands the significance of utilizing an interdisciplinary approach of care. The multidimensional aspect of being a human is not ignored in this phase of care. Skilled clinicians who work together to meet these multiple needs address the physical, emotional, and spiritual dimensions and together provide comprehensive coordinated care to reduce crisis and promote a holistic healthy experience—despite the gravity of knowing that the illness will ultimately take the patient to death.

The interdisciplinary team approach has been the basis of both hospice and palliative practices. Caring for patients and their families facing a limited life prognosis is often difficult and exhausting, and a single discipline cannot nor should attempt to provide all of the complex needs associated with the last phase of life (Berry & Kuebler, 2002). The interdisciplinary team works together with the patient and family to achieve optimal outcomes for all involved.

Palliative Care Assessment Tools

Palliative practices, not unlike other specialized areas, utilize psychometric reliable and valid assessment instruments to assist in the provisions of evidence-based interventions. In order to achieve a standardized dialogue between the interdisciplinary team and the patient the selection of specific instruments is important. A discussion of several palliative care assessment tools follows.

1. **The Edmonton Symptom Assessment Scale**
   The Edmonton Symptom Assessment Scale is used to assess and evaluate the intensity of multiple symptoms, such as pain, activity, nausea, depression, anxiety, drowsiness, appetite, well-being, and shortness of breath (Bruera & MacDonald, 1995; Bruera, Kuehn, Miller, Selmser, & MacMillan, 1991) (see **Figure 12.1**).

2. **The CAGE Questionnaire**
   The CAGE Questionnaire is used to screen for the presence of alcoholism and/or substance abuse. Two or more positive responses identify a history of alcoholism. Studies demonstrate that patients with pain and a positive history of substance abuse may tend to overuse medications in palliative care (e.g., opioids, benzodiazipines) (Bruera et al., 1995; Moore et al., 1989) (see **Figure 12.2**).

Figure 12.1 Edmonton Symptom Assessment Scale

Numerical Intensity	0	1	2	3	4	5	6	7	8	9	10
Pain											
Tiredness											
Nausea											
Depression											
Anxiety											
Drowsiness											
Appetite											
Wellbeing											
Dyspnea											
Date											

Used with permission (2002). Dr. Eduardo Bruera, M.D. Anderson Cancer Center. (Bruera, Kuehn, Miller, et al.).

3. **The Mini-Mental State Exam**
   The Mini-Mental State Exam is used to assess and evaluate the cognitive functioning in patients. This screening can pick up cognitive impairment that may reflect delirium or dementia (Yue, Fainsinger, & Bruera, 1994; Folstein, Folstein, & McHugh, 1975) (see **Figure 12.3**).

4. **The Home Care Assessment Tool**
   The Home Care Assessment Tool identifies a patient's realistic ability to die at home by asking a series of four questions. A negative answer on two or more questions can indicate that the patient or the primary care giver does not have adequate supports in place to ensure a home death (Cantwell, Turco, Bruera, Kneisler, & Hanson, 1998) (see **Figure 12.4**).

Figure 12.2 CAGE Questionnaire

CAGE assessment

1. Have you ever felt you should cut down on your drinking?   Yes   No

2. Have people annoyed you by criticizing your drinking?   Yes   No

3. Have you ever felt bad or guilty about your drinking?   Yes   No

4. Have you ever had a drink first thing in the morning or a drink to get rid of a hangover (eye opener)?   Yes   No

5. Have you ever had any problem with nonprescription or prescription medications? Please specify.   Yes   No

   _____

   _____

   _____

   _____

Two or more yes responses indicate a positive CAGE (2 of 5 = a positive CAGE).

Used with permission. Moore et al., 1989; Bruera, Magan et al., 1995.

Figure 12.3 Mini Mental State Examination

Maximum Score	Score	
5		What is the (year) (season) (day) (month) (date)?
5		Where are we (town) (state) (hospital) (floor)?
3		Name three objects:　　glass
		blanket
		pencil
5		Spell "World" backward.
3		Ask for the three objects repeated from above.
2		Name a pencil and watch.
1		Repeat the following: "no ifs, ands, or buts."
3		Follow a three-stage command: "Take a paper in your right hand, fold it in half, and give it to me."
1		Read and obey the following: **CLOSE YOUR EYES**
1		Write a sentence.
1		Copy a design (create two boxes).
30		**Total Score**

Assess level of consciousness along a continuum

Alert　　　Drowsy　　　Stupor　　　Coma

Number of years of schooling? _____

Lower Quartiles　Age

Schooling	< 39	40–49	50–59	60–89	70–79	> 80
0–4 years	20	20	20	19	18	16
5–8 years	24	24	25	24	23	22
9–12 years	28	28	27	27	26	23
College experience or higher degree	29	29	28	28	27	26

Used with permission (Folstein, Folstein, & McHugh, 1975).

Hospice Care

For those patients with a life expectancy of six months or less, a referral to a local hospice program may be considered. Oftentimes, patients and their families may fear that a referral to hospice care is "giving up" or that it means the "end" is near. Open and honest communication efforts are very important between the nurse and patient during this time so that family members are empowered and set realistic expectations. A patient who is actively seeking chemotherapy and who was newly informed by the oncologist that nothing more can be done to resolve his or her liver and bone metastasis may not be ready to enroll in a hospice program. This patient, however, can benefit from palliative interventions until he or she is ready to accept that death is forthcoming.

Enrollment Criteria

To enroll in a Medicare Hospice Program, the patient must have a terminal diagnosis with a prognosis of six months or less. The patient must also have two physicians (the patient's primary physician or referring physician [i.e., oncologist, cardiologist] and the hospice medical director) that agree with this life-limited prognosis. Most hospice programs require that the patient is identified with a primary care provider (family member and/or a significant other) who works with the interdisciplinary team to support the patient physically, emotionally, and spiritually until death. The referring physician, the patient, and the patient's family must be in agreement of a palliative plan of care versus seeking aggressive curative interventions that intend to prolong life (Vermillon, 1996).

Reimbursement

The Medicare Hospice Benefit established in 1983 for terminally ill patients provides palliative services for patients who opt to go for curative interventions. Patients seeking hospice services or the patient's legal representative must sign the hospice election form. This form provides informed consent and provides documentation to receive hospice care and contains an explanation of hospice services (Lattanzi-Licht, Mahoney, & Miller, 1998). Medicare beneficiaries who complete the hospice election form waive the right to standard Medicare benefits for healthcare related to their terminal illness (Lattanzi-Licht et al., 1998). However, standard Medicare remains in effect to cover healthcare costs unrelated to the patient's terminal diagnosis (Vermillon, 1996).

The Medicare Hospice Benefit provides payment for hospice beneficiaries directly to hospice programs based on a per diem rate, which is based on the "hospital market basket" index (Vermillon, 1996). The Medicare hospice benefit covers four levels of care, including the following:

- Routine home care
- Continuous home care
- General inpatient care
- Inpatient respite care

Routine home care per diem is designed to cover the cost of all hospice home visits, supplies, medications, and services. Medicare conditions of participation define necessary services that the

Figure 12.4 HOME CARE ASSESSMENT TOOL

	Yes	No
1. Does the patient have spiritual/religious support?		
2. Does the patient desire a home death?		
3. Does the primary caregiver desire a home death?		
4. Does the primary physician agree to a home death?		
5. Does the primary physician agree to regular home visits?		
6. Are there an adequate number of caregivers (two or more)?		
7. Are there physical barriers within the home that do not support a home death?		

Used with permission (2002). Dr. Bruera, M.D. Anderson Cancer Center. (Cantwell, Turco, Bruera, Kneisler, & Hanson, 1998).

hospice must provide regardless of setting and include the following:

- Interdisciplinary team involvement
- Medications and biologicals
- Laboratory services
- X-ray and radiation therapy
- Emergency services
- Ambulance and transport services
- Bereavement support
  (Vermillon, 1996; NHO, 1993)

Medicaid and private insurance plans often follow the Medicare Hospice Benefit, providing palliative care for those patients seeking hospice services.

Continuity and Coordination of Care

The ambulatory care nurse can play a key role when helping to coordinate the appropriate care for the patient living and dying from advanced illness. Establishing an understanding of how the patient and family perceive the illness is crucial when helping to direct appropriate care. For example, it would not be appropriate to set up hospice care when the patient has not considered his or her illness as being terminal. It may be better for this patient to receive palliative interventions while becoming more familiar with his or her limited prognosis.

The sensitivity that the nurse needs to have during this transition in the patient's healthcare planning should not be ignored. Facing the last chapter of one's life is met with many mixed emotions and is not an easy threshold to cross without the support of skilled clinicians and close family members. The nurse assisting the patient and family during this time should have a healthy sense of his or her own thoughts and feelings surrounding death and dying. Our society typically denies death; therefore, conversations that discuss one's desire and wishes regarding the last months of life are often very difficult to initiate. The nurse who is comfort-

able with these issues can gently lead the patient and family down the path of the unknown by gradually preparing them with the resources and supports that promote a healthy dying experience.

Reducing fragmented care and promoting a coordinated and continuous care approach throughout the disease trajectory until death should be the goal for this patient population. Patients who are introduced to hospice care days before death is ineffective. It is also difficult for patients and families to take on new professional relationships. Hospice care is the most effective when introduced earlier in the course of illness rather than weeks to days before death. Maintaining a constant relationship with one provider—whether it is the primary physician, nurse practitioner, or skilled home care nurse—will help to promote a coordinated care approach for the patient and family.

Case Study

The following example will help to demonstrate a coordinated and continuous approach to care from diagnosis until death. J.G.'s primary provider, while doing a routine physical examination, found an elevated prostate specific antigen. J.G. was sent for further diagnostic tests that included a total body bone scan, a chest X-ray, and additional laboratory tests. He was also referred to an urologist for evaluation. J.G. underwent a biopsy of his prostate, which returned positive for malignancy. Both his bone scan and chest X-ray were positive for metastatic disease. His primary physician and nurse practitioner collectively discussed the results of his diagnostic evaluations with the patient and his wife. J.G. was then referred to an oncologist, with planned follow-up visits to his primary provider. The oncologist, after surgical removal of his prostate, initiated chemotherapy despite his poor prognosis (stage 4).

J.G. entered his primary care provider's office and was seen by the nurse practitioner, who generally initiates palliative interventions within the practice. The nurse practitioner engaged J.G and his wife in discussion about how things were going at home and learned that J.G was not sleeping, had a poor appetite (weight loss of more than 6 pounds since his previous visit), was frequently nauseated, complained of moderate to severe somatic pain despite being on morphine, and was very depressed about not being able to make the planned trip that he and his wife had scheduled for their 45th wedding anniversary. J.G.'s wife was very emotional during the office visit and discussed her fears about the physical changes that she had observed in her husband since initiating chemotherapy. J.G. and his wife wanted to know what the benefit of chemotherapy had on prolonging his life, but were not willing to discontinue treatments.

The nurse practitioner initially focused on getting J.G.'s symptoms better controlled by adding dexamethasone 12 milligrams to control his somatic pain and nausea, to improve his appetite, and to help initially with his depression. She also initiated a taper of an antiemetic for breakthrough nausea, which could also be used to help J.G. sleep, but she believed his unmanaged symptoms were contributing to his insomnia. The nurse practitioner then opened the discussion surrounding advance directives and helped to put the focus on J.G.'s wishes and desires as they related to his healthcare planning as his disease progressed. J.G. and his wife were not ready to discuss his death. A referral was made to a social worker to address advance directives, depression, and anxiety related to his illness, prognosis, and future healthcare planning. During this meeting, J.G. made it a point that he did not want hospice care, believing that would mean he was giving up and he was still ready to fight back with chemotherapy. The plan after this meeting was to continue with his chemotherapy and then follow up in the office in two weeks.

During the next visit, the nurse practitioner noticed progressive weakness with improved symptom management. J.G. said he did not know how much longer he could continue with the treatment and felt that it was taking him down. His wife was finding it more difficult to manage his care at home. The nurse practitioner suggested skilled home care to help address J.G.'s physical care needs and to assess and evaluate his symptom management. A skilled homecare referral was made for nursing, social work, and home health aid interventions.

J.G.'s symptoms were well managed despite his progressive weakness. His wife called the nurse practitioner saying that her husband had decided to discontinue chemotherapy, and he now knew that this was the beginning of the end. The nurse practitioner arranged for a home visit to evaluate his physical status and invited the skilled home care nurse to also be present. Together with the patient and family, they discussed his plan of care. During the home visit, it was determined that J.G. would continue to qualify for skilled home care to support symptom management, and the social worker would continue to make visits to discuss the patient's fears related to his advanced illness and limited life expectancy. The plan of care was palliative, and when hospice was discussed, the patient remained adamant that he was not ready to receive "terminal care." The nurse practitioner agreed to continue home visits when J.G.'s symptoms exacerbated and would work collaboratively with the skilled home care team. J.G. continued with home care and occasional nurse practitioner visits and died comfortably at home without symptoms.

J.G. received palliative interventions throughout his disease from diagnosis until death with the support of an interdisciplinary team. J.G. directed the focus of his care with the support of a skilled nurse practitioner, and even though he chose to not have hospice care, he was still able to remain at home without symptoms using skilled home care services and frequent nurse practitioner reimbursable home visits. Both he and his wife did not experience fragmented care but rather participated in their plan of care together with his primary care provider and nurse practitioner who remained with him until his death. Had J.G. been accepting of hospice care, the nurse practitioner would have assisted in seeking a referral, but because she honored the patient's wishes, she chose to use available resources that would help support the patient and his wife through the dying process.

Conclusion

Palliative care provides patients and their families with many opportunities during the course of advanced illness. The ambulatory care nurse with a working knowledge of available services can help transition the patient who is living and dying from advanced illness to the appropriate provider. The field of palliative care strives to integrate palliative interventions earlier in the course of illness rather than reserving them for the final days and months of life. Palliative interventions are used to reduce symptoms and to promote improved quality of life. Providing and assuring coordinated continuous care are paramount for this fragile patient population. The ambulatory care nurse can help to hold the lantern to lighten the path and to provide guidance for the patient and family as they tread down the path of the unknown.

References

Bednash, G. & Ferrell, B. (2002). *Nursing Care at the End-of-Life. ANCC/AACN Continuing Education for Nurses.* Rockville, MD: American Nursing Credentialing Center.

Bennahum, D. (1996). The historical development of hospice and palliative care. In D. Sheehan & W. Forman (Eds.), *Hospice and Palliative Care* (pp. 1–10). Sudbury, MA: Jones & Bartlett Publishers.

Berry, P. & Kuebler, K. (2002). The advanced practice nurse in end-of-life care. In K. Kuebler, P. Berry, & D. Heidrich (Eds.), *End-of-Life Care Clinical Practice Guidelines* (pp. 3–12). Philadelphia: W.B. Saunders Company.

Bernard, S. & Bruera, E. (2000). Drug interactions in palliative care. *Journal of Clinical Oncology, 18,* 1780–1799.

Bruera, E., Kuehn, N., Miller, M., Selmser, P., & MacMillan, K. (1991). The Edmonton symptom assessment system (ESAS): A simple method for the assessment of palliative care patients. *Journal of Palliative Care, 7,* 6–9.

Bruera, E. & Lawlor, P. (1998). Defining palliative care interventions. *Journal of Palliative Care, 14,* 23–24.

Bruera, E. & MacDonald, S. (1995). Audit methods: The Edmonton symptom assessment system. In I. Higginson (Eds.), *Clinical Audit in Palliative Care.* (pp. 14–19) Oxford, UK: Radcliffe Medical Press.

Bruera, E., Moyano, J., Seifert, L., Fainsinger, R., Hanson, J., & Suarez-Almazor, M. (1995). The frequency of alcoholism among patients with pain due to terminal cancer. *Journal of Pain and Symptom Management, 10,* 599–603.

Brumley, R. (2002). Future of end-of-life care: The managed care organization perspective. *The Journal of Palliative Medicine, 5,* 263–270.

Cantwell, P., Turco, S., Bruera, E., Kneisler, P., & Hanson, J. (1998). Home death assessment tool: A prospective study. *Journal of Palliative Care, 14,* 104 (abstract).

Council on Scientific Affairs, American Medical Association. (1996). Good care for the dying patient. *JAMA, 275,* 474–478.

Davis, M., Walsh, D., LeGrand, S., & Lagman, R. (2003). "End-of-life care": The death of palliative medicine. *Journal of Palliative Medicine, 5,* 813–814.

Davis, M. & Homsi, J. (2001). The importance of cytochrome P450 monooxygenase CYP2D6 in palliative medicine. *Supportive Cancer Care, 9,* 442–451.

Doyle, D., Hanks, G., & MacDonald, N. (1998). Introduction. In D. Doyle, G. Hanks, & N. MacDonald (Eds.), *Oxford Textbook of Palliative Medicine* (2nd ed., pp. 3–8). Oxford: Oxford University Press.

Driver, L. & Bruera, E. (2002). *The M.D. Anderson palliative care handbook.* Department of Symptom Control and Palliative Care. Houston, TX: The University of Texas M.D. Anderson Cancer Center.

Emanuel, E. & Emanuel, L. (1998). The promise of a good death. *Lancet, 351,* S1121–S1129.

Farley, B. (1991). Ambulatory care services. In S. Baird, R. McCorkle, & M. Grant (Eds.), *Cancer Nursing a Comprehensive Textbook* (pp. 1011–1022). Philadelphia, PA: W.B. Saunders Co.

Field, M. & Cassel. C. (1997). *Approaching death: Improving care at the end-of-life.* Committee on Care at the End of Life, Division of Health Care Services, Institute of Medicine. Washington, DC: National Academy Press.

Finn-Paradis, L. (1985). *The development of hospice in America: The hospice handbook.* Rockville, MD: Aspen.

Folstein, M., Folstein, S., & McHugh, P. (1975). "Minimental state": A practical method for grading the cognitive state of patients for the clinician. *Journal of Psychiatric Residency, 12,* 189–198.

Friedman, B., Harwood, K., & Shields, M. (2002). Barriers and enablers to hospice referrals: An expert overview. *Journal of Palliative Medicine 5,* 73–81.

Introcaso, D. & Lynn, J. (2002). Systems of care: Future reform. *Journal of Palliative Medicine, 5,* 255–262.

Johnson, J., Herring, V., Wolfe, M., & Relling, M. (2000). Clinically significant drug interaction. *Postgraduate Medicine, 105,* 193–222.

Kuebler, K. & Heidrich, D. (2001). Perspectives on end-of-life care. In J. Black, J. Hawks, & A. Keene (Eds.), *Medical Surgical Nursing* (6th ed., pp. 447–460). Philadelphia, PA: W.B. Saunders Co.

Lo, B. (1995). *End-of-life care after termination of SUPPORT.* Hastings Center Report Special Supplement 25, S6–S8.

Lynn, J. (2000). Learning to care for people with chronic illness facing the end of life. *The Journal of the American Medical Association 284,* 2508–2511.

McHale, H. (2002). Palliative care. In K. Kuebler & P. Esper (Eds.), Palliative practices from A-Z for the bedside clinician (pp. 193–195). Pittsburgh, PA: Oncology Nursing Press.

Moore, R., Bone, L., Gellar, G., Mamon, J., Stokes, E., & Levine, D. (1989). Prevalence, detection and treatment of alcoholism in hospitalized patients. *JAMA, 261,* 403–407.

National Hospice Organization. (1993). *Standards of a Hospice Program of Care.* Arlington, VA: National Hospice Organization.

Ogle, K., Mavis, B., & Wyatt, G. (2002). Physicians and hospice care: Attitudes, knowledge and referrals. *Journal of Palliative Medicine, 5*, 85–92.

Scanlon, C. (1996). Nurses: Catalysts for improving end-of-life care. *ANA Communique, 5*, 1–2.

Singer, P., Martin, D., & Kelner, M. (1999). Quality end-of-life care. *JAMA, 281*, 163–168.

The SUPPORT Principal Investigators. (1995). A controlled trial to improve care for seriously ill hospitalized patients: The Study to Understand Prognoses and Preferences for Outcomes and Risks of Treatments (SUPPORT). *JAMA, 274*, 1591–1598.

Tilden, V., Drach, L., Tolle, S., Rosenfield, A., & Hickman, S. (2002). Sampling challenges in end-of-life research: Case finding for family informants. *Nursing Research, 51*, 66–69.

Tolle, S., Tilden, V., Rosenfield, A., & Hickman, S. (2000). Family reports of barriers to optimal care of the dying. *Nursing Research, 49*, 310–317.

Twycross, R., Wilcock, A., & Thorp, S. (Eds.). (1998). *Palliative Care Formulary*. Oxford, UK: Radcliff Medical Press.

United Kingdom Policy Framework for Commissioning Cancer Services. (1994). Calman report and recommendations for cancer services. Consultative Document. London, UK: Her Majesty's Stationary Office.

USA Today. (2000). Predictions mid-century. February, 22.

Vermillon, J. (1996). The referral process and reimbursement. In D. Sheehan & W. Forman (Eds.), *Hospice and Palliative Care: Concepts and Practice* (pp. 11–20). Sudbury, MA: Jones and Bartlett Publishers.

von Gunten, C., Ferris, F., D'Antuono, R., & Emanuel, L. (2002). Recommendations to improve end-of-life care through regulatory change in U.S. health care financing. *Journal of Palliative Medicine 5*, 35–41.

Woodruff, R. (2002). The problem of definition. Letter to the Editor. *Progress in Palliative Care, 10*, 17.

World Health Organization (WHO). (1986, 1990, 1996). Cancer pain relief and palliative care. Report of a WHO Expert Committed (WHO Technical Support Series, No. 804). Geneva: World Health Organization.

Yue, M., Fainsinger, R., & Bruera, E. (1994). Cognitive impairment in a patient with a mini-mental state examination (MMSE). *Journal of Pain and Symptom Management, 9*, 51–53.

Chapter 13

Oral and Dental Management For Cancer Patients

Sharon Elad

Joel B. Epstein

Cyril Meyerowitz

Douglas E. Peterson

Mark M. Schubert

Introduction

Radiotherapy, chemotherapy, hematopoietic stem cell transplantation (HSCT), and surgery are the most frequently selected options for treating cancer patients. Each modality is associated with a number of considerations related to the treatment of the cancer and the quality of life of the patient. This chapter is directed to oncology nurses, who are key members of the treatment team. It presents both an overview of the oral consequences associated with cancer treatment and an approach to their management. This chapter is intended to do the following:

- Increase awareness of the effects of cancer therapy on oral health
- Increase awareness of the effects of oral health on the efficacy and consequences of cancer therapy
- Provide guidelines for preventive and palliative oral health care
- Promote the maintenance of oral health after cancer therapy

The Treatment Team

An interdisciplinary team should provide comprehensive management of the cancer patient, including evaluation and treatment planning that incorporates the overall patient health, malignancy diagnosis, site and stage, and cultural/socioeconomic status. Assessment and education are crucial and should be performed by team members as appropriate in all stages of cancer therapy. The treatment team should include physicians, nurses, and pharmacists, as well as dentists and dental hygienists who are knowledgeable in oral medicine. Additionally, services of other healthcare workers, including physical therapists, social workers, and psychologists, enhance the patient's treatment experience. The oral/dental treatment team treating the cancer patient should have an expanded knowledge of oral medicine, the nonsurgical interface between dental medicine and medicine. Close collaboration should exist between the dental–oral medicine team and the other members of the interdisciplinary team. The dental–oral care team should participate in the hospital rounds to provide input into oral health issues related to cancer and its treatment. Outpatient follow-up by dental–oral care providers can provide continuity of oral care as deemed appropriate given the patient's ongoing oncology and oncology therapy status.

Patient Care

Cancer patients receiving different types of cancer therapy will have varying oral medicine–dental needs. Differences in the oral needs of cancer patients are related to pre-existing oral and dental conditions, which will need to be factored against the treatment modality that is selected in each case. For example, treatment of head and neck cancers with head and neck radiation or with head and neck surgery has a different impact on oral health than systemic treatments such as chemotherapy. Interventions such as surgery or irradiation that are directed to an organ remote from the head and neck have little or no impact on the oral tissues than interventions directed at the head and neck area. The major treatment modalities affecting oral tissues and oral health (head and neck radiation, chemotherapy, HSCT and head and neck surgery, and their effect on the oral tissues) are described here.

Head and Neck Radiation

Therapeutic radiation to the head and neck can result in both immediate (acute) and long-term (chronic) oral complications. Oral sequelae are related to the site, total radiation dose, and fraction rate. Solid tumors of the head and neck are commonly treated with 5,000–7,000 centi Gray (cGy) over a 4- to 7-week period. Hodgkin's and non-Hodgkin's lymphoma usually receive lower total doses (approximately 3,000–4,500 cGy). Ionizing radiation results in early death of cancer cells. It also concurrently damages or kills normal cells, thus resulting in both short- and long-term debilitating side effects.

The impact of radiation on oral tissues is due to effects on epithelial cells and connective tissue of the mucosa, taste receptors, bone, dental pulp, periosteum, and salivary glands. Early effects are mucosal injury and ductal and acinar salivary gland damage. Chronic effects include hypovascularity of irradiated tissue and increased fibrosis, resulting in salivary gland dysfunction, loss of tissue elasticity, and suppression of osteoblastic and osteoclastic activity that in turn results in decreased capacity for bone remodeling.

Mucositis, decreased salivary function, trismus, osteoradionecrosis, and soft-tissue necrosis are common oral side effects caused by head and neck radiation; however, hypogeusia/dysgeusia, dental caries, dental sensitivity, loss of periodontal attachment, taste dysfunction, and trismus are also important oral consequences of head and neck radiation. Nutritional deficiency and secondary side effects related to the loss of oral functions, including the risk for opportunistic infections caused by decreased salivary function, can further complicate the general oral health status of the patient.

Chemotherapy

Cancer chemotherapy is designed to destroy rapidly proliferating tumor cells by interfering with their metabolism. The drugs used are, however, also associated with numerous adverse side effects. Because of the nonspecific behavior of these agents, normal cells that have a high mitotic index, such as the oral mucosa and bone marrow, can also undergo cytolysis. The cytotoxic effect of the chemotherapy drugs can lead to damage of the oral epithelium and the vascular, inflammatory, and healing response of the oral cavity as well as changes in the oral ecology. In addition, damage to rapidly proliferating cells in the bone marrow can result in neutropenia, thrombocytopenia, and anemia, which in turn escalate the direct effect of drugs on oral tissue by increasing the propensity for infection or bleeding.

HSCT

With HSCT, the bone marrow is destroyed by intensive-dose chemotherapy or radiation therapy or a combination of chemotherapy and radiotherapy. The bone marrow is then repopulated by hemopoietic stem cells from either the patient (autologous transplant) or a donor (allogeneic or syngeneic transplant). In autologous and syngeneic transplantation, oral complications are most commonly related to conditioning regimen toxicities caused by chemotherapy (e.g., neutropenia increasing the risk for opportunistic infections) and/or total body irradiation (at relatively low dose than 1,200 cGy). In allogeneic transplant, the oral complications include those that are secondary to chemotherapy and radiotherapy as well as graft-versus-host disease (GVHD). In this latter toxicity, the grafted donor cells exert an immunologically based response against host tissues.

Recently, a hematopoietic transplant using nonmyeloablative protocols takes advantage of the potential killing of residual malignant disease by GVHD responses. Because less toxic conditioning regimens are used, there is less early post-transplant toxicity, including less oral toxicity. Oral GVHD does remain a significant concern.

Oral complications are more common in chronic GVHD than acute, and impaired oral function and quality of life can result. The clinical presentation of oral GHVD may be similar in both acute and chronic GVHD (Schubert, Peterson, & Lloid, 1999) and can effect multiple oral tissues: the mucosa, the lips, the salivary glands, the masticatory muscles, and the surrounding connective tissue (the later are more specific to sclerodermatous-like chronic GVHD during late stages).

Head and Neck Surgery

Surgery is employed as therapy for head and neck cancers where appropriate. Surgical techniques treat the primary site and the involved neck. The primary goal of head and neck cancer surgery is complete removal of the tumor. However, surgery may lead to compromised oral functions, including mastication, swallowing and speech, and cosmesis impairment. Repeated reconstructive surgical procedures may be required at later stages to restore the dentition and supporting jaw and facial structures, to prevent aspiration, and to restore cosmetic status and quality of life. Reconstruction options include primary closure, skin and bone grafts, local or regional flaps, and free tissue transfer. New modalities such as photodynamic therapy allow for more targeted therapy and thus damage oral tissues less intensely than traditional therapies.

Patient Evaluation and Assessment

Pretreatment

The pretreatment cancer period ranges from initial medical diagnosis and hospital admission to treatment by surgery, chemotherapy, bone marrow transplant conditioning therapy, and/or radiation therapy. The main emphasis of the oral care in this stage is the elimination of foci of infections and the establishment of preventive protocols to reduce the risk of therapy-related toxicities and complications. Therefore, all patients should receive a thorough dental evaluation, including necessary radiographs before radiation or surgical therapy to the head and neck, chemotherapy, or HSCT.

It is important to begin educating and motivating the patient regarding oral care as well as providing necessary dental treatment. The rationale of this concept is that patients who understand the potential risks of therapy and can be trained in appropriate self-care will reduce their risk for later therapy-related complications associated with oral infections and disease and may eliminate the future need for interventions or treatment.

The first step for dental providers is to obtain a complete and comprehensive medical history and to establish a line of communication with the medical–oncology team.

The information to be provided by the oncology team is as follows:

- The patient's current health status and the cancer diagnosis
- The planned cancer therapy regimen
- Patient prognosis
- In the case of chemotherapy, the anticipated number of treatment cycles and agents to be administered and the expected risk for myelosuppression
- Expected placement of chronic implanted and tunneled indwelling venous access lines (Hickman® CR Bard, Inc., Salt Lake City, UT; Groshong Port-A-Cath® Deltec, St. Paul, MN, etc.) that may require antibiotic premedication for dental treatment)
- Current hematologic data with attention to the white blood cell count and differential count (especially the absolute neutrophil count) and the platelet count
- In the case of radiation treatment, review of the cumulative dose and specific volume of tissue to be treated (i.e., treatment fields)
- In the case of HSCT, a review of the type of transplant and conditioning regimen and the anticipated timing of side effects

After pretreatment oral evaluation, the dental team should communicate effectively with the cancer treatment team by providing the following data:

- Recommended dental treatment/management plan and timeline
- Specific oral health issues that if unresolved may interrupt or complicate cancer treatment regimen and unresolved oral health issues that may significantly effect patient comfort during therapy
- Anticipated oral complications

An oral examination should be conducted, including examination of extraoral and intraoral tissues, soft and hard tissues, and appropriate radiographic evaluation. The dental–oral treatment plan should identify carious, pulpal, periapical, and/or gingival/periodontal pathology that is likely to affect cancer treatment adversely and necessitate immediate attention by restorative care, extractions, periodontal therapy, or pulpal treatment. Sources of intraoral trauma (such as fractured dental cusps or dental restorations, orthodontic appliances, ill-fitting dentures) and infection are eliminated. Potential complications caused by decreased salivary function should be addressed in the dental treatment plan (e.g., topical fluoride administration should be recommended). Limited mouth opening should be anticipated in radiotherapy-treated patients or in those with GVHD, and physical therapy should be recommended accordingly.

The treatment plan should be discussed with both the patient and oncologist, and the impact of oral health on the patient's oral and general health should be discussed. The oral treatment approach should be definitive and expeditious to achieve elimination of oral foci of infections and potential complications. The plan will incorporate the nature of the malignancy, diagnosis, and time constraints related to the cancer treatment plan. For example, for patients at risk for significant immunosuppression, dental extraction should be considered in cases of partially erupted third molars that are at risk for pericoronitis or periodontal abscesses, nonrestorable fractured teeth, unresolved periapical lesions, and advanced periodontal disease.

Dental treatment should be completed before initiation of the cancer treatment such as sufficient time exists the posttherapy healing of extraction sites (e.g., before myelosuppressive and risk for impaired wound healing). For example, sufficient healing of an alveolar socket after dental extraction may require 14–21 days before initiation of radiotherapy and 3–10 days before initiation of chemotherapy. Any invasive dental–periodontal treatment should be performed with minimal trauma. If the oral health of the individual scheduled to receive cancer therapy is such that it cannot be adequately treated to eliminate serious risk of infection from the oral cavity, delay of cancer treatment should be considered until oral health issues can be satisfactorily resolved.

Oral hygiene instruction will be an important part of the dental–oral treatment plan at this stage. Ideally, the patient's oral hygiene routine should be performed two to four times a day or within 30 minutes after meals and at bedtime. As the severity of oral complications increases, oral hygiene becomes increasingly important. Brushing should be performed slowly with gentle placement and with minimal pressure in order to avoid trauma. A soft brush and a nonabrasive minimally flavored toothpaste (e.g., non–mint-flavored toothpaste with high fluoride content) are suitable.

Instructions for mouth rinses will be in accordance to the oral care protocol accepted at the hospital and may include nonmedicated (e.g., normal saline solutions) and/or medicated (0.12% to 0.2% aqueous chlorhexidine solutions) mouthwashes, as indicated to help manage specific oral conditions. A protocol for denture care should also be established and should include daily cleaning of dentures with a toothbrush and by soaking in an appropriate antiseptic solution. Dentures should be worn as little as possible or not at all during periods in which oral tissues are at risk for mucositis.

Once the patient has begun cancer treatment, preventative therapies to manage oral complication may be instituted. These may include the administration of medication for the prevention of infections, prevention of GVHD in the case of HCST, and enhancement of salivary gland function. The preventive protocols administered by the medical team will address some of these expected complications, such as the GVHD, whereas other prophylactic measures should be delivered by the nurses and oral medicine team. New strategies for protection of salivary tissue from injury are needed; experimental protocols to reduce the salivary glands damage have been reported (Brizel et al., 2000; Zimmerman, Mark, Tran, & Juillard, 1997). The dental–medical staff should inform the patient of the currently available preventive protocols.

During Cancer Therapy

In chemotherapy and HSCT, the acute period of risk for myelosuppression and oral complications often extends up to 21 days after cytotoxic treatment. In radiation therapy, acute effects manifest within the first several weeks of starting therapy and continue several weeks after the end of treatment. The period, defined by significant myelosuppression and immunosuppression, in the case of chemotherapy, is a consequence of aggressive cancer treatment and can vary significantly from one protocol to another. The emphasis on oral care in this stage should be to prevent oral complications resulting from the cancer treatment (e.g., oral mucositis or infections related to the immunosuppression or stomatotoxic therapy). Additional objectives of the oral care during the cancer therapy are prevention and treatment of mucositis, infections, and bleeding complications. In order to accomplish this, the patient should be monitored regularly with respect to his or her subjective report of pain and the objective signs in the oral tissues. The principles of evaluation of pain and changes in oral tissues (teeth, mucosa, salivary glands, and periodontium) are described here.

Patient oral cavity complaints should be investigated as soon as possible, particularly in immunosuppressed patients, as oral infection may progress rapidly. Early assessment of even relatively minor complaints is particularly important, as tenderness and pain may be minimal but may be the most prominent sign of an oral infection, as redness and swelling may be muted because of myelosuppression. A common quantitative manner to describe oral pain uses a subjective scoring technique in which the patient is asked to rate the pain severity on a 0 to 10 scale (0 = no pain and

10 = the worst possible pain). The Visual Analogue Scale is an example of a data collection instrument for which the patient is asked to make a mark on a horizontal line between the two extremes of pain of no pain and worst possible pain. Because pain severity is a subjective sensation, complementary verbal description of the pain characteristics can be helpful in describing the nature of the pain. Examples of pain descriptors are pain location, pain duration, time of onset and its relationship to specific traumatic stimuli, disturbance of oral function and overall function, and pain response to the treatment.

Another oral complaint in cancer patients is related to taste change. The taste receptor cell is neuroepithelially derived. Damage to the receptors cells may relate directly to the direct cytotoxic effect of the cancer treatment, to the indirect effect on the red blood lineage, or to concurrent systemic and topical medications. With a turnover rate of approximately 10 days, it can regenerate if not irreversibly damaged, although recovery can take months (Schubert et al., 1999).

Dental tissues may be affected indirectly during the cancer treatment in several ways. For example, a common side effect of chemotherapy is gastrointestinal nausea and emesis. Frequent emesis can result in frequent exposure of the teeth to acidic gastric contents. The long-term effect of this exposure can result in erosion of palatal facets of the teeth, mainly the maxillary teeth. However, it is not typically clinically significant for patients receiving single or infrequent cycles of chemotherapy. Palliative treatment to reduce vomiting may decrease the severity and prevalence of this dental erosion. Additionally, immediate administration of antacid solutions may help to neutralize acidity, and the use of topical fluoride solutions and gels can help reduce potential damage to enamel. Another example occurs when "dental pain" is reported that is, in fact, independent of dental pathology and may be induced by the infiltration of malignant cells into the pulp or caused by neurologic disorders related

to the chemotherapy. A professional dental examination and appropriate radiographs will differentiate the cause of dental pain.

During cancer therapy, no dental treatment interventions should be initiated unless absolutely necessary, and only emergent and palliative oral care is provided. Should emergent dental procedures be necessary, they should be performed with great caution after the results of hematologic evaluation, blood chemistry, and coagulation tests are available and by experienced, knowledgeable persons. Although there is not scientific proof whether antibiotic prophylaxis is effective in reducing the risk for intravascular catheter-related infection, it is often empirically recommended when a vascular access device (central venous catheter) is in place (O'Grady et al., 2002). Although this recommendation remains empirically based, the American Heart Association endocarditis prophylactic antibiotic regimen is often recommended before invasive dental procedures (AHA Recommendations, 1985). It is important to remember that some individuals may receive myelosuppressive chemotherapy for several years on repeated schedules depending on the type of cancer and the protocol used. Every series of chemotherapy may result in the cycle of myelosuppression and immunosuppression. As long as patients remain on these types of protocols, the benefits of dental treatment must be weighted against possible complications and adjustments, and compensatory care must be considered to maintain oral health and also to prevent secondary complications.

A systematic examination of oral mucosal surfaces should be carried out during cancer therapy at regular intervals to identify signs of mucosal injury or infection, and depending on the differential diagnosis, microbiologic specimens may be taken from the oral lesions. This intraoral examination should include all surfaces; however, special attention should be directed at the ventral tongue, the floor of the mouth, buccal and labial mucosa, and the soft palate, as these manifest the most notable changes of mucosal injury, whereas the hard palate is least affected.

A number of scoring systems for mucositis can be used and include such scales as the World Health Organization score (Handbook for Reporting Results, 1979), the National Cancer Institute (NCI) score (Consensus Conference, 1989), and the Oral Mucositis Assessment Score (OMAS) (Sonis et al., 1999) discussed later here.

Evaluation of the salivary glands should be conducted, including documentation of enlargement, tenderness on palpation, lack or diminished saliva on palpation, and expression of pus on palpation. Salivary flow can be measured as stimulated or unstimulated whole or individual gland. On soft-tissue examination of patients with decreased salivary flows, dry, atrophic, fissured mucosa may be present. An examination of the dentition should be done and may reveal decalcification spots and caries, especially in the cervical surfaces of the teeth. If this occurs, attention to preventive agents, particularly topical fluoride, should be prescribed.

Cancer treatment commonly affects the gingiva and the periodontium. Infections may result in the rapid development of localized or generalized swelling, gingival recession, ulcerated gingiva, necrotic gingival papilla, loosen teeth, alveolar resorption, or alveolar bone exposure (Epstein & Stevenson-Moore, 2001; Raber-Durlacher et al., 2002; Wright, 1987). Such changes should be documented, diagnosed, and treated appropriately. In contrast to the obvious gingival and periodontal pathologies, occult sites of periodontitis may signal an increased risk for systemic infection as well. This has been well established by several studies (Greenberg, Cohen, McKitrick, & Cassileth, 1982; Laine et al., 1992) although systemic infection induced by generalized asymptomatic chronic infections may have been underestimated in the studies from the 1980s aimed at investigating the relationship between periodontal infection and systemic bacteremia in a leukemia patient (Raber-Durlacher et al.). Therefore, clinical evaluation should include visual examination and palpation to identify tender sites that may lead to diagnosis. In addition, cultures and speciation of microbial isolates from diseased periodontal pockets may be required in order to identify the source for bacteremia with a common periopathogen.

The periodontium may also present with pathologies related to the malignancy itself. Gingival hypertrophy caused by infiltrating leukemia (predominantly acute myelogenous leukemia) or lymphoma cells may change its contour before treatment or during the cancer treatment period. The response of the malignant cells to the cancer treatment may result in degradation of numerous cells in the tissue involved. Such a phenomenon in the gingival may result in shrinkage and various degrees of gingival and periodontal necrosis. Any other oral tissues that were infiltrated with the malignant cell may present similar changes if responding to the antineoplastic treatment. Alternatively, some of the symptoms associated with this tumor mass or leukemic infiltrate in the tissue will resolve, such as improvement of sensory deficiencies caused by perineural infiltration.

After Cancer Therapy

The postcancer treatment period is characterized by a reduced and altered immune response and a loss of organ functions related to tissue destruction. These changes can include liver dysfunction, renal dysfunction, central nervous system disorders, and salivary gland dysfunction. Clearly, the impact of loss of function depends on the type and location of the cancer. Furthermore, late complications of the cancer treatment and an adverse reaction to multiple chronic medications may occur. Accordingly, the oral medicine team will confront oral manifestations related to the immunocompromised state and late sequelae of the cancer treatment. These sequelae can be related to systemic disease, such as GVHD or loss of oral function, such as after head and neck surgery or radiation therapy.

Acute oral complications typically begin to resolve after completion of the cancer therapy. Patients should continue to follow an oral health self-care regimen to keep the teeth and gums healthy and to facilitate the repair of any residual oral damage. Close follow-up will facilitate the management of any chronic complications that may occur, such as decreased salivary function, mucosal sensitivity, increased risk of cavities, and candidiasis. All of these are described later here. Notable complications including osteoradionecrosis (ORN), trismus, oral GVHD, drug-related oral complications, risk for second cancers, and altered dental and maxillofacial growth are possible as well.

ORN results from an irreversible, progressive devitalization of irradiated bone characterized by necrotic soft tissue and results in bone that fails and is incapable of remodeling and is unable to heal spontaneously. Its principal causation is based on damage to the vascular bed. Most cases of ORN occur in the mandible where the vascularization is poor and bone density is high. Clinical manifestations of ORN may include pain, orofacial fistulas, exposed necrotic bone, pathologic fracture, and suppuration (Aitasalo, Grenman, Virolained, Niinikoski, & Klossner, 1995; Brown, Evans, & Sandor, 1998). Although one third of ORN cases may occur spontaneously, in those cases in which trauma initiates ORN, the majority of cases result from extraction of teeth. The incidence of ORN is doubled in dentate patients when compared with edentulous patients. Poor oral hygiene and the continued use of alcohol and tobacco also increase the risk and progression of ORN (Curi & Dib, 1997).

Therefore, tooth extractions should be avoided after radiotherapy. If absolutely necessary, tooth removal should be performed as atraumatically as possible, using antibiotic coverage. Pre-extraction hyperbaric oxygen should be considered as a preventive measure; however, these extractions should be performed by experienced clinicians, typically in specialized settings.

Prosthetic device such as dentures should be atraumatic; assessments of the denture tendency to produce excessive pressure over the bearing soft tissue should be done. Patient should be advised regarding maintaining good oral hygiene in order to avoid future dental extractions (oral hygiene recommendations are detailed later here).

Over the years, ORN has been treated by numerous methods with variable success rates (Laine et al., 1992). Hyperbaric oxygen therapy is considered an adjunctive treatment for ORN, often in conjunction with surgery, and has been associated with improved success rates (Aitasalo et al., 1995; Curi & Dib, 1997; David, Sandor, Evans, & Brown, 2001; McKenzie, Wong, Epstein, & Lepawsky, 1993; van Merkesteyn, Bakker, & Borgmeijer-Hoelen, 1995).

After radiotherapy to the head and neck, patients should be assessed for signs of trismus, which can be assessed by repeated measuring of maximum mouth opening and determining the relative flexibility of soft tissue, such as the muscles of mastication and oral tongue. Jaw exercises may limit the severity of trismus but will not mobilize fibrosis once it has occurred (Whitmeyer, Waskowski, & Iffland, 1997). Thus, stretching exercises must be instituted with the start of radiation therapy and should basically continue indefinitely.

After HSCT, patients commonly suffer from a unique complication, GVHD, which has acute and chronic forms (Schubert et al., 1999). Oral GVHD clinically mimics a number of naturally occurring autoimmune disorders, including lichen planus, lupus, and scleroderma. Symptoms of mouth dryness and sensitivity are often associated with evolving GVHD. The classic clinical presentation in the oral cavity includes mucosal erythema, atrophy, pseudomembranous ulcerations and hyperkeratotic striae, plaques, and papules, similar to oral lichen planus. Sclerodermatous changes can result in perioral fibrosis that decreases the oral opening and may affect tongue mobility, both interfering with oral function. Secondary oral infections caused by herpes simplex virus (HSV), cytomegalovirus (CMV), Candida, or trauma can be superimposed on the oral GVHD lesions and confound the diagnosis (Schubert et al.).

Postcancer treatment is complicated with chronic administration of medication, such as immunosuppressive drugs for GVHD management. The oral tissues may manifest reaction to these drugs. For example, both cyclosporine and niphedipine (often used to manage cyclosporine-induced hypertension) may result in gingival hyperplasia. Therefore, the etiology oral tissue change needs to include adverse drug reactions when the oral tissues are evaluated.

Patients should be closely monitored for recurrence of cancer as well as the increased possibility of a new primary cancer. The posttreatment cancer period includes long-term follow-up of the patient and needs to be considered as lifelong.

Children younger than 16 years who undergo chemotherapy or HSCT are at risk for abnormalities in developing dental and skeletal structures (Schubert et al., 1999). Damage to the tooth bud may result in enamel hypoplasia and root alterations. Delayed exfoliation of primary teeth and delayed dental eruption after HSCT are common. Altered skeletal development for craniofacial bones can result in orthognathic changes (Schubert et al.).

Despite the oral complications, the period after completion of cancer therapy is an excellent time for patients to resolve any oral concerns that were previously deemed nonmedically necessary and for which care had been deferred. Because patients with cancer are even more likely to develop a recurrence or new cancer and require further therapy, the resolution of any deferred necessary dental care should be a top priority.

Additional dietary counseling may also be appropriate for patients who must make long-term dietary adaptations to accommodate permanent changes to their oral cavity produced by surgery and radiation. The referral of patients to support groups may also be a useful adjunct to patients' return to optimal functioning.

Patient Education

Patient education is one of the most important elements of the oral care plan. Individual patient needs must be addressed in developing oral care regimens. Instructions should be given clearly and concisely. Written materials offering additional information are often helpful. Compliance with oral care procedures can have a considerable impact during the cancer treatment period. Stressing the importance of compliance will foster motivation of the patient to comply with the oral care protocol.

In addition to potential oral complications and their prevention, patients should be advised regarding oral hygiene care instructions and balanced diet recommendations. These instructions are important in respect to prevention of the oral complications.

Oral complications of the cancer treatment are very common. These oral complications are described here in the sections of "mucositis," "salivary glands dysfunction," "infections," and "patients evaluation and assessment." In addition, the patient should be informed about possible taste changes as a result of the cancer therapy or as a result of the supportive topical treatment. This information will help patients to cope with the oral symptoms and will facilitate the report of these symptoms to the treatment team so that early diagnosis can be made.

As with healthy patients, oral hygiene in cancer patients has a high importance. Dental plaque that covers the oral tissues and teeth consists of bacteria. Routine oral care reduces the amount of dental plaque and therefore the amount of bacteria. In an immune-suppressed individual, this is important so as to reduce the risk of infection. Moreover, good oral hygiene and compliance with specific oral care instructions reduce the risk, severity, or duration of the oral symptoms (Borowski et al., 1994).

Routine oral care consists of brushing, flossing, mouthrinses, and fluoride applications; unfortunately, however, adherence to sound basic oral hygiene protocols varies across various institutions. It is not uncommon to hear that patients have been told to "stop brushing and flossing because we don't want your gums to bleed." Nevertheless, by not brushing and flossing, gingival infection is promoted, and the risk of bleeding is actually increased. Basically stated, healthy gingival tissues do not bleed unless traumatized—routine flossing and brushing reduces the risk of infection. Patients should be instructed and supervised relative to appropriate mechanical oral hygiene practices.

Brushing

Patients should continue brushing as per prior instructions, at least twice a day. During neutropenia and thrombocytopenia, the patient should not use a traumatizing technique; a qualified staff's ongoing supervision is essential. If gingival bleeding occurs, continue dental brushing with an ultrasoft brush soaked in chlorhexidine and use cotton swabs and gauze sponges. The toothbrush should be rinsed frequently during the procedure to minimize the accumulation of bacteria and debris. After brushing, rinse the brush thoroughly, shake off extra water, and allow it to air dry.

Flossing

Waxed floss may reduce the risk for gingival bleeding and self-injury of the periodontium, leading to decreased risk for bacteremia secondary to oral flora. Patients who are not experienced with this technique should not do so during cancer therapy for the first time without care training and guidance. Alternatively, interproximal dental hygiene instruments (such as Stimudents® Johnson & Johnson, Raritan, NJ) and interproximal bushes can be used as long as the technique is not traumatic.

Frequent Rinsing

The purposes of rinsing is to cleanse and lubricate tissues, to prevent crusting and drying, to treat mucosal wounds, to hydrate and irrigate mucosal tissues, to remove debris, to prevent accumulation of debris, and to reduce bacterial plaque. The most common mouthrinses are presented in **Table 13.1**. Mouthrinses that are a combination of these agents and anesthetic agents are accepted widely. However, mixtures of various agents dilute the concentration of each, and agents may not be compatible, leading to inactivation of some of the compounds. Other rinses such as hydrogen peroxide and highly flavored and high-content alcohol commercial mouthwashes should be avoided.

Fluoride Applications

Dentate patients suffering from decreased salivary function need frequent fluoride applications. This can be using topical fluoride applications of different concentrations (1.1% neutral sodium fluoride topical gel or 0.05% neutral sodium fluoride mouthrinse). Fluoride gel applied in custom fluoride carriers achieves maximal fluoride incorporation into the dentition. Neutral pH fluoride is available and is suitable for patients suffering from mucosal erosions or ulcerations (see Salivary Gland Dysfunctions).

In addition, routine moisturizing of the lips is necessary to maintain comfort, especially in the presence of fever or mouth breathing, and may prevent fissures from secondary infection.

Nutritional support and recommendations for a balanced diet are especially important when mucositis develops, as oral intake may be limited because of pain. The patient should consume high-calorie foods that emphasize protein, increase water intake, and use liquid meal replacements. High-calorie, soft commercial products are available, but attention should be directed to reduction of sucrose-containing foods to reduce the risk of developing dental caries if

Table 13.1 MOUTHRINSES

Mouthrinses	Composition/ Instructions for Use	Uses/Functions	Disadvantages
Neutral rinse	1/4–3/4 tsp. salt 1/4 tsp. baking soda 1 qt. H_2O Use every two hours until soreness, nausea, or ropy saliva contraindicate Should not be swallowed	May be used during mucositis (omit salt) May neutralize acids after emesis Dissolves thick, mucinous salivary secretions Soothing to irritated tissues Dislodges debris	None
Saline rinse	1/4–3/4 tsp. salt eight oz. water	Not damaging to oral mucosa Helps reduce mucosal irritation Increases moisture in mouth Removes thickened secretions and debris Recommended for treatment of gingivitis and head and neck radiation	None
Caphasol	Calcium phosphate rinse Rinse four times a day or for one hour for mucositis	Remineralization of tooth surfaces	No published study in mucositis
Peridex	Chlorhexidine 0.12% Rinse with 15–30 cc for one minute, three times per day; apply directly to acutely inflamed site Allow 30 minutes before other oral hygiene procedure. Rinsing with water intensifies unpleasant taste Should not replace dental evaluation/treatment An alcohol-free, aqueous 2% solution can be compounded by the pharmacist Can be applied locally with cotton swab	Used in presence of poor plaque control, signs of inflammation, or decreased salivary flow Effective topical agent Has potent broad-spectrum anti-microbial activity, and mild antifungal activity Effective at a low concentration Minimal absorption from the gastrointestinal tract Results in fewer febrile days	May alter oral flora and promote a gram(-) overgrowth (e.g., *Pseudomonas*) May delay mucositis healing May contain alcohol Stains teeth and restorations Toothpaste and nystatin reduce its effectiveness Unpleasant taste Should not be used close to the time that topical fluoride is used

the patient is placed on long-term (approximately greater than three months) modified diet. Also, the patient should avoid acidic foods (such as citrus, tomato sauces/juice), spicy/salty/overly sweet foods, foods that require excess chewing (such as raw vegetables), abrasive foods (such as granola, toast, crackers, taco chips), and food temperature extremes. If decreased salivary function develops, similar difficulties while eating may appear. The patients will need to use adequate amounts of water drinking as part of any meal. Patients suffering from decreased salivary function are encouraged to avoid high sugar-containing foods.

Pain Relief

Pain has a significant impact on the quality of life in patients during and after cancer therapy. Oncologic patients may have pain because of the primary malignancy and/or as a result of the cancer therapy itself. Orofacial pain may be caused by oral mucositis (discussed in next section), oral infection, and an alteration in musculoskeletal and neurologic functioning (e.g., temporomandibular disorders associated with muscular fibrosis, scar formation, and limited jaw opening). Surgical management can result in acute postoperative pain and may lead to chronic musculoskeletal and neuropathic pain syndromes. Pain is aggravated by the stress, anxiety, and fear associated with cancer and its therapy (Barbasi et al., 2002; Chapman, Donaldson, Jacobson, & Hautman, 1997; Dodd et al., 2001; Epstein & Schubert, 1993; Schulz-Kindermann, Hennings, Ramm, Zander, & Hasenbring, 2002). The patient should be educated about these possible side effects of the treatment.

Oral mucosal pain is the most common source of oral source pain. Radiation or chemotherapy therapy can result in acute pain associated with mucositis that may persist throughout the course of therapy and several weeks after treatment. Mucositis pain can vary in frequency and severity across the range of cancer therapies. Prevention of

mucosal damage is a key to the prevention of this pain; however, when pain is present, mucositis pain management must be individualized. It is important that patients and staff are educated about the nature of mucositis and pain-management strategies.

When oral mucositis pain is present, assessment of severity, location, and character of pain is necessary before providing an analgesic recommendations. After the oral mucositis diagnosis is established, different topical or systemic treatments can be considered for relief of pain. The most common topical anesthetic used is lidocaine viscous. Topical rinsing with benzydamine has also been shown to have a pain relieving/analgesic effect when used topically (Epstein et al., 1989; Pederson, Parran, & Harbaugh, 2000). The patient should be informed that topical anesthetics provide temporary pain relief and that some agents may cause an initial burning discomfort. Topical anesthetics may potentially increase oral trauma during mastication and may provoke choking in conjunction with food. Gargling or swallowing of topical anesthetics can result in diminished gag reflex and thus increase the risk of aspiration as well as systemic toxicities. Whatever the active agent of the topical preparation is, it is suggested that alcohol-containing preparations should be avoided whenever possible. Alcohol, coloring agents, and dyes can be irritating to the oral mucosa.

The use of ice chips may reduce mucosal pain. Patients should allow the ice to melt in the oral cavity; chewing should be avoided in order to prevent trauma to the oral mucosa. Ice chips administered starting five minutes before and for 30 minutes after dosing of bolus 5-fluorouracil also reduces the prevalence of oral mucositis (Cascinu, Fedeli, Fedeli, & Catalano, 1994; Mahood et al., 1991).

Systemic analgesics can include opioids administered by a variety of routes, including an oral, intravenous drip or bolus, patient-controlled analgesics, transdermal or rectal morphine or methadone, or nonopioid analgesics. Nonsteroidal anti-inflammatory drugs, and cyclo-oxygenase type 2 inhibitors should be considered if topical treatment fails to provide sufficient pain control. The possible oral and systemic side effects of this treatment may interfere with other conditions as well as drug administration. For example, nonsteroidal anti-inflammatory drugs may cause inactivation of platelets that could exacerbate the thrombocytopenia-induced bleeding tendency in myelosuppressed patients.

Mucositis

Oropharyngeal mucositis is a prominent complication during cancer therapy, especially high-dose cancer chemotherapy and head and neck radiation. Mucositis and associated pain described in the previous section can be a highly distressing symptom that patients report when receiving head and neck cancer therapies or high-dose cancer chemotherapies (Bellm, Epstein, Rose-Ped, Martin, & Fuchs, 2000; Barbasi et al., 2002; Chapman et al., 1997; Dodd et al., 2001; Epstein & Schubert, 1993; Epstein et al., 1989; Pederson et al., 2000; Schulz-Kindermann et al., 2002). A significant increase in systemic complications and cost of care for patients with mucositis has been documented (Elting et al., 2003; Kline, Meiman, Tarantino, Herzig, & Bertolone, 1998; Sonis et al., 2001).

What Is Mucositis?

Direct cytotoxic effects of chemotherapy or radiotherapy affect cellular elements of the mucosal epithelium, connective tissue, and vasculature. These effects result in a decreased renewal rate of basal epithelium, leading to tissue damage that can progress to thinning of the epithelium and ulceration of oral soft tissues. The resulting mucositis is primarily evident for nonkeratinized tissues and will typically heal beginning approximately two weeks after discontinuation of the cancer therapy (DePaola et al., 1986; Peterson & D'Ambrosio, 1992). The oral sites most commonly involved include buccal and labial mucosa, and ventral and lateral surfaces of the tongue, soft palate, and floor of the mouth. The hard palate, attached gingiva, and dorsal surface of the tongue are rarely subject to mucositis but may become painful. Signs and symptoms of mucositis range from erythema with superficial degeneration or erosion to severe ulceration and from mild–to–severe pain requiring systemic analgesic treatment.

Pathophysiology of Mucositis

The current pathophysiologic hypothesis of development the mucositis presents a complex biologic process that occurs in at least four phases. The evolving nature of this model is expected to result in further adjustment of these phases to the new understandings.

1. Inflammatory/vascular phase: shortly after the administration of radiation or chemotherapy cytokines are released from the epithelial tissue. These include tumor necrosis factor-a, interleukin-1, and perhaps, interleukin-6.

   Ionizing radiation also incites cytokine release from the adjacent connective tissue. It is likely that these cytokines cause local tissue damage as the initiating event in mucositis. Increased vascularity caused by interleukin-1 may result in additional concentrations of cytotoxic drug in the mucosa. Increased submucosal cellularity is evident at this stage.

2. Epithelial phase: both radiation and chemotherapy adversely impact the dividing cells of the oral basal epithelium, resulting in reduced epithelial renewal, atrophy, and ulceration. The latter is most likely exacerbated by functional trauma and amplified by the flood of locally produced cytokines.

3. Ulcerative/bacteriological phase: the ulcerative phase is the most symptomatic. Localized areas of full-thickness erosions occur that often become covered by a fibrinous pseudomembrane. Secondary bacterial colonization of the lesion occurs with a mixed flora, including many gram-negative organisms, providing a source of endotoxin (lipopolysaccharides), which further stimulates cytokine release from connective tissue born around the cells. These cytokines, plus nitric oxide, serve to intensify the patient's condition. Importantly, the ulcerative phase generally occurs at the time of the patient's maximum neutropenia; this can lead to considerable morbidity or possible patient death.

4. Healing phase: the healing phase consists of a renewal of epithelial proliferation and differentiation, normalization of the peripheral white blood cell count, and re-establishment of the local microbial flora.

Incidence

Mucositis is a common cause of morbidity during chemotherapy and radiotherapy. The incidence of National Cancer Institute (NCI) grade 3–4 oral and mucositis derived from clinical trials of standard-dose chemotherapy is estimated to be between 5% and 15%. Chemotherapy with 5-fluorouracil or irinotecan is associated with rates of oral or gastrointestinal mucositis exceeding 15% (National Institutes of Health, 1989). Among patients receiving high-dose regimens or concomitant radiotherapy to the head, neck, thorax, chest wall, abdomen, or pelvis, rates may exceed 40% and may significantly affect quality of life (Epstein, Emerton, Le et al., 1999; Peterson, 1999; Trotti, 2000). Approximately one half of those individuals develop lesions of such severity as to require modification of their cancer treatment and/or require parenteral analgesia. However, rates of mucositis after most chemother-

apy regimens administered to patients with solid tumors are probably far lower. In contrast, the mucositis incidence is higher among patients undergoing conditioning therapy for HSCT, continuous infusion therapy for breast and colon cancer, and therapy for tumors of the head and neck. Among patients in high-risk protocols, severe mucositis occurs with a frequency in excess of 60% (McGuire et al., 1995; Schubert, Sullivan, & Truelove, 1991; Woo, Sonis, Monopoli, & Sonis, 1993).

The wide range in the reported rates of mucositis could be related to variability across diseases and therapies. Furthermore, reporting mucositis as a secondary endpoint of studies probably results in underreporting. A lack of good study design, small sample sizes, limited assessment of compliance, and limited use of validated measures of mucositis have resulted in the wide range in the reported rates of mucositis.

Risk Factors

The risk factors include treatment- and patient-related variables (Barasch & Peterson, 2003).

TREATMENT-RELATED VARIABLES

A large number of cytotoxic agents have been reported to produce oral mucositis (Wilkes, 1998). It is accepted that antimetabolites and alkylating agents produce a high incidence and severity of mucositis (Peterson, 1991; Peterson & Sonis, 1983; Seto, Kim, Wolinsky, Mito, & Champlin, 1985). However, conflicting evidence was reported in other studies (Barasch et al., 1995; Woo et al., 1993; Zerbe, Parkerson, Ortlieb, & Spitzer, 1992).

The type of HSCT may be related to the severity of the mucositis as well. Allogeneic HSCT results in increased frequency and severity of mucositis compared with autologous HSCT (Barasch & Peterson, 2003; Muller, Yeager, Hodgson-Woodruff, Peterson, & McGuire, 1991).

PATIENT-RELATED VARIABLES

It appears that younger age could be related to a lower incidence of mucositis; however, the reports are inconsistent (McCarthy, Awde, Ghandi, Vincent, & Kocha, 1998; Sonis, Sonis, & Lieberman, 1978; Zalcberg, Kerr, Seymour, & Palmer, 1998). However, the increased frequency may reflect the more common malignancies in children, which are more often treated with neutropenia-inducing aggressive chemotherapy. Variables of patient's gender, nutritional status, and inflammation status have not been proven to be consistently related to the prevalence and severity of mucositits (Barasch & Peterson, 2003). Although the oral microflora is conceptually linked to severity of mucositis, the specific role of the oral microflora in increasing severity of oral mucositis remains unclear. In microbial culture studies, topical antiseptic such as chlorhexidine and antibacterial and antifungal topical treatments were tested in relationship to mucositis parameters (Barasch & Peterson, 2003; Blijlevens, Donnelly, & de Pauw, 2001; Donnelly, Bellm, Epstein, Sonis, & Symonds, 2003). The first impression is that this variable may be a factor, but this is not supported in other studies and with a range of antimicrobial agents.

Intact salivary function is important for mucosal lubrication as well as delivery of antimicrobial proteins to oral tissues (Epstein, Tsang, Warkentin, & Ship, 2002; McCarthy et al., 1998). Quantitative salivary function has been reported to correlate with either increased or decreased prevalence of mucositis (Barasch & Peterson, 2003). However, it is not possible to conclude unequivocally from these studies that reduced salivary flow is a risk factor for oral mucositis.

Assessment and Grading

When oral mucositis pain is present, assessment of the severity, location, and character of pain is necessary. Conducting the oral assessment requires attention to detail and must be performed consistently. Several factors must be considered to allow for the collection of valid data.

The timing of assessments, both in terms of frequency and sequencing in relationship to eating and oral care, should be taken into account. If the assessments are performed too infrequently, they may not identify changes that were present but resolved as part of the normal healing process, and increased volume of data may not add to the goal of research or patient care. Completion of oral care before an oral assessment and the quality of that oral care may influence the findings. The length of time since the last cleansing and/or rinsing could effect the oral status, in terms of the presence of debris, and the amount of saliva present. In addition, selection and timing of interventions for pain will influence reports of pain intensity.

Appropriate lighting is critical to view all areas of the oral cavity adequately during an assessment. Halogen light sources are preferred and are the standard for consistent exams in research studies. Individuals performing regular assessments in the clinical setting can use an otoscope or ophthalmoscope as a light source if available. When these preferred light sources are not available or when assessments are conducted in the home, individuals may need to rely on a small portable flashlight. A tongue blade or dental mirror and gauze provide assistance for visualizating all areas of the oral cavity. The gauze can be wrapped around the tongue to allow retraction from side to side. For some patients, all areas may not be easily visualized because of mucosal pain or a sensitive gag reflex.

Determining interventions based on assessments of the presence of infection in the oral cavity is also complex. The thrush interferes with visualization of the extent of ulcerative lesions and can actually be present independent of ulcerative mucositis. Similarly, herpes virus infections in the aplastic patient can cause ulceration, changes in the appearance of the mucosal tissue, and extreme pain. Institutions also vary in terms of the scope of practice for the diagnosis prophylaxis and treatment of oral infections.

Selection of the most appropriate instrument to score mucositis severity requires an examination of the goals of the assessment and should consider which instrument to choose. Different tools should be selected for different purposes and with different types of therapy.

Studies have driven the development and testing of a number of assessment tools, including the Oral Assessment Guide (Eilers, Berger, & Petersen, 1988), the Oral Mucositis Assessment Scale (OMAS) (Sonis et al., 1999), the Oral Mucosa Rating Scale (Schubert, Williams, Lloid, Donaldson, & Chapko, 1992), and the Oral Mucositis Index (McGuire et al., 2002; Schubert et al., 1992). Additional scales that have been developed to assess mucositis in patients receiving head and neck radiation include Radiation Therapy Oncology Group (Cox, Stetz, & Pajak, 1995), and a detailed research scale (Spijkervet, van Saene, Panders, Vermey, & Mehta, 1989). Other scales that assess the physical, functional, and subjective status of the patients undergoing stomatotoxic therapy were reported (Parulekar, Mackenzie, Bjarnason, & Jordan, 1998). Clinical trial groups have routinely used the World Health Organization mucositis index (Handbook for Reporting Results, 1979) and the NCI Clinical Trials Common Toxicity Criteria (CTC) (**Table 13.2**) (Consensus Conference, 1989). Although commonly used, these toxicity scales have not been subject to validity and reliability testing.

Management

The management of oral mucositis pain begins with pretreatment assessment and management, with the goal of preventing or reducing severity of mucositis.

Current approaches to prevention consist of oral hygiene and topical agents. Some centers employ fluconazole prophylaxis to prevent or reduce fungal colonization and infections with

HSCT. Typical therapy is 200- to 400-mg fluconazole given orally beginning with conditioning chemotherapy and continuing through neutropenia. Oral nystatin rinses have not been shown to be effective in HSCT. Although nystatin troches have shown efficacy for prophylaxis in some patient populations, their effectiveness in immunosuppressed cancer patients receiving cancer therapy is not clear. These antifungal interventions when used, however, are not directed at the principal causes of mucosal injury.

Effective oral hygiene reduces the microbial load of the oral flora and can reduce the mucositis, reduces gingival inflammation and caries risk, and may reduce septicemia caused by oral pathogens, most commonly of periodontal origin (Epstein & Stevenson-Moore, 2001; Raber-Durlacher et al., 2002). Therefore, even though pain related to the mucositis often prevents patients from continuing oral care during the peak of mucosal injury, it is important to motivate patients to continue oral hygiene practices. Brushing should be continued as long as obvious gingival bleeding does not result from the brushing. If this occurs, the patient may soften the toothbrush with warm water or use cotton swabs or disposable sponge brushes soaked in chlorhexidine to reduce dental plaque build-up and increased oral colonization. If the patient is able to maintain flossing without damage to the gingiva, flossing should be continued. Frequent saline or bicarbonate rinses should be used in conjunction with the oral hygiene regimen, as previously described in **Table 13.1**.

Treatment directed at the cause of pain will generally have greater impact, and therefore, assessment of the potential cause(s) of pain is needed. The time of onset of symptoms relative to oral tissue damage and relative to cancer therapies may help guide the provider in determining the cause or causes of the pain. For example, if assessment leads to recognition that a sudden increase in oral pain is related to reactivation of viral agent or due to fungal or bacterial infection, specific treatment can be provided with greater assurance of effectiveness and control of the risk of progression of infection, rather than pain suppression with analgesics (Bubley, Chapman, Chapman, Crumpacker, & Schnipper, 1989; Epstein & Polsky, 1998). Topical agents for mucositis management generally have unproven efficacy, and treatment trials should be considered to determine the agents that help the patients. The discomfort of the mucositis may be reduced with use of coating agents, topical anesthetics, and topical analgesics, although systemic analgesics are frequently needed for moderate to severe mucositis (Carl, 1993). Milk of magnesia/Maalox® (Novartis Consumer, East Hanover, NJ) (aluminum hydroxide/magnesium hydroxide) and sucralfate have been suggested as coating agents for the oral mucosa (**Table 13.3**). Sucralfate suspension may also be helpful in the treatment of oral pain, although the effect on mucositis is not clearly documented (Allison, Vongtama, Vaughan, & Shin, 1995; Carter et al., 1999; Franzen, Henriksson, Littbrand, & Zackrisson, 1995; Makkonen, Bostrom, Vilja, & Joensuu, 1994; Merideth et al., 1997).

Topical anesthetics used in rinse form may result in intense but short-term anesthesia; however, as mentioned, early, indiscriminant use of the localized anesthesia can increase risk of trauma,

---

Table 13.2 COMMONLY USED MUCOSITIS SCALES

WHO score

Grade	Description
1	Soreness, erythema
2	Erythema, ulcers, can eat solids
3	Ulcers, requires liquid diet only
4	Alimentation not possible

NCI-CTC score

0	None
1	Painless ulcers, erythema, or mild soreness
2	Painful erythema, edema, or ulcers, but patient can eat solids
3	Painful erythema, edema, or ulcers, and patient cannot eat solids
4	Painful erythema, edema, or ulcers, and patient requires parenteral or enteral support

(continues)

Table 13.2 COMMONLY USED MUCOSITIS SCALES (CONT'D)

OMAS

Anatomic site	Erythema	Ulceration/pseudomembrane
Upper lip	0 1 2 3	0 1 2 3
Lower lip	0 1 2 3	0 1 2 3
Right cheek	0 1 2 3	0 1 2 3
Left cheek	0 1 2 3	0 1 2 3
Right ventral and lateral tongue	0 1 2 3	0 1 2 3
Left ventral and lateral tongue	0 1 2 3	0 1 2 3
Floor of the mouth	0 1 2 3	0 1 2 3
Soft palate	0 1 2 3	0 1 2 3
Hard palate	0 1 2 3	0 1 2 3
	0–none (no change in the color of the mucosa) 1–mild/moderate (increase in intensity of color of mucosa) 2–severe (mucosa color of fresh blood)	0–no lesions 1–cumulative surface area of a lesion(s) in a single site less than 1 cm^2 2–cumulative surface area of a lesion(s) in a single site greater than 1 cm^2 and less then or equal to 3 cm^2 3–cumulative surface area of a lesion(s) in a single site greater than 3 cm^2
Summarizing erythema and ulceration/pseudomembranes subscores at each site (possible score range 0 to 5) and then averaging these scores across all nine sites.		

reduction of the gag reflex, and aspiration. When oral mucosal pain is present, the patient can be prescribed benzydamine hydrochloride, Doxepin suspension 0.5%, or a mouthwash containing antihistamine such as diphenhydramine (Benadryl) (Epstein, Silverman et al., 2001; Epstein, Truelove et al., 2001; Turhal, Erdal, & Karacay, 2000). Benzydamine hydrochloride has shown in multicenter, double-blind, controlled studies to reduce mucositis and pain in head and neck cancer patients (Epstein, Silverman et al., 2001; Epstein, Truelove et al., 2001; Turhal, Erdal, & Karacay, 2000). Topical anesthetics, such as benzocaine and viscous lidocaine, can be applied locally to sites of pain with a swab (Carl, 1993).

In addition to agents commonly used for the management of oral mucositis, there are clinical trials of new agents and technologies under inves-

Table 13.3 TOPICAL ANESTHETICS/OCCLUSIVE AGENTS

Agents	Composition/Instructions for Use	Uses/Functions	Disadvantages
Viscous lidocaine	Rinse (30 seconds and spit) or apply topically Do not eat after application Consider dilution	Soothes oral mucosa	Risk of aspiration May promote emesis Potential for toxicity and systemic absorption Short duration of effect, stings with application on damaged tissue
Hurricaine® Topical Anesthetic (Beutlich)	20% Benzocaine topical gel Apply as needed for pain	Onset in 30 seconds 15 minutes in duration No systemic absorption	Short duration relief May promote emesis (as mentioned previously)
1-2-3 Mix	1.5 ml–50 mg/ml diphenhydramine 45-ml viscous xylocaine 2% 45-ml magnesium aluminum hydroxide solution Swish and hold 5 ml in mouth for 60–120 seconds Use up to four times a day Small amount may be swallowed	Combination of topical analgesic and coating effect, some add antifungal and antibacterial agents	Diphenhydramine extends therapeutic effect Composition may vary, each component causes dilution of the others; agents may interfere with function Relatively expensive to compound
Orahesive	Gelatin powder containing carmellose sodium Hold against oral site for 1–2 minutes Can remain in place for an average of 18 hours Relief up to 30 hours depending on location and application technique	Provides immediate relief Thin dressing that forms a protective coat Not harmful if swallowed	Unpleasant sensation
Zilactin® (Zila) Phoenix, AZ	Benzocaine 10% in occlusive film 7.5 g tube Apply prn Dry affected area and isolate until gel sets	Provides protective coating for up to 3 hours	Mild burning pain with application Can only be used for relatively small ulcerative lesions

(continues)

Table 13.3 TOPICAL ANESTHETICS/OCCLUSIVE AGENTS (CONT'D)

Agents	Composition/ Instructions for Use	Uses/Functions	Disadvantages
Carafate® (Aventis) King of Prussia, PA	Sucralfate 10 cc., gentle swirl, 4 times a day or every 2 hours if not swallowed Mixture must be refrigerated and shaken well before use Allow 30 minutes after oral hygiene care before using Sucralfate suspension: 8 crushed sucralfate tablets, 40-ml sterile water, 3 Ensure VariFlavor Pacs, 10-ml sterile water Add water to 120 ml Swish and hold 1 tsp. in mouth for 30 seconds	Cytoprotective effect in oral mucositis not documented May reduce microbial colonization May reduce pain Nonirritating and nondehydrating	Coats mucosa and therefore may mask infections; thus, the patient requires constant monitoring

ml = millimeters, g = grams, prn = as needed, tsp = teaspoon

tigation. Low-energy He/Ne laser, laser diode, granulocyte-macrophage colony-stimulating factor, and keratinocyte growth factor, prostaglandin, allopurinol, vitamin A, amifostine, antibiotic pastille or paste, benzydamine, camomile, chlorhexidine, clarithromycin, folinic acid, glutamine, and hydrolytic enzymes have been or are currently under study (Bensadoun et al., 1999; Clarkson, Worthington, & Eden, 2003; Mantovani et al., 2003; Schubert et al., 1999; Whelan et al., 2002; Worthington, Clarkson, & Eden, 2002a).

Salivary Gland Dysfunction

Dry mouth is a common and significant consequence of head and neck radiotherapy. Because of loss of saliva, patients suffering from dry mouth are more susceptible to rampant caries and oral fungal and bacterial infections. Patients complain of change in taste, difficulty with dentures, and speech and diet may be affected, with xerostomia being one of the primary enduring complications negatively impacting the quality of life of patients after cancer therapy.

Salivary Management

Systemic sialagogues may increase the production of natural saliva from functional glands. An optimal substitute for saliva for use when glands are nonfunctional is not available. Salagen (pilocarpine hydrochloride) has shown promising effects in increasing saliva but is only effective on salivary glands with residual function (Hawthorne & Sullivan, 2000). Evoxac (cevimeline hydrochloride), a new sialagogue approved for use in the United States for Sjögren's Disease, may also be used to increase salivary flow in head and neck radiation patients. Trials are currently underway to determine the effectiveness of this sialogogue for patients with GVHD-induced salivary gland dysfunction. Two alternate medications that may be beneficial in stimulating salivary glands include Bethanecol® (Merck) Whitehouse Station, NJ (urecholine) and Sialor® (Paladin Labs) Montreal, Canada (anethole trithione), although the latter agent is not available in the United States (Bagheri, Schmitt, Berlan, & Montastruc, 1997; Epstein, Decoteau, & Wilkinson, 1983; Epstein, Burchell, Emerton, Le, & Silverman, 1994; Hamada et al., 1999).

Although saliva replacements such as UniMist, Mouth Kote® (Parnell) Irvington, TX, and Oral Balance Gel® (Lacalede) Rancho Dominguez, CA are "poor salivary substitutes," patients may find that they offer some relief. Oral Balance Gel may be the best accepted by patients because of an extended duration of effect (Epstein, Emerton, Le, & Stevenson-Moore, 1999; Furumoto, Barker, Carter-Hanson, & Barker, 1998). Sugarless gum or lozenges may stimulate salivary secretion in patients with residual salivary gland function. Sugar-free popsicles, plain ice cubes, or ice water may be used to keep the mouth cool and moist. Eating foods high in ascorbic acid, malic acid, and citric acid will stimulate the glands to increase salivary flow but are not recommended in dentate patients because the acidity can further irritate oral tissues and contribute to the demineralization of teeth.

For prevention of rampant dental demineralization and caries, patients should apply a 1.1% neutral sodium fluoride gel daily (more than 5 minutes) using custom-fit vinyl trays. These trays should be fabricated based on diagnostic casts; it is important that the gingival third of the exposed tooth surface receive direct delivery of the fluoride compound. This practice may be started on the 1st day of cancer therapy and continued daily as long as salivary flow rates are low and the mouth remains dry. For patients who do not comply with use of fluoride carriers or in those in whom saliva production may be reduced but not eliminated, high-potency fluoride brush-on gels, mouthrinses, and dentifrices should be recommended. The lower salivary flow rate allows the fluoride to remain in the saliva medium for longer time. Therefore, the continuous effect of the fluoride, even in a lower concentration (0.05% sodium fluoride), may have a beneficial effect (Billings et al., 1988).

Infection

As reported in a National Institutes of Health consensus conference, the incidence of oral infections will vary among patients, depending on the type of cancer, the corresponding chemotherapy, and host susceptibility (National Institutes of Health, 1989). In leukemia patients, the incidence of oral infection may be as high as 35% because chemotherapy is designed to achieve myelosuppression. Particularly in myelosuppressed and immunosuppressed patients oral foci of infection may spread and expose the patients to systemic infections. Therefore, these oral infections should be diagnosed and treated meticulously.

Oral infections include

- Bacterial infection: Localized odontogenic infection of bacterial origin may be difficult to diagnose in neutropenic patients because signs and symptoms of infection such as swelling are often not present. In addition, the risk of spread of infections increases because of the loss of neutrophil function. Between 10% and 32% of cases of septicemia in neutropenic cancer patients may originate from oral infection (Bergmann, 1989). Infections in the oral cavity are associated with oral ulcers, periodontal disease, pulpal disease, and sinus infections. It was noted that there is a change in the oral microflora during and after immunosuppression and pathogens emerging include gram-negative mainly (e.g., *Pseudomonas aeruginosa*, *Klebsiella pneumoniae*) and for a lesser extend gram-positive (e.g., *Staphylococcus aureus*, *Staphylococcus epidermidis*, *Streptococcus pyogenes*) (Dreizen, Bodey, & Valdivieso, 1983; Dreizen, McCredie, Keating, & Bodey, 1982; Meurman, Pyrhonen, Teerenhvi, & Lindquist, 1997; Khan & Wingard, 2001). Oral infections caused by enterobacteriaceae were found to be responsible for a large proportion of positive cultures para-HSCT (Garfunkel et al., 1994).

- Viral infection: These include mainly the herpes virus family such as the Herpes Simplex Virus (HSV), Cytomegalio Virus (CMV), Epstein-Barr virus, and varicella zoster virus. HSV reactivation has serious local implications because of pain, impaired hydration, and nutrition when it results in widespread oral and perioral ulcers. Reactivation commonly occurs concurrently with neutropenia-inducing chemotherapy and results in oral ulceration involving any intraoral and perioral soft tissue surfaces. Because these patients are often expected to develop mucositis secondary to their chemotherapy, HSV reactivation may be overlooked as an etiology for the oral ulcers. Mucositis complicated by HSV reactivation tends to be more severe and lasts longer. In leukemia and bone marrow transplantation patients, reactivation of HSV occurs in 35% to 70% of HSV-seropositive patients (Anderson et al., 1984; Lam, Pazin, Armstrong, & Ho, 1981; Saral, Burns, Laskin, Santos, & Lietman, 1981; Saral et al., 1983). The systemic consequence of HSV infection is the disruption of the mucosal barrier, allowing a portal of entry for commensal oral micro-organisms that can lead to sepsis. Varicella zoster virus, CMV, Epstein-Barr virus, and human herpesviruses as well as community respiratory viruses, although much less common than HSV, have also proven problematic during the course of chemotherapy.

- Fungal infection: Candidal infections of the oral mucosa are the most common fungal infections in patients undergoing chemotherapy and can cause a burning or scalded sensation, distort taste, and interfere with swallowing. Spread to the esophagus or systemic dissemination is a serious consequence. Systemic fungal infection is a common cause of infectious death in neutropenic patients because established systemic infections may be difficult to recognize and can prove difficult to treat.

Infection Management

Healthcare providers should be concerned about preventing local and systemic infections in addition to managing oral symptoms. Treating infections as soon as they are detected will help to reduce pain, as well as to reduce the risk of spread of infection. A fungal, bacterial, or viral culture is recommended if infection is suspected.

Nystatin rinses are a widely prescribed treatment in North America for the onset of oral fungal infections, despite a lack of proven efficacy. Nystatin has an unpleasant flavor and may cause nausea and vomiting, and the high sucrose content in nystatin is a major concern in dentate patients (Ferber, 1995). For more severe infections, the use of a systemic antifungal medication such Diflucan® (Pfizer) New York, NY (fluconazole) or Fungizone (amphotericin B) is recommended (Carl, 1993). Systemic amphotericin B must be used with caution because of its potential to cause liver toxicity. Other topical antifungals to consider include clotrimazole, ketoconazole, and chlorhexidine (Clarkson, Worthington, & Eden, 2002; Worthington, Clarkson, & Eden, 2002b). In some countries, topical amphotericin B, as lozenges or as oral solution, is available.

Peridex (0.12% chlorhexidine gluconate), an antimicrobial rinse, has both antibacterial properties, which account for its antiplaque effects. It also has some antifungal; however, its value in infection management is not fully established except in settings of acute irritation of inflamed tissue. Its tendency to stain teeth and its alcohol content that can irritate inflamed tissues are drawbacks (Ferber, 1995). If chlorhexidine is used, it is important to note that Nystatin and chlorhexidine should not be used concurrently because chlorhexidine binds to Nystatin rendering both ineffective, and should be used at least 30 minutes before or after the use of any other topical agents with which it may bind (Ferber).

The decision of what type and form of antifungal prophylaxis and treatment is a matter of each department policy, and it is dependent on local microbiologic and microbial resistant surveys.

General guidelines for treatment of infections in cancer patients are available in the literature (Finberg, 2001). The specific antibiotic for bacterial infection that may originate from the oral cavity is dependent on the pathogen isolated. In general, penicillins are used for the sensitive species, and glycopeptide is used for the resistant species. *Streptococcus viridans bacteremia* is very common and will be treated this way. Enterococcus infection will be treated with ampicillin, amoxicillin, or penicillin G for a sensitive species. *Staphylococcus coagulase*-negative infection (such as *Staphylococcus epidermidis*) and *Staphylococcus coagulase*-positive infection (such as *Staphylococcus aureus*) will be treated with penicillinase-resistant penicillin for a sensitive species. Gram-negative rods infection (such as *Pseudomonas* species, *Klebsiella* species, and *Enterobacter* species) will be treated based on the antibiotic susceptibility of the particular organism as well as on the clinical setting. For *Pseudomonas aeruginosa*, (β-lactam plus an aminoglycoside-containing regimen is considered by many to be the standard of care (Strahilevitz & Engelhard, 2003).

In neutropenic patients, a broad-spectrum combined antibiotic regimen is widely accepted as soon as febrile neutropenia developed (Wingard, 1999).

In addition to antibiotic treatment, neu-tropenic patients with bacterial infection can be treated with growth factors, aiming at increasing the white blood count to enhance the self-immunity (Garcia-Carbonero & Paz-Ares, 2002).

For cancer patients with viral infections, such as HSV, Zovirax (acyclovir) or derivatives (e.g., valacyclovir; Valtres) are recommended for both prophylaxis and treatment (Anderson et al., 1984; Bubley et al., 1989; Saral et al., 1981, 1983). CMV will be treated with an antiviral agent (gancyclovir) that has a better affinity to CMV, (Epstein, Sherlock, & Wolber, 1993). Thus, because of this specificity, gancyclovir has a better efficacy in treating CMV infections. Denavir (penciclovir), a newer topical antiviral with increased tissue penetration, is now available, but in general, topical agents should not be considered for primary therapy or prevention in immunosuppressed cancer patients.

GVHD

As was described previously, GVHD may manifest as early as the stem cells are engrafted. Acute GVHD (until day 100 post-HSCT) and chronic GVHD (after day 100 post-HSCT) may involve the oral tissues. With chronic systemic extensive disease, the extent and severity of the oral lesions can become most disabling. Chronic GVHD is estimated to occur in 33% to 44% of allogeneic HSCT patients.

Differential diagnosis of GVHD is based on exclusion of other diseases. Cultures can be performed to exclude oral lesions caused by infections and can be combined with staining (potassium hydroxide or periodic acid-Schiff) to exclude fungal infection. Both oral labial mucosa and clinical examination can provide data supporting the diagnosis of GHVD. Minor salivary gland biopsy can assist in diagnostic confirmation of salivary gland GVHD. A correlation of systemic manifestations of oral changes should be noted.

GVHD Management

Several approaches to the local management of oral GVHD may be considered, including topical anti-inflammatory/immunosuppressive agents such as steroids (rinses and creams), azathioprine, cyclosporine, tacrolimus, and oral psoralen and ultraviolet A therapy (Schubert et al., 1999).

Systemic therapy is often required in conjunction with topical treatment. This treatment will include systemic steroids and immunomodulators (Woo, Lee, & Schubert, 1997). As GVHD encompasses numerous oral adverse effects, the treatment of oral GVHD must consider pain management, prevention of limitation of mouth opening, balanced nutrition, and surveillance for second malignancies. Other oral complications of GVHD should be diagnosed and managed, including xerostomia and related cavity risk, risk of candidiasis, and oral pain, which affect quality of life.

References

AHA recommendations. (1985). *The Journal of the American Dental Association, 110,* 664, 666, 668.

Aitasalo, K., Grenman, R., Virolained, E., Niinikoski, J., & Klossner, J. (1995). A modified protocol to treat early osteoradionecrosis of the mandible. *Undersea and Hyperbaric Medicine, 22,* 161–170.

Allison, R. R., Vongtama, V., Vaughan, J., & Shin, K. H. (1995). Symptomatic acute mucositis can be minimized or prophylaxed by the combination of sucralfate and fluconazole. *Cancer Investigation, 13,* 16–22.

Anderson, H., Scarffe, J. H., Sutton, R. N., Hickmott, E., Brigden, D., & Burke, C. (1984). Oral acyclovir prophylaxis against herpes simplex virus in non-Hodgkin's lymphoma and acute lymphoblastic leukaemia patients receiving remission induction chemotherapy. A randomised double blind, placebo controlled trial. *British Journal of Cancer, 50,* 45–49.

Bagheri, H., Schmitt, L., Berlan, M., & Montastruc, J. L. (1997). Comparative study of the effects of yohimbine and anetholtrithione on salivary secretion in depressed patients treated with psychotropic drugs. *European Journal of Clinical Pharmacology, 52,* 339–342.

Barasch, A. & Peterson, D. E. (2003). Risk factors for ulcerative oral mucositis in cancer patients: Unanswered questions. *Oral Oncology, 39,* 91–100.

Barasch, A., Peterson, D. E., Tanzer, J. M., D'Ambrosio, J. A., Nuki, K., Schubert, M. M. et al. (1995) Helium-neon laser effects on conditioning-induced oral mucositis in bone marrow transplantation patients. *Cancer, 76,* 2550–2556.

Barbasi, S., Cameron, K., Quested, B., Olver, I., To, B., & Evans, D. (2002). More than a sore mouth: Patients' experience of oral mucositis. *Oncology Nursing Forum, 29,* 1051–1057.

Bellm, L. A., Epstein, J. B., Rose-Ped, A., Martin, P., & Fuchs, H. J. (2000). Patient reports of complications of bone marrow transplantation. *Supportive Care in Cancer, 8,* 33–39.

Bensadoun, R. J., Franquin, J. C., Ciais, G., Darcourt, V., Schubert, M. M., Viot, M. et al. (1999). Low-energy He/Ne laser in the prevention of radiation-induced mucositis. A multicenter phase III randomized study in patients with head and neck cancer. *Supportive Care in Cancer, 7,* 244–252.

Bergmann, O. J. (1989). Oral infections and fever in immunocompromised patients with haematologic malignancies. *European Journal of Clinical Microbiology & Infectious Diseases, 8,* 207–213.

Billings, R. J., Meyerowitz, C., Featherstone, J. D., Espeland, M. A., Fu, J., Cooper, L. F. et al. (1988). Retention of topical fluoride in the mouths of xerostomic subjects. *Caries Research, 22,* 306–310.

Blijlevens, N. M., Donnelly, J. P., & de Pauw, B. E. (2001). Empirical therapy of febrile neutropenic patients with mucositis: Challenge of risk-based therapy. *Clinical Microbiology and Infection, 7 Suppl,* 47–52.

Borowski, B., Benhamou, E., Pico, J. L., Laplanche, A., Margainaud, J. P., & Haya, M. (1994). Prevention of oral mucositis in patients treated with high-dose chemotherapy and bone marrow transplantation: A randomized controlled trail comparing two protocols of dental care. *European Journal of Cancer. Part B, Oral Oncology, 30B,* 93–97.

Brizel, D. M., Wasserman, T. H., Henke, M., Strand, V., Rudat, V., Monnier, A. et al. (2000). Phase III randomized trial of amifostine as a radioprotector in head and neck cancer. *Journal of Clinical Oncology, 18,* 3339–3345.

Brown, D. A., Evans, A. W., & Sandor, G. K. (1998). Hyperbaric oxygen therapy in the management of osteoradionecrosis of the mandible. *Advances in Oto-rhino-laryngology, 54,* 14–32.

Bubley, G. J., Chapman, B., Chapman, S. K., Crumpacker, C. S., & Schnipper, L. E. (1989). Effect of acyclovir on radiation- and chemotherapy-induced mouth lesions. *Antimicrobial Agents and Chemotherapy, 33,* 862–865.

Carl, W. (1993). Local radiation and systemic chemotherapy: Preventing and managing the oral complications. *The Journal of the American Dental Association, 124,* 119–113.

Carter, D. L., Hebert, M. E., Smink, K., Leopold, K. A., Clough, R. L., & Brizel, D. M. (1999). Double blind randomized trail of sucralfate vs. placebo during radical radiotherapy for head and neck cancers. *Head & Neck, 21,* 760–766.

Cascinu, S., Fedeli, A., Fedeli, S. L., & Catalano, G. (1994). Oral cooling (cryotherapy), an effective treatment for the prevention of 5-fluorouracil-induced stomatitis. *European Journal of Cancer. Part B, Oral Oncology, 30B,* 234–236.

Chapman, C. R., Donaldson, G. W., Jacobson, R. C., & Hautman, B. (1997). Differences among patients in opioid self-administration during bone marrow transplantation. *Pain, 71,* 213–223.

Clarkson, J. E., Worthington, H. V., & Eden, O. B. (2002). Interventions for treating oral candidiasis for patients with cancer receiving treatment. *Cochrane Database of Systematic Reviews,* CD001972.

Clarkson, J. E., Worthington, H. V., & Eden, O. B. (2003). Interventions for preventing oral mucositis for patients with cancer receiving treatment. *Cochrane Database of Systematic Reviews, 3,* CD000978.

Consensus Conference. (1989). Oral complications of cancer therapies: Diagnosis, prevention and treatment. *Connecticut Medicine, 53, 393.*

Cox, J. D., Stetz, J., & Pajak, T. F. (1995). Toxicity criteria of the Radiation Therapy Oncology Group (RTOG) and the European Organization for Research and Treatment of Cancer (EORTC). *International Journal of Radiation Oncology, Biology, Physics, 31,* 1341–1346.

Curi, M. M. & Dib, L. L. (1997). Osteoradionecrosis of the jaws: A retrospective study of the background factors and treatment in 104 cases. *International Journal of Oral and Maxillofacial Surgery, 55,* 540–544.

David, L. A., Sandor, G. K. B., Evans, A. W., & Brown, D. H. (2001). Hyperbaric oxygen therapy and mandibular osteoradionecrosis: A retrospective study and analysis of treatment outcomes. *Journal of the Canadian Dental Association, 67,* 384.

DePaola, L. G., Peterson, D. E., Overholser, C. D., Suzuki, J. B., Minah, G. B., Williamson, L. T. et al. (1986). Dental care for patients receiving chemotherapy. *The Journal of the American Dental Association, 112,* 198–203.

Dodd, M. J., Dibble, S., Miaskowski, C., Paul, S., Cho, M., MacPhail, L. et al. (2001). A comparison of the affective state and quality of life of chemotherapy patients who do and do not develop chemotherapy-induced oral mucositis. *Journal of Pain and Symptom Management, 21,* 498–505.

Donnelly, J. P., Bellm, L. A., Epstein, J. B., Sonis, S. T., & Symonds, R. P. (2003). Antimicrobial therapy to prevent or treat oral mucositis. *The Lancet Infectious Diseases, 3,* 405–412.

Dreizen, S., Bodey, G. P., & Valdivieso, M. (1983). Chemotherapy-associated oral infections in adults with solid tumors. *Oral Surgery, Oral Medicine, and Oral Pathology, 55,* 113–120.

Dreizen, S., McCredie, K. B., Keating, M. J., & Bodey, G. P. (1982). Oral infections associated with chemotherapy in adults with acute leukemia. *Postgraduate Medicine, 71,* 133–138, 143–146.

Eilers, J., Berger, A. M., & Petersen, M. C. (1998). Development, testing, and application of the oral assessment guide. *Oncology Nursing Forum, 15,* 325–330.

Elting, L. S., Cooksley, C., Chanbers, M., Martin, C., Manzullo, E., & Rubenstein, E. (2003). The burdens of cancer therapy: Clinical and economic outcomes of chemotherapy-induced mucositis. *Cancer, 98,* 1531–1539.

Epstein, J., Emerton, S., Kolbonson, D., Le, N., Phillips, N., Stevenson-Moore, P. et al. (1999). Quality of life and oral function following radiotherapy for head and neck cancer. *Head & Neck, 21,* 1–11.

Epstein, J. B. & Polsky, B. (1998). Oropharyngeal candidiasis: A review of its clinical spectrum and current therapies. *Clinical Therapeutics, 20,* 40–57.

Epstein, J. B. & Schubert, M. M. (1993). Management of orofacial pain in cancer patients. *European Journal of Cancer. Part B, Oral Oncology, 29B,* 243–250.

Epstein, J. B. & Stevenson-Moore, P. (2001). Periodontal disease and periodontal management in patients with cancer. *Oral Oncology, 37,* 613–619.

Epstein, J. B., Burchell, J. L., Emerton, S., Le, N. D., & Silverman, S. Jr. (1994). A clinical trial of bethanechol in patients with xerostomia after radiation therapy. A pilot study. *Oral Surgery, Oral Medicine, and Oral Pathology, 77,* 610–614.

Epstein, J. B., Decoteau, W. E., & Wilkinson, A. (1983). Effect of Sialor in treatment of xerostomia in Sjogren's syndrome. *Oral Surgery, Oral Medicine, and Oral Pathology, 56,* 495–499.

Epstein, J. B., Emerton, S., Le, N. D., & Stevenson-Moore, P. (1999). A double-blind crossover trial of Oral Balance gel and Biotene toothpaste versus placebo in patients with xerostomia following radiation therapy. *Oral Oncology, 35,* 132–137.

Epstein, J. B., Sherlock, C. H., & Wolber, R. A. (1993). Oral manifestations of cytomegalovirus infection. *Oral Surgery, Oral Medicine, and Oral Pathology, 75,* 443–451.

Epstein, J. B., Silverman, S. Jr, Paggiarino, D. A., Crocket, S., Schubert, M. M., Senzer, N. N. et al. (2001). Benzydamine HCl for prophylaxis of radiation-induced oral mucositis: Results from a multicenter, randomized, double-blind, placebo-controlled clinical trial. *Cancer, 92,* 875–885.

Epstein, J. B., Stevenson-Moore, P., Jackson, S., Mohammed, J. H., Spinelli, J. J. et al. (1989). Prevention of oral mucositis in radiation therapy: A controlled study with benzydamine hydrochloride rinse. *International Journal of Radiation Oncology, Biology, Physics, 16,* 1571–1575.

Epstein, J. B., Truelove, E. L., Oien, H., Allison, C., Le, N. D., & Epstein, M. S. (2001). Oral topical doxepin rinse: Analgesic effect in patients with oral mucosal pain due to cancer or cancer therapy. *Oral Oncology, 37,* 632–637.

Epstein, J. B., Tsang, A. H., Warkentin, D., & Ship, J. A. (2002). The role of salivary function in modulating chemotherapy-induced oropharyngeal mucositis: A review of the literature. *Oral Surgery, Oral Medicine, Oral Pathology, Oral Radiology, and Endodontics, 94,* 39–44.

Ferber T. (1995). Mouth care for patients receiving oral irradiation. *Cancer Nursing, 10*, 666–670.

Finberg, R. (2001). Infections in patients with cancer. In Braunwald, Fauci, Kasper, Hawer, Longo, Jameson (Eds.), *Harrison's Principles of Internal Medicine* (pp. 552–553). New York: McGraw-Hill.

Franzen, L., Henriksson, R., Littbrand, B., & Zackrisson, B. (1995). Effects of sucralfate on mucositis during and following radiotherapy of malignancies in the head and neck region. A double-blind placebo-controlled study. *Acta Oncologica, 34*, 219–223.

Furumoto, E. K., Barker, G. J., Carter-Hanson, C., & Barker, B. F. (1998). Subjective and clinical evaluation of oral lubricants in xerostomic patients. *Special Care in Dentistry, 18*, 113–118.

Garcia-Carbonero, R. & Paz-Ares, L. (2002). Antibiotics and growth factors in the management of fever and neutropenia in cancer patients. *Current Opinion in Hematology, 9*, 215–221.

Garfunkel, A. A., Tager, N., Chausu, S., Chausu, G., Haze, C., & Galili, D. (1994). Oral complications in bone marrow transplantation patients: Recent advances. *Israel Journal of Medical Sciences, 30*, 120–124.

Greenberg, M. S., Cohen, S. G., McKitrick, J. C., & Cassileth, P. A. (1982). The oral flora as a source of septicemia in patients with acute leukemia. *Oral surgery, Oral Medicine, and Oral Pathology, 53*, 32–36.

Hamada, T., Nakane, T., Kimura, T., Arisawa, K., Yoneda, K., Yamamoto, T. et al. (1999). Treatment of xerostomia with the bile secretion-stimulating drug anethole trithione: A clinical trial. *The American Journal of the Medical Sciences, 318*, 146–151.

Handbook for reporting results of cancer treatment. (1979). WHO Offset Publication, *48*, 15–22.

Hawthorne, M. & Sullivan, K. (2000). Pilocarpine for radiation-induced xerostomia in head and neck cancer. *International Journal of Palliative Nursing, 6*, 228, 230–232.

Khan, S. A. & Wingard, J. R. (2001). Infection and mucosal injury in cancer treatment. *Journal of the National Cancer Institute. Monographs, 29*, 31–36.

Kline, R. M., Meiman, S., Tarantino, M. D., Herzig, R. H., & Bertolone, S. J. Jr. (1998). A detailed analysis of charges for hematopoietic stem cell transplantation at a children's hospital. *Bone Marrow Transplantation, 21*, 195–203.

Laine, P. O., Lindqvist, C., Pyrhonen, S. O., Strand-Pettinen, I. M., Teerenhovi, L. M., & Meurman, J. G. (1992). Oral infection as a reason for febrile episodes in lymphoma patients receiving cytostatic drugs. *Oral Oncology, 28*, 103–107.

Lam, M. T., Pazin, G. J., Armstrong, J. A., & Ho, M. (1981). Herpes simplex infection in acute myelogenous leukemia and other hematologic malignancies: A prospective study. *Cancer, 48*, 2168–2171.

Mahood, D. J., Dose, A. M., Loprinzi, C. L., Veeder, M. H., Athmann, L. M., Therneau, T. M. et al. (1991). Inhibition of fluorouracil-induced stomatitis by oral cryotherapy. *Journal of Clinical Oncology, 9*, 449–452.

Makkonen, T. A., Bostrom, P., Vilja, P., & Joensuu, H. (1994). Sucralfate mouth washing in the prevention of radiation-induced mucositis: A placebo-controlled double-blind randomized study. *International Journal of Radiation Oncology, Biology, Physics, 30*, 177–182.

Mantovani, G., Massa, E., Astara, G., Murgiam, V., Gramignano, G., Lusso, M. R. et al. (2003). Phase II clinical trial of local use of GM-CSF for prevention and treatment of chemotherapy- and concomitant chemoradiotherapy-induced severe oral mucositis in advanced head and neck cancer patients: An evaluation of effectiveness, safety and costs. *Oncology Reports, 10*, 197–206.

McCarthy, G. M., Awde, J. D., Ghandi, H., Vincent, M., & Kocha, W. I. (1998). Risk factors associated with mucositis in cancer patients receiving 5-fluorouracil. *Oral Oncology, 34*, 484–490.

McGuire, D. B., Altomonte, V., Peterson, D. E., Wingard, J. R., Jones, R. J., & Grochow, L. B. (1993). Patterns of mucositis and pain in patients receiving preparative chemotherapy and bone marrow transplantation. *Oncology Nursing Forum, 20*, 1493–1502.

McGuire, D. B., Peterson, D. E., Muller, S., Owen, D. C., Slemmons, M. F., & Schubert, M. M. (2002). The 20 item oral mucositis index: Reliability and validity in bone marrow and stem cell transplant patients. *Cancer Investigation, 20*, 893–903.

McKenzie, M. R., Wong, F. L., Epstein, J. B., & Lepawsky, M. (1993). Hyperbaric oxygen and postradiation osteonecrosis of the mandible. *European Journal of Cancer. Part B, Oral Oncology, 29B*, 201–207.

Merideth, R., Salter, M., Kim, R., Spencer, S., Weppelmann, B., Rodum, B. et al. (1997). Sucralfate for radiation mucositis: Results of a double-blind randomized trial. *International Journal of Radiation Oncology, Biology, Physics, 37*, 275–279.

Meurman, J. H., Pyrhonen, S., Teerenhovi, L., & Lindqvist, C. (1997). Oral sources of septicaemia in patients with malignancies. *Oral Oncology, 33*, 389–397.

Muller, S., Yeager, K. A., Hodgson-Woodruff, N., Peterson, D. E., & McGuire, D. S. (1991). Factors influencing the development and severity of oral mucositis in bone marrow and stem cell transplant patients. *Oral Surgery, Oral Medicine, Oral Pathology, Oral Radiology, and Endodontics, 87*, 458 (abstract).

National Institute of Health [NIH]. (1989). NIH consensus statement on oral complications of cancer therapies: Diagnosis, prevention, and treatment. *NIH Consensus Statement, 7*, 1–11.

O'Grady, N., Alexander, M., Patchen Dellinger, E., Gerberding, J. L., Heard, S. O., Maki, D. G. et al. (2002). Guidelines for the prevention of intravascular catheter-related infections. *Morbidity and Mortality Weekly Report, 51*,1–26.

Parulekar, W., Mackenzie, R., Bjarnason, G., & Jordan, R. C. K. (1998). Scoring oral mucositis. *Oral Oncology, 34*, 63–71.

Pederson, C., Parran, L., & Harbaugh, B. (2000). Children's perceptions of pain during 3 weeks of bone marrow transplant experience. *Journal of Pediatric Oncology Nursing, 17*, 22–32.

Peterson, D. (1999). Research advances in oral mucositis. *Current Opinion in Oncology, 11*, 261–266.

Peterson, D. E. (1991). Toxicity of chemotherapeutic agents. *Seminars in Oncology, 19*, 478–491.

Peterson, D. E. & D'Ambrosio, J. A. (1992). Diagnosis and management of acute and chronic oral complications of nonsurgical cancer therapies. *Dental Clinics of North America, 36*, 945–966.

Peterson, D. E. & Sonis, S. T. (1983). Oral complications of cancer chemotherapy. *Developmental Oncology, 12*, 801–818.

Raber-Durlacher, J. E., Epstein, J. B., Raber, J., van Dissel, J. T., van Winkelhoff, A. J., Guiot, H. F. et al. (2002). Periodontal infection in cancer patients treated with high-dose chemotherapy. *Support Care Cancer, 10*, 466–473.

Saral, R., Ambinder, R. F., Burns, W. H., Angelopulos, C. M., Griffin, D. E., Burke, P. J. et al. (1983). Acyclovir prophylaxis against herpes simplex virus infection in patients with leukemia. A randomized, double-blind, placebo-controlled study. *Annals of Internal Medicine, 99*, 773–776.

Saral, R., Burns, W. H., Laskin, O. L., Santos, G. W., & Lietman, P. S. (1981). Acyclovir prophylaxis of herpes-simplex-virus infections. *The New England Journal of Medicine, 9*, 305, 63–67.

Schubert, M. M., Peterson, D. E., & Lloid, M. E. (1999). Oral Complications. In E. D. Thomas, K. G. Blume, & S. J. Forma (Eds.), *Hematopoietic Stem Cell Transplantation* (pp. 751–763). Malden, MA: Blackwell Science.

Schubert, M. M., Sullivan, K. M. J., & Truelove, E. L. (1991). Head and neck complication of bone marrow transplantation. *Developmental Oncology, 36*, 401–427.

Schubert, M. M., Williams, B. E., Lloid, M. E., Donaldson, G., & Chapko, M. K. (1992). Clinical assessment scale for the rating of oral mucosal changes associated with bone marrow transplantation. Development of an oral mucositis index. *Cancer, 69*, 2469–2477.

Schulz-Kindermann, F., Hennings, U., Ramm, G., Zander, A. R., & Hasenbring, M. (2002). The role of biomedical and psychosocial factors for the prediction of pain and distress in patients undergoing high-dose therapy and BMT/PBSCT. *Bone Marrow Transplantation, 29*, 341–351.

Seto, B. G., Kim, M., Wolinsky, L., Mito, R. S., & Champlin, R. (1985). Oral mucositis in patients undergoing bone marrow transplantation. *Oral Surgery, Oral Medicine, and Oral Pathology, 53*, 32–36.

Sonis, S., Eilers, J. P., Epstein, J. B., LeVeque, F. G., Liggett, W. H., Mulagha, M. T. et al. (1999).Validation of a new scoring system for the assessment of clinical trial research of oral mucositis induced by radiation or chemotherapy. *Cancer, 85*, 2103–2113.

Sonis, S. T. (1998). Mucositis as a biological process: A new hypothesis for the development of chemotherapy-induced stomatotoxicity. *Oral Oncology, 34*, 39–43.

Sonis, S. T., Oster, G., Fuchs, H., Bellm, L., Bradford, W. Z., Edelsberg, J. et al. (2001). Oral mucositis and the clinical and economic outcomes of hematopoietic stem-cell transplantation. *Journal of Clinical Oncology, 19*, 2201–2205.

Sonis, S. T., Sonis, A. L., & Lieberman, A. (1978). Oral complications in patients receiving treatment for malignancy other than the head and neck. *The Journal of the American Dental Association, 97*, 476–482.

Spijkervet, F. K., van Saene, H. K., Panders, A. K., Vermey, A., & Mehta, D. M. (1989). Scoring irradiation mucositis in head and neck cancer patients. *Journal of Oral Pathology & Medicine, 18*, 167–171.

Strahilevitz, J. & Engelhard, D. (2003). Infections caused by gram-positive cocci and gram-negative rods. In J. R. Wingard & R. A. Bowden (Eds.), *Management of Infection in Oncology Patients* (pp. 147–163). Philadelphia: Martin Dunitz Taylor & Francis Group Plc.

Trotti, A. (2000). Toxicity in head and neck cancer: A review of trends and issues. *International Journal of Radiation Oncology, Biology, Physics, 47*, 1–12.

Turhal, N. S., Erdal, S., & Karacay, S. (2000). Efficacy of treatment to relieve mucositis-induced discomfort. *Supportive Care in Cancer, 8*, 55–58.

van Merkesteyn, J. P., Bakker, D. J., & Borgmeijer-Hoelen, A. M. (1995). Hyperbaric oxygen treatment of ORN of the mandible. Experience in 29 patients. *Oral Surgery, Oral Medicine, Oral Pathology, Oral Radiology, and Endodontics, 80*, 12–16.

Whelan, H. T., Connelly, J. F., Hodgson, B. D., Barbeau, L., Post, A. C., Bullard, G. et al. (2002). NASA light-emitting diodes for the prevention of oral mucositis in pediatric bone marrow transplant patients. *Journal of Clinical Laser Medicine and Surgery, 20*, 319–324.

Whitmeyer, C. C., Waskowski, J. C., & Iffland, H. A. (1997). Radiotherapy and oral sequelae: Preventive and management protocols. *Journal of Dental Hygiene, 71*, 23–29.

Wilkes, J. D. (1998). Prevention and treatment of oral mucositis following cancer chemotherapy. *Seminars in Oncology, 25*, 538–551.

Wingard, J. R. (1999). Bacterial infections. In E. D. Thomas, K. G. Blume, & S. J. Forma (Eds.), *Hematopoietic Stem Cell Transplantation* (pp. 537–549). Malden, MA: Blackwell Science.

Woo, S. B., Lee, S. J., & Schubert, M. M. (1997). Graft-vs.-host disease. *Critical Reviews in Oral Biology and Medicine, 8*, 201–216.

Woo, S. B., Sonis, S. T., Monopoli, M. M., & Sonis, A. L. (1993). A longitudinal study of oral ulcerative mucositis in bone marrow transplant recipients. *Cancer, 72*, 1612–1617.

Worthington, H. V., Clarkson, J. E., & Eden, O. B. (2002a). Interventions for treating oral mucositis for patients with cancer receiving treatment. *Cochrane Database of Systematic Reviews, 1*, CD001973.

Worthington, H. V., Clarkson, J. E., & Eden, O. B. (2002b). Interventions for preventing oral candidiasis for patients with cancer receiving treatment. *Cochrane Database of Systematic Reviews*, CD003807.

Wright, W. E. (1987). Periodontium destruction associated with oncology therapy. Five case reports. *Journal of Periodontology, 58*, 559–563.

Zalcberg, J., Kerr, D., Seymour, L., & Palmer, M. (1998). Hematological and non-hematological toxicity after 5-florouracil and leukovorin in patients with advanced colorectal cancer is significantly associated with gender, increasing age and cycle number. *European Journal of Cancer, 34*, 1871–1875.

Zerbe, M. B., Parkerson, S. G., Ortlieb, M. L., & Spitzer, T. (1992). Relationship between oral mucositis and treatment variables in bone marrow transplant patients. *Cancer Nursing, 115*, 196–205.

Zimmerman, R. P., Mark, R. J., Tran, L. M., & Juillard, G. F. (1997). Concomitant pilocarpine during head and neck irradiation is associated with decreased post-treatment xerostomia. *International Journal of Radiation Oncology, Biology, Physics, 37*, 571–575.

Chapter 14

Pharmacy Issues in Ambulatory Oncology

Valorie Wilkins

Introduction

Pharmacy is derived from the Greek word pharmakon, meaning medicine or drug (Cowen & Helfand, 1990). A pharmacist is therefore the expert on drugs. Other healthcare professionals use drugs in their practice, but only pharmacists are legally responsible for handling medications and professionally responsible for knowledge of medication use.

Pharmacy existed before language (Cowen & Helfand, 1990). Preliterate people used natural plants as medicines and had an extensive knowledge of plants and their therapeutic effects. Flowers and herbs have been discovered to be buried with Neanderthal man, and some of the earliest medication records are clay tablets written in Sumerian dating from 2100 B.C.

The profession of pharmacy has developed in parallel with science and our understanding of disease into the specialized, complex, and dynamic practice that it is today. Modern pharmacists provide patient care using vastly more sophisticated medication preparations, delivery formulations or devices, and knowledge of pathophysiology, but continue to use practices and concepts developed much earlier in history.

This chapter is intended to highlight some of the challenges and opportunities in providing pharmaceutical care to oncology patients, especially those in an ambulatory environment. Topics include the role and knowledge of pharmacists, challenges in clinical training and competence, and a discussion of how to evaluate the efficacy and utility of the pharmaceutical component of patient care services. Goals include highlighting the abilities and special training that pharmacists bring to the multidisciplinary healthcare team that benefit patients and providing tools to allow evaluation of the best way to provide pharmaceutical care to the patients in your practice environment. Medications in this chapter are generally referred to as chemotherapy, although the emphasis is on antineoplastics and similar cytotoxic or hazardous drugs.

The Role of the Pharmacist

The basis of pharmacy was, and still is, the provision of medications to patients—but it is also much more. In addition to traditional drug compounding or distribution activities, pharmacy is the science or body of knowledge about medications—their properties, actions, and clinical impact. Pharmacy is also an experimental science working to find new agents and delivery technologies. Diverse subspecialties continue to evolve and contribute to this body of knowledge (some examples are listed in Table 14.1).

Pharmaceutical Care

Central to the patient care provided by pharmacists is the concept of pharmaceutical care. Pharmaceutical care as defined by the American Society for Health-System Pharmacists (ASHP) is "the direct, responsible provision of medication-related care for the purpose of achieving definite outcomes that improve a patient's quality of life" (ASHP, 1993a).

Integral to the concept of the pharmaceutical care model is the fact that although "care" or service to patients includes the actual provision of medications, it also includes the fact that the pharmacist influences decisions about medication use for individual patients. This might include selection of a specific medication, dose, or route or even not to use the medication at all.

An emphasis on outcomes is also a key component of the model. Desired outcomes include (ASHP, 1993a) the following:

- Cure of the disease for the patient
- Elimination or a decrease in symptoms
- Stop or slow a disease process
- Prevention of a disease or symptoms

Pharmaceutical care requires a pharmacist to have access to timely patient-specific data to look for medication-related problems in development of a pharmaceutical care plan. Partnering with other members of the healthcare team to find information is critical. Nurses play a key role in this process because of their unique relationship with the patient, especially when seeking data about over-the-counter or alternative-medicine products.

Decisions are made based on data from the integration of medication-, disease-, laboratory test-, and patient-specific information. The patient's database should be assessed for any of the following medication–therapy problems (ASHP, 1993a):

- Medications with no medical indication

Table 14.1 SUBSPECIALTY SCIENCES IN PHARMACY

Pharmacoepidemiology	The study of the use of and effects of drugs in large numbers of people. Provides valuable information about additional drug risks or benefits, often during postmarketing surveillance.
Pharmacognosy	The study of drugs of natural origin, their nature, botany, properties, and effects on living organisms.
Pharmacokinetics	Discipline that describes the absorption, distribution, metabolism, and excretion of drug in patients. Used to individualize drug therapy for effectiveness and prevention of toxicity.
Pharmacoeconomics	Research that identifies, measures, and compares the costs and consequences of pharmaceutical products and services to healthcare systems and society using economic analysis tools (Bootman, Townsend, & McGhan, 1996).
Pharmacogenomics	Application of whole genome technologies (e.g., gene and protein expression data) for the prediction of the sensitivity or resistance of an individual patient's disease to a single drug or group of drugs (Ross & Ginsburg, 2003).

- Medical conditions for which there is no medication prescribed
- Medications prescribed inappropriately for a particular medical condition
- Inappropriate medication dose, dosage form, schedule, route of administration, or method of administration
- Therapeutic duplication
- Prescribing of medications to which the patient is allergic
- Actual and potential adverse drug events
- Actual and potential clinically significant drug–drug, drug–disease, drug–nutrient, and drug–laboratory test interactions
- Interference with medical therapy by social or recreational drug use
- Failure to receive the full benefit of prescribed medication therapy
- Problems arising from the financial impact of medication therapy on the patient
- A patient's lack of understanding of the medication therapy
- Failure of the patient to adhere to the medication regimen

The relative importance of medication-related problems must then be assessed on the basis of specific characteristics of the patient, the medication(s) being considered for use and the clinical goals of care. Preadmission medication regimens may require alteration to reflect the patient's current clinical status or circumstances.

Appropriate monitoring of the pharmaceutical care plan's effects is required, as is revising the regimen as the patient's condition changes and documenting the results (ASHP, 1996). An essential element of pharmaceutical care is that the pharmacist accepts responsibility for the patient's pharmacotherapeutic outcomes.

Pharmaceutical care can be practiced by any pharmacist, in any setting, and with any degree. It is not dependent on specific clinical pharmacy services or practice environment.

Pharmacists also have crucial roles in the selection of medications for routine use (formulary), drug delivery and administration devices, specific clinical services, patient and staff education, research, and patient safety (ASHP, 1997a, 1993b).

Education and Training

Pharmacy practice and licensure are state regulated. To practice, a pharmacist must become a licensed or registered pharmacist (RPh). In most states, this requires the individual to have graduated from an accredited school of pharmacy, participate in an internship program for a required number of hours, and pass both the National Association of Boards of Pharmacy Licensing Examination and the jurisprudence (law) examination for that state. Some states have additional testing requirements that may involve prescription assessment or a test of compounding skills.

Before 1992, schools of pharmacy graduated individuals with either a Bachelor of Science in Pharmacy degree (BS) or Doctor of Pharmacy (PharmD) depending on the program; both were acceptable for licensure. In 1992, however, a majority of pharmacy schools voted to offer only the PharmD degree as the entry-level professional degree (Keely, 2002).

Attaining a PharmD degree requires a minimum of 2 years of prepharmacy study, followed by 4 years of education in the school of pharmacy. Coursework includes study of disease management, physical assessment, pharmacology and physiology, pharmaceutical chemistry, pharmaceutics (the science of dispensing medicine), and microbiology. Specific clinical skills are taught, including pharmacokinetics, literature evaluation, drug information assessment, database management, documentation, and communication skills (written and verbal).

Pharmacy students also spend a required number of hours in actual practice settings with a preceptor. Tasks and learning objectives vary by program level and practice site, but the emphasis is on hands-on learning—a throwback to the old "apprenticeship" system in pharmacy history. This is intended to help pharmacy students integrate didactic learning with patient-focused practice patterns.

In our information-driven culture, new pharmacists will need to continue to learn new technologies to leverage their time and skills in assessment of new medications and therapies to implement their best practices in the complex industry that is healthcare.

Pharmacy leaders will need advanced training. This training includes their professional degree plus graduate degrees in business administration, public health, public administration, or health services administration or board certification (Knapp, 2002).

Specialization

The field of pharmacy, like that of medicine, is becoming large and diverse enough to make it difficult for any one pharmacist to be an expert in all areas of practice. In order to be useful, specialization must add value to the health-system and to patient care and outcomes. The most significant benefit of pharmacist specialization is the ability of the pharmacist to provide better and more comprehensive care to patients or selected groups of patients (Huckleberry, Thomas, & Erstad, 2003; Nester & Hale, 2002; Lesar, 2001). Complete care benefits the patient, other healthcare team members, the system generally, and payers of healthcare and pharmacy services (Clark, 2003; Commission on Workforce for Hospitals and Health Systems, 2002).

Beginning in 1976, the American Pharmaceutical Association created the Board of Pharmaceutical Specialties and began to recognize specialty areas of practice. Certification is voluntary and requires additional training and experience and passing the qualifying examination. Currently recognized specialty areas are as follows:

1. Nuclear pharmacy (1978)
2. Nutrition support pharmacy (1988)
3. Pharmacotherapy (1988)
4. Psychiatric pharmacy (1992)
5. Oncology pharmacy (1996)

Oncology pharmacy practice is a relatively new certified specialty and offers some significant advantages for patients and healthcare partners in this area. Oncology represents a diverse collection of disease states and therapies. Patients may require special pharmaceutical management to maximize their therapy and avoid toxicities. Side effects or adverse reactions can be severe and require immediate intervention from an experienced team of practitioners. Cancer treatment is expensive, complex, intense, and potentially toxic. Oncology pharmacists have opportunities to prevent adverse drug reactions, reduce costs, optimize drug regimens, and improve patient outcomes. Additional training in oncology pharmacy equips the pharmacist with the knowledge to manage pharmaceutical care for the comorbidities that these patients experience in addition to their specialized needs (Gourley, Fitzgerald, & Davis, 1997; Pon, 1996). Some elements of the additional training represented in an oncology pharmacy residency (ASHP, 1997b) are presented in Appendix 14A.

Team Participation

Acknowledging the responsibility of pharmacists for outcomes in pharmaceutical care is not intended to imply that pharmacists feel that they have exclusive authority for issues related to medication use. Pharmacists readily agree that other healthcare professionals have well-established and recognized roles in the medication use process. Nurses have a unique and trusting relationship with patients and play a crucial role in medication administration and in the coordination of pharmaceutical care into the overall care plan. A pharmacist's knowledge and skills should complement the professional skills of nurses and physicians (ASHP, 2003; Indritz & Artz, 1999; Leape et al., 1995).

Three main issues make collaborative practice a necessity:

1. The complexity of medication use
2. The importance of error detection and analysis
3. The respective roles of nurses and pharmacists in health-system medication use

Collaborative practice is also being driven by changes in pharmacy practice because of the pharmaceutical care model, the public demand for patient safety, and current economics that insist on value for investment. A 2001 survey by the American Hospital Association found a vacancy rate of 13% for both nursing and pharmacy (Bond & Raehl, 2000). Collaborative, not "solo," practice is the best available to maximize care of patients. The following discussions of medication distribution, pharmacy clinical services, and service evaluation all have elements of collaborative practice.

Drug Distribution

Medications are a major focus of many therapeutic modalities. In general, medications are less expensive than more invasive treatment strategies, are more available, are easier to administer, and have a wide therapeutic range. Medications used in oncology can be exceptions to these generalities because they can be both extremely expensive and have a narrow therapeutic window between the desired effect and toxicity.

Historically, the profession of pharmacy was centered on the production, management, and distribution of pharmaceutical agents. Early in the development of the profession this may have been due to the fact that so many medications were derived from natural resources. Today the pharmaceutical industry has taken over much of the primary packaging and production of medications, but preparation of patient-specific dosage forms is still an important role of the pharmacist.

Systems

Medication use systems are extremely complicated structures; between 80 and 200 steps can be associated with the administration of a single dose of medication in a hospital setting. Linear or written descriptions of the medication use process poorly reflect the system's variable responses to factors such as staff or materials shortages, new or unusual protocols, and failed technology. Steps in the medication use process are described in **Table 14.2**.

Although there may be limitations in using linear tools to describe the medication use process, a systems approach is vital because it can be designed to maximize outcomes and minimize errors. Put simply, it is hard to do a good job with a bad tool; it is important to depend on the system to be safe and effective and not a specific individual or group. Poorly designed systems waste resources and put patients at risk. For example, in an ambulatory care environment, efforts to create patient satisfaction may lead to a "hurry-up" focus for some team members; good system design can help to avoid overlooking critical steps in a rush and prevent errors.

Actual system design depends on the particular practice setting being discussed because ambulatory oncology services are delivered using multiple models (Woelkers, Jamieson-Baker, Hammon, & Einstein, 2002). From a pharmacy perspective, one of the most important is whether the facility is freestanding or part of a larger healthcare system and to what extent operations are shared. Will pharmacy services be provided from a central location, or does ambulatory oncology have dedicated staff and dispensing systems? Many combinations are also possible; drug distribution might be centralized, whereas clinical pharmacy functions are dedicated to the center.

Automation has become an important component in the design of medication use systems (Patel & Kaufman, 1998; Wise, Bostrom, Crosier, White, & Caldwell, 1996). Automation alone cannot prevent medication errors, but it has many

TABLE 14.2 MEDICATION USE PROCESS*

Prescribing	• Assessing the need for and selecting the correct drug • Individualizing the therapeutic regimen • Designating the desired therapeutic response
Dispensing	• Reviewing the order • Processing the order • Compounding and preparing the drug • Dispensing the drug in a timely manner
Administering	• Administering the right medication to the right patient • Administering medication when indicated • Informing the patient about the medication • Including the patient in administration
Monitoring	• Monitoring and documenting patient's response • Identifying and reporting adverse drug events • Re-evaluating drug selection, regimen, frequency, and duration of therapy
Systems management and control	• Collaborating and communicating among caregivers • Reviewing and managing patient's complete therapeutic drug regimen

* Adapted with permission from Nazdzam and Deborah (1991).

strengths. Automated processes do not get tired. They do not have a bad day, they do not take vacations, and they do not interpret handwriting incorrectly. Automation can be implemented in many of the steps in the medication use process and might include the following:

• Computerized physician order entry
• Interfacing with laboratory results to aid in individualizing therapy
• Transmitting the order to pharmacy staff
• Verifying appropriate laboratory parameters, schedule of the therapeutic regimen, or valid physician order prior to dispensing
• Bar coding of medications used in compounding and dispensing
• Bar coding of patient medication administration records and wrist bands
• Automated electronic charting of patient response
• Integration of patient data into an electronic chart to facilitate communication among health-team members
• Automatic billing

Automation has relieved pharmacists and pharmacy assistants of duplicate and repetitive work during the dispensing process and continues to develop at a rapid pace. Like the healthcare industry itself, however, automation is currently fragmented by differing providers and capabilities; its true value will be in standardization across healthcare settings.

Patient Safety

Drug distribution and medication safety are strongly linked and very much a public concern (Kohn, Corrigan, & Donaldson, 1999). Patient safety and errors in the delivery of healthcare services cause unnecessary patient harm and suffering, financial costs, and increased employee turnover. Provision of safe and effective pharmacy services involves both drug distribution systems and clinical services (clinical services are discussed in the next section).

Systems design and the use of automation are key elements of safe medication use. Patient advocacy groups and payers/employers are mandating the application of new technologies in situations that can benefit from them (Kohn et al., 1999). Healthcare is still a decade behind other industries in the application of available technology. Most medications in the United States are dispensed after a pharmacist reads and interprets a document handwritten by the physician. Implementing computerized physician order entry for medication orders eliminates handwriting as a source of error, but it should not imply that there is no potential for error in this process itself; it depends on clinical knowledge, human factors, and the safeguards programmed into the software. Patient safety cannot be mandated simply through the use of technology but involves good system design, trained clinicians, and a blame-free environment. A strategic plan for medication safety (Pathways for Medication Safety, 2002) is outline in **Table** 14.3; further detail on these issues is included in the chapter section on evaluation and control of services.

Patient safety is particularly important with medications used in oncology because many of them have a narrow therapeutic range—efficacy and toxicity are not far apart. In addition to patients, staff preparing medication doses and family members may also be at risk. Oncology medications have specialized dispensing concerns.

Oncology Medication Use

Oncology medication use is considered to be "high-alert" medications as defined previously; the use of appropriate pharmacy services as part of their use is a cornerstone for patient safety. Medication errors that occur with these agents can compromise therapy and the possibility of

Table 14.3 A STRATEGIC PLAN FOR MEDICATION SAFETY*

Process	Examples
Culture of safety	• Revise mission statement • Communicate safety commitment to staff and clients • Involve leadership in the process
Error detection	• Medication error reporting • Identify triggers or events to enhance error detection
Technology application	• Bar code applications • Computerized physician order entry
High alert medications (drugs with a higher risk of causing harm)	• Expand clinical pharmacy services with high/risk alert focus • Establish maximum doses of high alert medications and program into order-entry-processing computer system • 24 hour-7 day pharmacy IV admixture program
Blame-free environment	• Establish blame-free reporting program and review with staff • Provide education to all members of the healthcare team about how and why errors occur • Conduct system-based analysis of errors
Involve the community	• Communicate oncology center commitment to patients and visitors • Invite community members/patients to quarterly meetings at a medication safety forum
Controlled formulary	• Include error potential in discussion and evaluation of a medication being considered for use

* *Adapted from Pathways for Medication Safety, 2002.*

cure; they may also cause severe myelosuppression or even death. This section reviews some common steps in the medication distribution process with emphasis on their application to the ambulatory oncology environment. Pharmacists receive specialized training in skills that are of benefit in this area:

- Experience with drug administration devices and intravenous access may influence choice of the most appropriate system for a particular patient.
- Knowledge of solution compatibilities may facilitate timely administration of multiple agents when appropriate.
- Practiced dispensing skills may reduce staff occupational exposure to hazardous materials.

The medication use process for oncology (commonly called antineoplastic) medications begins with prescribing. Incorrect prescribing may be due to an error in dosage selection or calculation, ambiguity subject to interpretation, poor handwriting, or even selection of the wrong pen when using orders with carbon copies. Policies and procedures outlining prescribing guidelines can be developed to reduce errors in antineoplastic orders (ASHP, 2002; Beckwith & Tyler, 2000a). An example of prescribing guidelines is included in Appendix 14B, and an example of a Chemotherapy Order Forms in Appendix 14C.

Pharmacists and nurses should independently review chemotherapy orders after they are written and set aside time for this very important task. This involves not only the "five rights" of medication administration (patient, medication, dose, route, time), but also verification of intravenous access, scheduling administration times, and nurse availability for medication administration. General competencies for order review (Beckwith & Tyler, 2000b) are outlined in **Table 14.4**.

Procedures used during the dispensing process are critical because of the potentially toxic nature of many chemotherapy agents. A complete description of standards or procedures is outside the scope of this chapter, but there are several

excellent reviews and technical assistance bulletins already available (ASHP, 1990). The use of these procedures is not optional, however, as there is evidence that exposure to antineoplastic agents may result in danger to healthcare personnel. Studies examining this are not conclusive but demonstrate adequate evidence for caution as exposure and toxicity are considered to be cumulative; some personnel may prepare hundreds or even thousands of doses during their career. Other patients, their family members, and other staff in the ambulatory center must also be protected from harm.

Dispensing in an ambulatory oncology center is now more efficient because of increased use of technology and support personnel. A pharmacist's role has evolved into one in which they are a partner is providing care—assisting physicians, nurses, and consumers in making the most of drug therapy.

Clinical Services

Early European models of pharmacy practice show the pharmacist routinely rounding with the physician and even substituting for him in some cases (Cowen & Helfand, 1990). Later, pharmacy was separated from physicians by the guild systems, and it has remained an independent, specialized practice. Now modern clinical pharmacy again emphasizes collaborative and multidisciplinary practice.

Pharmacists have a subset of clinical skills that makes them valuable members of the healthcare team, but they must also have good communication skills and an appreciation for the talents of other team members. The ability to form professional "partnerships" with nurses and physicians is central to the care team concept as specialized but isolated clinical skills are not as effective in a multidisciplinary environment.

In hospital pharmacy practice, the presence of pharmacists, clinical versus dispensing staffing, and the presence of specific pharmacy services has

Table 14.4 PHARMACY COMPETENCIES FOR CHEMOTHERAPY ORDER REVIEW

Knowledge Focus	Tasks and Examples
Patient	Identify and retrieve patient-specific information such as demographics, diagnosis, height, weight, body surface area, general laboratory information, and diagnosis/therapy specific laboratory information.
Protocols	Be able to identify and retrieve standard regimens or research chemotherapy protocols. Identify and determine why a protocol may have been modified for a specific patient. Calculate all medication doses using an identified chemotherapy regimen and patient-specific data as a double check of the physician's order.
Clinical status	Know how to assess organ function as appropriate for the agent, protocol, and patient.
Process order	Select an appropriate delivery system, including solution, volume, and infusion rate or check those provided in the physician order. Enter and double check the order(s) into the pharmacy computer system.
Collaboration	Check with the patient's nurse to verify clinical information, intravenous access, and schedule of therapy. Collaborate with nursing staff for timing of blood samples for therapeutic markers or drug levels.
Preparation	Prepare or supervise preparation of the chemotherapy using safeguards and techniques appropriate for the agent and admixture environment.
Extravasation	Be able to identify which agents are vesicants or irritants and know how to manage extravasation of these agents. Ensure that needed agents for treatment of extravasation are available.
Chemotherapy spills	Know how to handle chemotherapy spills if they occur and train other staff in the use appropriate supplies.
Solution compatibility	Provide solution/medication compatibility information to staff of the center. Maintain in reference materials.

*** *Adapted from Beckwith and Tyler (2000).*

been correlated with decreases in patient morbidity and mortality, fewer medication errors, reduced medication costs, and reduced overall costs detailed here.

- An increase in the number of pharmacists is associated with a decrease in patient mortality (Bond, Raehl, & Franke, 1999a).
- Specific clinical pharmacy services are associated with decreases in patient mortality (Bond, Raehl, & Franke, 1999b).

- Higher numbers of clinical pharmacists (those not primarily associated with drug distribution) and specific clinical pharmacy services are associated with lower drug costs (Bond, Raehl, Pitterle, & Franke, 1999).
- Higher numbers of dispensing pharmacists, pharmacy technicians, and hospital pharmacy administrators are associated with higher drug costs (Bond, Raehl, Pitterle et al., 1999).

- Specific clinical pharmacy services are associated with a lower total cost of care (Bond, Raehl, & Franke, 2000).

These findings in hospital pharmacy demonstrate the value of a clinical pharmacist's service and abilities. The services detailed in this national-level, multiple-hospital survey are not specific to hospital pharmacy (Hatoum, Catizone, Hutchinson, & Purohit, 1986; Scarsi, Fotis, & Noskin, 2002; Schumock, 1999; Schumock, Meek, Ploetz, & Vermeulen, 1996). An oncology specialist pharmacist will have these same skills but also detailed knowledge about oncology patients, medications, and the ambulatory environment.

Dedicated Clinical Pharmacy Services

Not all ambulatory oncology practices have a pharmacist whose sole practice is at the ambulatory center. Pharmacist services have at least as many permutations, as do center service models. Many centers have pharmacy clinical services that may be partially or completely provided by a centralized institutional pharmacy. As is demonstrated by the Bond and Raehl data, it is the presence of the pharmacist in the patient care area that produces the benefits in patient outcomes and costs. Clinical pharmacy services, as represented by the pharmaceutical care model, cannot occur in the absence of patient care-specific data. These data are present in the patient care environment in written documentation or the knowledge of other caregivers.

Although a dedicated pharmacist is preferable, ambulatory oncology centers may not have a dedicated pharmacist for several reasons. They may be part of a larger organization that does not have the resources or available staff to assign a specific individual. The center may not have enough volume to justify a full-time position, requiring the pharmacist to also participate in other areas of practice.

Independent centers may also lack adequate volume or resources for a dedicated position.

In practice environments that do not have a dedicated pharmacist or where vacation staffing may be provided by another pharmacist who is not an oncology specialist, the emphasis on system design described earlier can more clearly be understood. Both drug distribution and clinical pharmacy services can be designed to maximize the use of available pharmacist resources.

Design of oncology clinical pharmacy services should include an evaluation of required services (discussed later in this chapter), documentation of service standards and procedures, and information on how to maintain competency. Replacing a specialized oncology pharmacist, even temporarily for vacations or other leave, should be well planned and covered by these service standards. Pharmacists who are providing service intermittently should at minimum demonstrate (ASHP, 1997b) the following:

- Basic knowledge of oncology diseases and treatment
- Basic knowledge of antineoplastic agents and their use
- Understanding of applicable policies and procedures
- Competency in safe handling practices used in dispensing
- Recognition of clinical resources and how to access them

In oncology as other pharmacy disciplines, all pharmacists retain the ability to seek and use appropriate information. In today's electronic environment, clinical support technologies might include simple reference texts and files or sophisticated electronic software or devices. The ability to research questions, evaluate the medical literature, and present conclusions is an important element of pharmacist education and training.

Patient-Focused Clinical Services

Clinical pharmacy services that contribute to patient care can be either generalized to all patients or specialized to oncology. Because medications or medication delivery methods commonly used in medical or surgical patients may not be appropriate or could even be harmful in ambulatory oncology patients, the pharmacist must use oncology-specific knowledge to tailor clinical services. Examples of clinical pharmacy services in an ambulatory oncology practice might include the following:

- Development of policies and procedures for medication orders, processing, handling of hazardous substances, and administration
- Collaborative input to establish maximum doses of high-alert medications
- Collaborative input to development or use of clinical pathways
- Routine meetings with physicians and nurses to plan and monitor pharmacotherapeutic care
- Collection and review of patient medication histories to facilitate care planning
- Use of pharmacokinetic analysis to dose-adjust medications when needed
- Conduct of medication use evaluations
- Overseeing of medication procurement and inventory management
- Participation in the selection of medications using an evidence-based approach and pharmacoeconomic analysis
- Maximizing therapeutic effectiveness of a pharmaceutical regimen by managing supportive medications for patient nausea and vomiting, fatigue, anemia, pain management, etc.
- Management of anticoagulation
- Education of patients in a multidisciplinary teaching plan for the practice
- Participation in research protocols

- Coordination of pharmaceutical care with providers at other sites or providers
- Provision of drug information
- Prevention of medication errors from dosage conversions when switching to a different route of administration
- Prevention of medication errors because of dose formulation issues, for example, sustained release versus immediate release products

Selection and implementation of clinical pharmacy services for a particular ambulatory practice will depend on the degree of pharmacist participation and multiple other practice parameters. Maximizing pharmacist integration into ambulatory oncology can benefit not only patients but their care partners. Expert systems in medication distribution and clinical services may assist the pharmacist in those areas but cannot replace the professional. One cannot automate clinical judgment (Wong & Ignoffo, 1996).

Evaluation of Pharmacy Services and Pharmaceutical Care

Tailoring Services to the Environment

Providing a service that is not needed or wanted is obviously a waste of resources. In order to match successfully pharmacy services to an ambulatory oncology practice, one must first assess how it functions and provides services. (These data will also be required to assess the impact of added services.) What is the organization's structure? How is the physician practice structured, and how well does it function?

One should assess the organization's financial status, the facility itself, and existing patient care protocols. How would pharmacy services contribute to patient care in this setting?

Also part of this analysis or practice assessment is an estimation of the resources needed by the pharmacist to function and whether or not they are already present. Is new technology needed? Are their adequate knowledge resources or access to them? What support staff are present in the organization? As discussed previously, using a pharmacist solely for drug distribution is a waste of resources and will not contribute significantly to patient care.

Outcomes, Control, and Change

After the addition of new clinicians or services, it is just as important to assess the results or impact on several parameters. These may include the following:

- Clinical (patient outcomes)
- Patient satisfaction
- Clinician job satisfaction
- Financial
- Organizational

Documentation and availability of data are essential to any of the previously mentioned analyses. Standards of practice and clinical guidelines should be used to establish the criteria by which outcomes will be judged. A complete discussion of service evaluation and control is outside the scope of this chapter. Awareness, vigilance, and dedication to continually improving the quality of patient care should be principal goals.

Conclusion

Pharmacists can make many important contributions to patient care in an ambulatory oncology practice. They have many abilities that make them complementary additions to services already provided by physicians and nurses. In today's intense clinical environment, the ability of healthcare team professionals to "take turns" in overlapping areas or tasks can substantially improve efficiency and ward off staff exhaustion or burnout.

As our population ages and individuals have multiple comorbidities, using medications appropriately is not only good clinical practice, but helps to meet the challenge of providing quality medical care at an affordable price. Pharmacists are trained to help make the most effective use of medications.

Author and clinician J.W. Hurst, MD, was frequently asked to define the most important attribute for someone who wishes to learn medicine. He believes it to be curiosity, the desire to find out and know things, and that the required sequence of thought and action in clinical learning cannot be achieved without it (Hurst, 2002). Curiosity is also an essential attribute for a good pharmacy clinician. Pharmacists are not ambulatory reference texts; instead, they have a combination of specific skills, knowledge, available clinical tools, and the curiosity to use them to benefit ambulatory oncology patients.

Appendix A Clinical Elements of Oncology Pharmacy Residency Training

Experience in Direct Patient Care in Neoplastic Diseases (Acute Care and Ambulatory Care)

- Breast cancer
- Colorectal cancer
- Leukemias, acute
- Lung cancer
- Lymphomas
- Ovarian cancer
- Prostate cancer

Experience in Managing Cancer-Related Disorders

- Anorexia
- Cachexia
- Disseminated intravascular coagulation
- Fatigue
- Hypercalcemia
- Malignant effusions
- Nausea and vomiting
- Pain
- Syndrome of inappropriate antidiuretic hormone secretion
- Superior vena cava syndrome
- Thrombosis
- Tumor compression syndromes

Experience in Managing Cancer Treatment-Related Disorders

- Anorexia
- Drug extravasation
- Infections in immunocompromised patients
- Infertility
- Nausea and vomiting
- Organ-specific toxicities (e.g., cardiotoxicity, hepatotoxicity, or nephrotoxicity)
- Mucositis
- Myelosuppression
- Secondary malignancies
- Syndrome of inappropriate antidiuretic hormone secretion
- Tumor lysis syndrome

Experience in Treatment Procedures

- Bone marrow transplantation, including high-dose chemotherapy with peripheral stem cell rescue or autologous bone marrow transplantation (experience with allogeneic bone marrow transplantation is also recommended)
- Immunotherapy
- Radiation therapy
- Surgery
- Gene therapy at participating institutions

Adapted from ASHP (1997).

Appendix B EXAMPLES OF PRESCRIBING GUIDELINE ELEMENTS FOR REDUCING ERRORS IN CHEMOTHERAPY ORDERS

- Write legibly or use computerized order entry.
- Use preprinted chemotherapy order forms.
- Use written orders only; verbal orders for chemotherapy are not accepted.
- Date and time each order.
- Verify the patient's full name and date of birth before writing the order.
- Patient information (height, weight, diagnosis) and protocol name should be included on the order form.
- Review current medication orders before writing additional orders and discontinue duplicate or conflicting therapies.
- Use the drug's generic name and avoid use of abbreviations.
- Establish and use standard terminology.
- Write the dosage calculation on the order and with the mg/kg or mg/m^2 basis used to calculate it. Round doses over 10 to the nearest whole number.
- Write "micrograms" or "mcg" clearly so that it is not mistaken for mg.
- Use a leading zero for doses less than a whole unit: .150 mg may be misinterpreted as 150 mg.
- Avoid trailing zeros: 2.0 mg may be read as 20 mg. Write 2 mg instead.
- Specify the drug dose or concentration, even if you believe there is only one formulation available.
- Specify the route of administration and the infusion rate for intravenous medications.
- Write the total daily dose to be given and the number of days, and then write the total dose for the entire treatment period.
- Review all elements of the order after it is written.
- Review all unusual orders with pharmacy and nursing to answer questions.

Adapted from Beckwith and Tyler (2000).

Appendix C AN EXAMPLE CHEMOTHERAPY ORDER FORM

Diagnosis _____   Protocol/Regimen _____

                                                                Cycle _____

Height _____ inches   Weight _____ kg Body Surface Area _____ m^2

- IV Access Required (check one)   ❏ Peripheral   ❏ Central

- Laboratory Orders _____

- Special Precautions/Other Orders _____

- Parameters that must be met prior to medication administration _____

  _____

- Medication Orders

  Premedications _____

  _____

Medication, Dosage Calculation, and Administration Sequence	Dose, Route, and Administration Schedule

MD _____ Date/Time _____

Patient Stamp Area _____

References

American Society of Health-System Pharmacists. (1990). ASHP technical assistance bulletin on handling cytotoxic and hazardous drugs. *American Journal of Hospital Pharmacy, 47,* 1033–1049.

American Society of Health-System Pharmacists. (1993a). ASHP statement on pharmaceutical care. *American Journal of Hospital Pharmacy, 50,* 1720–1723.

American Society of Health-System Pharmacists. (1993b). ASHP statement on the pharmacist's role with respect to drug delivery systems and administration devices. *American Journal of Hospital Pharmacy, 50,* 1724–1725.

American Society of Health-System Pharmacists. (1996). ASHP guidelines on a standardized method for pharmaceutical care. *American Journal of Health-System Pharmacy, 53,* 1713–1716.

American Society of Health-System Pharmacists. (1997a). ASHP guidelines on the pharmacist's role in the development of clinical care plans. *American Journal of Health-System Pharmacy, 54,* 314–318.

American Society of Health-System Pharmacists. (1997b). *ASHP supplemental standard and learning objectives for residency training in oncology Pharmacy practice.* Retrieved March 15, 2003 from *www.ashp.org/rtp/Oncology-stnd.cfm*

American Society of Health-System Pharmacists. (2002). ASHP guidelines on preventing medication errors with antineoplastic agents. *American Journal of Health-System Pharmacy, 59,* 1648–1668.

American Society of Health-System Pharmacists. (2003). Pharmacy-nursing shared vision for safe medication use in hospitals: Executive summary session. *American Journal of Health-System Pharmacy, 60,* 1046–1052.

Beckwith, M. C. & Tyler, L. S. (2000a). Preventing medication errors with antineoplastic agents, part 1. *Hospital Pharmacy, 35,* 511–526.

Beckwith, M. C. & Tyler, L. S. (2000b). Preventing medication errors with antineoplastic agents, part 2. *Hospital Pharmacy, 35,* 732–749.

Bond, C. A., Raehl, C. L., & Franke, T. (1999a). Clinical pharmacy services, pharmacist staffing, and drug costs in United States hospitals. *Pharmacotherapy, 19,* 1354–1362.

Bond, C. A., Raehl, C. L., & Franke, T. (1999b). Clinical pharmacy services and hospital mortality rates. *Pharmacotherapy, 19,* 556–564.

Bond, C. A., Raehl, C. L., Pitterle, M. E., & Franke, T. (1999). Health care professional staffing, hospital characteristics, and hospital mortality rates. *Pharmacotherapy, 19,* 130–138.

Bond, C. A. & Raehl, C. L. (2000). Changes in pharmacy, nursing, and total personnel staffing in U.S. hospitals, 1989–1998. *American Journal of Health-System Pharmacy, 57,* 970–974.

Bond, C. A., Raehl, C. L., & Franke, T. (2000). Clinical pharmacy services, pharmacy staffing, and the total cost of care in United States hospitals. *Pharmacotherapy, 20,* 609–621.

Bootman, J. L., Townsend, R. J., & McGhan, W. F. (1996). *Principles of Pharmacoeconimcs* (2nd ed.). Cincinnati, OH: Harvey Whitney Books Company.

Clark, T. R. (2003). A vision for pharmacy and how to get there–part 1. *Pharmacy Times.*

Commission on Workforce for Hospitals and Health Systems. (2002). *In our hands: How hospital leaders can build a thriving workforce.* Chicago: American Hospital Association.

Cowen, D. L. & Helfand, W. H. (1990). *Pharmacy: An illustrated history.* New York: Harry N. Abrams Inc.

Gourley, D. R., Fitzgerald, W. L., Jr., & Davis, R. L. (1997). Competency, board certification, credentialing, and specialization: Who benefits? *American Journal of Managed Care, 3,* 795–801.

Hatoum, H. T., Catizone, C., Hutchinson, R. A., & Purohit, A. (1986). An eleven-year review of the pharmacy literature: Documentation of the value and acceptance of clinical pharmacy. *Drug Intelligence & Clinical Pharmacy, 20,* 33–48.

Huckleberry, Y., Thomas, M. C., & Erstad, B. L. (2003). Dosage conversions as a potential cause of adverse drug events. *American Journal of Health-System Pharmacy, 60,* 189–191.

Hurst, J. W. (2002). A metaphoric equivalent for curiosity. *Medscape Cardiology, 6.*

Indritz, M. E. & Artz, M. B. (1999). Value added to health by pharmacists. *Social Science & Medicine, 48,* 647–660.

Keely, J. L. (2002). Pharmacist scope of practice. *Annals of Internal Medicine, 136,* 79–85.

Knapp, K. K. (2002). John Ogden talks about managed care in the Veterans Administration. *Journal of Managed Care Pharmacy, 8,* 91–93.

Kohn, L. T., Corrigan, J. M., & Donaldson, M. D. (Eds.). (1999). *To Err is Human: Building Safer Health System.* Washington, DC: National Academy Press.

Leape, L. L., Bates, D. W., Cullen, D. J., Cooper, J., Demonaco, H. J., Gallivan, T. et al. (1995). Systems analysis of adverse drug events: ADE Prevention Study Group. *Journal of the American Medical Association, 274,* 35–43.

Lesar, T. S. (2001). Medication errors related to dosage formulation issues. Medscape Pharmacists. Retrieved from *www.medscape.com*.

Nazdzam, D. M. (1991). Development of medication-use indicators by the Joint Commission on Accreditation of Healthcare Organizations. *American Journal of Hospital Pharmacy, 48*, 1925–1930.

Nester, T. M. & Hale, L. S. (2002). Effectiveness of a pharmacist-acquired medication history in promoting patient safety. *American Journal of Health-System Pharmacy, 59*, 2221–2225.

Patel, V. L. & Kaufman, D. R. (1998). Medical informatics and the science of cognition. *Journal of the American Medical Informatics Association, 5*, 493–502.

Pathways for Medication Safety: Leading a Strategic Planning Effort. (2002). American Hospital Association, Health Research and Educational Trust, Institute for Safe Medication Practices.

Pon, D. (1996). Service plans and clinical interventions targeted by the oncology pharmacist. *Pharmacy Practice Management Quarterly, 16*, 18–30.

Ross, J. S. & Ginsburg, G. S. (2003). The integration of molecular diagnostics with therapeutics: Implications for drug development and pathology practice. *American Journal of Clinical Pathology, 119*, 26–36.

Scarsi, K. K., Fotis, M. A., & Noskin, G. A. (2002). Pharmacist participation in medical rounds reduces medication errors. *American Journal of Health-System Pharmacy, 59*, 2089–2092.

Schumock, G. T. (1999). We've been shown the money, and we now know how to spend it. *Pharmacotherapy, 19*, 1349–1351.

Schumock, G. T., Meek, P. D., Ploetz, P. A., & Vermeulen, L. C. (1996). Economic evaluations of clinical pharmacy services—1988-1995: The Publications Committee of the American College of Clinical Pharmacy. *Pharmacotherapy, 16*, 1188–1208.

Wise, L. C., Bostrom, J., Crosier, J. A., White, S., & Caldwell, R. (1996). Cost-benefit analysis of an automated medication system. *Nursing Economics, 14*, 224–231.

Woelkers, J. F., Jamieson-Baker, P. A., Hammon, D. K., & Einstein, A. B. Jr. (2002). Effective strategic planning in clinical cancer services: A road map to success. *Oncology Issues, 17*, 22–28.

Wong, W. M. & Ignoffo, R. F. (1996). If there are expert systems and dose checks, why do we still need the clinical pharmacist? *Pharmacy Practice Management Quarterly, 16*, 50–58.

Chapter 15

Research and Clinical Trials in Ambulatory Oncology Care

Linda U. Krebs

Introduction

Clinical trials have been the pathway to increased survivorship and decreased morbidity and mortality from cancer. Through identification of new methods of treatment, strategies to prevent cancer or diagnose it early, and methods to manage symptoms and improve quality of life, clinical trials have altered the course of cancer for overall numbers of individuals surviving cancer and for increased length of survival. Additionally, with increased numbers of clinical trials focusing on palliative or end-of-life care, even those who succumb to cancer are doing so with decreased distress and increased quality of life.

According to Mulay (2001), "A clinical trial is a research method used to test in humans drugs that have shown positive activity in the laboratory and in animal studies." (p. 5) A clinical trial is designed to answer a specific scientific question. It begins with carefully controlled laboratory research and progresses to studies with people. In essence, it is the bridge between the basic research laboratory and the patient's bedside, with an ultimate goal of trying to find better ways to prevent, diagnose, and treat cancer and to help cancer patients and their families manage the experience of having cancer.

Even though great strides in cancer care have been made as a result of clinical trials, less than 5% of the individuals with cancer who are eligible to participate in a clinical trial do so. In addition, the percentage of minorities, women, and the medically underserved who participate in clinical trials is even lower (Lara et al., 2001). Low accrual to trials has many serious effects, including an increased length of time to answer pivotal treatment questions, early closing of studies (thus, research questions may never be answered), and the inability to make adequate generalizations of findings to the population at large. Healthcare providers and the public at large often have inadequate knowledge about clinical trials, making referral to and participation in a trial less likely. Because of their continuous patient and family interactions, oncology nurses have the opportunity to play an important role in facilitating the clinical trial process. Through their advocacy and education, oncology nurses can provide information about clinical trials, can support patients and families through the clinical trial process, and can provide the appropriate care and follow-up that will enhance quality of life for those participating in a clinical trial.

Historical Issues and Milestones

When looking at the milestones that have occurred in cancer care, three intertwining areas in relationship to clinical trials are identified (**Table 15.1**). The first of these is a historical perspective in relationship to the conduct of clinical trials (who, what, and when). The second relates to development of the clinical trial infrastructure, and the third relates to the identification of the ethical underpinnings of the clinical trial process. The first two areas are discussed here; the third is discussed under ethical issues.

Clinical trials have been documented in literature since the mid-1700s. The first documented clinical trial occurred in 1747 and evaluated patients with scurvy. The first randomized trial occurred in 1931, and the first randomized therapeutic trial occurred between 1946 and 1948. In this latter trial, patients with tuberculosis were randomized to either bed rest alone or streptomycin plus bed rest. The outcome of this trial influenced tuberculosis treatment for years to come (Chou & Liu, 1998; Green, Benedetti, & Crowley, 2003; Gullatte & Otto, 2001; Klimaszewski, Anderson, & Good, 2000; Klimaszewski et al., 2000; Wujcik & Fraser, 2000).

Along with these events in clinical trials, other milestones occurred, which created the infrastructure for and establishment of the ethical principles of the clinical trials of today. In terms of infrastructure, many events occurred to develop the capacity to conduct clinical trials. One of the most important was the establishment of the National Institutes of Health (NIH) in 1887, as eventually the NIH would become the focus from which much of the federally funded research emanates. In 1937, the National Cancer Institute Act was enacted, establishing the National Cancer Institute (NCI) as an agency within the Public Health Service. In 1955, the National Chemotherapy Program was founded, and the first cancer cooperative group was formed. In 1971, the National Cancer Act was enacted. This act was designed to expand the nation's cancer research programs and formally authorized the Cancer Centers Program, leading to the development of the clinical and comprehensive cancer centers located throughout the United States. The Cooperative Group Outreach Program was established in 1976 to extend clinical trial participation to individual community-based physicians, and in 1983, the Community Cancer Outreach Program was established to link groups of community-based physicians to a cancer cooperative group. Finally, in 1991, several minority Community Cancer Outreach Programs were established. These Community Cancer Outreach Programs were located in areas with high minority populations and were designed to increase minority recruitment and retention to clinical trials through providing access to quality cancer clinical trials within the target population's community (Chou & Liu, 1998; Green et al., 2003; Gullatte & Otto, 2001; Klimaszewski, Anderson, & Good, 2000; Klimaszewski et al., 2000; Wujcik & Fraser, 2000).

Overview of Clinical Research

Clinical Trials Conduct and Funding

Clinical trials are conducted and funded through a variety of mechanisms. Among these are cancer cooperative groups (e.g., Southwest Oncology group, Eastern Cooperative Oncology Group, Children's Oncology Group, Radiation Therapy Oncology Group), the National Cancer Institutes designated cancer centers, the community-based research programs (i.e., Cooperative Group Outreach Program, Community Cancer Outreach Program, and minority-based Community Cancer Outreach Programs), which receive funding

Table 15.1 CLINICAL TRIALS: HISTORICAL PERSPECTIVE

Year	Occurrence	Explanation/Outcome
1747	First documented clinical trial	Evaluated patients with scurvy
1887	National Institutes of Health founded	
1931	First randomization of patients in a clinical trial	
1937	Enactment of the National Cancer Institute Act, establishing the National Cancer Institute	Established as an agency within the Public Health Service
1944	First publication of the results of a multicenter clinical trial	
1944	Public Health Service Act	Consolidated nation's health efforts and designated the NCI as part of the National Institutes of Health
1946-48	First randomized therapeutic trial	Proved that for those with tuberculosis, streptomycin plus bed rest is better than bed rest alone
1947	Nuremberg Code established	Identified a code of ethics for research on human participants
1953	Warren Grant Magnuson Clinical Center established on the campus of the National Institutes of Health	Established for the conduct of basic and clinical research at the National Institutes of Health
1955	National Chemotherapy Program	Established to test compounds that might be effective antineoplastic agents
1955	Establishment of the first Cooperative Research Group	
1964	Helsinki Declaration	Established guidelines for physicians who are conducting human participant research
1966	Biomedical research regulations issued by Surgeon General	Mandated local review of all research protocols/establishment of Institutional Review Boards
1971	National Cancer Act	Designed to expand the nation's cancer research program; formally authorized the Cancer Centers Program
1974	National Research Act	Required all research protocols to be reviewed by an IRB before release of any federal funding
1976	Cooperative Group Outreach Program established	Designed to extend clinical trials participation to individual community-based physicians
1978	Belmont Report published	Identified guidelines and ethical principles for protecting humans participating in research
1983	Community Cancer Outreach Programs established	Groups of community-based physicians linked to cooperative groups

(continues)

Table 15.1	Clinical trials: historical perspective (cont'd)	
1988	High-priority Clinical Trials program established	Identified important phase III clinical trials for specific disease sites
1990	Office of Research on Women's Health created	Established to assure the safe inclusion of women in research activities
1991	Code of Federal Regulations (45 CFR) 46	Established protection for human subjects in research
1993	National Institutes of Health Revitalization Act	Mandated inclusion of women and minorities in clinical research
1993	Establishment of minority-based Community Cancer Outreach Programs	Located in areas that serve ethnic minorities and underserved populations
2000	Office of Human Research Protection Established	Responsible for guiding the medical community on research ethics/ implementing 45 CFR 46
2000	Central IRB pilot begun	Pilot project to centrally evaluate phase III cooperative group trials

Chow & Liu, 1998; Green et al., 2003; Gullatte & Otto, 2001; Klimaszewski, Aiken et al., 2000; Wujcik & Fraser, 2000; http://www.cancer.gov/clinicaltrials/conducting/informed-consent-guide.

through the National Cancer Institute; pharmaceutical and biomedical companies that support the conduct of their own trials; and more recently, insurance companies, health maintenance organizations, and private sources/funders that may focus on a particular research target or topic. This myriad of organizations that conduct research and funding sources to support the conduct of this research has resulted in more than 8,000 clinical trials being available for cancer treatment throughout the United States. Although this number of trials has the potential to offer treatment to a variety of individuals for whom standard treatment currently is not available or for those interested in participating in a clinical trial, there is much overlap and competition among institutions, organizations, and funders. In some instances, this competition actually decreases enrollment to any one trial, resulting in insufficient information both to provide an adequate understanding of the trial outcome or to make specific recommendations for cancer treatment/intervention for the population under study. A method currently in use to increase enrollment

across populations for a specific trial is the intergroup trial mechanism. Under this plan, a clinical trial is opened simultaneously in a variety of cooperative groups, and all data are collected and collated, resulting in decreased time to study completion and analysis and increased generalizability of findings. Collaboration, rather than competition, should enhance pivotal trial completion, getting results to consumers more rapidly without decreasing research quality (Gullatte & Otto, 2001; Klimaszewski, Anderson et al., 2000; Klimaszewski, Aiken et al., 2000).

Phases of Clinical Trial Research

The basis for the conduct of a clinical trial, particularly in the area of drug development, is laboratory and animal research in which new compounds are identified, screened, produced, and evaluated for toxicity, with the goal of eventual use in humans. A large number of compounds may be evaluated; however, only a very few will go on to clinical trials in humans. Before human evaluation, preclinical testing for drug toxicity occurs. The goal of preclinical testing is to identify the safest starting dose of a drug or compound that can be given in a clinical trial. Most commonly, initial testing for toxicity occurs in mice. A dose that is lethal in 10% of the mice (LD10) will be the initial dose used in the first phase of clinical testing in humans. Once preclinical testing is complete, the compound will go on to the clinical testing in humans. This testing consists of four phases that are outlined later here and in **Table 15.2**. These four phases are designed to determine systematically the safety, efficacy, and effectiveness of new compounds, treatments, procedures, and devices (Chou & Liu, 1998; Collichio, Griggs, & Rosenblatt, 2001; Gullatte & Otto, 2001; Klimaszewski, Anderson et al., 2000; Klimaszewski, Aiken et al., 2000; Krebs, unpublished; Whittemore & Grey, 2002; Works, 2000). It should be noted that with new compounds under development, new evaluation methods and measures to evaluate outcomes are actively being considered.

PHASE I

Phase I trials are designed to determine the maximum tolerated dose of a drug. These trials are considered to be safety trials because they are determining both the safest dose and best method of administration of the compound. Included in these trials are pharmacokinetics studies to evaluate absorption, excretion, distribution, and metabolism of the drug. Only a small number of patients, usually 15 to 20, will take part in a phase I trial. Those eligible to participate in phase I trials have been heavily pretreated, have no other standard treatment options, and are not expected to benefit from the treatment. Cohorts of three to six patients are given an initial dose of the drug, as determined in the preclinical testing, and then using a system to specify dose levels for each succeeding cohort, increasing doses of the drug are given until the maximum tolerated dose is reached. Before increasing the dose, the cohort at the given dose is watched for signs of toxicity. If no nonreversible or life-threatening toxicities occur, the next dose level can be given to a new cohort. If toxicities are seen, additional participants are added to the cohort, and if life-threatening toxicities are seen in a specified number of patients, the trial is stopped (Chou & Liu, 1998; Collichio et al., 2001; Gullatte & Otto, 2001; Klimaszewski, Anderson et al., 2000; Klimaszewski, Aiken et al., 2000; Krebs, Burnhansstiparov, Bradley, & Gamito, unpublished; Whittemore & Grey, 2002; Works, 2000).

PHASE II

Phase II trials are designed to determine in which tumor types a specific compound will be useful. These are efficacy trials, and they are intended to identify a specific tumor type that appears to respond to the drug. These trials use the dose and administration schedule identified in the phase I trial for treatment. Patients who can be enrolled are those who are likely to benefit but for whom no current effective therapy exists. Additionally, they may have been treated previously. Larger numbers of patients (15 to 30) are included (Chou & Liu, 1998; Collichio et al., 2001; Gullatte & Otto, 2001; Klimaszewski, Anderson, et al., 2000; Klimaszewski, Aiken et al., 2000; Krebs et al., unpublished; Whittemore & Grey, 2002; Works, 2000).

PHASE III

Phase III trials are designed to determine the value of a new treatment in relationship to the current standard. These trials include a large number of patients (100s to 1000s) who are usually randomized to one type of treatment or another. The primary end point is to improve on existing therapy. Those who may participate usually have received little or no treatment before entry. They must have adequate organ function and measurable disease. The inclusion of women, minorities, and the medically underserved are essential to these trials (Chou & Liu, 1998; Collichio et al., 2001; Gullatte & Otto, 2001; Klimaszewski, Anderson et al., 2000; Klimaszewski, Aiken et al., 2000; Krebs et al., unpublished; Whittemore & Grey, 2002; Works, 2000).

Table 15.2 PHASES OF CLINICAL TRIALS*

Phase	Purpose	Components	Eligibility
Phase I (safety)	Primary goal to determine the maximum tolerated dose in humans; secondary goals to identify the most effective administration schedule and to identify and quantify toxicities	• Pharmacokinetic studies for drug absorption, distribution, metabolism, and excretion • Includes specified dose escalations in small groups of 3–6 * Antitumor response not an endpoint	• Previously heavily pretreated patients • Life expectancy of at least 1–2 months • Major organ function must be adequate • Does not require measurable disease • Open to patients with a variety of tumor types
Phase II (efficacy)	Determines whether a compound or product has objective activity in a variety of cancers	• Focuses on identifying types of tumors that will respond • Uses the dose and administration schedule from the phase I study	• Patients likely to benefit for whom no effective therapy currently exists • Patient may or may not have been pretreated • Requires measurable or evaluable disease
Phase III (new vs. current standard)	Determines the value of a new treatment, product, or procedure in relation to the current standard	• Compares new drug/procedure with standard therapy • Includes large numbers of patients • Often includes randomization • Primary endpoint is to improve on existing therapy	• Must have measurable disease and adequate organ function • Usually have received little or no previous therapy • Inclusion of minorities, women, and the medically underserved being imperative
Phase IV (postmarketing)	Determines optimum use(s) after Food and Drug Administration approval	• Builds on previous research • Identify additional adverse events • Determine the effect of the drug on morbidity and mortality	• Often conducted on patient populations not previously studied in the phase I to phase III trials

* Includes evaluations of both treatment and cancer control studies as well as mechanical devices, specialized procedures, and tools to evaluate symptoms and outcomes.

(Chou & Liu, 1998; Green et al., 2003; Gullatte & Otto, 2001; Klimaszewski, Aiken et al., 2000; Krebs et al., unpublished; Wujeik & Froser, 2000).

PHASE IV

Phase IV studies are postmarketing studies that occur after Food and Drug Administration approval of the drug. These studies build on previous research and further investigate potential adverse events or reactions. Often these studies are undertaken in populations who were not part of the initial clinical trials that lead to Food and Drug Administration approval (Chou & Liu, 1998; Collichio et al., 2001; Gullatte & Otto, 2001; Klimaszewski, Anderson et al., 2000; Klimaszewski, Aiken et al., 2000; Krebs et al., unpublished; Whittemore & Grey, 2002; Works, 2000).

Pharmaceutical companies fund most phase IV studies. These are performed in the outpatient setting. Several issues surround patient accrual because physicians are often paid up to $5,000 per patient entered on a trial. Another concern is the increased workload for already overburdened outpatient nurses. Some pharmaceutical companies underwrite grants for salaries for additional staff for data management, but usually, the increased burden of additional patient care and documentation is the responsibility of the clinic nurse.

Types of Trials in Oncology Care

Multiple types of clinical trials are available. Although the focus of most discussions usually is on treatment trials, studies in other areas are essential for quality cancer care. As is noted in **Table 15.3**, in addition to treatment trials, there are trials to identify methods to prevent cancer or to diagnose cancer at an earlier stage than is currently possible; studies that evaluate new devices, procedures, and techniques for providing cancer care; trials that investigate specific methods of managing the symptoms associated with cancer

Table 15.3 TYPES OF CANCER CLINICAL TRIALS

Type	Focus
Treatment	Evaluate tumor response, overall survival, and disease-free survival
Prevention/early detection	Methods to either prevent cancer or to identify it earlier than currently possible
Devices/procedures/techniques	Evaluate new devices, procedures, or techniques used in providing cancer care (e.g., infusion devices, surgical techniques, radiation procedures)
Symptom management	Methods to prevent or manage symptoms related to cancer or cancer treatment
Quality of life	Evaluate the impact of cancer and its treatment on the patient's well-being, with focus on helping patients and families cope with cancer/treatment
Survivor/late effects trials	Investigate long-term effects of cancer and treatment
Phamacoeconomic	Evaluate of costs of a trial/treatment in relationship to benefit, effectiveness, or utility
Companion	Studies conducted either in conjunction with or parallel to an ongoing trial, often conducted by nurses in collaboration with other study investigators

(Klimaszewski, Anderson et al., 2000; Klimaszewski, Aiken et al., 2000; Krebs et al., unpublished).

and cancer treatment; and quality-of-life trials that evaluate the impact of cancer and/or cancer treatment on the patient's well-being. Additional trials may investigate the costs of the trial in relationship to its benefits, efficacy, or utility (i.e., the perceived usefulness or patient preference for one therapy over another), whereas other trials may evaluate the long-term effects of cancer or cancer treatment in survivors. Of major importance are companion trials that may occur either in conjunction with or parallel to an ongoing trial. These trials, conducted by nurses in collaboration with the investigators conducting the clinical trial and/or with other healthcare providers, often evaluate/identify strategies for management of symptoms or trial-identified side effects such as fatigue or nausea of the treatment currently being studied in the ongoing clinical trial (Krebs et al., unpublished; Rosse & Garcia, 2001).

The Research Protocol

The research protocol is the cornerstone of the clinical trial. The protocol is a blueprint or plan that specifically identifies how the trial is to be conducted. It details exactly how a trial will be carried out and how data will be collected and evaluated. Included in the protocol will be the study objectives or questions to be answered, the rationale for the study, who can and cannot be enrolled, what interventions will be tested and how they will be tested, what potential side effects occur related to the treatment, and how the data will be analyzed. Table 15.4 identifies the components of a clinical trial protocol. These components may be given different names or may be combined depending on institutional preferences. However, all components should be included for completeness and to ensure that those providing treatment will have a full understanding of what is to happen, how it is to be carried out, and how it should be monitored (Chou & Liu, 1998; Gullatte & Otto, 2001; Krebs et al., unpublished).

Issues in Clinical Trial Participation

Ethical Issues

When considering the ethical issues inherent in and associated with clinical trials, numerous topics must be included. In addition to identifying the milestones associated with clinical trials ethics, one must also identify the ethical principles that form the basis for clinical trials participation and the informed consent and have an understanding of institutional review boards (IRBs) and their conduct. In addition, of prime importance are the informed consent process itself and issues related to conflict of interest in the conduct of clinical trials. Finally, issues surround-

Table 15.4 Components of a Clinical Trial Protocol

Objectives

Background and rationale

Therapeutic information

Trial design

Study population (inclusion and exclusion criteria)

Pretreatment evaluation

Entry/randomization procedure

Treatment plan

Evaluation during and after protocol treatment

Criteria for measurement of study endpoints

Serious adverse event reporting

Protocol treatment discontinuation and therapy after stopping

Central review procedures

Statistical considerations

Publication policies

Ethical, regulatory, and administrative issues

References

Appendices (including sample consent forms)

ing what constitutes good clinical practice must be considered.

MILESTONES IN CLINICAL TRIALS ETHICS

Several events can be considered milestones in the development of the ethical underpinnings of clinical trials research (**Table 15.1**). Among these are the establishment of the Nuremberg Code in 1947 and the Helsinki Declaration in 1964, the enactment of the National Research Act in 1974, and the publishing of the Belmont Report in 1978. The Nuremberg Code identified a code of ethics for research on human participants. This code was a direct result of the Nazi atrocities in World War II and included the mandate that no individual could be experimented on without providing informed consent. The Helsinki Declaration established guidelines for physicians for the conduct of human participant research, whereas the Belmont report identified guidelines and ethical principles for protecting human subjects who are participating in research with a particular focus on the process of informed consent. Of additional importance was the National Research Act, which mandated that all research that was to receive federal monies must be reviewed by an IRB. This act further strengthened the Surgeon General's mandate in 1966 that all research studies undergo an internal review. In 1991, the Code of Federal Regulations Part 46 (45 CFR 46) formalized the protection of humans in research, whereas in 1993, the National Institutes of Health Revitalization Act mandated the inclusion of women and minorities in clinical research. Finally, in 2000, the Office of Human Research Protection was established to provide ethical guidance to the medical community and to promote the implementation of 45 CFR 46, and the Central IRB pilot was begun. The Central IRB pilot project is designed to evaluate whether a central reviewing body can be the IRB of record, assuring scientific integrity and participant safety for phase III cooperative group trials, thus eliminating the need for local IRB review and thereby decreasing the amount of time protocol generation to implementation.

ETHICAL PRINCIPLES

According to Jenkins (2001), "Basic ethical principles should form the cornerstone of any sound clinical trial." (p. 14) Numerous authors (Amdur, 2003; Jemec & Schi, 2000; Kim, 2002; Smith, 2000) have identified four primary ethical or moral principles that form the foundation of participation in clinical trials research. These principles evolved from a variety of sources, including the Nuremberg Code, the Helsinki Declaration (Getz & Borfitz, 2002; Sales & Folkman, 2000), and the Belmont Report (Sales & Folkman, 2000), and include the principles of *autonomy*, or respect for persons; *beneficence*, or the maximization of benefit coupled with minimization of risk; *nonmaleficence*, or do no harm; and *justice*, in which the burdens and benefits of research are equally distributed among research participants. To be autonomous means to be able to make decisions about those things that affect one's life and to be able to act on those decisions, whereas beneficence essentially means to "do no harm." Under the principle of autonomy, it is assumed that if appropriate and complete information is provided to a cognitively competent person, the individual will be able to make an informed choice about participation in a particular clinical trial, whereas under the principles of beneficence and nonmaleficence, the potential benefits of taking part in the clinical trial must be weighed against potential risks, whereas at the same time the overriding goal is to do no harm. The final principle, justice, means that there will be fairness within the research process, insuring that participants will be fairly selected from populations that are most likely to benefit and that patients in randomized trials will have an equal opportunity to be in any treatment group. It should be noted that when autonomy is diminished because of cognitive impairment or any other disabilities in a potential trial participant, special measures must be undertaken to assure that the principle of autonomy is not disregarded (Portney & Watkins, 2000).

Ezekiel et al. (2000) have further delineated what makes human subjects research ethical. They have identified seven ethical requirements of the clinical research program, including that the research have value, have scientific validity, include fair selection of subjects, have a favorable risk–benefit ration, be subject to an independent review through a designated IRB, include and assure informed consent of all participants, and maintain respect for all potential and enrolled participants. The authors believe that assurance of all of these requirements will assure that the clinical research proposed is ethical.

IRBs

According to Rosse and Garcia (2001), the function of the IRB is to protect the safety and welfare of patients who are participating in clinical trials by asking the following questions:

- "Do the benefits outweigh the risks?
- Is there adequate protection for the participants, including informed consent?
- Is the selection of participants equitable?" (p. 97)

In addition, IRBs are required to evaluate the scientific merits of the trial and to ensure that patient safety is maintained at all times.

A minimum of five individuals must be included in an IRB. These individuals must be from diverse backgrounds, race/ethnicities, and cultural perspectives, as well as include both genders. The IRB must include at least one nonmedical person and an additional person who has no direct relationship to the institution in which the trial will be conducted. Normal makeup of an IRB includes individuals such as physicians, nurses, pharmacists, ethicists, and clergy. In addition, those with special expertise may be included as either ad hoc or permanent members if the trials under review involve vulnerable populations (i.e., pregnant women, children, prisoners, or those who are cognitive impaired) or require specialized knowledge for accurate review.

IRBs must use the ethical principles of autonomy, beneficence, and justice to guide their reviews. The IRB must assure that the participant has voluntarily consented and signed an informed consent and that privacy and confidentiality are protected. In terms of beneficence, the IRB must assure that the benefits outweigh the potential risks to the participant, that the risks within the trial are minimized, and that any real or perceived conflicts of interest are appropriately managed. Finally, in relationship to the principle of justice, IRBs must assure that vulnerable populations are not targeted for inclusion because of convenience nor are those who might benefit from participation specifically and systematically excluded (Amdur, 2003).

INFORMED CONSENT

Daugherty (2000) described the informed consent as "a process of communication between a patient-subject and a clinician–investigator regarding an investigational or experimental protocol." (p. 78) The process includes both ongoing communication and the informed consent document that contains very specific components (**Table 15.5**), which serve to provide information about the trial while ensuring that the ethical principles needed to inform the potential participant fully about the conduct of a specific trial are incorporated.

The process of informed consent includes providing ongoing information about the clinical trial, including the objectives, rationale, study parameters, potential treatments, including their risks and benefits, and an ongoing dialogue of how the side effects will be managed or prevented. Factors that may impact the informed consent process include the timing of the discussion, the readability of the informed consent document, and who is available to advocate for and assist the patient in the informed consent process (Taylor, 1999; Lengacher et al., 2001). In addition, Taylor identified several additional patient factors that may affect informed consent, including the patient's physical and psychological status, the

Table 15.5 ELEMENTS OF THE INFORMED CONSENT DOCUMENT

Study title

Why is this study being done?

How many people will take part in the study?

What is involved in the study?

How long will I be in the study?

What are the risks of the study?

Are there benefits to taking part in the study?

What other options are there?

What about confidentiality?

What are the costs?

What are my rights as a participant?

Who do I call if I have questions or problems?

Where can I get more information?

Signatures

Ancillary study information with separate signatures

http://www.cancer.gov/clinicaltrials/conducting/informed-consent-guide/page1.

relationship between the provider and the patient, and potential blurring of the distinction between entering a clinical trial and receiving medical care for a life-threatening illness. Taylor also identified potential barriers that she called process-centered barriers, including the timing of the consent discussion, the time allocated for asking questions and making decisions about clinical trial participation, and readability and content of the informed consent. These latter barriers are of major concern because many organizations and institutions have specific information that they wish to include in the informed consent document and while incorporating this information may actually increase the reading level and therefore decrease the readability and understanding of the informed consent.

Specific concerns about the informed consent process are raised when vulnerable populations such as children, prisoners, pregnant women, the cognitively impaired, and the frail older people are considered for participation in a clinical trial. The potential for coercion constantly must be evaluated against the benefits from participation. Additionally, the potential for not being offered a trial that may be of benefit because of one's vulnerable position must be examined. In addition to parental consent for participation in a trial, children over the age of seven years must provide their assent. For the cognitively impaired, informed consent by proxy, in which those with legal power to make medical decisions for the patient, may occur; however, consent monitors may need to be present to assure the consent process is followed (Amdur, 2003) and a justification for offering the study to the particular participant must be included within the consent document (Klimaszewski, Anderson et al., 2000; Wendler & Prasad, 2001).

Meade (1999) provided specific suggestions for improving the understanding of the consent process and document. Among these are using principles of adult learning when developing and discussing the informed consent; evaluating the patient's literacy skills; using a variety of techniques to facilitate readability and comprehension of the document; simplifying the consent document and process verbiage by using plain language, being clear and concise, and summarizing concepts frequently; providing take-home materials about the trial, including a copy of the consent and protocol; and systematically evaluating the consent process and one's communication skills used in the consent discussion.

Nursing roles and responsibilities relative to the informed consent process are many and varied (Karigan, 2001; Rosse & Krebs, 1999). Rosse and Krebs divided the roles and responsibilities into those relevant to the informed consent document and those relevant to the consent process. The primary roles and responsibilities for the consent document focus on patient education, coordination, and advocacy, whereas the primary roles and responsibilities for the consent process focus on discussion, negotiation, advocacy, and problem solving.

Good (2003) stated that controversy exists over whether patients truly understand what is explained to them in the informed consent process and stated that nurses "have an obligation to stay abreast of informed consent issues and changes as well as ensure that patients are informed and making decisions appropriate to their needs." Providing information related to the informed consent must incorporate current knowledge that will help facilitate the patient's informed decision making while ensuring that the discussion and document are understandable to the potential participant are paramount. Joffe et al. (2001) have developed a standardized measure for assessing how adequately the informed consent document addresses the proposed research. The Quality of Informed Consent questionnaire measures both the actual and perceived understanding of the trial after informed consent. If understanding is less than optimal, additional information can be provided and questions asked and answered to assure that the consent to participate is truly an informed decision.

CONFLICT OF INTEREST

Much has been written about the potential for conflict of interest when the provider is also the principal investigator or actively involved in the conduct of a clinical trial. Cabriales (2000) defined conflict of interest in clinical research as "attempting to occupy dual roles that should not be performed together." (p. 221) The potential areas of conflict of interest include the situations in which the primary physician recommending the trial is also the investigator, leading to concerns of coercion in encouraging specific individuals to participate in a given trial, bias in those who are selected or not selected to be approached about participation, focusing on one trial over another, and the potential to exaggerate other patient's progress or status within a trial. An additional conflict may arise if the investigator is a member of the IRB that will review the trial, in which instance the investigator should recuse himself or herself from the discussion and voting. Particularly when financial incentives are involved, the potential for conflict of interest must be addressed. It should be noted that perceived conflict of interest, although different from actual conflict of interest, may be as important to patients, their families, other providers, and the scientific community at large as the existence of true conflict of interest. When the primary physician is also conducting the clinical trial, it is recommended that another healthcare provider should obtain the informed consent (Rakatansky et al., 2002).

GOOD CLINICAL PRACTICE

According to McFadden (1998), "The standards that define the conduct of clinical trials are known as the code of good clinical practice.... Good clinical practice represents standards by which clinical trials are designed, conducted, and reported insuring that the patients' rights have been protected throughout the course of the trial and that there is confidence in the integrity of the collected data and the published results of the trial." (p. 137) There are a variety of responsibilities that must be undertaken to assure good clinical practice at any given research site. Among these are IRB approval before trial implementation, fair and appropriate recruitment of patients to the trial, biases that are minimized, all eligible patients should be given the opportunity to participate and assurance that the potential participant has been accurately and fully informed and has consented to participate before study enrollment and the start of treatment. Additional responsibilities include assuring that protocol data are accurately collected and recorded, that adverse events are reported accurately and within the specified timeframes, and ensuring that there is compliance with all components (e.g., drug, dose, route, timing) of the protocol. Finally, there must be assurance of accurate ordering, storage, and administration of study compounds (McFadden, 1998).

Accrual and Adherence Issues

REPRESENTATION OF WOMEN, MINORITIES, AND THE UNDERSERVED

It has been noted that typical clinical trials participants are "white, have higher levels of education, are in the middle-to-upper socioeconomic class, and are male" (Lengacher et al., 2001, p. 1118). It has been well documented that minorities, the medically underserved, and women are less likely to be participants in a cancer clinical trial for a variety of sociocultural, economic, and logistical reasons. Although women were previously excluded from clinical trials because of the possibility of pregnancy and resulting teratogenetic and/or mutagenic complications, it has been suggested that many minorities and the underserved are not even offered the opportunity to participate in a clinical trial because of a perceived lack of interest or a lack of compliance on the part of the healthcare provider. In 2000, the sponsors of the Summit Series on Clinical Trials commissioned a survey of individuals with cancer to assess their participation in and beliefs about cancer clinical trials. Approximately 6,000 cancer patients were surveyed, including an over sample of Blacks and Hispanics. Study results showed that of those who responded to the poll, less than 25% recalled or knew that they had ever been talked with about cancer clinical trial participation. Of those who did not believe they had been approached, 75% said they would have considered participation had they known it was a possibility for the management of their cancers. An important finding, fewer minorities recalled discussing clinical trials with a provider, was that although interactive there were essentially no racial or ethnic differences in terms of willingness to consider participation (Harris, 2001) Additionally, a survey of participants in the National Native American Cancer Survivors' Support Network identified only five women from the network's first 100 members who had any type of discussion with their providers about a clinical trial. Significantly, the majority of cancer survivors attending the Native American Cancer Survivors/Thrivers Conference (N = 150+) did not understand the concept of a clinical trial, and only a few had been told about a trial as an option for their cancer treatment (Burhansstipanov, Gilbert, LaMarca, & Krebs, 2001).

The current National Institutes of Health policy, as mandated by the National Institutes of Health Revitalization Act of 1993, is that all clinical trials that are federally funded must include adequate numbers of women and minorities in the study population. Exclusion of a particular population must be clearly explained with appropriate rationale (e.g., a woman cannot by gender alone reasonably participate in a trial for those with prostate cancer). Outreach activities to assure inclusion are required, and a lack of finances is not a justifiable reason for exclusion (Collichio et al., 2001).

BARRIERS TO ACCRUAL

Barriers to accrual to clinical trials have been identified by numerous authors over the last 20 years. These barriers often are categorized into four different areas: barriers related to participants; providers; protocol or eligibility; and funding issues. Many of these barriers are overlapping, for if a patient is poor, he or she may be unable to afford transportation to participate in a clinical trial, or he or she may be perceived to be noncompliant, he or she may be culturally uncomfortable about participating in a clinical trial because of previous egregious experiences of his or her ethnic or racial group. Eligibility barriers have been the subject of much discussion (Clinical Trials Summits, personal communication), and methods to relax participant requirements without compromising the clinical trial currently are under investigation.

In addition to the well-known barriers of age, level of education, level of illness, and perception of treatment, many other factors may play a role in a decision to participate or remain in a clinical trial. Recent literature cites numerous patient-related barriers to recruitment (Amaro & de la Torre, 2002; Barker, 1992; Blumenthal, Sung Coates, Williams, & Liff, 1995; Bennet, 1993; Brawley, 1996; Brown, Fouad, Basen-Engquist, & Tortolero-Luna, 2000; Chen & Hawks, 1995; Chin, 1992; Clabots & Dolphin, 1992; Cornelius, Smith, & Simpson, 2002; Friedman et al., 1995; Giuiliano et al., 2000; Hodge, Weinmann, & Roubideaux, 2000; Joshi & Ehrenberger, 2001; Lengacher et al., 2001; McCabe, Varricchio, & Padberg, 1994; Merkatz et al., 1993; Millon-Underwood, Sands, & Davis, 1993; Musgrave, Allen, & Allen, 2002; Pinto, McCaskill-Stevens, Wolf, & Marcus, 2000; Ro, 2002; Swanson & Ward, 1995; Uba, 1992; Walters & Simoni, 2002). Included among these barriers are the following:

- A lack of knowledge about state-of-the-art cancer care
- A fear and distrust of the healthcare system
- A lack of access to cancer care trials
- Geographic isolation (distances from major treatment centers where phase I/II trials may be accessed)
- Socioeconomic factors such as age, education, income, family status, and lack of insurance
- Gender and race
- Fear of diagnostic tests, treatment, and treatment side effects (e.g., disfigurement, pain, nausea)
- Differing ethnic and cultural views of health and disease processes

Other barriers may be related to the type of cancer under study (the cancer may be less common in women or in a specific minority group), the site for the conduct of the study (Denver as opposed to a rural community hospital or clinic), or economic barriers to enrollment or protocol compliance (inability to travel or to pay for accommodations or medications) (Bennet, 1993;

Blumenthal et al., 1995; McCabe et al., 1994; Swanson & Ward, 1995). The literature also articulates additional barriers that may have particular cultural or ethnic relevance (Amaro & de la Torre, 2002; Barker, 1992; Blumenthal et al.; Bennet; Clabots & Dolphin, 1992; Cornelius et al., 2002; Frank-Stromborg & Rohan, 1992; McCabe et al.; Ro, 2002; Musgrave et al., 2002; Swanson & Ward; Uba, 1992; Walters & Simoni, 2002). These include the following:

- A delay of minority patients in seeking care and treatment until disease is in a later stage
- A lack of communication between communities of color and healthcare provider communities
- Information presented in a language that is not the first language of the targeted population
- Informed consent forms not written in the potential participant's first language or at an acceptable reading level
- The use of "traditional healers," herbal medicines, or complementary/alternative health practices before or during standard cancer care that may preclude or interfere with cancer care trial enrollment

Finally, barriers related to providers pose a major barrier to increased enrollment and must be addressed if changes to recruitment and retention are to be made. Included among these barriers are the following (Fromer, 2000; Glanz, Lewis, & Rimer, 1997; Karigan, 2000; Klein, 2000; Lengacher et al., 2001; Pinto et al., 2000):

- A lack of information about specific trials
- A lack of time to thoroughly discuss a trial
- A lack of staff for data management and support
- An inability to choose specific therapies
- Concerns about patient compliance
- Complicated protocols and consents
- A lack of access to trials in immediate practice area

- A loss of patients to other providers

STRATEGIES FOR ENHANCING ACCRUAL

What is probably much more important than listing all of the barriers that prevent individuals from participating in clinical trials is to identify strategies that may support a decision to participate in the clinical trial or for a provider to offer clinical trial to an individual. Less information is available about potential strategies to enhance accrual. However, a variety of strategies for both enhancing patient participation and assuring provider referrals have been postulated and include the following:

- Insure good communication between patients and providers and between referring physicians and those conducting the trial.
- Make consistent contact with participants and accommodate their needs whenever possible.
- Be culturally competent and have a good understanding of individual characteristics and cultural issues of those involved in trial.
- Involve special populations/ethnic/minority groups in the planning of the conduct of the clinical trial.
- Continually attempt to foster trust between minority participants and healthcare providers.
- Provide incentives and either small monetary incentives or small tokens of appreciation such as taxi cab vouchers, single-day bus passes, grocery store certificates, and telephone phone cards.
- Provide recognition for patient participation, including verbal thank yous, personal thank you notes, and formal thank you letters.
- Attempt flexible scheduling within confines of the trial and assist patients to meet trial schedule obligations.
- Conduct trials in facilities that are seen as trustworthy.

- Provide ongoing information to referring community providers and work with community providers to support patient follow-up.

FACTORS AND STRATEGIES ASSOCIATED WITH CLINICAL TRIAL RETENTION

As indicated by Davis and colleagues (2002) "Retention is defined as the continued involvement in a research project over the projected study duration." (p. 47) Numerous factors are correlated with remaining in the study, including such things as participant age, level of education, severity of illness, psychological distress, various sociocultural and demographic characteristics, and usual pattern of accessing and using healthcare facilities. In addition, in relationship to cancer clinical trials, the current rigors and complexities of trials influence an individual's decision to remain in the clinical trial (Ford, 2000). It is most common for participants to drop out of a trial in the first few months. In cancer treatment trials, the dropout rates appear to increase as treatment rigors and side effects increase, whereas in prevention trials, dropout rates increase as lengthy trials continue while the participant feels healthy or experiences side effects from treatments that focus on preventing a cancer that may never materialize. In order to enhance retention rates, a number of strategies have been put forth by Stasiewicz and Stalker (1999). They identified nine strategies to enhance retention:

- Establishing a project or trial identity through the use of stationery, logos, and other materials, thus ensuring that participants identify with the project and understand the project and its components. This may be particularly important for those enrolled in cancer control trials that tend to have long periods of treatment and follow-up during which participants may take treatments with or without side effects while having no evidence of any cancer-related disease.

- Emphasizing the significance of the study to participants has the potential to enhance retention through participant understanding of potential outcomes that may not be reached if there are significant numbers of dropouts.
- Conducting a run-in test will allow potential participants to gain some understanding of trial requirements and rigors before agreeing to take part in the full study. The concern with this strategy is the potential for decreasing the potential participant pool; however, this may be offset by the knowledge that the majority of individuals who agree to participate in the complete study are likely to complete all aspects of the study.
- Providing meaningful incentives has been shown to enhance retention even when the incentive is small. Among incentives that have been used are transportation vouchers, pay phone cards, grocery store coupons, or small (less than $25) monetary gifts.
- Developing an appealing control group treatment whenever possible so that the control group has some sense of actual meaningful participation in the trial.
- Maintaining contacts with participants between assessment contacts or visits enhances retention by promoting a sense of ongoing involvement and improving communication of issues that may be important to study outcomes.
- Providing interpersonal skills training for project staff enhances culturally appropriate communication between staff and participants and thus increases participant trust and fosters interactions about participant concerns/issues with the clinical trial.
- Individualizing data collection by being flexible with data-collection strategies (whenever possible, but without interfer-

ing with protocol compliance and quality) and assisting participants in scheduling appointments while working around their other obligations.
- Using a participant tracking database that includes a wide variety of methods to contact the patient will facilitate follow-up and data collection.

Ford (2000) identified additional strategies to enhance retention. These include the following:

- Patient reminders by phone, mail, or e-mail
- The use of protocol diaries or calendars to identify future protocol-related activities and to capture treatment medications and document treatment-related side effects
- Methods to minimize waiting for appointments and facilitate access to appointments
- Educational interventions to keep participants informed about the trial
- Consistent staff for treatment appointments, follow-up, and communications

Nursing Roles and Responsibilities

Nurses play pivotal roles in the facilitation of clinical trials and have many responsibilities that are vital to insure protocol compliance, accurate data collection, appropriate treatment administration, appropriate symptom management, and provide patient education and advocacy. Aiken (2000) identified five roles for nurses involved in clinical trials. These roles include research nurse, data manager, protocol treatment nurse, advanced practice nurse, and nurse researchers. These individuals may have a variety of different names and may also have roles that overlap or are consolidated to form a combined position. Whatever the name placed on the position or the combination of roles and responsibilities assigned to that position, each of the identified responsibilities is integral to the trial if the trial is to be completed under the code of good clinical practice. **Table 15.6** identifies nursing roles and responsibilities in the conduct of clinical trials.

The research nurse, also frequently identified as the clinical trials nurse, is responsible for the overall coordination of the clinical trial. The individual responsibilities of the research nurse may include patient recruiting, screening for clinical trial eligibility, managing medical and nursing-related participation issues, educating patient, family, and staff, administering treatment modalities, assuring compliance with protocol requirements, obtaining the informed consent and assisting with the informed consent process, and serving as a patient resource and advocate. A specific function of the research nurse is educating the staff and those involved in the administration of the clinical trials about the treatment and all components of the clinical trial protocol. Education of the staff includes assessment of current knowledge about the specific clinical trial and then specific educational interventions, including providing the objectives, rationale, and proposed treatment and follow-up plans for the trial, as well as providing protocol information materials, such as fact sheets, protocol summaries and schemas, and other instructions sheets that outline the essential components of the clinical trial. In addition, standing orders for symptom management and protocol treatment may be developed by the research nurse and, after approval of the trial's principal investigator, need to be a component of the clinical trials education process. After education, ongoing communication between the trained staff and the research nurse is crucial to assure protocol compliance.

Data managers are also known as clinical research associates. Although frequently a nurse,

Table 15.6 ROLES/RESPONSIBILITIES OF NURSES IN CLINICAL TRIALS RESEARCH*

Roles	Responsibilities
Research nurse/clinical trial nurse	Coordinates activities related to trial conduct including patient recruitment, adherence, and retention activities; participates in the informed consent process; educates patients, families, and staff about protocol; assures protocol compliance; may write treatment orders/establish standing orders; obtains and maintains IRB approval; patient advocate/resource
Data manager/clinical research associate	Collects and organizes all trial data, monitors accrual, provides reports, prepares for audits, may design forms for data collection, and may directly enter data into computer databases
Protocol treatment nurse	Administers treatment in compliance with protocol guidelines, communicates/collaborates with study team, and provides patient and family education; identifies and manages treatment-related symptoms; documents all aspects of treatment and reports any adverse events, patient advocate/resource
Advanced practice nurse	May function as research nurses, conduct patient evaluations, manage treatment, assess and manage symptoms/complications, promote clinical trials to others, consult with nurse researchers and treatment nurses, assist in new protocol development, and patient advocate/resource
Nurse researcher	Conducts companion studies in conjunction with current trials

* Depending on the institution, some roles may be combined.
Gullatte & Otto, 2001; Klimaszewski, Aiken et al., 2000.

depending on other clinical trials responsibilities, these individuals do not necessarily need to hold a nursing license. Data managers have the overall responsibility for gathering and organizing all data related to the trial, including evaluating original (or source) documents related to trial activities, entering data into case report forms or directly into computer programs, monitoring accrual, preparing audits, and assuring data quality through self-audits. Often the role of data manager and research nurse is combined, and the individual is identified as a clinical research associate. In this role, the nurse takes on not only the roles and responsibilities of the research nurse, including such activities as assessing toxicities and educating others about the clinical trial, but also maintains responsibility for ensuring that data are high quality and are accurately documented.

The protocol treatment nurse or oncology staff nurse has the responsibility for administering the relevant cancer treatment as outlined in the protocol. This nurse provides direct patient care, evaluates side effects and toxicities, provides education to patients and their families about potential side effects and management strategies, documents all of the aspects of the treatment process, and serves as both patient advocate and patient resource. These nurses are integral to the conduct of the trial and must be able to communicate and collaborate effectively with a clinical trials research team in order to ensure protocol compliance and quality cancer care outcomes for the patient (Edens & Safesak, 1998).

The advanced practice nurse may be either a nurse practitioner or a clinical nurse specialist. These individuals may have direct involvement in the conduct of clinical trials or may serve as consultants and collaborators with the protocol treatment nurse, research nurse, and data manager to assure appropriate management and care of patients undergoing a clinical trial. Responsibilities may include educating other healthcare providers about the clinical trial process or about a specific clinical trial, providing expert care in the

management of side effects and symptoms, educating staff about complex equipment and materials that will be used in a specific clinical trial, and/or providing direct patient care management to a patient who is participating in a clinical trial.

The final category is that of nurse researcher. The nurse researcher has an advanced degree and is responsible for conducting various types of clinical research. Clinical trials that nurse researchers conduct may include ancillary or companion studies, retrospective or secondary analyses of current data sets, or studies that are a subset of and are integral to the outcomes of the ongoing clinical trial. Ancillary independent studies are conducted prospectively along with the current clinical trial and may include evaluations of various aspects of quality of life or methods to manage an anticipated treatment-related side effect, whereas substudies are subcomponents of the overall trial. These trials often evaluate quality of life in relationship to the treatment under study.

Rice and Cheak (2000) noted that all nursing roles are vital to quality conduct of clinical trials. Because of role overlap and ambiguity, there may be conflict between the research nurse and the protocol treatment/oncology staff nurse, particularly if both have direct patient care responsibilities. They recommend that responsibilities be directly divided so that the research nurse has responsibility for those aspects of care that solely relate to the conduct of the trial (e.g., specific clinical procedures, treatment documentation, overseeing recruitment and obtaining the informed consent, and managing all protocol coordination and regulatory activities), whereas the oncology nurse facilitates the patient's complete care and serves as the patient's advocate. Ocker and Pawlik Plank (2000) further delineated these roles by identifying the function of the research nurse as protocol management with related patient care and the primary role of coordination of protocol activities, whereas the function of the protocol treatment nurse is in patient treatment management with primary responsibility for coordination of overall patient care.

Ambulatory Care Nurses

The role of the oncology nurse in managing clinical trials within the ambulatory care setting is complex. Many different issues face the nurse, who must provide expert care to the patient, all within the confines of the medical and nursing care parameters that the protocol mandated. The nurse has many roles in the management of the patient on a clinical trial, including such roles as administering treatments, providing education and ongoing information, participating in the informed-consent process, and facilitating adherence to protocol requirements for those who are only intermittently receiving care in the ambulatory care facility.

One of the most important roles of the ambulatory care nurse in providing care for a patient on a clinical trial is the thorough assessment and documentation of every aspect of care that the nurse provides. This includes information related to treatment administration, as well as assessment and documentation of expected and quite often unexpected side effects and toxicities. This role, in particular, is crucial in assuring that a complete picture of all aspects of the trial are understood and that adverse events are evaluated and catalogued for decisions about whether the treatment is of value and will be used in the future. Unfortunately, with patient care numbers and acuity at an all-time high, coupled with decreased numbers of registered nursing staff, it is often difficult for the nurse who has many patients, all with complex care, to assure that all of the assessments and documentation of events that occur with the patient on the clinical trial are adequately and accurately documented. Methods to assure understanding of this crucial role and strategies to facilitate assessment and documentation require that the ambulatory care nurse and the research team work closely together.

Another essential role of the ambulatory nurse is to facilitate adherence to the protocol. This is particularly difficult when the patient is seen only intermittently in the ambulatory care facility and

the nurse administering the protocol treatment is not always the same individual. Answering questions and providing the rationale for protocol requirements are essential for facilitating adherence. Providing comprehensive symptom management, communicating patient concerns, and advocating for quality care within the confines of the protocol are essential roles in enabling adherence and must be components of the care plan for the patient on a clinical trial in the ambulatory setting.

It is vital that the ambulatory care nurse receives complete information about the clinical trial. This information includes ongoing provision of specific protocol-related education, including protocol rationale, proposed treatments, administration issues, protocol follow-up requirements, and any new findings that might impact direct patient care, materials to facilitate providing patient education and answering questions, what to assess and document, who to directly communicate with about issues and concerns related to the protocol, and when and how to communicate this information. This requires the research team to consider and update constantly the ambulatory care staff who provide the treatments but may not have direct involvement with the team itself. Through collaboration, the ambulatory oncology nurse and the research team can make the complex care of the patient on a clinical trial much simpler while assuring that protocol is adhered to and that all necessary information is captured and documented.

It is essential that whatever the role and responsibilities, all nurses involved in the care of patients participating in a clinical trial collaborate and communicate effectively. These nurses are in the pivotal role of providing care, gathering data, assessing symptoms and toxicities, and providing ongoing care for protocol participants. Collaboration among all individuals is essential for assurance that all pertinent information necessary for final analysis and outcome determinations of the clinical trial is available.

Conclusion

Clinical trials are an essential component of quality cancer care. Unfortunately, too few eligible patients participate in clinical trials, prolonging the time to identify new treatments, methods, procedures, and devices that can be used to prevent, diagnose, treat, or manage cancer effectively. Efforts must be expended to increase participation while assuring that participants are fully informed and making informed decisions about participation relevant to their personal beliefs and values. The oncology nurse is pivotal to the clinical trial process, with responsibilities ranging from subject recruitment, informed consent, and patient and staff education to administering treatment medications, monitoring and documenting adverse events, and serving as the patients' advocate throughout the clinical trial process. Collaborating—as identified by Miller et al. (1997) and as evidenced by partnership, mutual respect and understanding, and effective communication that occurs laterally rather than hierarchically—is essential for quality research. As cancer treatment continues to be focused in the outpatient setting, the ambulatory oncology nurse will be even more integral to the clinical trial process, incorporating all aspects of his or her knowledge and skill to promote quality cancer care.

References

Aiken, J. L. (2003). Nursing roles in clinical trials. In S. E. Otto (Ed.), *Manual for Clinical Trials Nursing* (pp. 273–276). Pittsburgh: Oncology Nursing Press.

Amaro, H. & de la Torre, A. (2002). Public health needs and scientific opportunities in research of Latinas. *American Journal of Public Health, 92*, 525–529.

Amdur, R. (2003). Institutional Review Board Member Handbook (pp. 9–31). Sudbury, MA: Jones and Bartlett Publishers.

Barker, J. C. (1992). Cultural diversity—changing the context of medical practice. *Western Journal of Medicine, 157* (3-Special Issue, Cross cultural medicine - A decade later), 248–257.

Bennet, J. C. (1993). Inclusion of women in clinical trials - Policies for population subgroups. *New England Journal of Medicine, 329*, 288–292.

Blumenthal, D. S., Sung, J., Coates, R., Williams, J., & Liff, J. (1995). Mounting research addressing issues of race/ethnicity in health care. Recruitment and retention of subjects for a longitudinal cancer prevention study in an inner-city black community. *HSR: Health Services Research, 30*(1-April 1995, Part II), 197–205.

Brown, D. R., Fouad, M. N., Basen-Engquist, K., & Tortolero-Luna, G. (2000). Recruitment and retention of minority women in cancer screening, prevention, and treatment trials. *Annals of Epidemiology, 10* (8 Suppl), S13–S21.

Burhansstipanov, L., Gilbert, A., LaMarca, K., & Krebs, L. U. (2001). An innovative path to improving cancer care in Indian country. *Public Health Reports, 116*, 424–433.

Cabriales, S. (2000). Conflict of interest. In A.D. Klimaszewski, J. L. Aiken, M. A. Bacon, S. A. DiStasio, H. E. Ehrenberger, & B. A. Ford (Eds.), *Manual for Clinical Trials Nursing* (pp. 221–223). Pittsburgh: Oncology Nursing Press.

Chen, M. S. & Hawks, B. L. (1995). A debunking of the myth of healthy Asian Americans and Pacific Islanders. *American Journal of Health Promotion, 9*, 261–268.

Chin, S. (1992). This, that and the other. Managing illness in a first generation Korean-American family. *Western Journal of Medicine, 157*(3-Special Issue, Cross cultural medicine - A decade later), 305–309.

Chow, S. C. & Liu, J. P. (1998). *Designs and Analysis of Clinical Trials: Concepts and Methodologies* (pp. 1–46). New York: John Wiley & Sons.

Clabots, R. B. & Dolphin, L. (1992). The multilingual videotape project. Community involvement in a unique health education program. *Public Health Reports, 107*, 75–80.

Collichio, F., Griggs, J., & Rosenblatt, J. D. (2001). Basic concepts in drug development and clinical trials. In P. Rubin & J. P. Williams (Eds.), *Clinical Oncology: A Multidisciplinary Approach for Physicians and Students* (8th ed., pp. 160–167). Philadelphia: W.B. Saunders Company.

Cornelius, L. J., Smith, P. L., & Simpson, G. M. (2002). What factors hinder women of color from obtaining preventive health care? *American Journal of Public Health, 92*, 535–538.

Davis, L. L., Broome, M. E., & Cox, R. P. (2002). Maximizing retention in community-based clinical trials. *Journal of Nursing Scholarship, 34*, 47–53.

Daugherty, C. K. (2000). Informed consent, the cancer patient, and phase I clinical trials. In P. Angelos (Ed.), *Ethical Issues in Cancer Patient Care* (pp. 77–85). Norwell, MA: Kluwer Academic Publishers.

Ezekiel, E. J., Wendler, D., & Grady, C. (2000). What makes clinical research ethical? *JAMA, 283*, 2701–2711.

Ford, B. A. (2000). Compliance in clinical trials. In A. D. Klimaszewski, J. L. Aiken, M. A. Bacon, S. A. DiStasio, H. E. Ehrenberger, & B. A. Ford (Eds.), *Manual for Clinical Trials Nursing* (pp. 169–172). Pittsburgh: Oncology Nursing Press.

Frank-Stromborg, M. & Rohan K. (1992). Nursing's involvement in the primary and secondary prevention of cancer. *Cancer Nursing, 15*, 79–108.

Friedman, L. S., Simon, R., Foulkes, M., Friedman, L., Geller, N. L., Gordon, D. J. et al. (1995). Inclusion of women and minorities in clinical trials and the NIH Revitalization Act of 1993—The perspective of NIH clinical trialists. *Controlled Clinical Trials, 16*, 277–285

Fromer, M. J. (2000). Survey: Clinical trial participants report high degree of satisfaction with care received. *Oncology Times.*

Getz, K. & Borfitz, D. (2002). Informed consent: A guide to the risks and benefits of volunteering for clinical trials. Boston: CenterWatch.

Giuiliano, A. R., Mokuau, N., Hughes, C., Gortolero-Luna, G., Risendal, B., Ho, R. C. S. et al. (2000). Participation of minorities in cancer research: The influence of structural, cultural, and linguistic factors. *Annals of Epidemiology, 10* (8 Suppl), S22–S34.

Glanz, K., Lewis, B. F., & Rimer, B. K. (1997). *Health Behavior and Health Education: Theory, Research and Practice* (2nd ed., pp. 153–178). San Francisco: Jossey-Bass Publishers.

Good, M. J. (2003). Informed consent should include current issues. *Clinical Trials Nurses SIG Newsletter, 14*, 1, 2.

Green, S., Benedetti, J., & Crowley, J. E. (2003). *Interdisciplinary Statistics: Clinical Trials in Oncology* (2nd ed.). Boca Raton, FL: Chapman & Hall/ C. R. C.

Gullatte, M. M. & Otto, S. E. (2001). Cancer clinical trials. In S. E. Otto (Ed.), *Oncology Nursing* (4th ed., pp. 760–784). St. Louis, MO: C.V. Mosby.

Harris Interactive. (2001). *Health Care News, 1*, 3.

Hodge, F. S., Weinmann, S., & Roubideaux, Y. (2000). Recruitment of American Indians and Alaska Natives into clinical trials. *Annals of Epidemiology, 10* (8 Suppl), S41–S48.

Jemic, G. & Schi, P. (2000). Ethical considerations. In A. Cohen & J. Posner (Eds.), *A Guide to Clinical Drug Research* (2nd ed., pp. 113–125). Norwell, MA: Kluwer Academic Publishers.

Jenkins, J. (2001). Oncology nursing practice: The role of the nurse in support of progress in cancer treatment. In M. Barton-Burke, G. M. Wilkes, & K. Ingwerson (Eds.), *Cancer Chemotherapy: A Nursing Process Approach* (3rd ed., pp. 3–20). Sudbury, MA: Jones and Bartlett Publishers.

Joffe, S., Cook, E. F., Cleary, P. D., Clark, J. W., & Weeks, J. C. (2001). Quality of informed consent: A new measure of understanding among research subjects. *Journal of the National Cancer Institute, 93*, 139–147.

Joshi, T. G. & Ehrenberger, H. (2001). Cancer clinical trials in the new millennium: Novel challenges and opportunities for oncology nursing. *Clinical Journal of Oncology Nursing, 5*, 147–152.

Karigan, M. (2000). Obstacles to implementation. In A. D. Klimaszewski, J. L. Aiken, M. A. Bacon, S. A. DiStasio, H. E. Ehrenberger, & B. A. Ford (Eds.), *Manual for Clinical Trials Nursing* (pp. 63–66). Pittsburgh: Oncology Nursing Press.

Karigan, M. (2001). Ethics in clinical research. *American Journal of Nursing, 1001*, 26–31.

Kim, M. J. (2002). Ethics and clinical trials in a multicultural society. *Chart, 99*, 4, 6, 9.

Klein, J. (2000). Trial participation: Obstacles & misconceptions identified. *Oncology Times.*

Klimaszewski, A. D., Anderson, S., & Good, M. (2000). Informed consent. In A. D. Klimaszewski, J. L. Aiken, M. A. Bacon, S. A. DiStasio, H. E. Ehrenberger, & B. A. Ford (Eds.), *Manual for Clinical Trials Nursing* (pp. 213–219). Pittsburgh: Oncology Nursing Press.

Klimaszewski, A. D., Aiken, J. L., Bacon, M. A., DiStasio, S. A., Ehrenberger, H. E., & Ford, B. A. (2000). *Manual for Clinical Trials Nursing.* Pittsburgh: Oncology Nursing Press.

Krebs, L. U., Burhansstipanov, L., Bradley, A. M., & Gamito, E. *Clinical Trials Education for Colorado Providers 7Cs Curriculum.* (unpublished, work in progress, NCI, CA82714).

Lara, Jr., P. N., Higdon, R., Lim, N., Tanaka, M., Lau, D. H. M., Wun, T. et al. (2001). Prospective evaluation of cancer clinical trial accrual patterns: Identifying potential barriers to enrollment. *Journal of Clinical Oncology, 19*, 1728–1733.

Lengacher, C. A., Gonzalez, L. L., Giuliano, R., Bennett, M. P., Cox, C. E., & Reintgen, D. S. (2001). The process of clinical trials: A model for successful clinical trial participation. *Oncology Nursing Forum, 28*, 1115–1120.

McCabe, M. S., Varricchio, C. G., & Padberg, R. M. (1994). Efforts to recruit the economically disadvantaged to national clinical trials. *Seminars in Oncology Nursing, 10*, 123–129.

McFadden, E. (1998). *The Management of Data in Clinical Trials.* New York: John Wiley & Sons.

Meade, C. D. (1999). Improving the understanding of the informed consent process and document. *Seminars in Oncology Nursing, 15*, 124–137.

Merkatz, R. B., Temple, R., Sobel, S., Feiden, K., Kessler, D., & the Working Group on Women in Clinical Trials. (1993). Women in clinical trials of new drugs. A change in Food & Drug Administration policy. *New England Journal of Medicine, 394*, 292–296.

Miller, C., Johnson, J. L., Mackay, M., & Budz, B. (1997). The challenges of clinical nursing research: Strategies for successful conduct. *Clinical Nurse Specialist, 11*, 213–216.

Millon-Underwood, S., Sands, E., & Davis, M. (1993). Determinants of participation in state-of-the-art cancer prevention, early detection/screening and treatment trials among African Americans. *Cancer Nursing, 16*, 25–33.

Musgrave, C. F., Allen, C. E., & Allen, G. J. (2002). Spirituality and health for women of color. *American Journal of Public Health, 92*, 557–564.

Mulay, M. (2001). *A Step-By-Step Guide to Clinical Trials.* Sudbury, MA: Jones and Bartlett Publishers.

Ocker, B. & Pawlik Plank, D. M. (2000). The research nurse role in a clinic-based oncology research setting. *Cancer Nursing, 23*, 286–292.

Pinto, H. A., McCaskill-Stevens, W., Wolf, P., & Marcus, A. C. (2000). Physician perspectives on increasing minorities in cancer clinical trials: An Eastern Cooperative Oncology Group (ECOG) initiative. *Annals of Epidemiology: 2000, 10* (8 Suppl), S78–S84.

Portney, L. G. & Watkins, M. P. (2000). *Foundations of Clinical Research: Applications to Practice* (2nd ed.). Upper Saddle River, NJ: Prentice Hall Health.

Rakatansky, M. K., Riddick, F. A., Morse, L. J., O'Bannon, J. M. III, Goldrich, M. S., Ray, P. et al. (2002). Managing conflicts of interest in the conduct of clinical trials. *JAMA, 287*, 78–84.

Rice, J. & Cheak, T. L. (2000). The role of the nurse in hospital-based clinical research. *American Journal of Nursing, 100*, 24E–24G.

Ro, M. (2002). Moving forward: Addressing the health of Asian American and Pacific Islander women. *American Journal of Public Health, 92*, 516–519.

Rosse, P. A. & Garcia, M. T. (2001). Clinical trials. In R. A. Gates & R. M. Fink (Eds.), *Oncology Nursing Secrets* (pp. 97–102). Philadelphia: Henley & Belfus, Inc.

Rosse, P. A. & Krebs, L. U. (1999). The nurse's role in the informed consent process. *Seminars in Oncology Nursing, 15*, 116–123.

Sales, B. D. & Folkman, S. (Eds.). (2000). *Ethics in Research with Human Participants*. Washington, DC: American Psychological Association.

Smith, M. B. (2000). Moral foundations in research with human participants. In B. D. Sales & S. Folkman (Eds.), *Ethics in Research with Human Participants* (pp. 3–9). Washington, DC: American Psychological Association.

Swanson, G. M. & Ward, A. J. (1995). Recruiting minorities into clinical trials: Toward a participant-friendly system. *Journal of the National Cancer Institute, 87*, 1747–1759.

Stasiewicz, P. & Stalker, R. (1999). A comparison of three interventions on pretreatment dropout rates in an outpatient substance abuse clinic. *Addictive Behaviors, 24*, 579–582.

Taylor, H. A. (1999). Barriers to informed consent. *Seminars in Oncology Nursing, 15*, 89–95.

Uba, L. (1992). Cultural barriers to health care for Southeast Asian refugees. *Public Health Reports, 107*, 544–548.

Walters, K. L. & Simoni, J. M. (2002). Reconceptualizing native women's health: An "indigenist" stress-coping model. *American Journal of Public Health, 92*, 520–524.

Wendler, D. & Prasad, K. (2001). Core safeguards for clinical research in adults who are unable to consent. *Annals of Internal Medicine, 135*, 514–523.

Whittemore, R. & Grey, M. (2002). The systematic development of nursing interventions. *Journal of Nursing Scholarship, 34*, 115–120.

Works, C. R. (2000). Principles of treatment planning and clinical research. In C. Yarbro, M. H. Frogge, M. Goodman, & S. Groenwald (Eds.), *Cancer Nursing: Principles and Practice* (5th ed., pp. 259–271). Sudbury, MA: Jones and Bartlett Publishers.

Wujcik, D. & Fraser, M. C. (2000). The national cancer program. *Seminars in Oncology Nursing, 16*, 65–75.

Chapter 16

Symptom Management Programs: The Role of the Nurse in Ambulatory Care

Anna L. Schwartz

Lillian M. Nail

Introduction

Symptom management is an important element of nursing care that is provided to many different chronically ill populations in a variety of settings. In the ambulatory care setting, diabetes care was one of the earliest models of a nurse-run specialty clinic that included symptom management as a component of care (Backscheider, 1974). The diabetes care model has been extended to include computer-based monitoring services with nurse follow-up, an innovation built on the availability of new technologies that allow frequent monitoring without requiring face-to-face contact (Piette, Weinberger, Kraemer, & McPhee, 2001). Examples of other chronic illnesses with symptom-focused specialty nursing clinics include wound care, clotting problems, lipid disorders, inflammatory bowel disease, and neurologic disease (Connor, Wright, & Fegan, 2002; Crumbley, Ice, & Cassidy, 1999; Nightingale, Middleton, Middleton, & Hunter, 2000; Wahlquist, 1984).

Perhaps the most enduring model of outpatient symptom management by nurses caring for people with cancer originated in home care and continues today, primarily in end-of-life care. In their review of the research on home care for people with cancer, Milone-Nuzzo and McCorkle

(2001) pointed to the positive effect of nursing care on patient symptoms and function. Recognition of the important role that symptoms play in quality of life has encouraged the development of programs of research on symptom management and new ways of thinking about conceptualizing, measuring, preventing, and treating symptoms (Dodd et al., 2001). As symptom management continues to gain acceptance as a component of care during all phases of cancer experience, the integration of symptom-focused nursing care into active treatment settings and follow-up care will continue to expand.

Despite the long history of symptom management in oncology nursing practice, barriers to nurse-run practices remain. The public may not view nurses as primary resources for cancer symptom management; symptom management appears to be restricted to end-of-life care issues rather than side effects of active treatment and may cause other providers to have concern about competition for professional fees and practice resources. Additional challenges to building a symptom-management practice include funding, marketing, building and maintaining collaborative relationships, having regulatory compliance, obtaining backup coverage, establishing referral links, managing the practice, and acquiring space.

History

Several factors have influenced the development of nurse-run specialty clinics. The introduction of advanced practice nurses into oncology care, which began in the 1960s with the oncology clinical nurse specialist, was a critical element. The faculty practice movement that began in the mid-1970s brought an academic perspective to the emerging models of nurse-run specialty clinics. This perspective expanded the mission of the practices to include serving as a clinical laboratory for students and as a research resource (Fagin, 2000; Taylor & Marion, 2000). The preparation of oncology nurse practitioners in the 1980s added new dimensions to the role of the advanced practice nurse in cancer care. The availability of prescriptive practice for clinical nurse specialists and nurse practitioners in some states enhanced the services available to their clients. Both clinical nurse specialists and nurse practitioners provide symptom-management services in various cancer care settings within the direct care component of their respective roles (Brown, 2000). Examples of practice models in place today include the institution-based consultant model, the practice partner model, the independent practice model, and the institution-based nurse clinic model (Barger, 2001; Bruera et al., 2001; Escalante et al., 2001; Loftus & Weston, 2001). Patients may be seen for a one-time consultation, episodically depending on need, or regularly as part of an interdisciplinary team managing ongoing care, within the protocol of a case manager role; an advanced practice nurse may become the main provider of cancer care.

Issues in Developing Nurse-Run Symptom-Focused Clinics

Multiple issues can affect the success of a nurse-run clinic. The first is securing adequate funding for start up and then developing self-sustaining programs. Another significant issue that must be negotiated and developed is administrative support from the referring clinics and hospitals and an ability to bill for services and ultimately receive insurance reimbursement (Dougherty & Keller, 2000).

Challenges that are manageable but may be ongoing include developing an educated and independent staff that collaborates well with other healthcare providers and knows when referral is appropriate. A key to success may be a network of providers who refer patients into the clinic and specialists who refer patients out of the clinic. Developing this type of referral network happens over time, but at the inception of a clinic, lines of care for physical medicine, psychiatry, nutrition, neurology, physical therapy, and other common referral patterns must be established unless the clinic has specialists who are available to see patients on certain days of the week or month. Having a physician for backup in case a patient needs to be admitted or evaluated is extremely important; this individual may also be important in assisting with periodic long-term evaluation of patients who have challenging medical problems that do not respond to usual or creative management approaches.

The location of a clinic is an important feature related to not only visibility but also to accessibility for patients. An ideal symptom-management or long-term survivor clinic setting may be adjacent to a medical oncology suite, where medical backup is available in an emergency and access to laboratory, radiology, and other clinical services is convenient for both the nurse provider and the patient.

State licensing laws and policy have a direct impact on the extent of care that nurses provide in symptom-management clinics (Simpson, 2002). For example, some states do not have or restrict prescriptive practice for advanced practice nurses to certain classes of drugs, whereas others have liberal prescriptive practice laws that facilitate the provision of more comprehensive care. In states with liberal nurse practice acts, it may be reasonable to establish protocols for certain procedures that may be conducted in the clinic. Developing these protocols or guidelines in collaboration with a consulting physician may permit a broader range of offered services while permitting the collaborating or referring physicians to feel comfortable with the level of care that the clinic is providing. Nurses who are able to admit and care for patients in the hospital could provide a spectrum of services in collaboration with other medical specialists.

The Future of Ambulatory Cancer Care

Many types of nurse-run clinics may evolve, including symptom-focused clinics, late-effects or cancer survivor clinics, cognitive function clinics, rehabilitation clinics, and nurse-run administrative systems using telemedicine-type clinics for rural outreach and home-based care. With the rapid escalation of computer technology, Internet- and computer-based education will have more use for both patients and professionals so that side-effects and symptoms can be prevented during treatment and symptoms can be managed if they occur (Wilke et al., 2001). Of course this approach to patient management is limited to patients and facilities with computer and Internet access.

Our current healthcare model treats symptoms after they have occurred and often become problematic. The ideal goal for the future of nursing in ambulatory care is to be able to prevent symptoms before they occur. Although this may seem somewhat unrealistic and idealistic, statistical prediction models may be developed to help anticipate and identify which patient is the most likely to experience a particular side effect or symptom and how severe it may become. With this information, preventive strategies or early intervention plans can be implemented, ideally minimizing patient discomfort and overall cost to the healthcare system and society.

Technology is a strong factor in setting the future direction of nursing care in ambulatory care. Technological advances may help patients and providers become more aware and able to use techniques for early intervention. Computer and Internet-based programs will be available to help patients report their symptoms and learn a variety of skills to manage their symptoms (Wilke et al., 2001). These patient reports of side effects and symptoms may even be linked to a patient's medical record and may generate reports to inform an advanced practice nurse or physician of the patients current side-effect profile and suggest effective pharmacologic and nonpharmacologic treatment options. Computer programs can also be developed to link a patient's current medications and known allergies to a symptom report, which could then give a healthcare provider a directed, specific, and individualized management plan. Clearly, a one-size-fits-all computer program will not work for every patient, but it may be a means for healthcare providers to provide more easily state of the science evidence-based medicine.

Communication will be a critical component of a successful symptom prevention program. This includes communication in real time with people at the facility by telemedicine, tele-education, telecare, and Internet-based telesystems. Teleprograms may be broadcast via satellite to high-definition televisions that are available to medical staff through a local network. Telecommunication could be used to review patient electrocardiograms, labs, and radiographic scans. Internet-based telemedicine systems are being tested to improve healthcare in rural areas and for patients who need immediate access to an expert for a specialized consultation (Lowery, Hamill, Wilkins, & Clements, 2002). The Internet-based system allows a healthcare provider to see a patient or receive data from a patient and then transmit the data to a Website where a nurse, physician, or specialist could review the data and communicate back to the originating site.

References

Backscheider, J. E. (1974). Self-care requirements, self-care capabilities, and nursing systems in the diabetic nurse management clinic. *American Journal of Public Health, 64,* 1138–1146.

Barger, S. E. (2001). Nursing centers: A fit for the future. In N. Chaska (Ed.), *The Nursing Profession: Tomorrow and Beyond* (pp. 631–641). Thousand Oaks, CA: Sage.

Brown, S. J. (2000). Direct clinical practice. In A. B. Hamric, J. A. Spross, & C. M Hanson (Eds.), *Advanced Nursing Practice: An Integrative Approach* (2nd ed., pp. 137–182). Thousand Oaks, CA: Sage.

Bruera, E., Michaud, M., Vigano, A., Neumann, C. M., Watanabe, S., & Hanson, J. (2001). Multidisciplinary symptom control clinic in a cancer center: A retrospective study. *Support Care Cancer, 9,* 162–168.

Connor, C. A., Wright, C. C., & Fegan, C. D. (2002). The safety and effectiveness of a nurse-led anticoagulant service. *Journal of Advanced Nursing, 38,* 407–415.

Crumbley, D. R., Ice, R. C., & Cassidy, R. (1999). Nurse-managed wound clinic. A case study in success. *Nursing Case Management, 4,* 168–177.

Dodd, M., Janson, S., Facione, N., Faucett, J., Froelicher, E. S., Humphreys, J. et al. (2001). Advancing the science of symptom management. *Journal of Advanced Nursing, 33,* 668–676.

Dougherty, S. A. D. & Keller, J. M. (2000). Marketing and contracting considerations. In A. B. Hamric, J. A. Spross, & C. M. Hanson (Eds.), *Advanced Nursing Practice: An Integrative Approach* (2nd ed., pp. 655–677). Thousand Oaks, CA: Sage.

Escalante, C. P., Grover, T., Johnson, B. A., Harle, M., Guo, H., Mendoza, T. R. et al. (2001). A fatigue clinic in a comprehensive cancer center: Design and experiences. *Cancer, 15*(Suppl. 6), 1708–1713.

Fagin, C. M. (2000). Institutionalizing faculty practice. In C. M. Fagin (Ed.), *Essays on Nursing Leadership* (pp. 159–170). New York: Springer.

Loftus, L. A. & Weston, V. (2001). The development of nurse-led clinics in cancer care. *Journal of Clinical Nursing, 10,* 215–220.

Lowery, J. C., Hamill, J. B., Wilkins, E. G., & Clements, E. (2002). Technical overview of a web-based telemedicine system for wound assessment. *Advances in Skin & Wound Care, 15,* 165–169.

Milone-Nuzzo, P. & McCorkle, R. (2001). Home care. In B. R. Ferrell & N. Coyle (Eds.), *Textbook of Palliative Nursing* (pp. 543–555). New York: Oxford University Press.

Nightingale, A. J., Middleton, W., Middleton, S. J., & Hunter, J. O. (2000). Evaluation of the effectiveness of a specialist nurse in the management of inflammatory bowel disease (IBD). *European Journal of Gastroenterology Hepatology, 12,* 967–973.

Piette, J. D., Weinberger, M., Kraemer, F. B., & McPhee, S. J. (2001). Impact of automated calls with nurse follow-up on diabetes treatment outcomes in a Department of Verterans Affairs Health Care System: A randomized controlled trial. *Diabetes Care, 24,* 202–208.

Simpson, S. L. (2002). Issues in telemedicine: Why is policy still light-years behind technology? *Nursing Administration Quarterly, 26,* 81–84.

Taylor, D. & Marion, L. (2000). Innovative practice models: Uniting advanced practice nursing and education. In A. B. Hamric, J. A. Spross, & C. M Hanson (Eds.), *Advanced Nursing Practice: An Integrative Approach* (2nd ed., pp. 795–831). Thousand Oaks, CA: Sage.

Wahlquist, G. I. (1984). Impact of nurse managed clinic in multiple sclerosis. *Journal Neurosurgical Nursing, 16,* 193–196.

Wilke, D. J., Huang, H., Berry, D. L., Schwartz, A., Lin, Y., Ko, N. et al. (2001). Cancer symptom control: Feasibility of a tailored interactive computerized program for patients. *Family & Community Health, 24,* 48–62.

Chapter 17

Integrating Complementary and Alternative Medicine Therapies into an Oncology Practice: A Short History of Medicine

Georgia Decker

2000 B.C. — "Here, eat this root."

1000 A.D. — "That root is heathen. Say this prayer."

1850 A.D. — "That prayer is superstition. Drink this potion."

1940 A.D. — "That potion is snake oil. Swallow this pill."

1985 A.D. — "That pill is ineffective. Take this antibiotic."

2000 A.D. — "That antibiotic doesn't work anymore. Here, eat this root."

Author unknown

Introduction

From an historical perspective, alternative therapies have been defined "as practices that are not accepted as correct, proper or appropriate or are not in conformity with the beliefs or standards of the dominant group of medical practitioners in a society" (Gevitz, 1988, p. 1). These therapies encompass a spectrum of practices and beliefs (Murray & Rubel, 1992). In 1993, Eisenberg and colleagues defined alternative therapies as interventions that are neither taught widely in medical schools nor generally available in hospitals. This is no longer true, as more medical schools offer complementary and alternative medicine in their curricula. A recent survey of courses involving complementary and alternative medicine (CAM) therapies at U.S. medical schools was published in the 1998 *Journal of the American Medical Association* theme issue devoted to medical education (Wetzel, Eisenberg, & Kaptchuk, 1998). This article reported that 64% of the U.S. medical schools offer courses on CAM. Common topics included chiropractics, acupuncture, homeopathy, herbal therapies, and mind–body techniques. Ernst and colleagues (1995) contended that "complementary medicine is diagnosis, treatment and/or prevention which complements mainstream medicine by contributing to a common whole, by satisfying a demand not yet met by orthodoxy or by diversifying the conceptual frameworks of medicine" (p. 506). Current terminology used to describe these practices remains controversial. The term integrative medicine is being used with increased frequency. Several authors have addressed the challenges of labeling and describing this field (Kaptchuk & Eisenberg, 1998; Jonas, 1998; Angell & Kassirer, 1998). According to Eisenberg and colleagues (Letter, 1993b), commonly used labels (e.g., alternative or unconventional) are judgmental and inhibit collaborative research and the communication that is necessary to differentiate useful techniques from those that are useless. CAM is the language that the National Institutes of Health uses to describe this field. **Table 17.1** describes seven categories of CAM.

Until recently, relatively little was known about the safety, efficacy, cost, and mechanism of action of individual CAM therapies. Survey findings confirm the extensive use of those therapies in the United States and internationally, and peer-reviewed medical literature is increasingly including consensus conferences, systematic reviews, case studies, and randomized trials involving CAM therapies. In November 1998, the *Journal of the American Medical Association* and American Medical Association specialty journals published more than 80 articles that were devoted to CAM. Contained in these articles are those that suggest efficacy (Stephinson, Pittler, & Ernst, 2000; Linde et al., 1997; LeBars et al., 1997; Spiegel, Bloom, Kraemer, & Gottheil, 1989) and those that suggest a lack of efficacy (Park, White, & Ernst, 2000; Shlay et al., 1998).

CAM therapies have documented popularity for more than a decade. A 1998 study reported that physicians who were surveyed estimated that approximately 5% of patients are using CAM therapies (Landmark Healthcare, Inc., 1997). This same study reported that 40% of the U.S. population was regularly using CAM. Eisenberg, Kessler, and collegues (1993a) reported that in 1990, 60-million (33.8%) Americans used "alternative" therapies, with an out-of-pocket cost of approximately $14.6 billion. In 1997, this survey was replicated, with results revealing 83-million Americans (42.1%) spending $21.2 billion out of pocket on these therapies (Eisenberg et al., 1998). Historically, patients who sought alternatives were stereotyped as terminally ill, less educated, and members of cult-like groups. These surveys demonstrated that those seeking CAM therapies are primarily college-educated women who are between the ages of 35 and 49 years and who have annual incomes of more than $50,000 (Eisenberg

et al., 1993a). In 1990 and 1997, the most commonly used alternative therapies in both surveys included chiropractics, massage therapy, and relaxation techniques. The largest increases were seen in the use of herbal medicine (380%) and megavitamins (130%), with significant increases in the use of massage, self-help groups, folk remedies, energy healing, and homeopathy (Eisenberg et al., 1998).

1. The total visits to CAM providers (629 million) exceeded the total visits to all primary care physicians (386 million) in 1997.

2. More than 40% of those who used alternative therapies never mentioned it to their physicians.

3. The estimated expenditures for CAM for professional services increased by 45%, exclusive of inflation, and in 1997 were estimated at $21.2-billion dollars.

4. Out-of-pocket expenditures for CAM professional services in 1997 were estimated at $12.2 billion (this exceeded the out-of-pocket expenditures for all U.S. hospitalizations).

5. The current use of CAM services is likely to underrepresent use patterns if insurance coverage for CAM therapies increases in the future (Eisenberg, Kessler et al., 1993a; Eisenberg, Delblanco et al., 1993b; Eisenberg et al., 1998; Eisenberg, 2001a).

These therapies represent choice and control for many who are frustrated with and distrustful of traditional medicine. It is important to remember that these patients are not refugees from conventional therapy; rather, they value and seek a holistic patient-centered approach to their healthcare. In 1997, Eisenberg reported that those using CAM therapies tended to use more than one, and more than 70% of those who acknowledged using CAM therapies never mention it to their physicians.

Table 17.1 SEVEN CATEGORIES OF COMPLEMENTARY AND ALTERNATIVE MEDICINE

Categories	Description	Examples	Comments/Controversies
Alternative system of medical care	Stresses the prevention of disease and the promotion of health, including personal responsibility, and emphasizes self-healing	Traditional Chinese Medicine Naturopathy Ayurvedic medicine	These systems are a way of being and a way of living. They are not meant to be parceled into individual or separate modalities. However, Western medicine has begun to incorporate various aspects of these modalities.
Mind–body medicine	Known as behavioral medicine; unites biomedical, behavioral, and psychological strategies for the promotion of health	Meditation Guided imagery Visualization Relaxation Spirituality Art therapies Music therapy Biofeedback Yoga	Controversies exist over whether mind–body interventions prolong survival or merely enhance the quality of life and the sense of feeling healed. Imagery and visualization have been used by patients with cancer for relief of treatment- and disease-related symptoms, including pain control. Concerns have been raised regarding the use of guided imagery when patients have a psychiatric history. The idea that mental efforts can alter the course of cancer has not been proven by research and may induce feelings of guilt and inadequacy in patients whose diseases progress despite their best efforts.

(continues)

Table 17.1 SEVEN CATEGORIES OF COMPLEMENTARY AND ALTERNATIVE MEDICINE (CONT'D)

Categories	Description	Examples	Comments/Controversies
Bioelectromagnetic therapies	Based on the use of energy as a healing modality	Acupuncture Magnet therapy Cymatics	The contemporary use of magnets has stimulated discussion and research regarding the claims made that magnets reduce pain and may have health-promoting benefits. Acupuncture (taken from traditional Oriental medicine) has proven to be helpful for a variety of symptoms and is now recognized and accepted for pain relief.
Herbal medicine	Based on the Doctrine of Signatures, which states that a plant's characteristics or appearance provides a clue to medicinal implications	Herbs may be used as single agents or in combination. Examples of herbal remedies used to treat cancer are Essiac and Pau d'arco tea	Patients believe that "natural means safe" and that "if a little is good a lot is better." The concern for all patients is that possible and potential herb–drug interactions have been identified. More information about this will become available. To report an adverse event call 1-888-SAFE-FOOD or access the Website at http://www.fda.gov/medwatch/partner.htm. Because herbs are not regulated or standardized, safety issues related to these products must be scrutinized.

Table 17.1 SEVEN CATEGORIES OF COMPLEMENTARY AND ALTERNATIVE MEDICINE (CONT'D)

Categories	Description	Examples	Comments/Controversies
Pharmacological and biological therapies	Most often used as an alternative and has been described as having the "lure of the cure".	Laetrile Shark cartilage Oxidative therapies Antineoplastons PC-SPES (combination of 14 herbs for prostate cancer patients)	The concern with these therapies has always been that the patient will implement them instead of conventional therapies. Because we do not know many of the components of these therapies, any risk associated with use as a single agent or in combination therapy has yet to be identified.
Diet, nutrition, and lifestyle changes	Use of food or other supplements to prevent and treat illness. These therapies appeal to patients because they can be initiated immediately and patients have control over them.	Macrobiotics Gerson Program Kelley-Gonzalez High-dose vitamin therapies Antioxidants	Some of the controversies are related to the risk of malnutrition with restrictive dietary programs, effects of antioxidants and/or vitamins during certain therapies, and effects of soy in certain cancers.
Manual healing methods	Usually involve touch and are often thought of as complementary therapies	Reiki Chiropractics Reflexology Massage Therapeutic touch (actually a misnomer since actual touch is not involved).	Although touch is usually desirable, especially in our culture, the kind of touch has important implications. For example, the role of deep massage when there is risk of metastases has recently become controversial. Controversies related to the effect of therapeutic touch have been raised; however, it remains a very popular complementary therapy.

Reprinted with permission Gates, R. A. & Fink, R. M. (2001).

In Eisenberg and collegues (2001) recent publication describing perceptions about CAM therapies among adults who used both, the authors found the following:

- Seventy-nine percent perceived the combination of CAM and conventional care to be superior to either alone.
- Seventy percent saw a medical doctor before or at the same time as CAM provider visits.
- Sixty-three to 72% did not disclose CAM therapy use to their medical doctor.

Reasons for this nondisclosure include the following:

- Sixty-one percent reported that it was not important for the doctor to know.
- Sixty percent said that the doctor never asked.
- Thirty-one percent said that it was not the doctor's business.
- Twenty percent reported that the doctor would not understand.
- Fourteen percent felt their doctor would disapprove or discourage CAM use.

There is a concern with the interchangeable use of the terms complementary and alternative. In many surveys, subjects are typically asked about their use of these therapies without clarifying their understanding of these terms. It is the intent with which a therapy is used that describes it. Complementary describes a therapy that is used (to complement) with a conventional therapy, whereas alternative describes a therapy that is used instead of conventional therapy (Position of the Oncology Nursing Society (ONS), 2000; Cassileth & Chapman, 1996). Integrative care is more of a contemporary term and describes a combination of complementary and allopathic approaches to care.

Most complementary and alternative practitioners are family physicians, and typically, oncologists are not familiar with these therapies (Cassileth & Chapman, 1996). Studies that surveyed the use of CAM by patients with cancer revealed that a significant number, including those on clinical trials, use CAM (Richardson, Sanders, Palmer, Greisinger, & Singletary, 2000; Sparber et al., 2000; Cassileth, 1999; Cassileth & Chapman, 1996; Kaptchuk & Eisenberg, 1998; Montbriand, 1994; Mooney, 1987). Kaptchuk and Eisenberg (1998) have estimated that up to 85% of patients with cancer have at least considered CAM for the treatment of their disease and most often did not discuss this with their physician. In a 2000 study that surveyed 46 men receiving radiation therapy for prostate cancer, 37% used one or more complementary therapies during traditional therapy (Kao & Devine, 2000). A study presented at the 11th International Conference in Women's Health Issues reported that more than 70% of breast cancer survivors used at least one type of complementary therapy (Boon et al., 2000). **Tables 17.2** and **17.3** describe the use of CAM therapies by patients in clinical trials.

In 1992, the National Institutes of Health established the Offices of Alternative Medicine. The National Institutes of Health Center for Complementary and Alternative Medicine (NIH-NCCAM) was created in 1998 to "facilitate the evaluation of alternative medical treatment modalities" to determine their effectiveness (http://www.nccam.nih.gov). The NCCAM does not serve as a referral agency for CAM treatments or practitioners. It does conduct and support basic

---

Table 17.2 CAM/CLINICAL TRIALS RESEARCH

Eighty-two percent of patients surveyed used CAM at some time of their lives.

Fifty-seven percent of patients surveyed used CAM before and after cancer diagnosis.

Eighteen percent of patients surveyed did not use CAM before cancer diagnosis but did afterward.

Twelve percent of patients surveyed did use CAM before their cancer diagnosis but not afterward.

Source: Sparber et al., 2000.

and applied research and training and disseminates information on CAM to practitioners and the public (*http://www.nccam.nih.gov.*) Until recently, adequate research to establish safety and efficacy of most CAM therapies was reported to be lacking. Currently, a significant number of CAM research studies have been completed or are in progress at designated research centers, as well as at hospitals and academic institutions.

The NCCAM has generated interest in CAM research (Muscat, 2001). A 1998 issue of the *Journal of the American Medical Association* published the results of randomized, controlled clinical trials for a number of CAM therapies (Alternative Medicine, 1998). On July 13, 2000, President Clinton announced the appointments of a chair and members of the White House Commission on CAM policy. The group's mandate was "to develop legislative and administrative recommendations that would help public policy maximize potential benefits, to consumers and American health care, of complementary and alternative medicine (CAM) therapies—chiropractic, acupuncture, massage, herbs, and nutritional and mind-body therapies..." (Gordon, 2002, p. 1). The commission was to address specifically the following:

- "Education and training of healthcare practitioners in CAM
- Consideration of research to increase knowledge about CAM products
- Provision of reliable and useful information on CAM to healthcare professions

---

Table 17.3 CAM/CLINICAL TRIALS RESEARCH

Most Frequently Used Therapies After Diagnosis

Spirituality	Exercise
Relaxation	Lifestyle/Diet
Imagery	Supplements

Source: Sparber et al., 2000.

- Provision of guidance on the appropriate access to and delivery of CAM" (Gordon, p. 1).

There is increasing scientific research supported by acceptable methods, as well as anecdotal evidence and case studies that suggest the efficacy of these therapies (Eisenberg, 2001b). Ernst and colleagues (1995, p. 506), contended that complementary medical techniques "[complement] mainstream medicine by contributing to a common whole, by satisfying a demand not met by orthodoxy or by diversifying the conceptual frameworks of medicine." Oncology patients have reported that CAM therapies help to relieve the side effects of traditional cancer therapies (Shrock, Palmer, & Taylor, 1999). However, most oncology practices are not successfully integrating complementary therapies even though there are benefits for patients, improved patient satisfaction, and improved patient–doctor communication (Olendick et al., 2000).

Strategies for CAM Program Development

How to Begin: Assessment

Administrators may be reluctant to establish a CAM program because they lack practitioner accpetance. Practitioners who do not know about CAM will be understandably reluctant to recommend or prescribe them; however, now that patients (as consumers) are demanding access to these therapies and insurance companies are beginning to cover certain therapies, practitioners are being asked to recommend and/or prescribe them. Surveying patients and families as well as practitioners within a catchment area will provide documentation of interest and can establish priorities for program development.

Consider the following:

- What is the size of your institution/practice (patients, staff, potential space)?

- What is your catchment area?
- Are there any other programs that look like/sound like a CAM program?
- Were there any such programs? If they no longer exist, why?
- What do you have for start-up revenue?
- How do we develop an assessment survey (see **Figures** 17.1–17.3)?
- Do you have a program champion? Champions?

- Have you developed a model that is congruent with your institution/practice?

Developing a questionnaire to assess interest need not be a complicated or protracted process. Dissemination of a survey to the intended group and providing an envelope for return allow for anonymity (when indicated) and can encourage a higher rate of return. Conducting individual, confidential interviews is another strategy that may

---

Figure 17.1 SAMPLE INTERNAL CAM INTEREST SURVEY

APN	__
RN	__
MD	__
MSW	__
RD	__
Volunteer	__

What do you consider to be the most important therapies to be included in a / any Complementary Therapies Program? Choose from the list below or write suggestions in designated space:

Immediately:

Later:

__ Acupuncture	__ Fatigue Management	__ Music Therapy
__ Aromatherapy	__ Guided Imagery	__ Non-pharmacological pain
__ Biofeedback	__ Herbs	management
__ Cancer Risk Reduction	__ Hypnotherapy	__ Nutrition/Supplements
__ Chiropractic	__ Image Therapy: wigs,	__ Reiki
__ Counseling	prosthesis, cosmetics	__ Relaxation
__ Creative Arts	__ Lymphedema (maintenance)	__ Self-help
__ Energy Therapies	__ Massage	__ Smoking Cessation
__ Exercise	__ Meditation	__ Yoga
	__ Mind-Body	

Should the therapies be available to the staff as well as the patients and families?

How important is access to a Complementary Therapies Program to your practice/department?

Do you personally use any complementary/alternative medicine (CAM) therapies?

Which ones?

Additional comments/ suggestions?

Figure 17.2 SAMPLE ADDITIONAL QUESTIONNAIRE FOR STAFF

To prepare for the start-up of our Integrated Care Program, the planning committee and advisory council will schedule a series of CE/CME programs. You can help us <u>plan</u> these programs by completing the following questions:

Please rank the following topics according to your <u>personal</u> level of interest *(or list the top 10 CAM therapies determined by your assessment survey):*

__Acupuncture	__Fatigue Management	__Music Therapy
__Aromatherapy	__Guided Imagery	__Non-pharmacological pain
__Biofeedback	__Herbs	management
__Cancer Risk Reduction	__Hypnotherapy	__Nutrition/ Supplements
__Chiropractic	__Image Therapy: wigs,	__Reiki
__Counseling	prosthesis, cosmetics	__Relaxation
__Creative Arts	__Lymphedema (maintenance)	__Self-help
__Energy Therapies	__Massage	__Smoking Cessation
__Exercise	__Meditation	__Yoga
	__Mind-Body	

High Interest   Medium Interest   Low/No Interest

What time of day is best for you for an educational program?

7:00–8:30AM _____
12 Noon–2PM _____
4:30–6:30PM _____
Other–please be specific_____

Do you have any suggestions for speakers for these programs?

_____
_____
_____

---

prove helpful. Using a method that is familiar to the institution/practice is essential.

Discussing CAM therapies with patients remains a challenge for many practitioners. Concerns include the following:

- When patients ask about CAM, how do I respond?
- What do I know? What don't I know? What do I want to know?
- Am I (legally, morally, ethically) responsible if I do not ask?
- Am I (legally, morally, ethically) responsible if I do ask?
- Am I responsible for monitoring these therapies once I ask?
- Do I want to be involved?

Eisenberg (1997) suggested an algorithm for discussing and advising patients who seek CAM therapies. His algorithm assumes that there has been a complete medical evaluation and that conventional modalities have been discussed and offered to the patient. **Figure 17.4** suggests an approach for assessing and monitoring CAM therapy use. Eisenberg (2002) further contended that "don't ask, don't tell needs to be abandoned" (p. 423). At the 2002 Complementary and Integrative Medicine State of the Science and Clinical Applications Harvard Continuing Medical Education Program, Eisenberg presented a model for advising patients on the use of CAM therapies. He suggested that the provider ask this unanswered question: "have you used or consid-

Figure 17.3 Sample CAM Interest Community Survey

Have you used any of the following CAM Therapies?

Please put a √ in the box

	Have Used **If yes** →	How often?	Would like to	Not Interested
Acupuncture				
Chiropractic				
Herbal Therapies				
Homeopathy				
Massage Therapy				
Nutritional Supplements				
Reflexology				
Tai Chi				
Other- please specify				

You can use your top ten list here

Would you be interested in receiving these therapies at

_____

The name of your institution/ practice

Your name (optional)_____

ered using any other therapy for your (chief complaint)?" (Eisenberg, 2002, p. 412). The phrase "Safety Trumps Efficacy" (Eisenberg, 2002, p. 414) should be our mantra when discussing these therapies with patients. In his presentation, Eisenberg suggested a three-pronged approach: those therapies that we can (1) recommend and monitor; (2) tolerate, accept, and monitor; or (3) avoid and discourage. Evidence of efficacy and safety should be considered in each category. For example:

Recommend and monitor/evidence of efficacy is high/evidence of safety is high:

- Acupuncture for chemotherapy-induced nausea
- Mind–body techniques for chronic pain and insomnia

Tolerate/accept and monitor/evidence of efficacy is high, but inconclusive/evidence of safety is high:

- Massage for chronic lower back pain
- Mind–body techniques for cancer
- Dietary fat reduction for cancer
- Gingko biloba for dementia
- Chondroitin sulfate for osteoarthritis

Figure 17.4 Discussing CAM Therapies with Patients

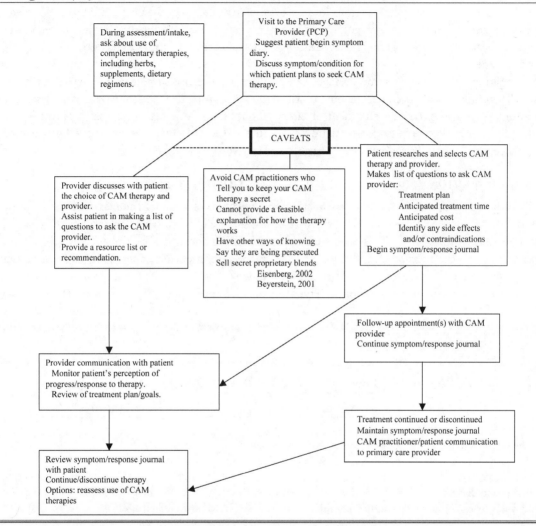

During assessment/intake, ask about use of complementary therapies, including herbs, supplements, dietary regimens.

Visit to the Primary Care Provider (PCP)
Suggest patient begin symptom diary.
Discuss symptom/condition for which patient plans to seek CAM therapy.

CAVEATS

Provider discusses with patient the choice of CAM therapy and provider.
Assist patient in making a list of questions to ask the CAM provider.
Provide a resource list or recommendation.

Avoid CAM practitioners who
Tell you to keep your CAM therapy a secret
Cannot provide a feasible explanation for how the therapy works
Have other ways of knowing
Say they are being persecuted
Sell secret proprietary blends
Eisenberg, 2002
Beyerstein, 2001

Patient researches and selects CAM therapy and provider.
Makes list of questions to ask CAM provider:
Treatment plan
Anticipated treatment time
Anticipated cost
Identify any side effects and/or contraindications
Begin symptom/response journal

Follow-up appointment(s) with CAM provider
Continue symptom/response journal

Provider communication with patient
Monitor patient's perception of progress/response to therapy.
Review of treatment plan/goals.

Treatment continued or discontinued
Maintain symptom/response journal
CAM practitioner/patient communication to primary care provider

Review symptom/response journal with patient
Continue/discontinue therapy
Options: reassess use of CAM therapies

Avoid and discourage/evidence of efficacy is low or disproven/evidence of safety is low or disproven:

- Laetrile for cancer
- Injections of any nonapproved substance
- Use of herbs known to be toxic

Professional education programs can expand practitioners' understanding and comfort with discussing these therapies. Within an institution or practice, a series of breakfast or lunch education programs can provide the information that prac-titioners seek. Adding questions to the assessment survey will provide data that you need to identify specific topics.

Program Champions

Central to your program development is identifying a champion(s) who believes in and is able to support your initiative. These individuals are typically administrators or physicians. Although it is not necessary to have a physician champion(s), it is helpful. CAM programs have been successful without unanimous support of the medical staff (Landmark Healthcare, Inc., 2002). Any resistance should decrease when there is visible evidence of the benefits to patients, patient satisfaction increases, and there is a realization that these therapies do not interfere with patient care but rather enhance it (Landmark Healthcare, Inc.). Champions may become visible at the beginning of your program development or later in the process. Do not overlook patients and family members as potential program champions.

Implementation

A CAM therapy program is most successful when a model that is familiar to the practice or institution is used as a framework. This will maintain consistency with the mission and a vision of the institution. As an exercise, insert CAM therapies into your practice/institution's mission statement.

Example:

Old: Our mission is to prevent disease and promote the health of the people we serve. We pledge to provide state-of-the-art diagnostic techniques and care for all of those in our care.

New: Our mission is to prevent disease and promote the health of the people we serve. We pledge to provide state-of-the-art diagnostic techniques and care for all of those in our care. This includes CAM therapies that have been demonstrative as safe and effective.

Choosing a Model

The choice of a model is dependent on the physical setting of the institution or practice, as well as the vision and mission. Your survey will provide pivotal information identifying the appropriate model(s) for your program. Some institutions/practices prefer a satellite location, whereas others want only an onsite program. A number of models can be considered. Examples include those

Table 17.4 PHYSICAL PLANT MODELS OF IMPLEMENTATION

Models	Advantages	Disadvantages
SATELLITE MODEL The CAM therapies are provided at a location other than that of the institution or practice.	• Separate identity can be given. • Sometimes separate budget can be done. • You can offer services to families and community. • Practitioners benefit from group marketing. • You can market outside the system as well as inside the system. • It is easier to explain out-of-pocket expenses to patients because it is not at the healthcare location where insurance coverage may be assumed. • Patients may not wish to return to a location equated with treatment after they have completed traditional therapy.	• Financially sustaining the program can be difficult. • Referrals may be delayed or never occur because there is a tendency to keep patients on site. • Patients may like one-stop care.

Table 17.4 PHYSICAL PLANT MODELS OF IMPLEMENTATION (CONT'D)

Models	Advantages	Disadvantages
MOTHER SHIP MODEL The CAM therapies are provided at a location where administrators and staff can monitor all activities.	• Geographical proximity to other departments • Geographical proximity to patients	• Blurring of identities can happen when traditional practitioners become CAM providers (e.g., a nurse who is also a licensed massage therapist). • Because all referrals are made department to department, favoritism can enter into the process. • There are difficult to explain out-of-pocket payment to patients because insurance covers other therapies provided there. • It is difficult to market to families and community.
INTEGRATED MODEL This model provides CAM therapies at the primary institution and a satellite location.	• It has onsite and satellite visibility. • The budget is integrated. Profits can be used to maintain other sites. • There are department to department referrals. • There is easy access for patients, families, and community.	• Budget is integrated. • Some confusion regarding covered and noncovered services may occur.

described in **Tables** 17.4 and 17.5. It may be desirable or necessary to mix models. For example, in your institution, an integrated physical plant model may implement the patient choice model at its satellite location so that services may be offered to the community whereas a specialty practice model would be used on site.

Table 17.6 is a sample of a mixed model CAM program. This integrated physical plant model program has one room on site where patients and families may access CAM therapies that are available based on a survey that patients, family, staff, and members of the community complete. There is a small, offsite, free-standing building where CAM therapies will be offered to the community at large, as well as to the patients, family, and staff of the primary institution. This hypothetical practice has chosen to integrate certain cancer-prevention programs (smoking cessation) as well as an extended lymphedema program into its CAM program.

Staffing Models

CAM healthcare practitioners can be hired as employees or contracted independent practitioners. These options pose advantages and disadvantages and should be discussed with human resources, attorneys, and/or risk management to identify the implications for your program (**Table** 17.7).

Table 17.5 PRACTICE MODELS

Models	Advantages	Disadvantages
PATIENT CHOICE MODEL Referral may be made by any practitioner, or the patient may self-refer.	• All disciplines are equal. • Patients have a choice (of therapy) and control (over dollars spent). • CAM specialties are organized as any other specialty. • Focus is on those therapies most often chosen/used by patients, family, and community. • Satisfaction survey drives therapy/practitioner choice. • Builds teams when it works.	• Billing is separate; each practitioner is responsible for his or her own. • Patient's therapies can get lost in the system because they can enter the system at any point. • Practitioners may have conflicts that will impact patient satisfaction. • Team building does not occur when it does not work.
SPECIALTY MODEL (DIAGNOSIS MODEL) This program is used for and located within a specialty area (e.g., oncology) and is available to only these patients.	• Communication is easily accomplished. • Treatments are specific to a particular diagnostic group. • Fees are more easily controlled.	• Choice and use of therapies are vulnerable to the preference of the referring practitioner and not the patient(s). • Referral flow becomes unidirectional.
OASIS MODEL This has become possible as providers become more familiar with CAM therapies and increase expertise with a particular therapy (for example, the nurse-licensed massage therapist, nurse-licensed acupuncturist or physician-licensed acupuncturist). Examples are Dean Ornish's cardiovascular program and Keith Block's cancer program.	• These programs have a core concept that is central to all of its therapies. • There is a supervising provider. • The program is built on staff cohesiveness (team building). • It can put direct pressure on those who may not support the program.	• A lack of multidisciplinary healthcare teams and credentialed practitioners exists. • If the program director has limited vision, so does the program. • There is competition between providers. • It can be sabotaged by those who do not support the program.

Table 17.6 SAMPLE OF MIXED MODEL CAM PROGRAM

		Mon	Tue	Wed	Thur	Fri	Sat	Sun
Room 1 On site	a.m. ----- 7:30–11:30	Smoking cessation program	Fatigue-management program	11-2 Chair massage	Nutrition, supplements, and herb counseling	Counseling	11-2 Chair massage	11-2 Chair massage
	p.m. 1 ----- 12–4	Nutrition, supplements, and herb counseling	Nutrition, supplements, and herb counseling	Counseling	Acupuncture	Nutrition, supplements, and herb counseling	Nutrition, supplements, and herb counseling	2-5 Acupuncture
	p.m. 2 --- 4:30–8:30	Counseling	Counseling	Acupuncture	Massage	Open	Open	5:30–8:30 Open
Room 2 Satellite	a.m. ----- 7:30–11:30	Open	Nutrition, supplements, and herb counseling	Counseling	Lymphedema (maintenance)	Open		
	p.m. 1 ----- 12–4	Counseling	Smoking cessation program	Nutrition, supplements, and herb counseling	Counseling	Acupuncture		
	p.m. 2 --- 4:30–8:30	Massage	Acupuncture	Support groups	Massage			
Room 3 Satellite	a.m. ----- 7:30–11:30	Open	Open	Open	Open			
	p.m. 1 ----- 12–4	Massage	Massage	Lymphedema (maintenance)	Acupuncture			
	p.m. 2 --- 4:30–8:30	Support groups	Acupuncture	Support groups	Massage			

Key:
Chair Massage: These 10- to 15-minute massages were identified by the survey and planning committee as important to their program.
Massage: The most requested therapy in their survey.
Acupuncture: Frequently requested.
Nutrition/supplements/herbal counseling
Counseling: Proximity.
Fatigue.
Lymphedema (maintenance) Lymphatic drainage is billable to insurance as long as possible from the physical medicine department. Patients are encouraged to continue on a maintenance program. When insurance coverage is no longer possible, the patient is referred to the CAM program (off site) to emphasize the uncovered status. It is imperative that the maintenance be accomplished in a different room in an environment that distinguishes itself from covered lymphedema services.

Table 17.7 PRACTITIONER MODEL

CAM Practitioner's Position	Advantages	Disadvantages
Employee	• Periodic evaluations and other performance measurements are available. • Employer has the ability to control and monitor practitioners.	• Many institutions have difficulty meeting institution orientation requirements and other standardized programs required of all employees. • You may have to pay for hours scheduled when there are no patients/clients. • An employer may be responsible for CE, malpractice insurance, and other state requirements.
Independent contractor	• The employee does not have to pay for hours not worked. • He or she can pay on a percentage basis in most states.	• There is less control over practice issues. • Contractors are known to schedule patients and family at other sites to build a private practice. • Contractors must monitor insurance coverage, CEs.
Employee/CAM practitioner (e.g., nurse, licensed massage therapist-LMT)	• The employee has already demonstrated loyalty to the institution/practice.	• Patients can become confused about role. • How to reimburse staff, e.g., an RN employee as a licensed massage therapist—independent contractor. • How to schedule (e.g., mixed model) as RN—primary institution/practice as LMT at satellite. • Contractor responsible for continuing education, insurance.

Forms and Communication

Create CAM forms that are consistent with institution/practice forms for referral and communication. **Figure 17.5** is an example of a CAM referral form. The interval between communication should be consistent with the patient's diagnosis, condition, and the CAM therapy. For example, medical massage for chronic pain management may not need to be reported after every appointment. Reports can be made monthly or with any change in condition, whereas herbal therapies might require a shorter interval between communications (**Figure 17.6**).

Figure 17.5 CAM Program Sample Referral Form

Date:_____

Referred to:_____ Therapy:_____

Patient name: _____ Date of birth:_____

Address:_____ Diagnosis:_____

Time frame requested   Type of service
❏ As soon as possible (less than   ❏ Consultation only
  48 hours)
❏ Within____ Days ____Weeks   ❏ Consult and treat
                                ❏ See specifics below

Specific information:_____
_____
_____

Legal Issues and CAM Therapies

Organizations and practitioners must consider what is needed to allow integration of CAM therapies while addressing the potential risk for liability. The perceptions and politics of medicine have created the legal environment for CAM therapies (Cohen, 2002). The state's authority to regulate health, safety, and welfare is well established. Courts have been consistent in enforcing the state's power in health regulations. Under the Constitution, states can decide which providers (conventional or CAM) "lawfully may practice or be excluded from practice" (Cohen, 2002, p. 375).

In U.S. vs. Rutherford (1977–1986), courts held that individuals "who may die of cancer nonetheless" have no constitutional privacy right to their choice of treatment.

Rationale

Congress could have intended to protect even terminally ill patients from cures that a government agency did not approve (Cohen, 2002, p. 375–376). History has been key in determinations made. Regulatory structures are changing, and the previously clear parameters that separated conventional and CAM therapies are less clear. This results in confusion. Clear legal, regulatory, and policy guidelines are lacking. Cohen suggested seven interrelated areas of law that affect integrating CAM therapies:
- Credentialing and licensure
- Food and drug law
- Scopes of practice
- Professional discipline
- Malpractice
- Third-party reimbursement
- Healthcare fraud

Figure 17.6 CAM PROGRAM SAMPLE COMMUNICATION FORM

Date:_____

Name of practitioner: _____   Phone/extension: _____

Patient name: _____

Modality: (list those that you offer)

Acupuncture   Massage   Herb consult   Nutrition/supplement   Counseling
                                                   consult

Reason for referral/comments: _____

_____

Treatment plan: _____

_____

Additional information: _____

_____

Next appointment: _____   Practitioner's signature _____

LICENSURE

"Any CAM provider who lacks health care licensure could be prosecuted for the unlicensed practice of medicine" (Cohen, 2002, p. 364). In the United States, CAM providers who are licensed include (1) acupuncturists, (2) chiropractors, (3) MD Homeopaths, (4) naturopathic physicians, and (5) massage therapists. Examples of CAM providers not separately licensed include (1) aromatherapists, (2) herbalists, (3) hypnotherapists, (4) nonphysician homeopaths, and (5) spiritual healers/energy healers.

SCOPES OF PRACTICE

Licensed providers who exceed their legally authorized scope of practice can be prosecuted for unlicensed medical practice (e.g., chiropractors who make nutritional recommendations, naturopathic physicians who prescribe drugs or perform minor surgery, or acupuncturists who recommend Western medicine supplements).

MALPRACTICE — INSTITUTION — DIRECT LIABILITY

The institution is directly negligent, causing patient injury.

VICARIOUS LIABILITY

The institution is liable because a negligent provider is deemed an agent of the institution.

PROVIDER

The general rule is that a physician is not liable for making a referral to another physician or specialist, but there are exceptions: when the referral delays or defers necessary medical treatment, when the physician knew or should have known that the referral to the provider was incompetent, and when the referral to provider is considered the physician's agent.

PROFESSIONAL DISCIPLINE

"Unprofessional Conduct" includes obtaining a license fraudulently, practicing with gross negligence, practicing while impaired (alcohol or drugs), and "any departure from prevailing and acceptable medical standards" (Cohen, 2002, p. 366) A physician may not be found guilty of unprofessional conduct on the basis of providing a complementary integrated therapy unless the therapy has a demonstrated safety risk that is unreasonably greater than the conventional therapy. (Cohen, 2002; Standards for Physicians Practicing Integrated and Complementary Medicine, Texas Administration Code S200. 1-200.3)

Creating a legally defensible CAM program/practice can do the following (Cohen, 2002):

- Provide and document adequate informed consent.
- Keep files of medical literature justifying choices involving CAM therapies.
- Create policies and procedures for each of the therapies offered.
- Continue conventional monitoring.
- When referring or co-managing a patient's care, know the CAM provider.

Presenting Your CAM Proposal

The introduction provides historical information for preparation of your proposal. Your proposal should include answers to the questions mentioned previously in this chapter, as well as any others you can anticipate. Before the day of your presentation, provide every meeting participant with a copy of your proposal, including the background information and copies of any supportive information. On the day of your presentation, be prepared with as much information as possible. Bring all supportive information with you: all survey results; your business program/plan, including any equipment costs, space costs, practice encounters (this should be a conservative number so that you can exceed expectations); and all of the ego strength that you can muster. CAM programs may remain controversial, but preparation can help you to be proactive and successful.

References

Alternative Medicine (Theme Issue). (1998). *JAMA, 280,* 1569–1651.

American Health Consultants (pub.). (1999). *The Physician's Guide to Alternative Medicine.* Atlanta: American Health Consultants.

Angell, M. & Kassirer, J. P. (1998). Alternative medicine—the risks of untested and unregulated remedies [editorial]. *New England Journal of Medicine, 339,* 839–841.

Beyerstein, B. L. (2001). Alternative medicine and common errors of reasoning. *Academic Medicine,76,* 230–237

Boon, H. M., Stewart, M. A., Kennard, R., Gray, C., Sawka, J. B., Brown, C. L. et al. (2000). Use of complementary/alternative medicine by breast cancer survivors. *Journal of Clinical Oncology, 18,* 2515–2521.

Cassileth, B. (1999). Evaluating complementary and alternative therapies for cancer patients. *Cancer Journal for Clinicians, 49,* 362–375.

Cassileth, B. & Chapman, C. (1996). Alternative and complementary cancer therapies. *Cancer, 77,* 1026–1033.

Cohen, M. H. Medical Liability and Complementary and Alternative Medicine in Eisenberg. (2002). Complementary & Integrative Medicine State Of The Science And Clinical Applications, Harvard Medical School Department of Continuing Education, March 24–26, Boston, MA. Syllabus.

Decker, G. & Cleveland, M. J. (2001). Complementary and Alternative Therapies. In R. Fink & R. Gates (Eds.), *Oncology Nursing Secrets* (2nd ed.). Philadelphia: Hanley & Belfus, Inc.

Eisenberg, D. (1997). Advising patients who seek alternative medical therapies. *Annals of Internal Medicine, 127.*

Eisenberg, D. M. (2001). Complementary & Integrative Medicine Clinical Update And Implications For Practice. Presentation at Harvard Medical School Department of Continuing Education, February 10–13, Boston, MA.

Eisenberg, D. M. (2002). Complementary & Integrative Medicine State Of The Science And Clinical Applications, Harvard Medical School Department of Continuing Education, March 24–26, Boston, MA. Syllabus.

Eisenberg, D. M., Davis, R. B., Ettner, S. L., Appel, S., Wilkey, S., Van Rompay, M. et al. (1998). Trends in alternative medicine use in the United States 1990-1997: Results of a follow-up national survey. *Journal of the American Medical Association, 280,* 1569–1575.

Eisenberg, D. M., Delblanco, T. L., & Kessler, R. C. (1993). Letter to the editor. *New England Journal of Medicine, 329,* 1023.

Eisenberg, D. M., Kessler, R. C., Foster, C., Norlock, F. E., Calkins, D. R., & Delblanco, T. L. (1993). Unconventional medicine in the United States. Prevalence, costs, and patterns of use. *New England Journal of Medicine, 328,* 246–252.

Eisenberg, D., Kessler, R. C., Van Rompay, M. I., Kaptchuk, T. J., Wilkey, S. A., Appel, S. et al. (2001). Perceptions about complementary therapies relative to conventional therapies among adults who use both: Results from a national survey. *Annals of Internal Medicine, 135,* 344–351.

Ernst, E., Resch, K. L., Mills, S., Hill, R., Mitchell, A., Willoughby, M. et al. (1995). Complementary medicine—a definition. *British Journal of General Practice, 45,* 506.

Gevitz, N. (1988). Other healers; unorthodox medicine in America. Baltimore: Johns Hopkins University Press.

Gordon, J. (2002). The Chairman's vision in The White House Commission on Complementary and Alternative Medicine Policy Final Report. Accessed at *http://www.whccamp.hhs.gov/finalrepor.html*

Jonas, W. B. (1998). Alternative medicine—learning from the past, examining the present, advancing to the future [editorial]. *JAMA, 280,* 1616–1618.

Kao, G. D. & Devine, P. (2000). Use of complementary health practices by prostate carcinoma patients undergoing radiation therapy. *Cancer, 88,* 615–619.

Kaptchuk, T. J. & Eisenberg, D. M. (1998). The persuasive appeal of alternative medicine. *Annals of Internal Medicine, 129,* 1061–1065.

Landmark Healthcare, Inc. (1997). The Landmark Report on Public Perceptions of Alternative Care. Sacramento: Landmark Healthcare, Inc.

Lawlis, G. F. & Bowman, M. (2001). Complementary and Alternative Medicine Management. Gaithersburg, MD: Aspen Publishers.

LeBars, P. L., Katz, M. M., Berman, N., Itil, T. M., Freedman, A. M., & Schatzberg, A. F. (1997). A placebo-controlled, double blind, randomized trial of an extract of gingko biloba for dementia. North American Egb Study Group. *JAMA, 278,* 1327–1332.

Linde, K., Clausius, N., Ramirez, G., Mulrow, C. D., Pauls, A., Weidenhammer, W. et al. (1997). Are the clinical effects of homeopathy placebo effects? A meta-analysis of placebo-controlled trials. *Lancet, 350,* 834–843.

Montbriand, M. (1994). An overview of alternate therapies chosen by cancer patients. *Oncology Nursing Forum, 21,* 1547–1554.

Mooney, K. (1987). Unproven cancer treatment usage in cancer patients who have received conventional therapy. *Oncology Nursing Forum, Supp2,* 112.

Murray, R. H. & Rubel, A. J. (1992). Physicians and healers–unwitting partners in health care. *New England Journal of Medicine, 326,* 61–64.

Muscat, M. (2001). Report–Alternative medicine in health and medicine. National Center for Complementary and Alternative Medicine. Bethesda, MD: NCCAM, 7, 22, 23.

Olendick, R., Coker, A. L., Wieland, D., Raymond, J., Probst, J., Schell, B. et al. (2000). Population-based survey of complementary and alternative medicine usage, patient satisfaction and physical involvement. *Southern Medical Journal, 93,* 375–381.

Park, J., White, A. R., & Ernst, E. (2000). Efficacy of acupuncture as a treatment for tinnitus: A systematic review. *Archives of Otolaryngology, Head and Neck Surgery, 355,* 134–138.

Position of the Oncology Nursing Society on the use of Complementary and Alternative Medicine (CAM) Therapies in Cancer Care, 2000.

Richardson, M. A., Sanders, T., Palmer, J. L., Greisinger, A., & Singletary, S. E. (2000). Complementary/alternative medicine use in a comprehensive cancer center and the implications for oncology. *Journal of Clinical Oncology, 18,* 2505–2514.

Schrock, D., Palmer, R. F., & Taylor, B. (1999). Effects of psychosocial intervention on survival among cancer patients with Stage I breast cancer and prostate cancer: A matched case-control study. *Alternative Therapies in Health and Medicine, 5,* 49–55.

Shlay, J. C., Chaloner, K., Max, M. B., Flaws, B., Reichelderfer, P., Wentworth, D. et al. (1998). Acupuncture and amitryptyline for pain due to HIV-related peripheral neuropathy: A randomized controlled trial. *JAMA, 280,* 1590–1595.

Sparber, A., Bauer, L., Curt, G., Eisenberg, D., Levin, T., Parks, S. et al. (2000). Use of Complementary Medicine by Adult Patients Participating in Cancer Clinical Trials. *Oncology Nursing Forum, 27,* 623–630.

Spiegel, D., Bloom, J. R., Kraemer, H. C., & Gottheil, E. (1989). Effect of psychosocial treatment on survival of patients with metastatic breast cancer. *Lancet, 2,* 888–891.

Standards for Physicians Practicing Integrative and Complementary Medicine, Texas Administrative Code s.200.1–s.200.3.

Stephinson, C., Pittler, M. H., & Ernst, E. (2000). Garlic for treating hypercholesterolemia: A meta analysis of randomized clinical trials. *Annals of Internal Medicine, 133,* 420–429.

Wetzel, M. S., Eisenberg, D. M., & Kapchuk, T. J. (1998). Courses involving complementary and alterative medicine at U.S. medical school. *JAMA, 280,* 784–787.

Chapter 18

Community-Based Survivorship Programs

Barbara J. Murphy

Christine Rimkus

Betsy Patterson

Approximately 9-million people in the United States are living with cancer (National Coalition of Cancer Survivors, 2003a). It is estimated that the 5-year survival rate for all cancers is 62% (American Cancer Society, 2002). Advances in early detection, broader understandings of cancer biology leading to more aggressive treatments, improved supportive care, and an increased focus on rehabilitation have contributed to the improved survival (Rowland et al., 1984). Many patients with cancer are not being cured; instead, they are living with the disease, which when controlled sometime renders cancer a chronic disease. In 1986, an advocacy group, the National Coalition for Cancer Survivorship (NCCS), began to address treatment issues for cancer survivors. Previous literature on cancer survivorship focused on the time period immediately after completion of therapy. More recent literature has described cancer survivorship as part of a trajectory that starts at diagnosis through the treatment and the issues of late effects of cancer and its treatment. Literature is just beginning to mature from the childhood cancer databases.

Healthcare professionals have traditionally placed most of their time and energy into giving patients and their caregivers information at the time of the diagnosis regarding treatment and the subsequent side effects of treatment. Very little information is provided to the patients about the psychosocial issues and long-term effects. Patients often seek information from a multitude of sources. Many of the resources are legitimate, such as the Internet, free reading material, purchased books on cancer and treatment, friends and/or family members, community lectures, and nonprofessionals, but others may provide inaccurate or misleading information. It becomes the nurse's responsibility to help the patient identify appropriate educational material. Cancer patients also have several avenues that are available to them to help them cope with the illness, including support groups, both traditional as well as online support programs, individual counseling, and telephone counseling. With the vast amount of information and resources available to patients with cancer, as well as the varied needs of the individual with cancer, it becomes necessary for the nurses in the ambulatory setting to help the patient navigate the system of resources.

Impact of Cancer Diagnosis

A cancer diagnosis is a highly stressful and traumatic event (Zabora et al., 1997). It can cause chaos in the most stable life of an individual and family. Fear, anxiety, shock, disbelief, anger, bitterness, hostility, self-pity, and depression are common and "normal" reactions to the situation. The cancer experience is a series of events and experiences that are far beyond the initial impact of diagnosis and across the continuum of time. Zabora et al. provided a review of the literature, outlining three points of highest distress or stages throughout the continuum of the cancer experience (Zabora et al., 1997). Most studies of stress levels and adjustment focus on the initial diagnosis, and few studies have focused on disease recurrence as a phase of illness.

Stage I is the time of diagnoses and initial treatment. This stage may last six months to two years. This is a time of acute distress, including treatment-related anxiety and discomfort, as well as deep concerns about disease progression and potential for a fatal outcome. A time of major crisis for the patient and family is often associated with a need for education and support. This is the beginning of the journey of living with and through the cancer experience.

Stage II is often referred to as "watchful waiting"—learning to live life in remission while the fear of a relapse remains strong. Today, patients and families are more educated than in the past and have developed some strategies to maneuver through the healthcare system. Personal relationships have become deeper and stronger, or barriers are built that isolate the patient and family members. Support groups can be particularly healing to the patient and family so that positive coping and communication skills can be developed or improved. Because defenses and old habits are difficult to break once built, prevention is a key strategy for averting further deterioration.

Stage III is often considered the chronic disease state. In this stage, the individual may be a survivor who has been cured of their disease but is now experiencing the late effects of treatment. More commonly, this stage is associated with the patient who is not curable but continues to have treatment options. At this point, a degree of comfort with the disease and the patient's ability to cope with long-term side effects have developed.

Mahon & Donovan reported in 1970 that the patients who were most distressed at disease recurrence were those experiencing more physical symptoms, more outside stressors, and fewer support systems (Cella, Mahon, & Donovan, 1990). In a later study, Mahon et al. found that in a convenience sample of 40 patients, 31 diagnosed with recurrent cancer reported that the recurrence was more upsetting than the initial diagnosis (Cella, Mahon, & Donovan). At this time, many patients use denial as a defense mechanism, whereas others channel their anxiety into the search of proven or unproven new treatment methods (Krumm, 1982). Emotional distress and physical symptoms accompanied by the fear of pain and dying are associated with the terminal stage of cancer. Portenoy et al. reported that high distress is clearly associated with the fear of uncontrolled pain in the final stages of cancer and the fear that death itself will be excruciatingly painful (Portenoy et al., 1994). In the terminal phase of the disease, the patient may have come to an attitude of acceptance. Often this acceptance of the terminal outcome has come to the patient long before it comes to the family, friends, and even the healthcare providers.

At any given time, all of these stages of illness will be evident in patients and families in cancer support groups. These diverse groups' needs and various coping styles can be brought together with communication, education, and compassion. Frequently, the experience of simply having "been there" allows for and creates the group interaction.

To target the appropriate intervention, healthcare providers must understand the impact on the level of distress and provide the appropriate support. Much depends on where the patient and family members are in the disease trajectory. Healthcare professionals routinely teach patients to anticipate the emotional highs and lows that are described as the "roller coaster effects" frequently common to the cancer experience. A cancer diagnosis poses obstacles to be negotiated through the challenging and complex healthcare system.

Bushkin was eloquent in her description of her experiences as a cancer survivor. She suggested that her trek was similar to that of a traveler who was "confronting life-challenging and life-changing sarcoma" on a journey. She invited patients to take on the role of traveler and to face the many roads to be negotiated and signposts encountered in their personal and professional life (Bushkin, 1993). In an epilogue, Ellyn Bushkin's husband described that despite having a career as an oncology nurse, being experienced with caring for the dying, and having multiple academic credentials, she was unprepared for the end of her own road. He cautions that to the tourist her journey is complete, but to those who serve as guides or caregivers or who are fellow travelers, the journey continues through teaching insight and caring to patients with cancer. This is a powerful message to those who are in a position to provide supportive care.

History of Cancer Survivor Support Groups

Support groups in general have been traced to the development of social work and group psychotherapy at the turn of the 20th century (Fobair, 1997). Early group work was begun in settlement houses and tuberculosis wards. Jane Adams, a social worker, was awarded the Nobel Peace Prize for her innovative work on Chicago's West Side at the Hull House in 1889. She addressed the needs of the immigrants and the poor and unemployed by forming educational groups and community action programs to assist them with social, economic, and personal problems. Nurses are credited with recognizing the need for social support while delivering health messages (Stuart, 1992).

Early emphasis focused on providing patient and caregiver education to assist with coping with the cancer experience. In a pioneering textbook Bouchard (1967) emphasized that the nurse needs to create an atmosphere in which the patient or family can feel free to talk about problems "without feeling that they are causing too much trouble." The author offered that the individual nurse "should be able to advise, counsel, and teach the patient ways of adapting" (1967, pp. 25–26). There is little mention of community or group support other than in areas of financial concerns and public assistance. The multiple services of the American Cancer Society are highlighted, and other organizations that might offer individual services are mentioned; however, any discussion of a formal support/survival group, as we know it today, is lacking.

Mention of support groups for patients with cancer first appeared in the literature in the 1970s. Reports of initial efforts to bring groups of patients and their families together on a cancer ward and in outpatient areas focused on educational or financial concerns and treatment options. Early on, it became clear that these groups evolved into meeting psychosocial needs (Fobair, 1997). Johnson and Flaherty redefined the role of the oncology nurse as an educator who is responsible for patient education. They defined patient education as "any combination of learning opportunities designed to affect the knowledge level, skills attitudes, or other behaviors and persons closely associated (Johnson & Flaherty, 1980)."

"I Can Cope" is an educational program that was developed in 1978 and adopted by the American Cancer Society in 1979. It is now offered in more than 1,000 locations in the United States. I Can Cope provides information to cancer patients, families, and friends to help cope with a cancer diagnosis and the physical and psychological sequelae (McMillan, Tittle, & Hill, 1993). Pillon and Joannides described a "Living with Cancer" program established in 1979, that met weekly with the inpatient population and families to provide informal discussions (Pillon & Joannides, 1991). No set agenda existed, but issues included treatment concerns, financial problems, emotional issues, and the general effects of cancer. Soon the program developed subgroups to look at family- or disease-specific issues, children/adolescent concerns, and bereavement issues.

The growth of self-help groups in the oncology population can be traced to the many changes in the fabric of our society. The consumer movement is a prime example of individual actions that have led to widespread actions, advocacy, and support. Ever-growing numbers of chronically ill are dealing with incredible problems and challenges of daily living. Despite advances in scientific and medical research that have expanded treatment options, we have increased confusion in the average person who is overwhelmed by multiple decision-making tasks. The current healthcare delivery system is often perceived as an impenetrable maze, lacking in support from busy, overworked, and understaffed professionals. It was estimated in the year 2000, that more than 25-million Americans have been involved in some type of self-help group and that groups are effective for a variety of problems (Wituk, Shepherd, Slavich, Warren, & Meissen, 2000).

Effectiveness of Support Groups

There are multiple groups devoted to providing education and support and many reported successes. A study that the Department of Health and Kinesiology at Texas Agriculture and Mining University completed on social support networks indicated that health professionals did not provide information regarding social support groups to patients with cancer at the time of diagnosis (Guidry, Aday, Zhang, & Winn, 1997). Fewer than half of the respondents were asked whether they would be interested in joining a formal social support group.

Other surveys of health professionals have found that they are usually favorable toward self-help groups. A favorable attitude does not always translate into making referrals or having contact with groups (Gray & Fitch, 2001). Leis investigated the beliefs of medical and radiation oncologists regarding their use of psychosocial groups and routine referrals to groups (Leis, Haines, & Pancyr, 1994). The survey asked 16 of 20 oncologists about perceived harm or benefit that they expected from psychosocial groups. Although harm to the patient was not a major concern, the participants did not expect much benefit. The oncologists were only minimally concerned about the possibility that programs would interfere with their treatment plan. One half of the oncologists selected depression, anxiety, anger, and compliance with medical treatment as appropriate reasons to refer patients to psychosocial groups.

Matthews et al. reported that despite much work that has been accomplished in the areas of patient support, many individuals lack the support and information needed (Matthews, Baker, & Spillers, 2002). A multidisciplinary random sample of physicians, nurses, and social workers (n = 1,180) was surveyed. Of the total sample, 44% were physicians, 24% nurses, and 32% social workers. The sample spanned 49 of the 50 states and a comprehensive representation of practice settings. A list of American Cancer Society (ACS) and National Cancer Institute (NCI) programs and services were used as part of the Health Care Professional Awareness Questionnaire. Among those who did refer patients to cancer organizations, the ACS (83%), the NCI (55%), and the Leukemia and Lymphoma Society (formally the Leukemia Society; 42%) were ranked at the top. Although a large number of participants were aware of the available support services, fewer reported recommending or satisfaction with the listed services. Those services found most helpful included Reach to Recovery (63%), Look Good, Feel Better (60%), and I Can Cope (55%).

How well a program is perceived or how often it is used is relevant but does not necessarily address any given program's effectiveness. In a frequently quoted early study, Spiegel et al. reported the effectiveness of support groups in a prospective study of 86 women with metastatic breast cancer. Those women who participated in weekly supportive group therapy (n = 50) survived for a mean of 36.6 months, whereas the control group (n = 36) survived for a mean of 18.9 months. Both groups received routine oncological care (Speigel, Bloom, Kraemer, & Gottheil, 1989). Because statistical analysis of survival had not been a planned outcome, further research was warranted.

Several randomized subsequent studies did not support Spiegel's findings (Edelman, Lemon, Bell, & Kidman, 1999). Goodwin et al. attempted to replicate the results of Spiegel's study (Goodman et al., 2001). In a multicenter trial, 235 women with metastatic breast cancer who were expected to survive at least three months were randomly assigned to an intervention group that participated in a weekly support group (n = 158) or a control group (n = 77). All women were provided with educational material and received any medical or psychosocial care required. Although the women assigned to the support group had a greater improvement in psychological symptoms and reported less pain than in the control group, their survival was not prolonged. The median survival in the support group was 17.9 months compared with 17.6 months in the control. The authors concluded that group therapy's effectiveness is not an issue of survival but rather quality of life. Mood was improved, and the perception of pain was decreased, particularly in women who were initially more distressed.

A meta-analysis of 116 studies was done in 1995 (Devine & Westlake, 1995) to determine how educational and psychosocial care affected

seven outcomes: anxiety, depression, mood, nausea, vomiting, pain, and knowledge. A comprehensive literature search was done, and the interventional studies used were published between 1976 and 1993. The studies were based on data from 5,326 patients with cancer. Across all the types of care provided, statistically significant, beneficial effects were found in relationship to all seven of the outcomes. The researchers reported, however, that being able to differentiate between the effectiveness of various types of psychoeducational care was difficult to determine, concluding that more research is required.

Survival may not be prolonged, but there is a growing body of knowledge that indicates that the modulation of immunologic activities relevant to cancer by behavioral factors may influence disease progression. Behavioral factors include stress, depression, and social support. It has also been reported that social support (friends, neighbors, and groups) may influence the progression of ovarian cancer. Lutgendorf et al. noted that greater support appears to be associated with a reduced level of vascular endothelial growth factor in patients with ovarian carcinoma. The study showed that an association between vascular endothelial growth factor and social well-being was " sufficiently robust" for a significant correlation. Vascular endothelial growth factor has been labeled as a key cytokine that can stimulate tumor angiogenesis and is associated with reduced survival. Although there were many stated limitations, this study may open new pathways relating biobehavioral factors to tumor growth and disease progression (Lutgendorf et al., 2002).

Emergence of Support/Survivor Groups

All humans are fundamentally social creatures who derive much of our sense of well-being, importance, and value through the daily response of others. It is rare for humans to live alone or even spend much time alone. A diagnosis of cancer or another life-threatening illness disrupts social contact in many ways. It removes people from customary contacts because of absence from work, school, and family. Newly diagnosed cancer patients suddenly enter a new and strange social system. Furthermore, the isolation is bidirectional. Friends and family are awkward about the illness, not knowing what to say, and are fearful for the ill person and for their own selves. The cancer patient has a new set of norms, as comfortable old ones disappear (Spiegel & Glassen, 2000).

Although dramatic progress has been made in curing some cancers and although it is reasonable in other circumstances to be optimistic, people with cancer have reason to worry. The purpose of support groups is to help people learn from each other, to feel sustained at a time when illness makes them feel alone, and allow them to express and deal with feelings that they may never have coped with before. A supportive atmosphere can assist patients, friends, and family feel less alone and helpless when fears are shared with those who are in a similar situation. This conviction is rooted in studies of group therapy in women with advanced breast cancer (Yalom, 1980).

Yalom found that the women benefited from the coping skills used to master other parts of their life and could use these same tools when the prospect of dying is presented. He concluded that such a confrontation with death can be a stimulus to a new prospective of life, devoid of the daily routine in which we hide from existential dread.

What Is a Support Group?

A support group should ideally provide a safe, supportive environment that is free from prejudice and judgment and a place where the following patient and family goals can be reached:

- Become aware of their fears and feelings about the disease and its treatments.
- Acknowledge depression, anxiety, and excessive emotional outbursts.
- Express their fears and feelings in positive ways.

- Achieve effective stress-management skills.
- Acquire a sense of optimism and empowerment.
- Acquire a sense of control and self-efficacy.
- Achieve competence in communication and assertiveness skills and learn to use them effectively with family, friends, and healthcare providers.
- Restore or establish positive family and other interpersonal relationships.
- Identify and promote use of support systems.
- Acquire information about their disease and treatment options.
- Learn ways to reduce the aversive side effects of cancer treatment.
- Maintain a self-concept in the face of the disease and its treatment.
- Approach spiritual or existential issues related to cancer and potential for death.
- Maximize quality of life with the promotion of a healthy and rewarding lifestyle while living with illness.
- Find effective coping skills to deal with recurrence and even death (Seligman, 1996).

Several successful support networks have been mentioned earlier in this chapter. Such groups are often established as a foundation, managed by a board of directors who share a prime goal related to major fund-raising activities. For example, the Leukemia/Lymphoma Society has national chapters that provide educational forums for patients, physicians, and other healthcare providers. The society also provides limited but meaningful financial assistance to patients with the hematologic cancers. The Society trains healthcare professionals as facilitators to organize and manage monthly meetings. The Society allows for much freedom at the local levels, but gives direction on specific educational programs and activities on the national or state level. The leukemia/lymphoma support group can be defined as a survivor group, a support group, and an advocacy group.

Locating international and national support agencies via the Internet is easily accomplished. Simply log in the organization's name and almost any search engine will get you to a link for the organization or society (**Table 18.1**).

What Is a Survivor Group?

A definition of cancer survivor group as a pure form does not exist. "Survivor" refers to one who has continued to exist after a specific physical threat or a perception of a serious life-threatening experience. The NCCS defines a cancer survivor as "anyone with a history of cancer, from the time of diagnosis and for the remainder of life." Many organizations use the term "survivor group," whereas others use the more generic term "support group." To define the term survivor group, the support process must be prepared to deal with issues from diagnosis to death. Family or friends (often referred to as cosurvivors) are a part of the cancer patient's support team. These important team members attend group sessions to provide support to the patient and themselves. To have survived a near-death or potential for near-death situation permits the term to be used appropriately for rape, domestic violence, holocaust, or AIDS, and of course, cancer. The term "survivor" is the accepted term used in lay and professional publications to identify people who have or who had cancer. The value of this definition of cancer survivor is that it confers more hope and dignity than "cancer victim" or "cancer patient" (Harpham, 1998).

The term cosurvivor is used to include the most significant other or others to the patient. The cosurvivor is often the spouse, partner, or the one most likely to be the full-time caregiver. Studies have suggested that those emotionally connected to the cancer survivor suffer from the same levels of distress, anxiety, and isolation as the actual patient undergoing diagnosis and treat-

ment (Schimmel, 1999). The unique character of these individual members within the group develops the dynamics of any group. (**Table 18.2**)

Types of Groups

Peer-to-Peer

Peer-to-peer groups match cancer survivors with others with the same types of cancer and within the same stage of illness. These groups are homogeneous and create a sense of belonging easily and rapidly. Homogeneous groups enhance a member's sense of safety and allow for openness and sharing of more private or delicate issues. For example, a women recovering from a mastectomy might feel more comfortable discussing sexual or body image issues in a group composed of women recovering from similar procedures. The ACS's "Reach to Recovery" program is an example. These volunteers provide new breast cancer survivors with education and support.

Closed Membership

Closed membership, or time-limited support groups (structured support groups), are often organized by a hospital, oncology practice, or a national cancer support network. The group meets every week for a predetermined number of the meetings, typically six to 12 weeks. New members are not invited to join after the second session. These groups allow emotional sharing and support, but the prime purpose evolves around education.

Advantages of the closed membership are in the amount of information that is gained in a series of scheduled sessions and the trust among members. Disadvantages include patients who are ready for information who need to wait until the group's next starting point. These groups lack flexibility for those with responsibilities such as shift work, children, and/or family emergencies (Seligman, 1996). The I Can Cope program that the ACS supports is an example.

Table 18.1 NATIONAL ORGANIZATIONS

Organization	Mission	Mailing Address	Phone Number	Website
The Leukemia/Lymphoma Society	Provides advocacy, support, education, and financial assistance to those with hematologic malignancies. Provides funding for research.	1311 Mamaroneck Avenue White Plains, NY 10605	800-955-4572	www.leukemia-lymphoma.org
American Lung Association	Provides education on lung cancer and resources to quit smoking.	1740 Broadway New York, NY 10019	800-586-4872	www.lungusa.org
International Myeloma Foundation	Helps to improve the quality of life for people with multiple myeloma and helps work toward a cure and prevention. Provides information about joining a patient-to-patient directory.	12650 Riverside Drive, Suite 206 North Hollywood, CA 91607	800-452-2873	www.myeloma.org
The Skin Cancer Foundation	Provides patient materials, including books, brochures, and newsletters focused on the prevention, detection, and treatment of skin cancer.	245 Fifth Avenue, Suite 1403 New York, NY 10016	800-754-6490	www.skincancer.org
Ovarian Cancer National Alliance	Provides information for patients, family, and caregivers about clinical trials, tips on dealing with the disease, research, education, awareness, and advocacy and legislation.	910 17th Street, NW, Suite 413 Washington, DC 20006	202-331-1332	www.ovariancancer.org
Pancreatic Cancer Action Network	Works to focus national attention on the need to find the cure for pancreatic cancer. Provides information about advocacy efforts and patient and liaison services.	P.O. Box 1010 Torrance, CA 90505	877-272-6226	www.pancan.org

Table 18.1 NATIONAL ORGANIZATIONS (CONT'D)

Organization	Mission	Mailing Address	Phone Number	Website
US TOO! International, Inc.	Assists survivors of prostate cancer and prostate disease and their families with coping with the physical, emotional, and spiritual aspects of this disease. Provides updated medical information, treatment options, peer counseling, support groups, and links to other Websites.	5003 Fairview Avenue Downers Grove, IL 60515	800-808-7866	www.ustoo.org
The United Ostomy Association	A volunteer-based health organization dedicated to assisting people who have had or will have intestinal or urinary diversions. Provides educational information and available services.	19772 MacArthur Boulevard, Suite 200 Irvine, CA 92612-2405	800-826-0826	www.uoa.org
Make-A-Wish Foundation	Grants wishes of children with terminal or life-threatening illnesses.	3550 North Central Avenue, Suite 300 Phoenix, AZ 85012	800-722-wish (9474)	www.wish.org
American Brain Tumor Association	Provides advocacy, support, education, and funding for research.	2720 River Road Des Plaines, IL 60018	800-886-2282	www.abta.org

Table 18.2 CHARACTERISTICS OF SURVIVORSHIP AND SUPPORT GROUPS

Characteristics of Survivorship Groups

• There is potential for terminal outcome.

• They provide a shared reality.

• Participants have had a major disruption of one's routine that poses a sudden and intense life threat, burdens, and potential losses.

• Participants are often involved for the long haul or for intermittent disease related stressors.

• The facilitator is often a cancer survivor.

• The most important purpose is to give emotional support to persons with a common problem.

• Groups tend to be much more cohesive with strong emotional bonds.

• Follow-up will occur when a member of the group is missing.

• Groups often have a similar cancer diagnosis and/or experience: bone marrow transplant group, ovarian cancer, breast cancer, or prostate cancer.

• When cosurvivors are encouraged to attend, they are considered to be the most significant support to the actual survivor and by definition have the most to lose.

• Groups are closed to other "outsiders" unless otherwise invited as a guest or speaker.

• Groups meet on a regular schedule, and the group continues indefinitely as long as members continue to attend.

• Members are encouraged to share as much or as little as they wish. Insight occurs from gentle acceptance, not from in-depth probing.

• The members are the experts on the feelings and life experiences shared in the group.

Characteristics of Support Groups

• They are associated with a group that needs support and education for a very diverse group of illnesses, syndromes, 12-step programs, or health problem management.

• They are often used for discreet disease related stressors: ostomy group, lymphedema group.

• The facilitator is often a committed healthcare professional.

• Support groups can be much more open to education and advocacy while still providing support, encouragement, and hope.

• Groups are much more relaxed about attendance; often members come and go dependent on their need for support and information.

• Often one of the goals of the group is to encourage change in members.

• Members usually meet ongoing, but there can also be a specific time table allotted for the support like the I Can Cope program or Look Good, Feel Better program.

Open Membership

Open membership or open-ended groups are the most commonly used method of providing cancer support in communities. All types of cancer and staging participate, and they include family and friends. The groups are ongoing with no established ending point. Frequently, these groups meet once monthly with attendance fluctuating. Generally, there is a core group that attends with regularity, and these individuals tend to develop close personal ties. The advantages include the opportunity for diversity in disease type and in coping skills. New members can join at any time, allowing the group to be more available to those who seek immediate support and attention. Disadvantages of open-ended group can be related to the degree of flexibility allowed. Members that might benefit from a longer time with the group may end their association prematurely. Members may become disruptive within the group process or have individual needs that can overpower neophyte members. Leaders new to the group facilitation may find open-ended groups more difficult because of the many unknowns and diverse needs of the group. Members may feel that they are always "starting over" as new members arrive.

Cancer support can come in many forms, and no support network is cast in stone. Frequently, the terms "survivor group" and "support group" are used interchangeably. The individual group and its members will define the format, characteristics, and dynamics as the group evolves. Each group will experience change as the participants adjust and adapt. The new, emotionally fragile member will over time become a source of strength and encouragement to someone else in the future. Members of the group come to realize that while trying to help themselves, they are also helping others. This give-and-take relationship of support groups is a very important part of the healing process (Kurtz-Farris, 1997).

Despite the many differences in individuals that seek out support groups, there are some physical, emotional, and spiritual similarities. The typical support group member is between the ages of 34 and 65 years, is white, has 12 years or more of education, has a moderate income, and has the ability to read and write English. In Coriel and Behal's study, the demographics of a man-to-man prostate support group were surveyed. Facilitators and participants alike were typically retired, white males in their 60s and 70s from well-educated, professional backgrounds (Coriel & Behal, 1999).

In emotional terms, group members shared several common characteristics. Determined to be of importance was the search for kindred souls; finding support through others that had made the same journey. Finding a safe place to evaluate and to explore their feelings was another need that was consistent in members. Finding meaning within the illness and finding hope for a future were also common denominators in cancer patients that chose support groups (Klein, 2000). The patients who chose not to attend support groups stated that their faith and support came from their churches and family. However, when support groups have questioned participants, over 70% reported being affiliated with a church or religious organization.

Those at risk for not attending support groups are, unfortunately, often the patients and families that need it most. The low incidence of minority population representation in cancer support groups continues to be a concern and is an important area of future research (Legislative Action Center, 1999b).

Special Populations

Although support groups are offered to many patients, the majority of patients choose not to participate. Krizek et al. reported the results of a study comparing the behavior of men diagnosed with prostate cancer and women diagnosed with breast cancer. One hundred and thirty women with breast cancer and 87 men with prostate cancer completed a structured telephone interview. The interview included questions about patients' choices regarding support group participation. The interview findings showed that men are less likely to join a support group, but those men who did join did attend meetings for about one year, as did the women who joined support groups. Although more women than men join support groups, the majority of both populations (67% for women and 87% for men) did not attend any support group meetings (Krizek, Roberts, Ragan, Ferrara, & Lord, 1999).

Specific Cultural Groups

The importance of feeling accepted and allowing a sense of shared reality are very important components to the healing nature of support groups. When individuals feel isolated from the group because of race or culture, the group dynamics and personal support are compromised. It is not always possible to provide special groups for those of different cultures; however, it is essential that every measure be taken to include all members equally within the group. Facilitators need to attempt to enter the world of those that they are trying to help. This means learning their unique cultures, family histories, languages, customs, values, and priorities.

Blacks, as with many minorities, have typically been underrepresented and underserved in the support group setting. Research indicates that not only do Blacks seek therapy less often, but also those that seek out support groups tend to discontinue after a few meetings (Kurtz-Farris, 1997). The Black experience is replete with examples of repression and exploitation. Facilitators cannot allow the group dynamics to isolate or minimize issues unique to this population. For further information and for a search for minority physicians, visit the organization Black Health Net at *www.blackhealthnetwork.com/*.

The Hispanic population has the largest growth rate in the United States in the last 10 years of all minority groups. With this growth comes a responsibility to provide culturally sensitive cancer information and support. Additional information and support can be reached via the Office of Minority Health at www.omhrc.gov. The Office of Minority Health is responsible for public health program activities affecting American Indians, Alaska Natives, Blacks, Asian Americans, Pacific Islanders, and Hispanic populations. Its goal is to promote improved health among these racial and ethnic minority populations.

Gay and Lesbian Groups

The literature suggests that gays and lesbians may face challenges that are different from those who experience cancer as a heterosexual patient. In a study by Matthews et al., experiences of lesbian and heterosexual patients with breast cancer were explored (Matthews, Peterman, Delaney, Menard, & Brandenburg, 2002). The study findings suggested that lesbians reported higher stress associated with the diagnosis, lower satisfaction with care received from physicians, and a trend toward lower satisfaction with the availability of emotional support. Although breast cancer is a crisis for any woman (or man), few studies are available about the needs of the lesbian population. Discussions of sexual orientation to medical providers was found to be difficult and a concern to the lesbian sample in this study. It is necessary for the members of any support group to feel comfortable, safe, and free to express feelings without judgment and rejection. For additional resources and support for the gay and lesbian patient, see **Table 18.3**.

Pediatric Support Groups

The stress and psychological difficulties of pediatric patients with cancer are enormous. Children need support from their peers just as adults do. Pediatric support groups are infrequent because of the relative rareness of the condition and the severity of the illness and treatment. Specialized pediatric oncology units can meet these needs, but small community hospitals and communities often do not have this resource available. Peer support in this age group is important, and it becomes critical that the school and the child's friends, classmates, and teachers become involved in the supportive therapy for the child.

Siblings of the patient must be included. Siblings cope with a myriad of emotions: separation from family and the routine of family life. Therefore, a need exists to include this often forgotten group. Heiney et al. used a quasiexperimental design to determine the effects of participation in a support group on the social adjustment of siblings of children with cancer (Heiney, Goon-Johnson, Ettinger, & Ettinger, 1990). Conclusions suggest that a support group provides siblings with the opportunity to decrease

Table 18.3 CANCER WEBSITES

Organization	Website
American Cancer Society	www.cancer.org
Asian American Health	www.baylor.edu/~Charles_Kemp/asian_health.html
Cancer Care	www.cancercare.org
CancerNet	www.cancernet.nci.nih.gov
Candlelighters Childhood Cancer Foundation	www.candlelighters.org
Children's Hospice International	www.chioline.org/
Foundation for the Children's Oncology Group	www.nccf.org
GayHealth.com	www.gayhealth.com
Lance Armstrong Foundation	www.laf.org
Lung Cancer Awareness Campaign	www.lungcancer.org
National Asian Women's Health Organization	www.nawho.org
National Breast Cancer Coalition	www.natlbcc.org
National Cancer Institute	www.nci.nih.org
National Coalition for Cancer Survivorship	www.canceradvocacy.org
National Cervical Cancer Coalition	www.ncc-online.org/
National Family Caregivers Association	www.nfcacares.org
National Hospice and Palliative Care Organization	www.nhpco.org
Native American Cancer Research	www.members.aol.com/natamcan/
Office of Minority Health	www.omhrc.gov
Patient Advocate Foundation	www.patientadvocate.org
The Childhood Brain Tumor Foundation	www.childbraintumor.org
The Childhood Leukemia Center	www.patientcenters.com/leukemia/
The Intercultural Cancer Council	www.icc.bcm.tmc.edu/
The Lesbian Community Cancer Project	www.lccp.org/index.html
The Mautner Project for Lesbians with Cancer	www.mautnerproject.org/
The Susan G. Komen Breast Cancer Foundation	www.komen.org/

their sense of isolation, to vent negative feelings, and to learn from each other. Additionally, data suggest a need for ongoing follow-up with siblings to help them manage the stresses emerging from the impact of the diagnosis and treatment on the family unit.

Parents also suffer from multiple stresses and financial concerns. Research has shown that the financial burden is more pronounced in the younger patient. The potential of having a child die is of such grave importance that individual and couple counseling is highly encouraged. The strain on the marital relationship and the conflict that can occur if the parents are unable to share and work together are enormous. In addition to professional counseling, these parents can benefit from talking with others who are going through a similar experience. The diagnosis is typically a shock and unexpected, filling parents with fear, guilt, and helplessness as they watch their child undergo painful and sometimes futile treatments. Parents' initial reaction to the diagnosis in a child has been described as anticipatory mourning; they may assume the child will die even if the prognosis is encouraging (Seligman, 1996).

Advocacy Groups

"Out of suffering have emerged the strongest souls, the most massive characters are seared with scars" (Klein, 2000). As this quote so clearly states, out of suffering comes great character. This has been the impetus of much of the advocacy movement. Unfortunately, sometimes only through struggles and obstacles can change occur. Advocacy groups are cancer support groups that have a mission about making change through awareness, education, and empowerment. Becoming an advocate on a larger level may increase an individual's feeling of power over cancer. Cancer Care (*www.cancercare.org*), a national organization that provides advocacy as well as information and support to those with cancer, suggests that the following actions can be done by individual patients or groups of patients, and by healthcare professionals:

- Contacting legislators through letters, phone calls, meetings, and email on issues of concern to the cancer patient population
- Acting as an information resource in the community through media or community organizations
- Having a voice in what research should be funded and how new treatments should be implemented and helping researchers, local internal review boards, and government agencies recognize the importance of involving people with cancer on committees reviewing research
- Testifying at government hearings
- Being involved in "THE MARCH coming together to conquer cancer" (for further information call 1-877-THE-MARCH)

There are many respected and powerful advocacy organizations for those desiring to be involved at the national level. These organizations have united to support public policy that affects and hopefully protects the rights of those with a cancer diagnosis. Issues that are concerned with public policy and legislation are often the primary missions of managed-care practices, speedier review and approval of drugs through the Food and Drug Administration, and easier access to new drugs and insurance coverage for clinical trials.

Psychological Effects of Survivorship

Cancer treatment can cause psychological trauma, including the loss of security and control over the happenings of one's body. There are several themes of psychosocial distress that patients with cancer encounter; they have been documented in the literature. These effects include emotional well-being, employment and insurability, lifestyle and relationships, and the physical effects of cancer and its treatment (Quigley, 1989; Welch-McCaffrey, Hoffman, Leigh, Loescher, & Meyskens, Jr, 1989).

Emotional Well-Being

Patients who recently completed treatment have higher anxiety and depressive symptoms than healthy control subjects. These symptoms were found to decrease over time, eventually equaling that of the general population (Quigley, 1984). The incidence of depression among cancer survivors was approximately 6% to 30% as compared with 6% in the noncancer population (Sellick & Crooks, 1999).

Posttraumatic stress disorder resulting in high anxiety levels has also been identified as a delayed effect from cancer and treatment. One study concluded that 4% to 10% of patients with cancer experienced this stress disorder after treatment. The study found that posttraumatic stress disorder occurred more readily in those patients who did not accept the disease (Alter et al., 1996).

Feelings of anxiety and depression after treatment of cancer can lead to a decreased feeling of well-being, as reported on quality-of-life surveys. One theory for why these feelings occur is the concept of "uncertainty" after the treatment is completed. Losing contact with the healthcare team, fear of recurrence, and uncertainty about the future are a few of the concerns that have been described (Mullan, 1985). The tale of the Sword of Damocles, from Greek mythology, describes the tale of a man who was invited to the king's palace. He was placed in the vulnerable position of lying under a sword only held in place by a horse's hair. This story is not unlike the patient, happy to be done with treatment, yet vulnerable to the concerns and issues of survivorship that must be faced without the support of the health-care team (Koocher & O'Malley, 1981). A major-ity of breast cancer patients still worried and had major cancer-related concerns up to five years after treatment. These concerns affected their emotional well-being and view of life overall (Fredette, 1995). The concerns of breast cancer patients up to six months after radiation therapy included issues surrounding work and socializa-tion, which were classified as adaptation to sur-vivorship (Dow & Lafferty, 2000).

Economic Issues

Work and insurance discrimination are common issues. Re-entry into "normal life" has been iden-tified as a stressor for cancer survivors. The Americans with Disabilities Act was passed in 1992, protecting the rights of persons with dis-abilities. This legislation protects the rights of patients with cancer also. Although this legisla-tion exists, cancer patients continue to fear dis-crimination. Feldman (1986) in a classic trilogy of studies reported cancer patients' difficulties in the workplace. The issues included overt discrim-ination from coworkers and employers, workplace attitudes about cancer, and the patient's own atti-tudes about cancer. Although this literature is dated before the disability legislation, many patients still report these feelings, and current reports still refer to these studies.

Although the thoughts of cancer patients rest primarily on health, recovery, and the fear of death, issues concerning finances are also of grave importance. Even with health insurance, most cancer patients fear that the illness will drain the family's financial reserves. Many patients have concerns about being able to work while going through treatment and/or the ability to go back to work after the treatment is over. Will they be able to do their job? Will their job still be there when they recover? If the patient is single, the financial concerns may be greater than those who are in a partnership or marriage. Most people can-not financially afford to have a life-threatening illness and the additional stress that can come from financial insecurity. The energy used for healing is often used instead for fighting for care and finding ways to pay for it. The number of uninsured and underinsured Americans continues to rise. Minorities again are at the greatest risk. Many people who do not have the ability to pay for healthcare will not seek medical care when needed. Many people with a cancer risk do not receive adequate screening or prevention because of inability to pay (Schimmel, 1999).

There is much controversy about access to treat-ments for cancer patients. Although everyone wants to constrain the present healthcare costs, no one wants to be denied access to appropriate test-ing or treatments. It has now become part of the ambulatory care center responsibility to help patients obtain as much financial support as possi-ble. Many ambulatory cancer centers no longer have the availability of a social worker. Case managers are often seen in only the hospital setting. Often this places the nurse in the position to find assistance for the patient. Finding ways to obtain patient sup-portive care is an additional burden to an over-stressed and overworked staff. Third party payers often will not pay for many components of the patient's care. Even with insurance copays, reim-bursement for office visits and medications can be costly. Over-the-counter home prescriptions are not paid for by Medicare and can cost thousands of dol-lars a year. When patients come to the initial con-sultation, they need to bring documents that include their work history, insurance coverage, and prescription coverage. Their ability to pay should be discussed at the initial consultation as well.

Every opportunity for economic assistance should be considered, including pharmaceutical drug assistance programs. Having a skilled and diplomatic billing specialist provides assistance to patients who are having problems with insurance coverage or managed-care corporations and is beneficial to both the patient and the oncology practice. Providing medication samples can relieve some of the prescription costs. Encouraging participation in appropriate clinical trials may offer patients an opportunity to obtain free investigational medications.

Early in the cancer treatment, patients and families require sequential education. Side effect and symptom management is essential for optimal functional and cognitive rehabilitation. Many patients report that the ability to continue working while receiving treatment provides the patient with a sense of normalcy and independence (Dendreon Corporation, 2003b). Being able to return to work is different for every patient, and patient counseling may be considered before entering the work setting. Most oncologists underestimate the time that it requires to recover from chemotherapy and/or radiation. Returning to work depends on the nature of the patient's occupation, type and toxicities of treatment, level of recovery, their emotional stability, job flexibility, and their financial need (Hersh, 1997). The concerns over job security, long-term health insurance, life insurance, and disability insurance are continued threats to the survivor.

Insurance Coverage

Insurance companies are a for-profit business. Many patients and healthcare providers often feel intimidated when claims are denied. However, healthcare providers must advocate and empower patients in communications with their insurance providers for adequate coverage for their care. Encourage patients to review insurance policies and to familiarize themselves with the stipulations of their policy. Patients need to keep careful records of all expenses related to medical treatment, including transportation costs, housing, and other out-of-pocket expenses. Uncovered medical expenses are tax deductible if they exceed a certain percentage of the patient's adjusted gross income. Have patients follow-up with the insurance company any questions that they have about filed claims. The logistics, time, and place of future coverage are to be determined before their current insurance is changed or cancelled. Reinforce to patients and families not to allow the insurance coverage to expire.

Life insurance is difficult to obtain for someone with a history of cancer. The following suggestions come from the National Coalition for Cancer Survivorship:

- Try large companies that carefully grade type and stage of cancer.
- Obtain estimates from several companies. Patients can get a list of all licensed insurance brokers in their area from their state insurance department.
- If a patient is unable to obtain a life-insurance policy with full death benefits, consider a graded policy. If the patient dies from cancer within the first few years of the policy (usually three years), a graded policy returns only your premium plus part of the face value of the policy to the beneficiaries. If the patient should die after the waiting period has passed, the company will pay the full face of the policy.
- Encourage patients to obtain life insurance through a work or group plan. Most group plans do not make an individual answer questions or evaluate the health of each member in a large group.
- The American Council on Life Insurance at 1001 Pennsylvania Avenue, NW, Washington, DC 20004 provides information about brokers who specialize in high-risk life insurance.

Spirituality

Spirituality is the relationship between a person and their surroundings, people, and higher beings. "Spiritual well-being is the ability to maintain hope and derive meaning from the cancer experience that is characterized by uncertainty." (Ferrell, 1996). Patients who have been diagnosed with cancer are faced with their own mortality. It is with this experience that many cancer patients report the ability to accept successfully death as unavoidable, yet not imminent, thereby moving forward past the fears that death evokes (Ferrell, Grant, Dean, Funk, & Ly, 1996). Spirituality fosters hope and provides meaning to a devastating disease (Highfield, 2000). Spiritual care is a new discipline that is considered a separate domain of quality of life. Previously, spirituality was included in the psychological, well-being domain. Bone marrow transplant recipients were the first to describe how spirituality helped them survive what they termed as the "Holocaust." Other cancer survivors described how relationships with others and higher beings helped them to transcend the challenges of the disease and survivorship (Ferrell et al., 1996). Healthcare providers, although aware of spirituality issues, seldom discuss or refer patients and/or caregivers to spiritual care specialists (Highfield, 2000).

Quality of Life

Impaired role performance was found to have both a direct and indirect effect on cancer survivorship (Lancee et al., 1994). Illness may shift an individual's role within the family or work place. Relationships with family and friends have been reported to be both positively as well as negatively effected by cancer. The impact often has to do with the relationships before the cancer diagnosis. Hirshberg and Barash , found that survivors of life-threatening cancers who had long-lasting partnerships of 20 to 30 years had a positive survival benefit over those who did not have this relationship (Hirshberg & Barash, 1995). Social isolation is a common complaint of cancer patients while undergoing treatment. Cancer patients often form strong relationships with

office staff, nurses, phlebotomists, and other patients who are undergoing treatment in the office or hospital. Separation anxiety and a sense of abandonment may accompany the completion of therapy. There is a lack of research on interventions for the late effects of treatment. Many pediatric oncology centers have created long-term follow-up clinics to address the issues of survivorship, but it is rare in the adult oncology population. The challenge is to create this new dimension of ambulatory oncology care. Transitioning the patient into the survivorship role can be difficult but offers a challenge and opportunity (**Table 18.4**).

How to Establish a Survivor Group

Support groups are useful, cost-effective methods of providing service to a large number of patients and family members. All groups are not necessarily successful. Groups may not be successful if they fail to "gel," and a cohesion or bonding is not achieved. Absenteeism, dropouts, and personality clashes may cause internal conflict. Personality types may disrupt the flow of conversation (the monopolizer) or stall the direction (the silent type). Others may fail as limited resources either from the sponsoring organization (budget cuts or personnel reshuffling) or skill and experience level of the facilitators. Some issues can be avoided, however, with careful initial planning. The following sections will provide information to help start a support/survivor group.

Assessing the Need

As more individuals become convinced of the benefits of support groups, hospitals, clinics, or other healthcare facilities have started or have been directed to start programs to meet the growing need. Often the initial impetus of forming support groups was recurring requests from patients or family members struggling to deal

Table 18.4 EDUCATIONAL TOOL DEVELOPMENT FOR PATIENTS FINISHED WITH TREATMENT

1. Provide the patient with a written statement with the type of disease, stage, and any prognostic indicators.

2. Make a list of drugs received and list potential long-term physical risks associated with each drug; give cumulative doses of appropriate agents.

3. Educate patient on the risk of secondary malignancy (risk of getting cancer from the drugs/treatment received).

4. Educate patient on the risk of second/third malignancies related to general population risk or carcinogen exposure.

5. Educate patients on the risks of chronic diseases such as osteoporosis and thyroid dysfunction.

6. Include assessment of physical and psychological effects of cancer survivorship on follow-up appointments (include specific questions about how patient is coping, insurance and work issues as well as fatigue, sexuality, and cognitive dysfunction).

7. Offer support groups specifically for survivors of cancer.

8. Refer to survivorship organizations such as the NCCS.

9. Offer information regarding subscriptions to survivor derived magazines such as Coping, Cure, and Bone Marrow Transplant Newsletter.

10. Develop a transition program to assist patients from the frequent office visit schedule to the less frequent follow-up mode after the completion of treatment. Phone calls can be made at frequent intervals that decrease over time and based on patient need.

11. Initiate a "graduation" ceremony to celebrate the completion of treatment and the start of a new phase of care.

12. Identify which physician is appropriate to call for specific issues (when to call oncologist and when to call primary-care physician).

13. Do a celebration of life ceremony yearly in conjunction with the NCCS's survivor day: the first Sunday in June each year.

14. If you cannot put on a celebration, send a card or put up a banner.

---

with a specific situation or issue. Healthcare providers may observe an increased need for patients with a particular tumor type, that is, ovarian cancer, or a persistent problem across multiple tumor types, that is, symptom management or multiple telephone calls from anxious caregivers.

Gaining a perspective of existing community resources is essential. Calls to the local chapter of the ACS, churches, county agencies, hospitals, and/or clinics will shed light on programs that may be formally or informally in place. Many locations may offer support groups, but it is important to note that the nature of the group may vary greatly depending on the population served, time and space constraints, and a myriad of other factors. The number of patients in a given geographic location should be considered, as well as the urban, suburban, or rural area represented and the existing community culture regarding the use of support groups. Conducting a needs assessment survey may provide valuable insight into gaps in community services.

Identify a Group

Once a need is established, groups of participants that share similar concerns could be "evaluated" as potential members. Screening patients offers the opportunity to initiate dialogue and begin to establish a working relationship with the individual group member. An initial meeting helps to alleviate any nervousness that a person may have about entering the group and may allow the facilitator to interact in a personal way. General goals and expectations can be discussed, and any inappropriate people can be excluded. Although individual reasons to join a group may be diverse, common goals include meeting for the expressed needs of mutual help, information, and discussion of concerns.

Resources

Despite what may seem an overwhelming need and community outcry for a support group, without adequate resources, the project may be destined to fail. To establish and maintain a viable program, a wide variety of resources are essential. Resources can be broken down into system, personnel, and fiscal.

System resources include the cooperation of administration in planning and staffing for a new group. Administration needs to allocate appropriate personnel full-time equivalents to staff the management of a support group. These include secretarial support to field queries and register participants, duplication of materials, and arrange meeting space and scheduling. Qualified nurses and social workers to facilitate the programs are usually the best combination to address both clinical-/treatment-related questions and psychosocial concerns. Public relations and marketing of programs, brochure/flyer development, and distribution are all vital in communication and recruitment, both in the community and among other departments and disciplines.

Logistical resources include location, which should be chosen carefully. The composition of a particular group may function with a more relaxed atmosphere in a location away from the clinic setting. The physical environment is vital to planning a comfortable setting for symptomatic patients. Room temperature and ventilation are considerations for patients experiencing cold intolerance or frequent hot flashes. Comfortable chairs with supporting armrests and a supply of cushions are necessary to facilitate the relaxation of the patient with pain or fatigue issues. The consistent location, time, and schedule (weekly, monthly) are to be consistent because switching sites or times may confuse an already stressed or cognitively impaired individual. Easy access for the physically impaired or quickly fatigued must also be considered.

Personnel resources include the caliber and quality of staff selected to plan, implement, and facilitate the group(s). A multidisciplinary staff possesses excellent communication skills and a proficiency in listening and raises appropriate questions. Group facilitation is an inherent component of social worker preparation, but not necessarily of nursing; however, this learned skill can be acquired via a team approach.

Fiscal resources include budgeted monies to initiate and sustain the support group. Facilitator salaries provide for the time spent in preparation and actual time spent at group meetings. Marketing costs often cover the artwork, typesetting, printing, and mailing of pamphlets, brochures, and posters. Such publications are necessary to alert potential group members and potential sources of referral to the group about the existence of the group. Allocating room space may be easily done within the healthcare organization, but there may be circumstances that prohibit such accommodations. It may be necessary to locate an off-site conference room at a community center, school, or church. Off-site locations may require a rental fee.

Members of the group may appreciate the provision of healthful and nutritious snacks. Refreshments encourage additional fluid and calorie intake for those who may be in need of additional supplements. Various pharmaceutical companies obtain sponsorship funding for refreshments. A resource library of books, relaxation tapes, or informational audiocassettes suitable for home use by group members is an excellent supplement to enhance learning. Videotapes specific to survival issues may be purchased or rented to provide information or spark discussion. Inviting various healthcare professionals to speak to the group and/or to answer specific questions or areas of concerns is informative. Consultants can range from dieticians to address nutritional concerns or childcare experts to discuss behavioral issues or hospital administrators to discuss diagnosis-related groups and other reimbursement issues.

Recruitment

Marketing a survivorship program begins with communication with all those groups that may have expressed an initial interest. Posters, flyers, and the mailing of an invitation to physicians' offices will help to alert potential members and staff that may provide referrals. Newspapers, radio stations, and local or cable television stations are frequently willing to feature information of community interest. Marketing to special populations should include use of newspapers that are targeted to a particular cultural or religious group. Providing a speaker for a specific group meeting in a community church or gathering place may assist in recruitment efforts.

Size of Support Groups

According to Cella and Yellen, a minimum of five and a maximum of twelve form an ideal group size (Cella & Yellen, 1993). Groups limited in size are large enough to permit good interaction yet small enough to allow members to work on individual problems and offer all an opportunity to participate. Groups can also be large, but this venue requires a different structure. Usually large groups include an invited speaker, followed by a question-and-answer period. Members can break into smaller groups for sharing and support. Facilitators of large groups have a responsibility to assess frequently the needs of individual members so that members who need more attention or assistance with a specific problem can be directed to an alternate source of help.

Setting the Environment

Establishing trust is the most initial task in setting the environment of the group. Basic ground rules regarding confidentiality, medical advice, and physician "bashing" are usually discussed as part of the introduction. Confidentiality provides the individual to share personal information without fear of names or stories used outside of the confines of the meeting. Group decisions about the establishment and sharing of a group roster of telephone or e-mail addresses need to be made. Often questions are raised, and medical information and advice are shared. Checking with one's own physician is always recommended before implementing any change in an attendee's medical care. Controversy and physician distrust of the group process can be avoided if there is an early recognition of the differences in medical practice styles and treatment protocols.

Starting and stopping on time provide boundaries that helps an individual feel secure. It also provides validation that their time is important and valued. Because many may have never joined a support group before, it is important to acknowledge their nervousness. Sensitivity is required to identify those who appear frightened or overwhelmed. It is helpful for everyone to introduce himself or herself and share something about their own experiences or what they hope to gain from the group. Early disclosure of even the most basic information helps to establish the experiences and feelings that they have in common and immediately develops cohesion.

Cultural Considerations

In our increasingly diverse communities, it is important to address the unique needs of various cultures and special populations. Special populations include people who are socioeconomically disadvantaged, people of different cultural or ethnic groups, or people with sexual differences. Basic skills described earlier apply, but each group has unique concerns.

These ideas will help to improve communication in the group setting:

- Acknowledge the similarities within the group.
- Acknowledge the differences within the group.
- Provide frequent opportunities for the group to tell individual stories about their culture and family history.
- Encourage as appropriate information regarding ways of seeing the world (Moursund & Kenny, 2002).

The Internet as a Resource

Patients seek information from many sources. Baby boomers have a different attitude about their role in the healthcare arena. They view themselves as leaders in a partnership with their physician. In light of this view, they often seek information before office visits to be prepared for information given and to offer questions to their physician. Patients and their families usually seek information from the Internet because they lack information from other sources (Clark, 1999). Patients report overall satisfaction with the information obtained, the ability to seek out information that is important to them based on their own needs, and the convenience of information seeking from home at times needed (Voluntary Hospital Association, 1999a). Of the estimated 349-million people worldwide that used the Internet in the year 2000 (Lawrence, 2000), 45% searched the Internet for health-related topics. In 1998, 52% were searching for disease-specific information, with one third of those surveyed seeking cancer-related content (Miller et al.,

1992). A disproportionate number of Internet users are White. Blacks and Hispanics compromise 28% of online access. Blacks were more apt to seek online access at academic and public locations (Cyberdialogue, 1999c).

Evaluating Sites

Gaining information from the Internet requires finding credible sources with reliable information. Nurses need to keep in mind and remind patients that not all Websites are reliable or contain correct information. There are many ways to evaluate Websites (Biermann, Golladay, Greenfield, & Baker, 1999). The Health on the Net Foundation is an organization based in Geneva, Switzerland and has published a code of conduct for Websites. Within the code of conduct are principles of appropriate Internet content. These principles include authority, complementarily, confidentiality, attribution, justifiability, transparency of authorship, transparency of sponsorship, and honesty in advertising. If the Website meets all of these principles, they are given a seal of approval that can be found on the home page of the Website (Health on the Net Foundation, 2000). Information sought from credible organizations and their links can be considered reliable. Such sources include the Oncology Nursing Society, the NCI, and the ACS (**Table 18.5**).

Nurses can recommend to patients and family that sites should be chosen if there is a reputable organization or institution to back the site. Information quoted should be timely (within the last year) and reveal the source of sponsorship. Although it is difficult for the uninformed to determine whether a site is fair balanced, other areas such as technical support for site problems occur, and a glossary of terms for difficult terminology (Clark, 1999) may be helpful. Websites should be viewable regardless of the computer software or computer memory. The acceptable reading level for patient education material is eighth grade. The readability of several sections of

NCI's Cancer Net site revealed that the average reading level was 12th grade, with some sections within the same site being more difficult than that (Wilson, Baker, Brown-Syed, & Gollop, 2000).

Information Sites Versus Chat Rooms

There are several sites that offer education alone. However, Websites do not offer the patient the ability to exchange information with other patients or healthcare personnel. Online support groups are held at a certain time of the day of the week and are moderated by a nurse or social worker. These programs allow the patients to exchange issues and have the benefit of a group facilitator to answer questions and manage group dynamics. The Internet can also be used to communicate to the healthcare provider via e-mail, and specialized reporting mechanisms are being developed to have the patient report specific symptoms to the doctor or primary nurse. E-mail has inherent concerns, namely confidentiality and response time. As medical practices become more busy and patients and healthcare providers become more computer savvy, these forms of interactions will

likely be daily occurrences (Clark & Gomez, 2001) (**Table 18.6**).

Patients and family members should be cautioned about the use of chat rooms that are not moderated by healthcare professionals. Although anecdotal information may provide a novel or unconventional complementary therapy, many horror stories exist (Fogel, 2002) about patients who ignore standard therapy and follow the "expert" they met online.

Sample Programs

There are many online support programs that are available to patients. Diseases such as the chronic lymphocytic leukemia and myelodysplastic syndrome have their own list serves and chat rooms to post questions and issues as well as communicate with patients with like diseases. University of Iowa Hospitals and Clinics is a rural setting with a low attendance to traditional support services. They started an online support group that is free and confidential and is facilitated by an oncology nurse and oncology social worker (Abbott, Sutter, & Felkner, 2000). Another interesting program that was developed by a multidisciplinary care team at City of Hope is based on a

Table 18.5 CHARACTERISTICS OF SELECTED WEBSITES HELPFUL FOR PATIENTS EXPERIENCING CANCER

Web Address	Sponsor	Medical Information	Psychological/ Coping Information	Personalization Option	Online Support Group
www.cancer.org	American Cancer Society	Yes	Yes	Yes	Yes
www.webmd.com	WebMD Health	Yes	Yes	Yes	Yes
www.susanlovemd.com	Dr. Susan Love	Yes	Yes	Yes	No
www.komen.org/	The Susan G. Komen Breast Cancer Foundation	Yes	Yes	No	No
www.cancer.gov	National Cancer Institute	Yes	Yes	No	No
www.ivillage.com	ivillage	Yes	Yes	Yes	Yes
www.oncolonk.com	Oncolink (University of Pennsylvania)	Yes	Yes	Yes	No

Fogel, 2002. Reprinted with permission from Medscape, WebMD, Inc.

needs-assessment survey. This program offered a Website that linked the patient to 302 agencies across six counties (Mercurio & Rhodes, 2000). A comprehensive listing of educational and support programs for prostate cancer patients was highlighted in a professional publication. This listing gave the Internet resources for prostate cancer information and support. Thirty-three Websites were listed, with three of them including online support, as well as several others offering links to online support programs (Davis, 2000). The Internet is becoming the newest form of communication for patients with cancer, and nurses in the ambulatory setting will need to familiarize themselves with these, as well as be prepared for patients to bring in information from this source.

Survivorship Issues

This section of the chapter on support groups and survivorship programs focuses on the physiologic as well as the psychological issues cancer survivors confront with any cancer diagnosis. It is important to identify these issues to successfully develop support programs and education that will reflect the needs of this unique population. "Late effects" are symptoms that appear after treatment is complete, ranging from months to many years after treatment. "Persistent symptoms" are symptoms that present during treatment and continue on after treatment has completed. See **Table 18.6**.

Late Effects of Cancer Treatment

Cancer treatment is multidimensional, often employing several toxic treatment modalities with effects on healthy as well as cancerous tissue. Effects can be short term, lasting only as long as the treatment, or long term, lasting beyond cure or control of the disease. Effects can be clinically obvious, minimally observable, or even subclinical in nature. Unlike acute symptoms of cancer therapy, late effects of cancer treatment tend to affect slower growing cells such as organs and arise and persist long after the treatment is complete (Ruccione & Weinberg, 1989). Over the last decade, acute symptoms have been studied, resulting in interventions that decrease these effects. Interventions for late effects of cancer treatment are scarce and have not improved over the last decade (Ganz, 2001). The latent effects are more evident as patients live longer past treatment and studies continue to mature. The majority of the data compiled on long-term survivors of cancer come from the pediatric literature. There are only small subsets of adult patients such as those with Hodgkin's lymphoma, testicular cancer, and non-Hodgkin's lymphoma who have been studied (Ruccione & Weinberg, 1989; Ganz, 2001). Familiarization with the long-term effects of treatment will prepare nurses to assess patients and develop educational material or programs to encourage the patients to survive and thrive.

Table 18.6 ONCOLOGY NURSING INTERNET INTERVIEW

Have you used the Internet for medical information or support?

Can I recommend some Websites that may be helpful to you regarding your medical condition?

Have you been following any treatment recommendations that you read on a Website or heard about from an online support group?

Is there any information that you read on a Website or heard about from an online support group about treatment that you would like to discuss?

Fogel, 2002. Reprinted with permission from Medscape, WebMD, Inc.

Cognitive Dysfunction

Cognitive function is "a mental process by which one becomes aware of ideas." It involves perception, thinking, reasoning, and remembering (Glanze, 1985). Cognitive dysfunction is a vague concept that describes a number of neuropsychological dysfunctions (O'Shaughnessy, 2000). Cognitive dysfunction is thought to be a sequelae of chemotherapy and cranial irradiation. The symptoms include difficulty concentrating (Schagen et al., 1999) and short-term memory loss.

Cognitive dysfunction has been studied most extensively in breast cancer survivors. Several studies have concluded that breast cancer patients who undergo chemotherapy have changes in cognition and lower IQ scores as compared with those who do not undergo chemotherapy. This effect was worse during chemotherapy but continued for years after treatment. Even two years past treatment, moderate impairment in cognition, which impacted their performance in work and home activities, was reported (Schagen et al., 1999). Cognitive dysfunction has also been evaluated in patients with lung cancer and non-Hodgkin's lymphoma, resulting in findings similar to those of breast cancer (Meyers, Weitzner, Valentine, & Levin, 1998).

Many studies have evaluated the cognitive impairments in children receiving cranial irradiation prophylactically for acute lymphocytic leukemia (Pui, 2000). These studies found a significant decrease in IQ scores among patients who received cranial irradiation and/or intrathecal chemotherapy. Another study evaluated the difference between those children who received cranial irradiation versus intrathecal chemotherapy alone and found that those who received cranial irradiation had more severe deficits in word recognition, spelling, and math (Rowland et al., 1984). This cognitive dysfunction increases over time (Twaddle, Britton, Craft, Noble, & Kernahan, 1983). Cognitive dysfunction occurs in patients undergoing cranial irradiation for small-cell lung cancer (Chak et al., 1986) for primary brain tumors (Corbett, 1999). Patients who underwent cranial irradiation for acute lymphocytic leukemia and small cell lung cancer and were found to have abnormal CAT scans and magnetic resonance imaging. Atrophy was the most common abnormality found with leukoencephalopathy, and calcifications were found less often (Peylan, Ramu, Poplack, Pizzo, Adornato, & Di Chiro, 1978). Biologic response modifiers have also been shown to cause cognitive impairment (Curt et al., 2000).

With the growing body of knowledge about cognitive dysfunction, there has been increased interest in researching interventions to prevent or compensate for these impairments. One interesting finding studied in rodents is the effect of epoetin alfa on cognition. Erythropoietin receptors are found in the brain and are thought to have a protective effect on damaged brain tissue. Several preclinical murine studies have concluded that by giving erythropoietin before or immediately after brain damage or injury, there was a decrease in the necrosis or brain damage (Cerami, Brines, Ghezzi, & Cerami, 2001) compared with those mice that did not receive erythropoietin. Natural restorative interventions have been shown to have an impact on attention. The interventions included walking or sitting outdoors in natural surroundings, tending to plants or gardening, watching birds, and caring for pets. Patients who received this intervention strategy showed significant improvement in attentional capacity over the patients who did not perform the intervention (Cimprich, 1993). Other interventions have been found to be beneficial, although no formal clinical trials evaluating the benefits have been completed. These interventions include exercising, making lists and keeping a journal, keeping reminders from friends and family, sleeping, managing stress, challenging the brain by doing crossword puzzles or math problems, and eating nutritious foods (Cimprich, 1995). Meyers et al. evaluated the potential benefit of methylphenidate to improve cognition in brain tumor patients and concluded that 10 mg twice a day improved cognition and daily functioning with minimal adverse effects (Meyers et al., 1998).

Vision and Hearing

Visual changes have been identified with patients who have undergone cranial irradiation, total-body irradiation, corticosteroid therapy, and tamoxifen (Wharam, 1983).

During the National Surgical Adjuvant Breast and Bowel Project trial comparing estrogen receptor positive and progesterone receptor negative patients on tamoxifen to placebo, it was found that there was a significant increase in cataracts in the tamoxifen arm as compared with the placebo arm of the trial. Cataracts are the most common long-term visual effects of cancer treatment (Ruccione & Weinberg, 1989).

High-pitched hearing loss has been associated with use of cisplatin. The neurotoxic effect of cisplatin results in this persistent effect. The symptom begins during treatment and if cisplatin is continued, the hearing loss will become permanent (Nielsen & Brant, 2002). Other toxic agents are antibiotics such as amikacin, gentamycin, and vancomycin. The best treatment for visual and hearing deficits is prevention. Pretreatment evaluation of vision and hearing is beneficial to determine baseline function. Vision and hearing deficits should be assessed throughout treatment, as well as after treatment. When deficits occur, stopping treatment is the only way to decrease the severity of symptoms.

Cardiac Effects

Cardiac damage has been reported extensively in the acute setting after the administration of a cumulative dose of anthracyclines and high doses of cyclophosphamide. Late effects of treatment on the heart have been studied for many years. It has been found that cardiac damage can occur as late as 2.5 to 7 years after anthracycline administration (Freter, Lee, Billingham, Chak, & Bristow,

1986). The muscle fibers are damaged by drug administration but may not cause any effect until a stressful event or advancing age occurs. It has been reported that patients who have undergone treatment for Hodgkin's disease as a child/adolescent have lower cardiac reserve when undergoing vigorous exercise or even pregnancy several years after mediastinal radiation treatment (Hancock & Hoppe, 1996). A report of deaths caused by congestive heart failure, dysrhythmias, and sudden death as late as six years after treatment with anthracyclines for pediatric tumors has been documented (Welch-McCaffrey et al., 1989). Radiation therapy causes an increased risk of myocardial fibrosis to the pericardium. The damage is progressive and surfaces several years after completion of radiation therapy. Late effects of radiation therapy have been repeatedly documented in the young adults with Hodgkin's disease. Cardiovascular abnormalities have been seen ranging from coronary artery disease to myocardial infarction, with resulting bypass surgery in patients five years after treatment (Pohjola-Sintonen, Totterman, Salmo, & Siltanen, 1987).

Treatment has been refined to include alternative dosing schedules: lengthening administration times and development of unique delivery systems such as liposomal doxorubicin that have resulted in decreased cardiac toxicity (Keefe, 2001). Radiation techniques have been improved to include shielding the heart to protect it from the damaging effects of radiation. Cardioprotective agents such as dezrazoxane are available to decrease the cardiotoxic effect of anthracyclines on the heart muscle (Wilkes, Ingwersen, & Barton-Burke, 2001). Despite improvements to treatment, long-term follow-up is necessary for those patients who received any cardiotoxic drugs and/or mediastinal radiation therapy because as many as 5% will have chronic cardiotoxicity (Camp-Sorrell, 1999). Suggested follow-up includes physical examination assessing for a third heart sound or gallop, an annual echocardiogram, and clinical symptom evaluation. If symptoms do occur, a cardiology consultation is recommended. Treatment may include angiotensin-converting enzyme inhibitors, diuretics, fluid volume monitoring, and reduction of salt intake. If the cardiac disease progresses to the point of irreversible cardiomyopathy, heart transplantation may be a viable option (Keefe, 2001).

Pulmonary Toxicity

Pulmonary toxicity can occur from both chemotherapy and radiation therapy. Chemotherapy affects the endothelial cells in the lining of the lung tissue, causing permanent damage to the lung parenchyma. There appear to be two types of reactions: an inflammatory reaction causing pneumonitis and an allergic-type reaction. Continued administration of pulmonary toxic chemotherapeutic agents can cause changes in the connective tissue, causing alveolar damage and pulmonary fibrosis, resulting in an increased effort to breathe (Lund et al., 1995). Drugs known to cause pulmonary damage include Bleomycin, nitrosureas, alkylating agents, and methotrexate (Camp-Sorrell, 1999). Symptoms can occur as early as six weeks after treatment or can take several years to present. The symptoms usually include a dry, nonproductive cough, shortness of breath, and dyspnea on exertion (Keefe, 2001).

Radiation to the chest results in alveolar damage and can have the same effect on the lung tissue as chemotherapy. Fibrosis will evolve over the next several months to years after radiation therapy because of endothelial damage. The degree and duration of radiation pneumonitis and fibrosis are dependent on the dose of radiation. The greater the dose and more lung tissue radiated the greater the damage (Loescher, Welch-McCaffrey, Leigh, Hoffman, & Meyskens, Jr., 1989).

Treatment of pulmonary toxicity is prevention and early identification. Patients should be monitored closely for signs and symptoms of pulmonary fibrosis. Patients should contact the healthcare team immediately for any symptoms of cough, shortness of breath, and/or restrictive airway. Corticosteroids have been shown to have some benefit in reducing the symptoms. Oxygen therapy at conservative doses may be beneficial in reducing hypoxia. Referral to a pulmonologist is often beneficial (Ruccione & Weinberg, 1989).

Genitourinary Effects

Late renal failure has been reported with nitrosureas and cisplatin as well as radiation therapy. Glomerular sclerosis, tubular atrophy, and necrosis often progress to renal failure (Schilsky, 1984). Renal impairment has been shown to begin 2 months to two years after treatment of both cisplatin and the nitrosoureas (Fjelborg, Sorensen, & Helkjaer, 1986). Radiation's toxic effect to the kidney appears to be worse when given in doses of more than 2,000 gray and when given with radiation enhancing chemotherapy (Tefft et al., 1976). Latent bladder toxicity has been associated with the administration of ifosfamide and cyclophosphamide. The byproduct acrolein can cause hemorrhagic cystitis and long-term effects on the bladder, potentially leading to cystectomy. The use of mesna and vigorous hydration has greatly reduced this risk (Loescher et al., 1989; Ruccione & Weinberg, 1989).

The risk of renal dysfunction can be diminished with vigorous hydration during treatment and monitoring renal function via blood and urine testing. At the completion of treatment, monitoring patients who have had cisplatin closely for signs of renal insufficiency is warranted. Patients who are on other nephrotoxic drugs such as antibiotics, immune suppressants, nonsteroidal anti-inflammatory drugs, and cyclooxygenase-2 inhibitors should also be monitored for renal dysfunction.

Reproductive Effects

"Sexuality includes feelings about one's body, the need for touch, interest in sexual activity, communication of one's sexual needs to a partner, and the ability to engage in satisfying sexual activities" (Thaler-DeMers, 2001). Although patients have reported sexuality as an important issue, healthcare professionals infrequently address the topic. Cognitive, emotional, and physical circumstances can affect sexuality (Thaler-DeMers, 2001). A study of the sexual effects of breast cancer patients found that 49% of the patients reported the onset of sexual dysfunction to be after chemotherapy or surgery. It was also noted that none of the study participants identified the nurse as a person with whom to discuss sexuality issues (Barni & Mondin, 1997). Another study found that sexuality as well as family distress had a greater negative influence on social well-being than any other measure (Ferrell & Dow, 1997).

Women often are placed into a premature menopausal state, depriving them of estrogen. Estrogen is necessary for the health of the vaginal mucosa. Without estrogen, a woman has atrophy of the vagina and vaginal dryness, often leading to painful intercourse. There also may be a decrease in the libido related to body image, stress, and fatigue, as well as this estrogen deprivation (Bush & Griffen-Sobel, 2002).

Males can also be negatively affected sexually after cancer therapy. Patients with prostate and testicular cancer have been the most widely studied. Prostate cancer patients have approximately 20% risk of erectile dysfunction after surgery (Stanford et al., 2000). Other issues after surgery or radiation therapy include dry ejaculation, nerve damage causing diminished sensation, and orgasm intensity. Hormonal therapy can cause gynecomastia, penile atrophy, or testicular atrophy, all of which can cause altered sexual image (Thaler-DeMers, 2001).

Chemotherapy, radiation therapy, surgery, and hormonal therapy can have an adverse effect on gonadal function and result in infertility (Check, Brown, & Check, 2000). Infertility rates are hard to determine because of a lack of long-term follow-up. Case reports of two male bone marrow transplant patients who received total body irradiation found that both fathered a child. The chemotherapy treatments affect spermatogenesis, oogenesis, as well as physical function.

Fertility after cancer treatment is a concern for those survivors of childbearing age. The alkylating agents have been extensively studied regarding their effects on reproduction. Alkylators have been shown to cause gonadal impairment with resultant azoospermia or oligospermia. Patients with testicular cancer, lymphoma, and leukemia have also been shown to have decreased sperm counts pretreatment, identifying that the disease itself may cause dysfunction (Meirow & Schenker, 1995). Radiation therapy below the diaphragm has resulted in infertility in both men and women. It has also been shown to induce premature menopause (Byrne, 1999). Surgical removal of the ovaries and testicles render the patient infertile after surgery. Some abdominal and pelvic surgeries will cause adhesion that can cause infertility.

Many advances have been made both in the fertility specialty as well as in the field of oncology to preserve fertility as often as possible (Thaler-DeMers, 2001). Chemotherapy drugs with the highest rate of infertility such as nitrogen mustard have been eliminated from treatments if fertility is a viable option for the patient. Ovaries have been suspended out of the radiation field to protect them from the effects of radiation (Thaler-DeMers, 2001; Ganz, 2001). Surgeries have been modified to preserve reproductive function without compromising cure (Low, Perrin, Crandon, & Hacker, 2000).

Radiation and chemotherapy have been shown to cause chromosomal damage to the ovarian and testicular tissue (Chatterjee, Haines, Perera, Goldstone, & Morris, 2000). Studies are limited but have shown no increased risk for congenital malformations or childhood cancer among the offspring of survivors. Although this is true, there has been shown to be a higher rate of spontaneous abortion, low birth weight babies, and neonatal deaths among females who had previously undergone chemotherapy or radiation therapy. This effect may be from damage to the uterine tissue.

Interventions for reproductive effects include a multidimensional approach, including both the psychosocial issues and the reproductive issues. One study found that patients had a desire to learn more about sexuality issues but were not offered the information (Thaler-DeMers, 2001).

Interventions for infertility should be considered before the start of treatment. Sperm cryopreservation is an easy way to attempt to preserve fertility after treatment. Sperm collection can be done before treatment or early in the treatment cycle before a decline in sperm counts (Zapzalka, Redmon, & Pryor, 1999). Intracytoplasmic sperm injection is a new procedure that has shown promise for those who have pretreatment suboptimal sperm counts. Women have fewer options to preserve ovaries. Cryopreservation of ovarian tissue is promising but has a high failure rate and holds a risk of harboring malignant cells. Hormonal stimulation of oocytes and fertilization at time of harvest with subsequent cryopreservation has improved conception rates (Newton, 1998). Once pregnant, whether it be natural or from cryopreserved ova, the woman should be referred to a high-risk obstetrician.

Fatigue

Fatigue is a symptom that has recently received much attention as a long-term effect (Curt, 2000). There is growing evidence that fatigue is a long-term consequence of cancer and its treatment, but the etiology remains unknown. Treatment-related fatigue is caused by anemia, infection, dehydration, hormonal deficiency, malnutrition, and sleep disturbances as well as cytokine release. Many of these effects last for several months after treatment (Nail, 2001). Thyroid dysfunction, ovarian failure, and cardiopulmonary abnormalities must also be considered (Harpham, 1998). The typical scenario is that initially the fatigue is highest after treatment, with a rapid decline over the first several months. Fatigue then slowly declines and plateaus months to years post treatment (Schwartz et al., 2000). Long-term breast, ovarian, and thyroid cancer survivors (n = 910) found that fatigue remained a negative impact on all aspects of quality of life (Ferrell, 1996). Survivors of Hodgkin's disease and non-Hodgkin's lymphoma found that at even 32 months after treatment, a lack of energy was evident and impacted daily living (Devlen, Maquite, Phillips, Crowter, & Chambers, 1987). Fatigue has been the most consistently reported symptom after bone marrow transplantation (Haberman, Bush, Young, & Sullivan, 1993). Fatigue may prevent patients from returning to work, engaging in social activities, or even being able to care for himself or herself (Nail, 2001).

Thyroid Dysfunction

Thyroid dysfunction can occur as late as 15 to 20 years after treatment and thus may be misdiagnosed (Samaan et al., 1987). Patients who receive radiation therapy to the head, neck, and mantle are at greatest risk. The incidence has been reported as 4% to 79% of those who received radiation to the neck region (Ramsay, Kim, & Coccia, 1978). Hypothyroidism can occur from direct radiation damage to the thyroid or from damage to the anterior pituitary or hypothalamus, resulting in decrease production of thyroid hormones. Symptoms include lethargy, extreme fatigue, weight gain, hair loss, dry skin, bradycardia, anemia, as well as poor intellectual development in children (Ingbar, 1985). The body compensates for the damaged thyroid gland by elevating the level of thyroid stimulating hormone. This elevation can stimulate the damaged thyroid to produce normal levels of thyroid hormones for a period of time. Patients who have this compensatory hypothyroidism may be asymptomatic. The replacement of thyroid hormone results in a rapid improvement of symptoms.

Secondary Malignancies

Secondary malignancies can be defined as tumors that occur after the initial cancer that are not metastatic disease. Second tumors can be due to natural history risk factor (i.e., women have a 1:8 chance of developing breast cancer by the age of 85 after cure of cervical cancer at the age of 30) or due to exposure to a common carcinogen. Patients who develop bladder cancer followed by the development of lung cancer often have been exposed to the common carcinogen of smoking. There may be a genetic trait that predisposes a person to more than one form of cancer, as is the case in breast and ovarian cancer. Finally a secondary malignancy may occur as a result of the toxic effects of treatment (Fraser & Tucker, 1989).

Chemotherapy effects DNA synthesis in both healthy and cancerous tissue. Healthy cells have the ability to repair the damage. If the damage is not repaired, cell mutation may occur, which can start a proliferative process (Fraser & Tucker, 1988). Alkylating agents bind directly to DNA, causing damage to the cancerous as well as normal cells (Chabner & Myers, 1985).

Epidemiologic studies of patients with cancer have evaluated the risks of secondary malignancies. There has been a clear relationship between patients with Hodgkin's disease, multiple myeloma, ovarian cancer, non-Hodgkin's lymphoma, breast cancer, gastrointestinal cancers, lung cancers, and testicular cancer and secondary leukemias (Fraser & Tucker, 1988). Hodgkin's disease has been the most extensively studied. There has been said to be a 77-fold increased risk of developing acute myeloid leukemia in Hodgkin's disease survivors within the first four years after treatment. Secondary malignancy occurrence range has been shown to be between 1 to 20 years after treatment (Tucker, Coleman, Cox, Varghese, & Rosenburg, 1988; Whedon, Stearns, & Mills, 1995). The drugs most likely to cause secondary malignancies are melphalan, mechlorethamine, procarbazine, and cyclophos-phamide (Fraser & Tucker, 1989). A study done at St. Jude's Children's Research Hospital found an increased risk of secondary malignancies after treatment with doxorubicin, dactinomycin, and etoposide. Sarcomas of the bone and soft tissue have been reported after radiation therapy. These tumors can develop as early as five months after treatment, but they more commonly occur 10 years after radiation therapy (Tucker et al., 1987) (**Table 18.7**).

Table 18.7 LONG-TERM PHYSICAL EFFECTS OF CANCER TREATMENT

Long-Term Effect	Cause	Assessment	Interventions
Cardiac	Anthracyclines Chest irradiation	Monitor cumulative dose of anthracyclines. Assess for signs and symptoms of heart failure (i.e., shortness of breath, edema, etc.). Periodic EKG and CXR. Ejection Fraction evaluation.	Refer to cardiologist for heart failure. Administer anthracycline via continuous infusion or liposomal formulation. Administer cardioprotectant, Zinecard if appropriate.
Cognitive dysfunction	Radiation to the brain Chemotherapy Biotherapy	Assess memory. Assess IQ tests. Assess ability to function on the job.	Treat possible underlying causes (i.e., anemia, electrolyte imbalance). Use of mental puzzles. Mental restorative interventions. Brain damage rehabilitation. Stress relief.
Fatigue	Chemotherapy Biotherapy Radiation Surgery	Assess fatigue level each visit during treatment and after completion. Develop a fatigue assessment that works for your ambulatory setting.	Treat underlying causes of fatigue (i.e., anemia, thyroid dysfunction, dehydration, malnutrition). Offer intervention strategies (i.e., energy conservation, energy restoration, good nutrition).
Hearing	Radiation to the brain Cisplatin–dose dependent	Professional assessment of hearing before the start of therapy. Periodically assess during and at completion of treatment.	Refer to audiologist if needed for interventions (i.e., hearing aids).
Pulmonary	Alkylating agents Nitrosureas Chest or total body irradiation	Assess all lung fields. Assess for dry hacking cough. Periodic chest X-ray.	Corticosteroids. Low-dose oxygen therapy. Refer to pulmonologist.
Renal	Cisplatin	Hydrate while receiving the drug. Monitor renal function periodically for several years after treatment.	Refer to nephrologist if needed. Dialysis. Avoid additional nephrotoxic drugs.

Table 18.7 LONG-TERM PHYSICAL EFFECTS OF CANCER TREATMENT (CONT'D)

Long-Term Effect	Cause	Assessment	Interventions
Reproductive	Alkylating agents Radiation to pelvis	Assess patient's desire to have children after entering into treatment. Shield reproductive organs during radiation if possible.	Refer to reproductive specialist as soon as possible before or early into treatment. Educate patient and partner on sexuality as well as reproductive issues. Educate patient and partner about safe handling issues related to secretions 48 hours after each treatment.
Thyroid dysfunction	Radiation to the head and neck	Assess thyroid function periodically after treatment.	If thyroid deficiency, give supplementation.
Vision	Radiation therapy Biotherapy Tamoxifen	Professional assessment before treatment. Intermittent assessment during and after treatment completion.	Refer to ophthalmologist for specialized testing (i.e., split lamp evaluation, surgical removal of cataracts).

EKG – electrocardiogram
CXR – chest X-ray
IQ – intelligence quota

References

Abbott, L., Sutter, J., & Felkner, J. (2000). On-Line support group: The wave of the future. Oncology Nursing Society's 25th Annual Congress. San Antonio, TX.

Alter, C. L., Pelcovitz, D., Axelrod, A., Goldenberg, B., Harris, H., Meyers, B. et al. (1996). Identification of PTSD in cancer survivors. *Psychosomatics, 37*, 137–143.

Barni, S. & Mondin, R. (1997). Sexual dysfunction in treated breast cancer patients. *Annals of Oncology, 8*, 149–153.

Biermann, J. S., Golladay, G. J., Greenfield, M. L., & Baker, L. H. (1999). Evaluation of cancer information on the Internet. *Cancer, 86*, 381–390.

Bouchard, R. (1967). *Nursing Care of the Cancer Patient*. St. Louis: C.V. Mosby Company.

Bush, N. J. & Griffin-Sobel, J. P. (2002). Management of mood changes related to treatment-induced menopause. *Oncology Nursing Forum, 29*, 1269–1272.

Bushkin, E. (1993). The Mara Mogensen Flaherty memorial lecture. Signposts of survivorship. *Oncology Nursing Forum, 20*, 869–875.

Byrne, J. (1999). Infertility and premature menopause in childhood cancer survivors. *Medical and Pediatric Oncology, 33*, 24–28.

Camp-Sorrell, D. (1999). Surviving the cancer, surviving the treatment: Acute cardiac and pulmonary toxicity. *Oncology Nursing Forum, 26*, 983–990.

Cella, D. F., Mahon, S. M., & Donovan, M. I. (1990). Cancer recurrence as a traumatic event. *Behavioral Medicine, 16*, 15–22.

Cella, D. F., Mahon, S. M., & Donovan, M. I. (1970). Cancer recurrance in a traumatic event. *Behavorial Medicine, 16*, 15–22.

Cella, D. F. & Yellen, S. B. (1993). Cancer support groups: The state of the art. *Cancer Practice, 1*, 56–61.

Cerami, A., Brines, M. L., Ghezzi, P., & Cerami, C. J. (2001). Effects of epoetin alfa on the central nervous system. *Seminars in Oncology, 28*(2 Suppl 8), 66–70.

Chabner, B. A. & Myers, C. E. (1985). Clinical pharmacology of cancer chemotherapy. In V. T. DeVita, S. Hellman, & S. A. Rosenberg (Eds.), *Cancer: Principles and Practice of Oncology* (2nd ed., pp. 156–197). Philadelphia: J.B. Lippincott.

Chak, L. Y., Zatz, L. M., Wasserstein, P., Cox, R. S., Kushlan, P. D., Porzig, K. J. et al. (1986). Neurologic dysfunction in patients treated for small cell carcinoma of the lung: A clinical and radiological study. *International Journal of Radiation Oncology, Biology, Physics, 12*, 385–389.

Chatterjee, R., Haines, G. A., Perera, D. M., Goldstone, A., & Morris, I. D. (2000). Testicular and sperm DNA damage after treatment with fludarabine for chronic lymphocytic leukaemia. *Human Reproduction, 15*, 762–766.

Check, M. L., Brown, T., & Check, J. H. (2000). Recovery of spermatogenesis and successful conception after bone marrow transplant for acute leukaemia: Case report. *Human Reproduction, 15*, 83–85.

Cimprich, B. (1993). Development of an intervention to restore attention in cancer patients. *Cancer Nursing, 16*, 83–92.

Cimprich, B. (1995). Symptom management: Loss of concentration. *Seminars in Oncology Nursing, 11*, 279–288.

Clark, P. M. (1999). How can we coach patients to become critical consumers of information and the Internet? *ONS News, 4*, 8.

Clark, P. M. & Gomez, E. G. (2001). Details on demand: Consumers, cancer information, and the Internet. *Clinical Journal of Oncology Nursing, 5*, 19–24.

Corbett, T. C. (1999). Mental fatigue: A patient shares her story. *Fatigue Forum Newsletter, 3*, 5.

Coriel, J. & Behal, R. (1999). Man to man prostate support groups. *Cancer Practice, 7*, 122–129.

Curt, G. A. (2000). Impact of fatigue on quality of life in oncology patients. *Seminars in Hematology, 37*(4 Suppl 6), 14–17.

Curt, G. A., Breitbart, W., Cella, D., Groopman, J. E., Horning, S. J., Itri, L. M. et al. (2000). Impact of cancer-related fatigue on the lives of patients: New findings from the Fatigue Coalition. *Oncologist, 5*, 353–360.

Cyberdialogue. (1999). While digital gap remains, 4.9 million African-Americans now online (press release). Retrieved from *http://www.cyberdialogue.com/resource/press/release/1999/12-06-ic-afro_am.html*

Davis, L. E. (2000). Internet resources for prostate cancer information. *Highlights in Oncology Practice, 18*, 77–84.

Devine, E. C. & Westlake, S. K. (1995). The effects of psychoeducational care provided to adults with cancer: Meta-analysis of 116 studies. *Oncology Nursing Forum, 22*, 1369–1381.

Devlen, J., Maquite, P., Phillips, P., Crowter, D., & Chambers, H. (1987). Psychological problems associated with diagnosis and treatment of lymphomas. I: Retrospective study. *British Medical Journal Clinical Research Edition 295*, 953–954.

Dow, K. H. & Lafferty, P. (2000). Quality of life, survivorship, and psychosocial adjustment of young women with breast cancer after breast-conserving surgery and radiation therapy. *Oncology Nursing Forum, 27,* 1555–1564.

Edelman, S., Lemon, J., Bell, D. R., & Kidman, A. D. (1999). Effects of Group CBT on the survival time of patients with metastatic breast cancer. *Psycho-oncology, 8,* 474–481.

Feldman, F. L. (1986). Female cancer patients and caregivers: Experiences in the workplace. *Women Health, 11,* 137–153.

Ferrell, B., Grant, M., Dean, G., Funk, B., & Ly, J. (1996). "Bone tired": The experience of fatigue and its impact on quality of life. *Oncology Nursing Forum, 23,* 1539–1547.

Ferrell, B. P. (1996). The quality of lives: 1,525 voices of cancer. *Oncology Nursing Forum, 23,* 909–916.

Ferrell, B. R. & Dow, K. H. (1997). Quality of life among long-term cancer survivors. *Oncology, 11,* 565–576.

Fjeldborg, P., Sorensen, J., & Helkjaer, P. E. (1986). The long-term effect of cisplatin on renal function. *Cancer, 58,* 2214–2217.

Fobair, P. (1997). Cancer support groups and group therapies: Part 1. *Journal of Psychological Oncology, 15,* 63–81.

Fogel, J. (2002). Internet use and advanced practice oncology nursing. *Topics in Advanced Practice Nursing eJournal, 2.*

Fraser, M. C. & Tucker, M. A. (1988). Late effects of cancer therapy: Chemotherapy-related malignancies. *Oncology Nursing Forum, 15,* 67–77.

Fraser, M. C. & Tucker, M. A. (1989). Second malignancies following cancer therapy. *Seminars in Oncology Nursing, 5,* 43–55.

Fredette, S. L. (1995). Breast cancer survivors: Concerns and coping. *Cancer Nursing, 18,* 35–46.

Freter, C. E., Lee, T. C., Billingham, M. E., Chak, L., & Bristow, M. R. (1986). Doxorubicin cardiac toxicity manifesting seven years after treatment. Case report and review. *American Journal of Medicine, 80,* 483–485.

Ganz, P. A. (2001). Late effects of cancer and its treatment. *Seminars in Oncology Nursing, 17,* 241–248.

Glanze, W. D. (1985). *The Mosby Medical Encyclopedia.* New York: New American Library.

Goodwin, P. J., Leszcz, M., Ennis, M., Koopmans, J., Vincent, L., Guther, H. et al. (2001). The effect of group psychosocial support on survival in metastatic breast cancer. *New England Journal of Medicine, 345,* 1719–1726.

Gray, R. E. & Fitch, M. (2001). Cancer self-help groups are here to stay: Issues and challenges for health professionals. *Journal of Palliative Care, 17,* 53–58.

Guidry, J. J., Aday, L. A., Zhang, D., & Winn, R. J. (1997). The role of informal and formal social support networks for patients with cancer. *Cancer Practice, 5,* 241–246.

Haberman, M., Bush, N., Young, K., & Sullivan, K. M. (1993). Quality of life of adult long-term survivors of bone marrow transplantation: A qualitative analysis of narrative data. *Oncology Nursing Forum, 20,* 1545–1553.

Hancock, S. L. & Hoppe, R. T. (1996). Long-term complications of treatment and causes of mortality after Hodgkin's Disease. *Seminars in Radiation Oncology, 6,* 225–242.

Harpham, W. S. (1998). Long-term survivorship: Late effects. In A. M. Berger, R. K. Portenoy, & D. E. Weissman (Eds.), *Principles and Practice of Supportive Oncology* (pp. 889–907). Philadelphia: Lippincott-Raven.

Health on the Net Foundation. (2000). HON code of conduct. Retrieved from *http://www.hon.ch/HON code/*

Heiney, S. P., Goon-Johnson, K., Ettinger, R. S., & Ettinger, S. (1990). The effects of group therapy on siblings of pediatric oncology patients. *Journal of Pediatric Oncology Nursing, 7,* 95–100.

Hersh, S. P. (1997). *Beyond Miracles: Living with Cancer.* Chicago: Contemporary Books.

Highfield, M. E. (2000). Providing spiritual care to patients with cancer. *Clinical Journal of Oncology Nursing, 4,* 115–120.

Hirshberg, C. & Barasch, M. I. (1995). *Remarkable Recovery.* New York: Riverhead Books.

Ingbar, S. H. (1985). The thyroid gland. In J. Wilson & D. Foster (Eds.), *Williams Textbook of Endocrinology* (7th ed., pp. 682–815). Philadelphia: W.B. Saunders Company.

Jemal, A., Tiwari, R. C., Murray, T., Ghafoor, A., Semels, A., Ward, E. et al. (2001). Cancer Statistics, 2004. CA: *Cancer Journal for Clinicians, 54,* 8–29.

Johnson, J. & Flaherty, M. (1980). The nurse and cancer patient education. *Seminars in Oncology, 7,* 63–70.

Keefe, D. L. (2001). Anthracycline-induced Cardiomyopathy. *Seminars in Oncology Nursing, 28,* 2–7.

Klein, L. (2000). *The Support Group Sourcebook.* New York: John Wiley & Sons.

Koocher, G. P. & O'Malley, J. E. (1981). *The Damocles Syndrome: Psychosocial Consequences of Surviving Childhood Cancer.* New York: McGraw-Hill.

Krizek, C., Roberts, C., Ragan, R., Ferrara, J. J., & Lord, B. (1999). Gender and cancer support group participation. *Cancer Practice, 7,* 86–92.

Krumm, S. (1982). Psychosocial adaptation of the adult with cancer. *The Nursing Clinics of America, 17,* 729–737.

Kurtz-Farris, L. (1997). *Self-Help and Support Groups: A Handbook for Practitioners.* Thousand Oaks, CA: Sage.

Lancee, W. J., Vachon, M. L., Ghadirian, P., Adair, W., Conway, B., & Dryer, D. (1994). The impact of pain and impaired role performance on distress in persons with cancer. *Canadian Journal of Psychiatry, 39,* 617–622.

Lawrence, S. (2000). The net world in numbers. *Industry Standard, 3,* 219.

Legislative Action Center. (1999). Cancer Care, Inc. Retrieved from *http://www.cancercare.org*

Leis, A. M., Haines, C. S., & Pancyr, G. C. (1994). Exploring oncologists' beliefs about psychosocial groups: Implications for patient care and research. *Journal of Psychosocial Oncology, 12,* 77–87.

Loescher, L. J., Welch-McCaffrey, D., Leigh, S. A., Hoffman, B., & Meyskens, F. L., Jr. (1989). Surviving adult cancers. Part 1: Physiologic effects. *Annals of Internal Medicine, 111,* 411–432.

Low, J. J., Perrin, L. C., Crandon, A. J., & Hacker, N. F. (2000). Conservative surgery to preserve ovarian function in patients with malignant ovarian germ cell tumors. A review of 74 cases. *Cancer, 89,* 391–398.

Lund, M. B., Kongerud, J., Nome, O., Abrahamsen, A. F., Bjortuft, O., Forfang, K. et al. (1995). Lung function impairment in long-term survivors of Hodgkin's Disease. *Annals of Oncology, 6,* 495–501.

Lutgendorf, S. K., Johnsen, E. L., Cooper, B., Anderson, B., Sorosky, J. I., Buller, R. E. et al. (2002). Vascular endothelial growth factor and social support in patients with ovarian carcinoma. *Cancer, 95,* 808–815.

Mahon, S. M., Cella, D. F., & Donovan, M. I. (1990). Psychosocial adjustment to recurrent cancer. *Oncology Nursing Forum, 17*(3 Suppl), 47–52.

Matthews, A. K., Peterman, A. H., Delaney, P., Menard, L., & Brandenburg, D. (2002). A qualitative exploration of the experiences of lesbian and heterosexual patients with breast cancer. *Oncology Nursing Forum, 29,* 1455–1462.

Matthews, B. A., Baker, F., & Spillers, R. L. (2002). Healthcare professionals' awareness of cancer support services. *Cancer Practice, 10,* 36–44.

McMillan, S. C., Tittle, M. B., & Hill, D. (1993). A systematic evaluation of the "I Can Cope" program using a national sample. *Oncology Nursing Forum, 20,* 455–461.

Meirow, D. & Schenker, J. G. (1995). Cancer and male infertility. *Human Reproduction, 10,* 2017–2022.

Mercurio, A. & Rhodes, M. (2000). From clutter to computer: Creation of a community resource web-site for cancer patients and their caregivers. Poster session presented at the Oncology Nursing Society's 25th Annual Congress. San Antonio, TX.

Meyers, C. A., Weitzner, M. A., Valentine, A. D., & Levin, V. A. (1998). Methylphenidate therapy improves cognition, mood, and function of brain tumor patients. *Journal of Clinical Oncology, 16,* 2522–2527.

Miller, C. B., Platanias, L. C., Mills, S. R., Zahurak, M. L., Ratain, M. J., Ettinger, D. S. et al. (1992). Phase I-II trial of erythropoietin in the treatment of cisplatin-associated anemia. *Journal of the National Cancer Institute, 84,* 98–103.

Moursund, J. & Kenny, M. (2002). *The Process of Counseling and Therapy* (4th ed.). Upper Saddle River, NJ: Prentice Hall.

Mullan, F. (1985). Seasons of survival: Reflections of a physician with cancer. *New England Journal of Medicine, 313,* 170–173.

Nail, L. N. (2001). Long-term persistence of symptoms. *Seminars in Oncology Nursing, 117,* 249–254.

National Coalition of Cancer Survivors. (2003). Retrieved from *www.canceradvocacy.org*

Newton, H. (1998). The cryopreservation of ovarian tissue as a strategy for preserving the fertility of cancer patients. *Human Reproduction Update, 4,* 237–247.

Nielsen, E. & Brant, J. (2002). Chemotherapy-induced neurotoxicity: Assessment and interventions for patients at risk. *American Journal of Nursing, 102* (Suppl 4), 16–19.

Peylan-Ramu, N., Poplack, D. G., Pizzo, P. A., Adornato, B. T., & Di Chiro, G. (1978). Abnormal CT scans of the brain in asymptomatic children with acute lymphocytic leukemia after prophylactic treatment of the central nervous system with radiation and intrathecal chemotherapy. *New England Journal of Medicine, 298,* 815–818.

Pillon, L. R. & Joannides, G. (1991). An 11-year evaluation of a living with cancer program. *Oncology Nursing Forum, 18,* 707–711.

Pohjola-Sintonen, S., Totterman, K. J., Salmo, M., & Siltanen, P. (1987). Late cardiac effects of mediastinal radiotherapy in patients with Hodgkin's disease. *Cancer, 60,* 31–37.

Portenoy, R. K., Thaler, H. T., Kornblith, A. B., Lepore, J. M., Friedlander–Klar, H., Coyle, N. et al. (1994). Symptom prevalence, characteristics and distress in a cancer population. *Quality of Life Research, 3,* 183–189.

Pui, C. H. (2000). Acute lymphoblastic leukemia in children. *Current Opinion in Oncology, 12,* 2–12.

Quigley, K. M. (1989). The adult cancer survivor: Psychosocial consequences of cure. *Seminars in Oncology Nursing, 5,* 63–69.

Ramsay, N., Kim, T., & Coccia, P. (1978). Thyroid dysfunction in pediatric patients after mantle field radiation therapy for Hodgkin's Disease. *Proceedings of the American Society of Clinical Oncology, 19.*

Rowland, J. H., Glidewell, O. J., Sibley, R. F., Holland, J. C., Tull, R., Berman, A. et al. (1984). Effects of different forms of central nervous system prophylaxis on neuropsychologic function in childhood leukemia. *Journal of Clinical Oncology, 2*, 1327–1335.

Ruccione, K. & Weinberg, K. (1989). Late effects in multiple body systems. *Seminars in Oncology Nursing, 5*, 4–13.

Samaan, N. A., Schultz, P. N., Yang, K. P., Vassilopoulou-Sellin, R., Maor, M. H., Cangir, A. et al. (1987). Endocrine complications after radiotherapy for tumors of the head and neck. *Journal of Laboratory and Clinical Medicine, 109*, 364–372.

Schagen, S. B., van Dam, F. S., Muller, M. J., Boogerd, W., Lindeboom, J., & Bruning, P. F. (1999). Cognitive deficits after postoperative adjuvant chemotherapy for breast carcinoma. *Cancer, 85*, 640–650.

Schilsky, R. L. (1984). *Renal and Metabolic Toxicities of Cancer Treatment*. Orlando, FL: Grune & Stratton.

Schimmel, S. R. (1999). *Cancer Talk: Voices of Hope and Endurance from "Group Room," The World's Largest Cancer Support Group*. New York: Broadway Books.

Schwartz, A. L., Nail, L. M., Chen, S., Meek, P., Barsevick, A. M., King, M. E. et al. (2000). Fatigue patterns observed in patients receiving chemotherapy and radiotherapy. *Cancer Investment, 18*, 11–19.

Seligman, L. (1996). *Promoting a Fighting Spirit: Psychotherapy for Cancer Patients, Survivors, and Their Families*. San Francisco: Jossey-Bass.

Sellick, S. M. & Crooks, D. L. (1999). Depression and cancer: An appraisal of the literature for prevalence, detection, and practice guideline development for psychological interventions. *Psycho-oncology, 8*, 315–333.

Spiegel, D., Bloom, J. R., Kraemer, H. C., & Gottheil, E. (1989). Effect of psychosocial treatment on survival of patients with metastatic breast cancer. *Lancet, 2*, 888–891.

Spiegel, D. & Glassen, C. (2000). *Group Therapy for Cancer Patients*. New York: Basic Books.

Stanford, J. L., Feng, Z., Hamilton, A. S., Gilliland, F. D., Stephenson, R. A., Eley, J. W. et al. (2000). Urinary and sexual function after radical prostatectomy for clinically localized prostate cancer: The Prostate Cancer Outcomes Study. *JAMA, 283*, 354–360.

Stuart, M. (1992). Nurse Marjorie Heeley and the Mother's Club. *Nursing Research, 41*, 190.

Tefft, M., Lattin, P. B., Jereb, B., Cham, W., Ghavimi, G., Rosen, G. et al. (1976). Acute and late effects on normal tissues following combined chemo- and radiotherapy for childhood rhabdomyosarcoma and Ewing's sarcoma. *Cancer, 37*(2 Suppl), 1201–1217.

Thaler-DeMers, D. (2001). Intimacy issues: Sexuality, fertility, and relationships. *Seminars in Oncology Nursing, 17*, 255–262.

Tucker, M. A., Coleman, C. N., Cox, R. S., Varghese, A., & Rosenberg, S. A. (1988). Risk of second cancers after treatment for Hodgkin's Disease. *New England Journal of Medicine, 318*, 76–81.

Tucker, M. A., D'Angio, G. J., Boice, J. D., Jr., Strong, L. C., Li, F. P., Stovall, M. et al. (1987). Bone sarcomas linked to radiotherapy and chemotherapy in children. *New England Journal of Medicine, 317*, 588–593.

Twaddle, V., Britton, P. G., Craft, A. C., Noble, T. C., & Kernahan, J. (1983). Intellectual function after treatment for leukaemia or solid tumours. *Archives of Disease in Children, 58*, 949–952.

Voluntary Hospital Association. (1999). 43% of consumers turn to Internet for answers about their health care (press release). Retrieved from *http://www.vha.com/NEWS/releases/1999/4_5_99.shtml*

Welch-McCaffrey, D., Hoffman, B., Leigh, S. A., Loescher, L. J., & Meyskens, F. L., Jr. (1989). Surviving adult cancers. Part 2: Psychosocial implications. *Annals of Internal Medicine, 111*, 517–524.

Wharam, M. D. (1983). Radiation therapy. In A. J. Altman & A. D. Schwartz (Eds.), *Malignant Diseases of Infancy, Childhood and Adolescence* (p. 103). Philadelphia: W.B. Saunders Company.

Whedon, M., Stearns, D., & Mills, L. E. (1995). Quality of life of long-term survivors of autologous bone marrow transplantation. *Oncology Nursing Forum, 22*, 1527–1553.

Wilkes, G. M., Ingwersen, K., & Barton-Burke, M. (2001). *Oncology Nursing Drug Handbook*. Sudbury, MA: Jones and Bartlett Publishers.

Wilson, F. L., Baker, L. M., Brown-Syed, C., & Gollop, C. (2000). An analysis of the readability and cultural sensitivity of information on the National Cancer Institute's Web site: CancerNet. *Oncology Nursing Forum, 27*, 1403–1409.

Wituk, S., Shepherd, M. D., Slavich, S., Warren, M. L., & Meissen, G. (2000). A topography of self-help groups: An empirical analysis. *Social Work, 45*, 157–165.

Yalom, I. (1980). *Existential Psychotherapy*. New York: Basic Books.

Zabora, J. R., Blanchard, C. G., Smith, E. D., Roberts, C. S., Glajchen, M., & Sharp, J. W. (1997). Prevalence of psychological distress among cancer patients across the disease continuum. *Journal of Psychological Oncology, 15*, 73–87.

Zapzalka, D. M., Redmon, J. B., & Pryor, J. L. (1999). A survey of oncologists regarding sperm cryopreservation and assisted reproductive techniques for male cancer patients. *Cancer, 86*, 1812–1817.

Chapter 19

The Building of a Cancer-Related Fatigue Clinic

Carmen P. Escalante

Rosalie U. Valdres

Introduction

Cancer-related fatigue (CRF) is commonly reported and is often distressing in patients with active cancer as well as those with a history of cancer. Its incidence has been reported to be from 60% to 90%, with variation caused by the definitions used and the specific populations studied (Cella, Davis, Breitbart, & Curt, 2001; Cella, Peterman, Passik et al., 1998; National Comprehensive Cancer Network, 2003). It may be present well beyond the initial time of cancer treatment regardless of whether the cancer is in remission or widely metastatic. This is particularly difficult for patients who are cured but who are unable to work because of unremitting fatigue and for healthcare providers who lack the scientific knowledge and treatment options for this debilitating symptom. The National Comprehensive Cancer Network defines CRF as a persistent, subjective sense of tiredness related to cancer or cancer treatment that interferes with the usual functioning. CRF may have physical and mental components.

Patients with CRF commonly report to the clinic for routine follow-up or restaging of their malignancy. They frequently relate the fatigue experienced to evidence of recurrence or worsening of their cancer. Diagnostic testing and their physical examination may be normal and not indicative of why they are fatigued. This may be very perplexing for the patient, family, and healthcare provider.

CRF may be inadequately addressed because of several reasons. The patient may refuse to alert family members or healthcare providers of the impact that it has on their well-being because of the fear that he or she will be labeled a "whiner." In part, he or she may begin to question whether this symptom is actually real. The patient may also fear that if this symptom is discussed with the healthcare provider and is relevant, the cancer treatment may be modified or abated, and this may decrease their chances for improvement or cure. Healthcare providers may feel uncomfortable discussing this symptom because the pathophysiology is unknown and it is a subjective symptom that is often difficult to measure with limited treatment options. In addition, healthcare providers are often very busy and may target more treatable symptoms such as pain and nausea and vomiting during the patient evaluation.

The CRF clinic at our institution was developed after considering many of these factors, including the high incidence of fatigue in our patient population and the impact that it has on our patients' and their families' well-being. In addition, we wanted to develop better strategies to deal with this very common but difficult to treat symptom and hoped that this would also stimulate both laboratory and clinical research.

CRF Clinic Objectives

Originally, the objectives of the clinic were to improve the quality of life of patients by decreasing fatigue; to educate the healthcare providers, patients, and patients' families about this phenomenon; to develop methods for clinical and diagnostic evaluation of this symptom; to correlate objective measures with the clinical evaluation; and to develop innovative treatments. Since initiating the clinic over five years ago, we have modified the initial objective based on our experiences. Today we have accepted that although we may not eradicate the symptom, we have often improved the patient's quality of life by reducing or stabilizing the level of fatigue. It is important to discuss and evaluate the symptom because even partial improvement may be significant for some. In addition, the validation of the symptom as being real may substantially decrease anxiety and improve life quality for both the patient and caregivers. In that aspect, our initial objective is modified to "improve our patients' quality of life" by addressing fatigue. We have worked incessantly on innovative treatments but face significant challenges because of a restricted treatment spectrum and scant funding options.

CRF Clinic Profile

The CRF clinic offers multidimensional symptom management ranging in patient spectrum of supportive to palliative or curative goals. Sophisticated methods of evaluating CRF and commonly associated aspects such as depression or sleep were implemented using validated and reliable tools. This process assists the healthcare team by aiding identification of contributing factors. By addressing some of these influences, CRF may

be decreased or stabilized, enabling the patient to potentially improve their daily quality of life. During CRF evaluation, it is important to evaluate the patient in a global perspective rather than simply the symptom alone. The multidisciplinary CRF clinic team is comprised of professionals who address the medical, emotional, physical, psychologic, and spiritual needs of the patient and family.

CRF Clinic Framework

The ambulatory CRF clinic is based on exceptional and collaborative teamwork. During the early planning stage, it is extremely important to identify interested persons in multiple disciplines that are willing to participate in planning, implementation, and continual reassessment. Each team member be committed to the project and be willing to dedicate the required time for a successful outcome. These team members may include physicians in various specialties (internal medicine, psychiatry, physical medicine, and rehabilitation, nutritionists, oncology nurses, social workers and case managers, physical and occupational therapists, and psychologists. A leader should be identified who is dedicated and accepts responsibility for team vision and guidance. The range of the proposed project with realistic objectives are to carefully planned in an early phase.

The CRF clinic was begun in 1998 and designed based on already available resources. A physician leader and oncology nurse who understood the challenges in assessment and management of fatigue and were committed to clinic development were identified. The nurse performed all of the preclinical screening using the Brief Fatigue Inventory to measure the fatigue level objectively. We first targeted breast cancer patients and the CRF clinic nurse went to the Breast Center and screened patients for fatigue while they were waiting to see their oncologists. Patients with moderate or severe levels of fatigue were asked if they would like to be evaluated in the CRF clinic. Those patients who were screened and had only mild fatigue were educated concerning energy-conservation techniques.

The CRF clinic is housed in the Internal Medicine Center at our institution. Appropriate accommodations each cancer center can identify will meet their project objectives. This will vary depending on the project scope unique to an institution. Presently, the CRF clinic has two general internists who evaluate every patient for fatigue at their initial consultation. An oncology nurse practitioner is assigned and is an integral part of this clinic. The CRF clinic also uses the services of available clinic nurses and clerical support routinely who are assigned to each physician. A similar combination of healthcare workers address specific needs and will be responsible for clinical evaluation should be identified during the early planning phase.

An oncology NP can be is an essential member of the clinic team. He or she is the key provider involved in early patient contact and performs the initial screening and patient evaluation. The functions of the NP may vary depending on the objectives of the project (**Table 19.1**) At our institution, the NP developed the CRF follow-up clinic. Here she evaluates patients after their initial fatigue consultation under guidance that a supervising physician provided. The interaction with the physician varies and is dependent on the medical complexity of the individual patient at the follow-up appointment. Each patient continues to see a physician on an intermittent basis while being evaluated by the NP between physician visits. We believe that our NP is experienced and very capable of providing excellent patient care. Because of the frequent medical complexities of this patient population, an experienced NP with previous oncology exposure is recommended for this role.

The physician is the leader of the clinic and is responsible for performing a comprehensive patient evaluation and formulating an assessment and treatment plan. The physician requires excellent communication skills, which are essential in the development of patient and family rapport.

Table 19.1 FUNCTION OF THE NP IN THE CRF CLINIC

Before appointment	Appointment day	After appointment
• Screens patient for fatigue	• Reviews assessment packet with patient	• Contacts patient in 1–2 weeks to assess therapies
• Obtains appropriate physician referral	• Conveys results to physician	• Follows and notifies physician of workup results
• Contacts patient and arranges appointment scheduling	• Gathers history	• Receives patient calls and consults with physician as necessary
• Mails clinic assessment packet	• Verifies medications and allergies	• Sees patient in follow-up with physician supervision
• Facilitates scheduling of initial diagnostic workup	• Reviews systems	
• Reminds patient 1–2 days before appointment	• Records data on consultation record	
	• Initiates patient education	
	• Facilitates prescription writing	
	• Answers patient/family questions	
	• Facilitates scheduling of an additional workup	

Also, the physician may need to build alliances within his/her facility so that appropriate referrals and necessary resources are made available during the development and implementation of the project. The role of the physician in our CRF Clinic is outlined in **Table 19.2**.

CRF Clinic Patient Selection

Initially, the patient selection process for our clinic was based on fatigue severity. Because of limited resources, a decision was made to focus on those patients who might benefit the most. The "cutoff" was six or more on the Brief Fatigue Inventory. Patients can also be referred by their primary care physician for fatigue consultation. In cases in which patients initiate the clinic contact, we contact the primary clinic physician and obtain a referral. In those situations, physicians are typically grateful to have our clinic manage this aspect of the patient's care. It is extremely important that all healthcare providers manage various aspects of the patient's care understand the treatment plans because there is commonly overlap with some treatments, to other medical problem that may affect the patients fatigue levels. On occasion, we have evaluated self-referred patients who are external to our institution and who are having an oncologist who is not affiliated with our institution provide their cancer management.

The clinic is available for all patients, from those with active cancer to those who have been cured. Initial diagnostic evaluation at the time of the initial consultation includes a comprehensive metabolic profile (chemistry and electrolytes), a complete blood count, and thyroid-stimulating hormone. We have developed appropriate testing times for each test to eliminate any redundancy and appropriately use patient data already available. Specialized testing is ordered on an individualized basis, as determined by the physician after obtaining the history and performing the patient examination.

CRF Clinic Assessment Packet

The CRF clinic assessment packet provides additional objective data that aid in patient evaluation. It is important to chose tools that were easy for patients to comprehend and are not excessively lengthy but were reliable. This packet was

---

Table 19.2 FUNCTION OF PHYSICIAN IN THE CRF CLINIC

Day of Appointment	Appointment
• Reviews medical record and fatigue scores from clinic assessment packet	• Reviews additional follow-up evaluations when completed
• Reviews patient data with NP	• Discusses findings with NP
• Discusses patient data with NP before evaluation	
• Evaluates and examines patient	
• Formulates and discusses treatment plan with patient, family, and NP	
• Answers patient/family questions	
• Orders additional diagnostic workup and refers as necessary	
• Prescribes medications as appropriate	
• Discusses overall patient findings and plans with NP after evaluation	

devised to help measure difficult symptoms such as sleep, nutrition, and depression and allow a way of assessing prescribed treatments at follow-up visits. In our experience, these tools are extremely helpful and often guide the provider in directing the evaluation. For example, if a patient has extreme difficulty with sleep or pain, the clinician often probes into these aspects while taking a patient history.

The CRF clinic assessment packet includes nine survey instruments. The CRF clinic assessment packet is described in **Table 19.3**.

CRF Clinic Operations

The main aspects involved in the clinic operation include patient appointment scheduling, NP review and scoring of the survey tools, the physician consultation and discussions of a treatment plan, patient education, and scheduling additional diagnostic testing, referrals, and follow-up appointments.

The consultation appointment is scheduled for 1.5 hours. The first 0.5 hour is allotted for NP evaluation and scoring of the tools. The remaining 60 minutes are available for a comprehensive physician evaluation. This time is extremely important in order to complete a thorough history and physical examination and to allow adequate time for listening to patient and family concerns. In our experience, this time allotment is necessary because of the complexities of the patient population. In addition, time for reassurance and answering of questions is best performed in a relaxed atmosphere.

A clinic service coordinator schedules referred patients for a consultation with one of two general internists who are experienced in CRF management. At this time, a CRF clinic assessment packet composed of various survey tools is usually mailed to the patient. Occasionally, the survey may be available in the institution for the patient to fill at home before the appointment. It is imperative that every question is answered in order to assist the clinician in identification of significant aspects that may be contributing to fatigue. If the patient has difficulty in completing the tools, the NP assists but does not complete the tools for him or her during the NP interview time. Results of the surveys are reviewed with the physician before the evaluation.

The patient data that the NP collected are discussed with the physician. A comprehensive history and physical examination are performed. We have developed a consultation form to ensure review of all relevant aspects of fatigue. An accurate history is important and includes cancer history and treatment, extent of the disease and response to treatment, current medications, other comorbidities, and functional performance status. The history also addresses specific aspects of fatigue such as the onset of fatigue, duration, frequency, pattern, factors affecting fatigue, and other associated symptoms. The physician discusses results of objective measures (diagnostic testing, physical examination, and scores of various tools) with the patient and family and formulates a treatment plan. A customized approach is necessary, and further testing or other referrals may be required. Patients with an identifiable and reversible abnormality, such as hypothyroidism, hypokalemia, hypomagnesemia, or anemia, should have appropriate treatments prescribed.

The majority of patients usually do not have easily remedied abnormalities and require multiple treatment modalities. Nonpharmacologic managements that may be prescribed include exercise programs. This may include walking, water exercise therapy, or other physical activities that the patient may enjoy. Deconditioned patients should be carefully assessed when being prescribed exercise regimens. For some, cardiac evaluation may be necessary. In certain patients, a referral to physical therapy or rehabilitation medicine may be appropriate. Patients with decreased

Table 19.3 CRF CLINIC ASSESSMENT PACKET

Assessment tool	Entity assessed	Description
Brief Fatigue Inventory (Mendoza et al., 1999)	Fatigue	Nine questions Score of more than 6 considered severe fatigue
Brief Pain Inventory (Cleeland & Ryan, 1994)	Pain	Fifteen questions Score 0, no pain; 10, worst pain
Beck Depression Inventory II (Steer et al., 1987)	Depression	Twenty-one groups of statements Score 0–13, minimal depression; 14–19, mild; 20–28, moderate; more than or equal to 29, severe
Patient-Generated Subjective Global Assessment of Nutrition	Nutrition	Developed for the CRF clinic; Easy checklist for patients to answer
Brief Sleep Disturbance Scale	Sleeping habits	Developed by Pain Research Group at University of Texas M.D. Anderson Cancer Center; Six questions Score 22–29, mild sleep disturbance; 30–34, moderate; more than or equal to 35, severe
M.D. Anderson Cancer-Related Symptom Inventory (Cleeland et al., 2000)	Multiple cancer-related symptoms	Each symptom rated on 11-point scale (0–10) to indicate severity
Functional Status Index (Harvey & Jellinek, 1981)	Physical function or mobility	Eighteen-item questionnaire Score of 54 is normal; a score of more than 97 indicates significant decrease in function
SF-12 Health Survey Standard Scoring (Stewart, Hays, & Ware, 1988)	Patient opinions on his/her health	Eleven questions
Beck Anxiety Inventory (Beck et al., 1988)	Anxiety	Twenty-one item scale Score of 0–7 is minimal; score 8–15, mild; 16–25, moderate; 26–63, severe

Mendoza, 1999; Cleeland & Ryan, 1994; Steer et al, 1987; Cleeland et al, 2000; Harvey et al, 1981; Harvey et al, 1983; Steward et al, 1998; Beck et al 1988.

physical activity and other treatment effects, such as neutropenia, thrombocytopenia or osteoporosis, should be cautioned and may need to avoid certain physical activities. Deconditioned patients should slowly increase their exercise program as stamina is improved. This will avoid significant injury. Realistic exercise goals may better motivate patients.

Energy conservation should be reviewed with all patients. Stress reduction and distraction techniques are taught and may be helpful in managing fatigue. Available resources regarding activities to decrease fatigue such as use of our institutional Wellness Center, which offers relaxation and self-hypnosis classes, meditation, pilates and yoga classes, and support groups, are made available to the patient. Friends and family members are encouraged to offer support, which may include helping with grocery shopping, cleaning, or preparing meals in advance.

Sleep hygiene is especially important for those with sleep disturbances. Sleep disturbances are common and are extremely challenging. They may be influenced by daytime naps, depression, anxiety, certain medications, and caffeine and beverage intake. Patients with significant sleep issues should be queried for snoring or increased nighttime movement, which may indicate sleep apnea or another sleep disorder. These patients may require a sleep study.

The pharmacologic armamentarium for CRF is limited. Pharmacologic therapies may be used in selective patients with CRF. The use of stimulants may be necessary to boost the patient's energy. Caution must be used when prescribing stimulants, especially for patients with uncontrolled hypertension, known cardiac arrhythmias, or underlying cardiac ischemia. The timing of daily dose administration must be outlined because taking the drug later in the afternoon or evening may disrupt nighttime sleep and worsen fatigue. There are no well-designed clinical trials with sufficient patients to support stimulants in CRF; however, anecdotal evidence has shown improvement of energy levels for some patients. We have had mixed results in our experiences, with some patients having significant improvement and others having little or no change. In some cases, patients may stop the drug after one dose because of complaints of feeling "jittery and wound up."

Educating the patient and patient's families regarding CRF plays a major role in the planned therapy. Educational materials are made available to the patient at the initial encounter. Education and teaching frequently cultivate self-assurance in the patients and their families. A patient who has the knowledge and an understanding of this symptom often has better compliance and patience with any treatment modality prescribed. The physician discusses with the patient a reasonable timeline to assess treatment response, overall patient care experiences, and some background relating to the clinic at the initial encounter. Also, the physician frequently discusses treatment modalities and the level of clinical evidence with the patient and family.

Follow-up is important. Patients are usually scheduled for follow-up at specified intervals, depending on the needs of the patient and the treatment plan implemented. Coordination of a follow-up schedule is especially important if patients are not local residents. In these situations, coordination of appointments on a returning visit is imperative, and often telephone conversations are helpful. Telephone follow-up is routine for all patients and provides reassurance and trust. Patients who are prescribed medications receive a telephone call from the NP to assure compliance and to assess effectiveness. Dose adjustments may be done via the telephone based on the patient's condition. This gesture fosters a genuine interest for the patient and helps to eliminate some clinic visits, which maybe extremely taxing for these patients. **Figure 19.1** outlines a pneumonic that may be useful.

CRF Clinic Wisdom

From our clinic observations we have learned valuable lessons. For many patients, CRF is a long-term symptom and is an issue for many, including those with active or stable cancer and those cured of the malignancy. It is especially a problem for those who are cured of the disease and who are trying to return to their lives at the same functional capacity as before their diagnosis and treatment. Many have difficulty coping with the fact that they may no longer be able to perform at pretreatment levels. In addition, it is often difficult for those with a significant disability to obtain long-term disability benefits. It is extremely important that the clinicians

Figure 19.1 A HELPFUL FATIGUE PNEUMONIC

- *F* — Fatigue is a fact.
- *A* — Assurance is important.
- *T* — Time for improvement should be discussed.
- *I* — Interdisciplinary care is necessary.
- *G* — Good communication is essential.
- *U* — Unplanned activities should be avoided.
- *E* — Energy conservation is encouraged.

who are managing these patients not only educate patients and their families but also continue to educate colleagues and insurers about this entity. Because there is no diagnostic test available to measure CRF, many do not believe that it is a valid entity and will deny benefits. This often causes extreme financial stress for patients and their families.

It is so very important to communicate with the patient and family about this entity. Providing a realistic timeline and discussing the benefits of various treatments are essential. Continued education of the patient and family is required at all visits, not just at the initial consultation.

It is important to use valid and reliable measurement tools in the evaluation of fatigue and commonly associated symptoms. Because many patients continue to have various treatments and fluctuations in fatigue levels are commonly influenced by treatments administered, it is important to correlate objectively the level of fatigue with the current treatments and other life influences on the patient at specific time points.

It is often necessary for the clinician to ask the patient at the initial interview whether he or she believes that the fatigue is related to recurrence or worsening of the malignancy. In some cases, the patient or family may ask, but often it remains unsaid and once queried is frequently a significant concern generating much anxiety and stress. Most

of the CRF that our patients experience is not due to this factor but rather to the effects of treatment. When possible, the patient should be reassured.

Although not common in our experiences, easily reversible causes of fatigue such as hypothyroidism or anemia should be corrected. It is imperative that a thorough history and physical exam with appropriate diagnostic testing be completed to eliminate such factors. In most cases, a multitude of factors are contributing, and by carefully addressing each, CRF may be decreased and in a few cases totally eliminated.

It is essential that a multidisciplinary group of clinicians be committed to the effort of a CRF clinic. The success of the program is dependent on the work of many individuals in various specialties.

It is extremely important that we continue to study CRF objectively in both laboratory and clinical settings. Understanding the pathophysiology of this symptom will help develop targeted therapies that may be effective in control or elimination of this symptom. As we develop more aggressive cancer therapies and these therapies are more successful in controlling or curing cancer, patients will likely experience CRF more frequently.

In summary, CRF is extremely common and distressing for patients. It may be improved with appropriate evaluation and treatment management. Institutions should devise ways to address this suitably for patients. The type of CRF program developed will be influenced by available resources, specific patient factors (cancer diagnosis, disease extent, treatment response, treatment administered, comorbidities, etc.), and patient volume. CRF education should occur early and be continuous. This alone may help to alleviate patient worry. In addition, our best hope may be to encourage funding for both basic and clinical investigations so that improved management of this very challenging symptom is readily accomplished.

References

Beck, A. T., Epstein, N., Brown, G., & Steer, R.A. (1988). An inventory for measuring clinical anxiety: Psychometric properties. *Journal of Consulting Clinical Psychology, 56,* 893–897.

Cella, D., Davis, K., Breitbart, W., & Curt, G. (2001). Cancer–related fatigue: Prevalence of proposed diagnostic criteria in a United States sample of cancer survivors. *Journal of Clinical Oncology, 19,* 3385–3391.

Cella, D., Peterman, A., Passik, S., Jacobsen, P., Breitbart, W. (1998). Progress toward guidelines for the management of fatigue. *Oncology (Huntingt), 12,* 369–377.

Cleeland, C. S. & Mendoza, T. R., Wang, S. X., Chou, C., Harle, M. T., Morrisey, M. et al. (2000). Assessing symptom distress in cancer patients. The M. D. Anderson Symptom Inventory. *Cancer, 89,* 1634–1646.

Cleeland, C. S. & Ryan, K. M. (1994). Pain assessment: Global use of the brief pain inventory. *Annals of the Academy of Medicine, Singapore, 23,* 129–138.

Harvey, R. F. & Jellinek, H. M. (1981). Functional performance assessment: A program approach. *Archives of Physical Medicine and Rehabilitation, 62,* 456–461.

Harvey, R. F. & Jellinek, H. M. (1983). Patient profiles: Utilization in functional performance assessment. *Archives of Physical Medicine and Rehabilitation, 64,* 268–671.

Mendoza, T. R., Wang, X. S., Cleeland, C. S., Morrisey, M., Johnson, B. A., Wenolt, J. K. et al. (1999). The rapid assessment of fatigue in cancer patients. *Cancer, 85,* 1186–1196.

NCCN Cancer-Related Fatigue Panel Members and Writing Committee. (2003). Cancer–Related Fatigue–Clinical Practice Guidelines in Oncology. *Journal of National Comprehensive Cancer Network, 1,* 308–331.

Steer, R. A., Beck, A. T., Brown, G., & Berchick, K. J. (1987). Self–reported depressive symptoms that differentiate recurrent–episode major depression from dysthymic disorders. *Journal of Clinical Psychology, 43,* 246–250.

Stewart, A. L., Hays, R. D., & Ware, J. E., Jr. (1988). The MOS short–form general health survey. Reliability and validity in a patient population. *Medical Care, 26,* 724–735.

Chapter 20

The Future of Ambulatory Nursing in the Oncology Setting

Catherine Glennon

Introduction

Ambulatory care nursing is a unique practice that is characterized by rapid, focused assessment and triage of patients. Ambulatory nursing spans all ages of patients with cancer and related healthcare needs. This includes individuals who are seeking prevention counseling and intervention, screening, detection, diagnosis, treatment of the acute and chronic states of disease to terminal care—a broad continuum. Ambulatory care is a specialty practice in which high volumes of patients are cared for directly, or indirectly, by limited numbers of registered nurses. There is a high patient-to-nurse ratio, and frequently, the patients' conditions and outcomes are not always predictable. The need for ambulatory care nursing will increase as many interventions in oncology care continue to shift to the outpatient setting and as the numbers of oncology patients continue to increase.

Jemal et al. (2004) stated that 1,368,030 new cancer cases and 563,700 cancer deaths are expected in the United States in 2004. In the United States, one in four deaths is due to cancer. Cancer is second to heart disease in mortality, accounting for 22.9% of total deaths; heart disease claims 29%. Lung and bronchus cancer remains the number one cause of cancer death in both males and females and the second in incidence in both genders in 2004. The relative 5-year survival rates for most of the selected cancer sites and all cancer sites combined have improved over time; however, the survival rates for African Americans remain substantially lower than survival for whites. These statistics demonstrate the need for oncology nurses, not only to treat and manage patients but also to assist with prevention, education, and advocacy.

The future of nursing in the ambulatory setting is impacted by factors affecting not only healthcare but society in general. To ensure quality care to oncology patients, the profession of nursing must acknowledge and position itself to confront and embrace what lies ahead. The environmental scan that the Oncology Nursing Society (ONS) performed in 2002 highlighted trends and associated implications that will be helpful for strategic planning for oncology nurses. Trends in society, associations, industry, and the profession itself were analyzed (Mafrica et al., 2002).

Aging

A key trend noted in nursing's future is that the United States is an aging nation, with people older than 65 making up the fastest growing segment of the population (**Figure 20.1**). By 2050, individuals older that 80 years are expected to comprise 36% of the population, and 1.1-million people in the United States will be older than 100 years (Mafrica et al., 2002). Aging is noted as a high risk factor for cancer. NCI Surveillance Epidemiology and End Results data reveal that nearly 60% of all cancers and 70% of all cancer deaths occur in persons aged 65 years and over. The age-adjusted incidence rate for persons aged 65 years and older is 10 times greater than the rate for persons aged under 65 years. Peak rates occur in persons aged 70 years and older. The age-adjusted cancer mortality rate for persons aged 65 years and older is over 15 times greater than the rate for persons aged under 65 years (National Institute on Aging, National Cancer Institute, 2004).

Generation Mix

The current adult population is inclusive of five distinct generations, each with its own challenges and strengths. They include the World War II, Swing, Baby Boomer, X, and Y generations. The millennial generation, generation Y, includes those born between 1977 and 1994 and currently makes up 11.3% of the population. This group is the first to grow up with advanced technology. It would be rare for a member of this generation to have never lived in a setting without computers or cell phones; therefore, they are well equipped to handle future technology. There are, however, indications that they may be the least healthy, with a large percentage as cigarette smokers and less physically fit. The majority of the future workforce will be comprised of this generation.

Diversity

Diversity, both racially and ethnically, is on the rise. The majority of the population remains pri-

---

Figure 20.1 U.S. POPULATION 65 YEARS AND OLDER

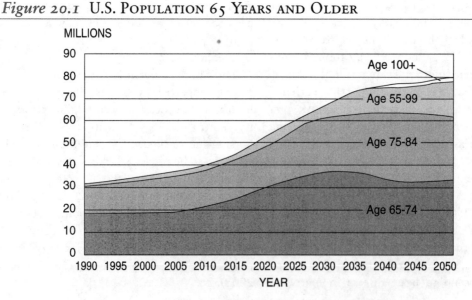

Source: U.S. Census Bureau, Population Projections of the United States by Age, Race, and Hispanic Origin: 1993—2050, P 25-1104, 1993.

marily white and non-Hispanic; however, the Hispanic, African American, Asian, and Native American populations are growing at rates that far exceed that of the population.

Terrorism

The terrorist attack on September 11, 2001, is considered one of the most significant events in American history. The threat of terrorist attacks and bioterrorism has changed how individuals prioritize what is important to them, which in turn influences how they spend their work and discretionary time. It also changed how healthcare institutions prepare for such catastrophic events, either structurally and staff preparedness. The impact of this event is profound, touching almost every entity in some manner.

Impact on Oncology Nursing

The influence of these societal factors on nursing in the ambulatory setting is evident. Nurses will be caring for an older group of patients with associative comorbidities and frailties that add to the complexity of treatment and care. The number of conditions and prevalence increase with advancing age for both women and men. Forty percent of each gender has five or more comorbidities, such as hypertension, anemia, arthritis, and heart and gastrointestinal problems (National Institute on Aging, National Cancer Institute, 2004).

The older population will not only have intense healthcare needs, but also social and daily care needs that will impact healthcare. They may need extended family/friends or professional services to attend to them; the caregiver burden is another consideration. This patient population may have an increased requirement for transportation to and from the ambulatory setting for appointments. Financial aspects of their care will require a greater understanding of the limited Medicare and supplemental third-party payer coverage. The recent Medical prescription Drug Improvement and Modernization Act of 2003 is only now beginning to confound experts on its implications and true benefits (Altman, 2004). Ambulatory care settings will especially need staff that is expert in understanding the applications of public policies and legislative changes not only to the older population but also to clinical administrators. A burgeoning business of adult daycare settings for the older patient with cancer will require a new way of delivering care in either ambulatory or home care settings.

Ambulatory oncology nurses will care for patients with diverse backgrounds and cultural considerations. It is critical that patients are treated respectfully and that differences are appreciated and acknowledged, especially as it relates to areas such as prevention in cancer care, where culture dictates importance of interventions and degree of compliance; however, diversity in the profession of nursing is quite limited. Eighty-six percent of professional nurses are white, which is not reflective of the U.S. population, which comprises 12% of the black and 12.5% of the Hispanic populations. Blacks comprise 4.9% of the nursing population, and Hispanics nurses make up 2%. The representation of minority nurses increased from 7% in 1980 to 12% in 2000. Despite these increases, the diversity of the registered nurse population remains far less than the general population, where minority representation was greater than 30% in 2000 (Health Resources and Services Administration, 2000). The largest population gap is between males and females. Men continue to comprise a very small percentage of the total registered nurse population at 5.4%; however this is an increase from 2.7% in 1980 (U.S. Department of Health and Human Services, Health Resources and Services Administration, 2000).

In the midst of threats of bioterrorism, healthcare settings are assessing the emergency preparedness of staff and environment for instant readiness, which has changed the training and education priorities from the nurse's practice specialty. President Bush's budget in 2003 included $60 million to provide training for healthcare professionals to be able to identify quickly and correctly the indications of a bioterrorist event and ensure that all healthcare professionals have the knowledge and skills to recognize and treat patients involved in such an event (U.S. Department of Health and Human Services, The Registered Nurse Population, 2004). National funding of homeland security is a priority. Agencies and organizations, such as the Centers for Disease Control, are involved in supporting disease surveillance and communication in response to the threat of bioterrorism. Technology for rapid and urgent communication will become more important. Commonplace activities such as mailing patient appointment information and records may take another form of communication if the postal system continues to be threatened with anthrax and other chemicals.

Future

Future considerations in the healthcare industry deal with advancements and pronounced changes in genetics, telehealth, technology, pharmaceutical industry, and healthcare costs and access. Genetic discoveries will influence nursing through the entire continuum of care; from prevention to treatment of disease. Technology will influence the patient care delivery system with features to enhance accuracy, safety, and efficiency in the ambulatory systems to the delivery of patient care beyond the nurse's view. Through the use of such measures as video conferencing, geographic boundaries will be transcended. Healthcare spending continues to rise for various reasons such as the costs of technology and pharmaceuticals, increased number of uninsured recipients of care, including children, and limited reimbursement by third-party payers. Healthcare spending is projected to total $2.3 trillion of 15.5% of the gross domestic product in 2008,

which represents an increase of 4.3% per year from 1999 through 2010. By 2005, the number of people covered by health maintenance organizations will increase 25% from 78 million in 1998 to more than 100-million people. Employers insuring employees will decrease from 59% in 1997 to 56% in 2010. Simultaneously, the number of Medicare recipients will increase from 38 million in 1998 to 45 million in 2007. Additionally, 15% of the population will be uninsured in 2007. Healthcare organizations and institutions will assess employment opportunities for assistive personnel to deliver patient care because they are lower cost workers. Four of the highest growth occupations for 1998 to 2008 in healthcare and human services will be personal care and home health aides, medical assistants, social and human service assistants, and physician assistants, each predicting a 48% to 58% increase (Mafrica et al., 2002; Centers for Medicare & Medicaid Services, 2004).

Nursing Shortage

Characteristics of the nursing profession itself will influence the future most dramatically. Mafrica et al. (2002) identified key facts about ONS's members. The largest segments of ONS member demographics, along with other observations, include the following:

- Approximately 19% of ONS members are 45 to 49 years of age. Sixty percent of members are older than 40 years.
- Twenty-one percent of ONS members earn $40,000 to $50,000 annually.
- Patient care is the largest functional area, at 67%.
- ONS members' largest patient population is in adult care at 85.5%.
- ONS members are primarily employed on oncology specialty units, and 52.5% work in direct patient care.
- As of January 2002, members' primary specialty is in hematology–oncology

(33%), with chemotherapy and biotherapy falling second (25.25%). In 1997, these numbers were reversed.

- ONS members work primarily in a hospital or multihospital system (43%). The number of members in this setting in 2002 is almost the same as it was in 1997, although the number of members in physicians' offices has almost doubled, and the number in home care has decreased by almost half.
- Currently, ONS members have worked, on average, for 20 years in nursing and 10 years in the field of oncology. The number of members with more than 20 years in oncology is five times what it was in 1997, and the number of members with more than 20 years in nursing is almost twice what it was in 1997.

Acknowledgment that approximately 19% of ONS members are 45 to 49 years of age is imperative. Sixty percent of members are older than 40. Replacement of the workforce is critical. **Figure 20.2** demonstrates the future supply and demand

of nurses. Coupled with the global nursing shortage and the growing aging of the nursing and general population, this is a very complex issue. The factors influencing the shortage are multiple; increased opportunities for women, causes fewer enrollments in nursing schools. With those who do enroll, there are a decreased number of nurses passing the national registered nurse licensing examination. Nurses complain of mandatory overtime, increased paperwork, and decreased time with patients because of workload and patent's shorter length of stay. Employers, institutions, policy makers, and professional organizations such as the ONS, in efforts to attract and retain individuals in the field of nursing, are addressing these issues aggressively. For example, Johnson & Johnson has developed a nationwide campaign in support of the nursing profession. Working with healthcare leaders and nursing organizations such as the National Student Nurses Association, the National League for Nursing, the American Nurses Association, the American Organization of Nurse Executives, and Sigma Theta Tau International, the company hopes to bring more people into nursing, develop

Figure 20.2 NATIONAL SUPPLY AND DEMAND

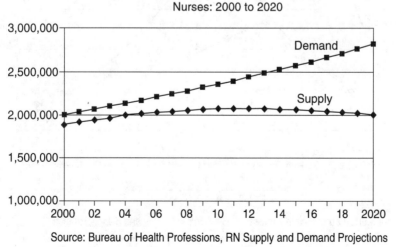

Chart 1: National Supply and Demand Projections for FTE Registered Nurses: 2000 to 2020

Source: Bureau of Health Professions, RN Supply and Demand Projections

more nurse educators, and retain the talent already in the profession (Campaign for Nursing Future, 2003). Similarly, colleges of nursing are addressing creative courses to capture those with college degrees in fields other than nursing. The northwest Advanced Practice Nursing Immersion Program is an accelerated path for non–nurse-holding undergraduate degrees in other fields. The Advanced Practice Nursing Immersion prepares graduates to be primary-care nurse practitioners. The first program was launched in 2003 and accepted 25 students. Over 250 applications came forth (personal communication, Mary Walker, February 23, 2004). These and other programs are emerging throughout the United States.

Aging of the registered nurse workforce is critical to recognize. The average age for registered nurses has climbed steadily in recent years, result-

ing in a greater proportion of nurses in the older age brackets who are approaching retirement age. Three factors contribute to this aging of the registered nurse workforce: (1) the decline in number of nursing school graduates, (2) the higher average age of recent graduating classes, and (3) the aging of the existing pool of licensed nurses. Graduates of associate degree programs, the largest source of new registered nurses, are on average 33 years old when they graduate, considerably older than in 1980 when the average age of a new associate degree graduate was 28 years. The result has been a significant decline in the proportion of registered nurses under the age of 30 years. Between 1980 and 2000, that proportion declined from 25% to 9% as noted in **Figure 20.3**. This slowing of new, young entrants coupled with an accelerating retirement rate for older registered nurses will produce a national supply of

Figure 20.3 AGE DISTRIBUTION OF REGISTERED NURSES

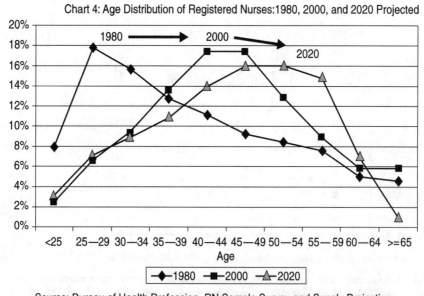

Source: Bureau of Health Profession, RN Sample Survey and Supply Projections.

U.S. Department of Health and Human Services, The Registered Nurse Population (2004).

nurses that in 2020 will not only be older but no larger than the supply projected for 2005. The number of new licenses in nursing is projected to be 17% lower in 2020 than in 2002, whereas the loss from the registered nurse license pool because of death and retirement is projected to be 128% higher (U.S. Department of Health and Human Services, The Registered Nurse Population, 2004).

Conclusion

The future holds much promise and opportunities for oncology nurses, especially in the ambulatory care setting. The ongoing vitality of the oncology nurse will assure that the individuals with cancer will receive the highest quality of care available. The nurse will use this information of trends and implications to influence and manage changes required and ultimately to advocate for the patient.

References

Altman, E. (2004). The new Medicare prescription drug legislation. *New England Journal of Medicine, 350,* 9–10.

Campaign for Nursing Future. (2003). Retrieved on February 29, 2004 from *http://www.jnj.com/our_company/advertising/discover_nursing*

Centers for Medicare & Medicaid Services (CMS). (2004). Retrieved on February 29, 2002 from *http://www.cms.hhs.gov/media/press/release.asp?Counter=961*

Jemal, A., Tiwari, R., Murray, T., Ghafoor, A., Samuels, A., Ward, E. et al. (2004). Cancer Statistics, 2004. *CA: A Cancer Journal for Clinicians, 54,* 8–29.

Mafrica, L., Ballon, L., Culhane, B., McCorkle, M., Murphy, C., & Worrall, L. (2002). ONS 2002 Environmental Scan: A Basis for Strategic Planning, Oncology Nursing Society Online Exclusive 29, 9. Retrieved February 29, 2004.

National Institute on Aging–National Cancer Institute. (2004). Exploring the Role of Cancer Centers for Integrating Aging and Cancer Research. Retrieved on February 27, 2004 from *http://www.nia.nih.gov/health/nianci/intro.asp*

U.S. Department of Health and Human Services, Health Resources and Services Administration. (2000). The Registered Nurse Population.

U.S. Department of Health and Human Services, The Registered Nurse Population. (2004). Retrieved on February 19, 2004 from *http://www.bhpr.hrsa.gov/healthworkforce/reports/rnproject/report.htm#table7*

Index

A

AAACN (American Academy of
Ambulatory Care Nurses), 2
AANP (American Academy of Nurse
Practitioners), 66
AARP (American Association of
Retired Persons), 40
academic outpatient departments, 82
accountability, outpatient surgery
centers, 130
accreditation, 146
accrual to clinical trials, 339–342
accuracy of websites, 51, 61–62
acute side-effects. *See* side-effects
management
ADA (Americans with Disabilities
Act), 391
addresses, e-mail. *See* e-mail
adherence to clinical trial guidelines,
339–342
administrative responsibilities, 75
ICs (infusion centers), 108–109
outpatient surgery facilities, 131,
133
radiation oncology centers, 151
admission criteria for patients. *See also*
assessing patient health
clinical trials, 331–332, 339–342
CRF (fatigue) clinics, 416–418
hospice care, 272
outpatient surgery, 121–122
presurgical testing and surveys,
124–126

radiotherapy treatment centers,
179–186, 199
survivorship group membership,
395
transplant therapy, 217, 223–224
advanced practice nurses. *See* APNs
Advanced Practice Nursing Immersion
Program, 428
advocacy groups, 389–390
African Americans, support groups for,
388
age and aging, 4–5, 93, 424–425
eligibility for outpatient surgery,
122
longevity and death (U.S.),
263–265. *See also* palliative care
mucositis and, 293
registered nurses, 428
alcoholism and palliative care, 271
alkylators, 403
allogenic transplants, 213
alternative therapies, 26, 355–373
categories of, 357–359
clinical trials, 360–361
defined, 360
program development, 361–373
assessing interest in, 361–365
forms and communications,
370–371
legal issues, 371–373
models for, 366–370
proposing program for, 373
ambulatory care, 99–100. *See also specific
type of care*

alternative therapies with. *See*
CAM therapies
care requirements, 3
clinical trials. *See* research and
clinical trials
current issues and trends, 7–23
cost-effectiveness. *See* economics
and finances
evidence-based practice, 14
informatics. *See* informatics
leadership, 16
legal issues. *See* legal issues
nutrition and psychosocial
standards, 22–23
patient and caregiver education,
11–14
patient safety, 8–11
triage nursing, 15
defined, 6
economics of. *See* economics and
finances
eligibility for. *See* admission
criteria for patients
history and trends, 1–6, 26,
115–116, 423–429. *See also*
future issues and trends
pharmaceuticals. *See* pharmaceuticals
surgery. *See* outpatient surgery
ambulatory care settings, 2–6, 82–83
clinical trials. *See* research and
clinical trials
economics of. *See* economics and
finances

facility design. *See* facility design

fatigue clinics (CRF clinics), 413–421
   operations of, 417–419
   patient selection, 416–418

history and trends, 2–6, 81, 141, 423–429. *See also specific care setting*

infusion centers. *See* ICs

Internet access in, 51–59

office practice settings, 81–97
   economics and reimbursement, 90–92
   history of, 81
   patient classification systems, 89–90
   role of oncology nurses, 83–89
   surgical care in, 120
   trends and nursing shortages, 92–95
   types of, 82

pain clinics and centers, 254–258

palliative and hospice care. *See* palliative care

radiotherapy treatment centers, 139–209
   demographics, 142–143
   economic issues, 178–179
   history and trends, 139–144
   multidisciplinary collaboration, 150–179
   patient assessment (pretreatment), 179–186
   patient education, 187–188
   practice models and operational structures, 141–150
   services available, 148–150, 179–186, 204–206
   side-effects management, 188–194
   special considerations, 188–198

services available in, 83

surgery facilities. *See* outpatient surgery

survivorship. *See* survivorship programs and support groups

amenities for ambulatory care settings, 25

American Academy of Ambulatory Care Nurses, 2

American Academy of Nurse Practitioners, 66

American Association of Critical Care Nurses, 60

American Association of Retired Persons, 40

American Lung Association, 384

American Medical Informatics Association, 22

American Society for Health-System Pharmacists, 310

Americans with Disabilities Act, 391

AMIA (American Medical Informatics Association), 22

analgesics for oral pain, 290, 295–297

ancillary support staff, radiation oncology centers, 152

anesthesia
   postanethesia recovery score form, 128
   risks from, 117, 124

annual earnings. *See* salaries for service providers

antiemetic drug therapy, 45

antineoplastic medications, 316

anxiety, patient. *See* emotional issues; psychosocial services

APCs (Ambulatory Payment Classifications), 37, 43, 133
   J codes, 41, 92

APNs (advanced practice nurses), 145, 153, 167–174, 428
   Advanced Practice Nursing Immersion Program, 428
   clinical trials, 343–344

appointment scheduling. *See* scheduling

architectural design, 25–26. *See also* facility design

ASHP (American Society for Health-System Pharmacists), 310

assessing pain. *See* pain management

assessing patient health
   for admission to care. *See* admission criteria for patients
   cultural assessment, 186, 188
   documentation of, 196, 199
   mucositis, 293–294
   oral health and dental care, 281–287
   pain management, 250–252, 258
   palliative care, 266–269
      tools for, 269–271
   spiritual, 186, 188–189
   triage. *See* triage nursing

vision and hearing evaluation, 401

assistance (financial) to patients, 46–47, 145

associations, professional
   nursing, 2, 40. *See also specific organization by name*
   survivorship programs and support groups, 384–385

ASTRO task force, 173

attitude, patient. *See* education, patient

auditing patient notes, 72

autologous transplants. *See* transplant therapy

automation in medication system design, 313–314

autonomy (ethical principle), 335

available services. *See* services available in outpatient cancer care

B

bacterial infection, oral, 299

barriers to learning (patients), 88

BAT Ultrasound Unit, 206

bathrooms, accessibility from waiting area, 102

battery requirements for PDAs, 57

beds in waiting area, 102

behavioral factors and immunology, 381

belief systems of patients, 186, 188. *See also* culture

beneficence (ethical principle), 335

benzydamine, 290

best practice guidelines, 14–15

billing. *See also* economics and finances
   abuses, Medicare, 70
      CPT codes, 70–72
      maximizing payment for services, 39–43
   for pharmaceuticals, 40–43
   reimbursement. *See* reimbursement
   software for PDAs, 56

bioelectromagnetic therapies, 356

biological therapies, 359

biopsychosocial model in cancer care, 182

biotechnology. *See* technology

bioterrorism, 425–426

biotherapy. *See* chemotherapy and biotherapy

birth and birthing defects, 403–404

Blacks, support groups for, 388
blood product procedures, 88–89
BMTs (bone marrow transplants), 213
brain cancer, websites about, 52, 385
breast cancer, 232–234
    clinics for, 229–243
        developing, checklist for,
            239–241
        quality and development
            resources, 235–237
    lesbian support groups, 388
    Web-based resources, 52
breast-related side-effects, 190
Brief Fatigue Inventory, 414
brushing teeth, 288. *See also* oral health
    and dental care
budgeting. *See* economics and finances
bypassing PACU, 127

C

CAGE Questionnaire, 269, 271
calculators, medical, 56
CAM therapies, 26, 355–373
    categories of, 357–359
    clinical trials, 360–361
    program development, 361–373
        assessing interest in, 361–365
        forms and communications,
            370–371
        legal issues, 371–373
        models for, 366–370
        proposing program for, 373
cancer care settings. *See* ambulatory care
    settings
cancer pain. *See* pain management
cancer prevention programs, 26
cancer-related fatigue. *See* fatigue
cancer research. *See* research and clinical
    trials
cancer survivorship. *See* survivorship
    programs and support groups
Caphasol, 289
capitation, 35–36, 135
Carafate, 298
cardiac pacemaker malfunction, 194
cardiac-related side-effects to cancer
    therapy, 401–402, 406
cardiovascular services, salaries for, 28
care eligibility. *See* admission criteria for
    patients

care settings. *See* ambulatory care
    settings; job settings for nurse
    practitioners; outpatient models
careers for nurse practitioners. *See*
    employment issues; responsibilities
    of nurse practitioners
caregivers
    cosurvivor, defined, 383
    educating. *See* education, caregiver
    emotional issues, 273. *See also*
        psychosocial services
    fatigue management, 420
    pain management and, 249
    palliative care and, 266, 270
    patient advocacy, 87
    radiotherapy treatment planning,
        149–150
    role in transplant theory, 216–218
    side-effects management, 189
    stages of cancer experience, 378
    surgery eligibility and, 122
    therapy with, 183
    transplant therapy, role in, 219,
        225–226
CARING organization, 20
case management responsibilities, 77
cast technicians for radiotherapy, 151
Cat Scan Simulator, 204
CAT scan unit on rails, 204
cavities, oral. *See* oral health and dental
    care
Center for Medicare and Medicaid
    Services, 37, 69–70, 133. *See also*
    Medicare and Medicaid programs
Central IDB pilot, 335
central line management, 88
certification to practice, 74–77
chairs in waiting area, 102
champions to CAM program
    development, 365
charitable care services, 82
charting by exception, 89. *See also*
    documentation
chat rooms for support groups, 398
chemotherapy and biotherapy
    high-dose therapy, 220
    infusion centers. *See* ICs
    long-term physical effects of
        cancer therapy, 406–407
    nurse education, 14
    in office settings, 88–89

ongoing physical assessment, 181
oral health and dental care, 280,
    287
    care during treatment, 283–285
    infection, 299–301
pharmacy errors, guidelines for
    reducing, 322–323. *See also*
    medical errors
pulmonary side-effects, 402, 406
reimbursement issues, 112
reviewing orders for, 316–317,
    322–323
secondary malignancies, 405
transplant therapy. *See* transplant
    therapy
chest-related side-effects, 191
children. *See* pediatric care
chronic disease state, 378
chronic illness. *See* palliative care
cisplatin, 401
classes of controlled substances, 72
classification of patients, 56, 89–92
    ICs (infusion centers), 107
clinical competencies, implementing,
    85
    chemotherapy order review, 317
    pain management, 258
    radiation nurses, 160–163
clinical nurse coordinator. *See* nurse
    administration
clinical nursing, 109, 153
clinical pharmacy services. *See* pharma-
    ceuticals
clinical practice. *See* ambulatory care
    settings; job settings for nurse
    practitioners
Clinical Practices, University of
    Pennsylvania, 38
clinical responsibilities. *See* responsi-
    bilities of nurse practitioners
clinical settings. *See also* ambulatory
    care settings
clinical trials. *See* research and clinical
    trials; research nurses
clinics. *See* ambulatory care settings
closed-membership support groups,
    383
CMMS (Center for Medicare and
    Medicaid Services), 37, 69–70, 133.
    See also Medicare and Medicaid
    programs

CNS (clinical nurse specialist), 153, 167–174
coding
  diagnosis codes, 37–38
  J codes, 41, 92
  reporting patient services, 90–93
cognitive impairment, 390, 400
  informed consent issues, 337
collaboration between nurses, 16
  clinical trials, 330, 334, 345
  CRF (fatigue) clinics, 414–416
  pain management, 253–254
  pharmacy, 312–313
  radiotherapy treatment centers, 167, 171–172
color requirements for PDAs, 57
colorectal cancer, websites about, 52
communicating with patients. *See also* telephone-based communication
  before and after surgery, 122–123
  chat rooms for support groups, 396
  e-mail vs. phone, 57–58. *See also* e-mail
  effects of survivorship, 390
  fatigue, 420
  language barriers, 186
  pain management checklist, 252
  responsibilities of nurse practitioners, 76
  symptom prevention programs, 353
community, role in support programs, 394
community clinics, 82
  interest in CAM therapies, 364
  survivorship programs. *See* survivorship programs and support groups
  transplant therapy, 213
community hospital outpatient centers, 82
community outreach, 89
comorbid diseases, 4
competencies. *See* clinical competencies, implementing
complementary medicine, 360. *See also* CAM therapies
complications in outpatient surgery, 127–129
computers. *See* Internet technologies

concurrent review of care, 36
confidentiality. *See* privacy and confidentiality
conflicts of interest in clinical trials, 338
consultations with patients, 179. *See also* patient assessment
  CRF (fatigue) clinics, 417
  over Internet, 58
continuing education, 60, 85
continuity of care, 273–275
contractors, Medicare, 37
controlled substances, classifications for, 72
cooperative care, transplantation vs., 226
copay, with insurance programs, 35
costs. *See also* economics and finances
  to care provider. *See* outflow, financial
  cost-effectiveness, 15, 135
  to patients. *See* patient costs for care
cosurvivor, defined, 383
counseling, financial, 46–47, 145
couples, cancer experience for, 183. *See also* psychosocial services
CPT codes, 70–72
CRF clinics. *See* fatigue
criteria for admission. *See* admission criteria for patients
critical care providers, salaries for, 28
culture. *See also* demographics
  barriers to accrual to clinical trials, 340
  community outreach, 89
  diversity, 424–425
  hospice care, underuse of, 264
  longevity and death (U.S.), 263–265. *See also* palliative care
  patient assessment by nurses, 186, 188
  profile of U.S. population, 4–6
  psychosocial services. *See* psychosocial services
  shifts in healthcare system priorities, 231–232
  social context of patient lives, 182
  surgery eligibility and, 122
  survivorship programs, 381–382, 387–390, 396–397

cure, expectation for, 265
customized patient education, 51, 54

D

data managers, clinical trials, 343–344
databases of medical knowledge, 51
day hospitals. *See* ICs
death and longevity (U.S.), 4, 263–265. *See also* palliative care; survivorship programs and support groups
dedicated clinical pharmacy services, 318
deductibles for insurance programs, 35
delayed side-effects. *See* side-effects management
demographics, 424–425. *See also* culture
  aging and social shifts, 4–6, 93
  alternative therapies, 356
  clinical trials, patients in, 331, 339–342
    informed consent issues, 337
  longevity and death (U.S.), 263–265. *See also* palliative care
  mucositis, incidence of, 293
  nurses, 93–95
  ONS members, 426–427
  pharmacokinetics, 269
  profile of U.S. population, 4–6
  radiotherapy treatment centers, 142–143
  survivorship programs, 380–381
  special populations, 387–390
  typical, 387
denial as defense mechanism, 378
dental care. *See* oral health and dental care
dentures, 286
depression. *See* emotional issues
dermatologic side-effects, 193, 201–202
desquamation, 193
detection services, 99
diagnosis, impact of on patient, 182, 378–379
diagnosis codes, 37–38
diagnosis model of CAM therapy, 368
diagnostic testing, 68
dietary counseling. *See* nutrition and dietary counseling
digest mode (mailing lists), 60

direct costs of cancer care. *See* outflow, financial
direct liability with CAM therapies, 372
discharge from care facilities
after surgery, 127–128
pain management and, 249
discipline, CAM therapy and, 373
discontinuous care model, 265
dispensing medications. *See* pharmaceuticals; prescriptions
distance education, 60. *See also* entries at education
distress. *See* emotional issues
distribution e-mail messages, 58
distribution of pharmaceuticals. *See* pharmaceuticals
diversity, 424–425. *See also* demographics
documentation, 89
auditing, 70
of care, 16
clinical competency, 85
clinical trials, 328
data management, 343–344
informed consent, 337
complementary and alternative medicine (CAM), 360
interest questionnaires, 361–365
dental care in pretreatment, 281–282
educational materials and resources, 88, 187
survivorship programs and support groups, 377
evaluating patient understanding, 88, 198
clinical trials, 336–338
radiation therapy, 180, 180–182
transplant therapy, 218
HIPPA. See HIPPA
infusion logs, 18–19
instructions for patients. *See also* documentation; education, patient
informed consent, 337
outpatient surgery, 117–118
postoperative instructions, 123
outpatient surgery facilities, 117–118, 133

patient profiles and tracking, 56
patient records. *See* patient records
pharmaceuticals, 318
medication descriptions, 313
prescriptions, 315, 316
radiation nurse responsibilities, 154–160
radiotherapy treatment centers, 195–196, 199–202
reliability of Web-based information, 51, 61–62, 397–398
telephone and e-mail communication, 57–58, 87
dose fractionation, 140–141. *See also* radiotherapy treatment centers
dosimetrics, 149, 151. *See also* radiotherapy treatment centers
phase I clinical trials, 331
quality assurance and documentation, 195–196
side-effects management, 192
dry desquamation, 193
dry mouth. *See* salivary function
dying, 4, 263–265. *See also* palliative care; survivorship programs and support groups

E

e-consultations, 58
e-mail, 55, 58. *See also* Internet technologies
mailing lists for nurses, 61
mailing lists for survivorship group members, 396, 398
mailing lists of patients, 58
validity of information received by, 51, 61–62
e-prescription software, 56
early-discharge model of outpatient care, 212
earnings of nurse practitioners. *See* reimbursement; salaries for service providers
eating before surgery, 118
economics and finances, 33–48
bioterrorism threats and, 426
clinical trials, 17. *See also* research and clinical trials
conflicts of interest, 338
funding, 328, 330

incentives for patient retention, 342
complementary and alternative medicine (CAM), 356, 373
cost-effectiveness, 15, 135
costs to patients. *See* patient costs for care
earnings and salaries. *See* salaries for service providers
expenses (outflow), 34–35, 43–45
ambulatory surgery facilities, 118–121
profitability, quantifying, 242
transplant therapy, 224–225
financial assistance and counseling, 46–47, 145
growth of ambulatory care, 2, 4
marketing centers for outpatient surgery, 132
office practice settings, 90–92
outpatient surgery facilities, 133, 135
pharmacy services, 319
quantifying profitability, 242
radiation oncology centers, 178–179
reimbursement. *See* reimbursement
revenue sources (inflow), 34–43
billing software for PDAs, 56
e-consultations, 58
freestanding clinics, 148
maximizing payment for services, 39–43
outpatient surgery facilities, 132, 135
profitability, quantifying, 242
reimbursement. *See* reimbursement
survivorship programs, 391–392, 395
transplant therapy, 224–225
Edmonton Symptom Assessment, 269–270
education, caregiver, 12–14
advocacy groups, 389–390
fatigue management, 419, 420
financial assistance and counseling, 46–47, 145
orientation sessions, 12–13, 146, 149
radiotherapy treatment, 146, 149
recovery issues, 394

responsibilities of nurse practitioners, 77

survivorship, 379, 392

Internet as resource, 397–399

transplant therapy, 217–218

education, nurse, 14, 26

advocacy groups, 389–390

clinical trials, 345

complementary and alternative medicine (CAM), 365

drug costs, 42–43, 45

Internet-based learning, 59–62

MSN (Masters of Science in Nursing) programs, 65–66

office practice settings, 85

patient education and, 51

radiation therapy, 152

recruitment requirements, 111, 176–178

self-development responsibilities, 76

survivorship programs, 382

university hospital outpatient departments, 82

validity of Web-based information, 51, 61–62

education, patient, 11–14, 26, 87–88. *See also* communicating with patients

advocacy groups, 389–390

clinical trials, 336–338, 343

complementary and alternative medicine (CAM), 363

customized, 51, 54

e-consultations, 58

ethical right to, 198

fatigue management, 419, 420

financial assistance and counseling, 46–47, 145

fluid and electrolyte imbalances, 21

ICs (infusion centers), 105

medical instructions. *See also* documentation; education, patient

informed consent, 337

outpatient surgery, 117–118

postoperative instructions, 123

misconceptions of radiation therapy, 181–182

nurse education and, 51

oral health and dental care, 281, 287–291

orientation sessions, 12–13, 146, 149

outpatient surgery, 117–118, 133

postoperative instructions, 123

radiotherapy treatment, 146, 149, 187–188

recovery issues, 394

responsibilities of nurse practitioners, 77

survivorship, 377, 379, 392

closed-membership support groups, 383

Internet as resource, 397–399

transplant therapy, 217–218

validity of Web-based information, 51, 61–62

in waiting room, 58–59

websites for. *See* Web-based resources

education, pharmacist, 311, 321

education, physicians, 38, 82

education, student. *See* students

educational materials, 88, 187. *See also* instructions for patients

survivorship programs and support groups, 377

elective surgery. *See* outpatient surgery

electrolyte imbalances, self-care tool for, 21

electronic documentation. *See* documentation

electronic mail. *See* e-mail

eligibility for cancer care. *See* admission criteria for patients

emergency service providers, salaries for, 27

emergency situations resulting from surgery, 127–129

emotional issues. *See also* psychosocial services; quality of life (QOL)

assessing for CRF (fatigue) clinics, 418

barriers to accrual to clinical trials, 340

diagnosis, impact of on patient, 182, 378–379

end-of-life care. *See* palliative care

facility design, 25–26, 102. *See also* facility design

pain. *See* pain management

stress. *See* stress

support services. *See* psychosocial services

survivorship programs, 390. *See also* survivorship programs and support groups

employment issues. *See also* responsibilities of nurse practitioners

job settings, 66–69, 75. *See also* ambulatory care settings

patient health insurance and, 34

recruitment and retention, 111, 176–178

registered nurses in office settings, 93–95

enabling operations, clinical settings, 86

end-of-life care. *See* palliative care

endoscopic ambulatory surgery centers, 121

energy conservation guidelines, 418

environment design, 25–26. *See also* facility design

clinical trials, barriers to, 340

ICs (infusion centers), 101–103

pharmacy services, 319

surgery eligibility and, 122

survivorship programs and support groups, 395–396

transportation issues. *See* transportation

equipment and supplies

costs of, 45

ICs (infusion centers), 104

outpatient surgery facilities, 131

erectile dysfunction, 403

errors. *See* medical errors

erythema, 193

erythropoietin, 400

esophagus-related side-effects, 191

estrogen dysfunction, 403

ethics

clinical trials, 328, 334–339

complementary and alternative medicine (CAM), 373

radiation therapy, 197

survivorship advocacy groups, 389–390

evaluating patient health. *See* assessing patient health

evaluating patient inclusion. *See* admission criteria for patients

evaluating patient understanding, 88, 198
   clinical trials, 336–338
   radiation therapy, 180, 180–182
   transplant therapy, 218
evidence-based practice, 14–15
examination, physical, 68, 71
expenses for healthcare. *See* economics and finances
expert nurses. *See* APNs
eye cancer, websites about, 52
eye-related side-effects to cancer therapy, 407

F

facial pain. *See* oral health and dental care; pain management
facility design, 23–26
   breast cancer clinics, 235–237, 239–240
   CAM therapy models, 366–367
   freestanding radiotherapy treatment centers, 146–147
   ICs (infusion centers), 100–105
   medication safety plan, 315
   oncology clinical pharmacy services, 318
   orienting patients to physical layout, 12–13, 146, 149
   outpatient surgery facilities, 129–135
      example of surgery center, 133–135
   survivorship programs and support groups, 395–396
family. *See* caregivers; education, caregiver
fast tracking (PACU bypass), 127
fatigue, 189–193, 390, 404
   clinics for (CRF clinics), 413–421
      operations of, 417–419
      patient selection, 416–418
      mnemonic for, 420
fear, patient. *See* psychosocial services
federal healthcare systems, 82
federal legislation. *See* legal issues
fee-for-service systems, 35
feelings, patient. *See* emotional issues; psychosocial services
Feng Shui, 25

fertility and reproductive effects, 402–404
fibrosis, 402
financial assistance to patients, 46–47, 145
financial issues. *See* economics and finances
fixed equipment, defined, 131
flossing teeth, 288. *See also* oral health and dental care
fluid imbalances, self-care tool for, 21
fluoride applications, 288–290. *See also* oral health and dental care
food and diet. *See* nutrition
form-based facility design, 25–26
forms (printed) for CAM programs, 370
fractionation, 140–141
freestanding clinics, 82
   complementary and alternative medicine (CAM), 366
   health insurance advantages, 147
   ICs as. *See also* ICs
   independent pharmacy centers, 318
   outpatient surgery facilities, 119
   pharmacy services, 313
   postoperative recovery units, 121
   radiotherapy treatment centers, 144, 146–148
   surgical care in, 120
function-based facility design, 23, 130
funding issues. *See* economics and finances
fungal infection, oral, 300
future issues and trends, 26, 112, 353, 423–429
   ambulatory care settings, 141
   healthcare costs, 33–34. *See also* economics and finances
   ICs (infusion centers), 112
   longevity and death (U.S.), 263–265. *See also* palliative care
   nursing shortage. *See* nursing shortage
   office practice settings, 92–95
   outpatient surgery, 116, 135
   radiotherapy treatment centers, 143–144
   role of nurse practitioners, 78, 173–174
   shifts in healthcare system priorities, 233–234

survivorship programs, 381–382

G

gamma knife stereotactic radiosurgery, 194
gastrointestinal procedures, 121
gastrointestinal-related side-effects, 191
gays, support groups for, 388
genitourinary-related side-effects, 191, 402, 406
geriatric oncology, 4–5
gingiva, cancer treatment and, 285. *See also* oral health and dental care
GOC (Generic Oncology Consortium), 5
government-sponsored health insurance, 34, 36–40
   chemotherapy reimbursement, 112
   Medicare contractors, 37
   reimbursement from, 69–70
graduates and graduate students. *See* students
graft-versus-host disease. *See* GVHD
group e-mail distribution, 58
group practices. *See* office practice settings
guidelines for quality practice. *See* standards of practice
GVHD (graft-versus-host disease), 281, 283, 286–287, 301–302
gynecologic-related side-effects, 192

H

handheld computing (PDAs), 54–57
HCFA. *See* CMMS
HCPCS coding levels, 92
HDR equipment, 205
head and neck
   cancer in, Web-based resources for, 52
   radiation and oral care, 280, 281
   side-effects management, 190
health and medical insurance, 35–43. *See also* economics and finances; reimbursement
   advantages of freestanding clinics, 147
   employment and, 34
   fee-for-service systems, 35

government-sponsored, 34, 36–40
  chemotherapy reimbursement, 112
  Medicare contractors, 37
  reimbursement from, 69–70
  HMOs (health maintenance organizations), 15, 36
  nurse practitioner reimbursement, 70
  managed-care programs, 35–36
  pharmaceuticals billing, 41–42
  survivorship programs, 380, 391–392
  Tricare program, 70
Health Care Financing Administration. *See* CMMS
health maintenance organizations. *See* HMOs
Health Plan Employer Data and Information Set, 36
healthcare economics. *See* economics and finances
healthcare worker shortage. *See* nursing shortage
hearing-related side-effects to cancer therapy, 401, 406
heart problems, 194, 390, 401–402
hematopoietic stem cell transplant. *See* transplant therapy
herbal medicine, 358
herpes simplex virus (HSV), 301
high-dose therapy, 220
high-dose-rate equipment, 205
high-tech procedures in office settings, 88–89
HIMSS (Healthcare Information and Management Systems Society), 18
HIPPA (Health Insurance Portability and Accountability Act), 56
Hispanics, 5, 388
history, patient. *See* patient records
history taking, 71
HMOs (health maintenance organizations), 15, 36, 70
Hodgkin's lymphoma, side-effects related to, 192
home care
  palliative care, 270, 272
  symptom management, 351
  transplant therapy, 219
  trends, 425

Home Care Assessment Tool, 270, 272
homosexuals, support groups for, 388
hospice care, 271–273. *See also* palliative care
  continuity and coordination of care, 273–275
  underuse of, 264
hospital-based programs, 100
  CAM therapy models, 367
  closed-membership support groups, 383
  ICs as. *See also* ICs
  pharmacy practice, 316–317
  pharmacy services, 313
  radiation oncology centers, 144–146
  surgery facilities, 119
hospital satellite facilities. *See* freestanding clinics
HSCT (hematopoietic stem cell transplant). *See* transplant therapy
HSV (herpes simplex virus), 301
Hurricaine, 297
hygiene
  oral, 283, 287
  sleep, 419
hyperbaric oxygen therapy, 286
hypothyroidism, 404

I

"I Can Cope" program, 379–380
ice chips to reduce pain, 290
ICs (infusion centers), 99–114
  issues and trends, 112
  managers and administrators, 108–109
  nursing roles, 108–111
  planning, 100–104
  practice models, 106–107
  UAP (unlicensed assistive personnel), 108, 110
  workload analysis, 107
immobilization of patient (radiotherapy), 151, 205
immunology
  behavioral factors and, 381
  immunotherapy, 88–89
  oral care and, 283, 285
  oral hygiene and, 287
  oral infection and immunosuppression, 299–301

impact of cancer diagnosis, 182, 378–379
implanted pumps, managing, 88
independent clinics. *See* freestanding clinics
indirect costs of cancer care. *See* outflow, financial
infections, oral. *See* oral health and dental care
infectious patients, 102
infertility and reproductive effects, 402–404
inflow, financial, 34–43
  billing software for PDAs, 56
  e-consultations, 58
  freestanding clinics, 148
  maximizing payment for services, 39–43
  outpatient surgery facilities, 132, 135
  profitability, quantifying, 242
  reimbursement. *See* reimbursement
  survivorship programs, 391–392
informatics, 17–22
informed consent, 180, 336–338
infusion centers (ICs). *See* ICs
infusion logs, 18–19
ingestion. *See* nutrition and dietary counseling
initial physical assessment, 180–181
inpatient settings, shift toward outpatient, 2–6
institutional affiliated centers. *See* hospital-based programs
institutional liability with CAM therapies, 372
institutional review boards. *See* IRBs
instructions for patients. *See also* documentation; education, patient
  informed consent, 337
  outpatient surgery, 117–118
  postoperative instructions, 123
insurance. *See* health and medical insurance
integrated model of CAM therapy, 367
integrative medicine, 355, 360. *See also* CAM therapies
International Myeloma Association, 384
Internet technologies
  chat rooms for support groups, 398

e-mail. *See* e-mail
educational opportunities for
　nurses, 59–62
influence on patient trust, 51–54,
　61–62
PDAs (personal digital assistants),
　54–57
resource websites. *See* Web-based
　resources
survivorship programs, 397–399
telemedicine systems, 353
validity of content, 51, 61–62
waiting room access, 58–59
interventions, nursing, 15
　cognitive impairment, 400
　impact of cancer diagnosis,
　　378–379
　infertility and reproductive effects,
　　402–404
　mucositis, 293–294
　pain management checklist, 252
　psychosocial, 183
　survivorship programs, 393
intraoperative care of surgical patients,
　124
intraoperative radiation, 150
intravenous care costs, 45
IPA (Independent Practice Association),
　36
IRBs (institutional review boards), 336
　Central IDB pilot, 335
isolating infectious patients, 102

J

J codes, 41, 92
jaw exercises, 286
JCAHO (Joint Commission of
　Association of Hospital
　Organizations), 11, 22, 119, 186
　pain management standards,
　　248–251
job description
　complementary and alternative
　　medicine (CAM), 367–370
　CRF (fatigue) clinics, 415–416
　radiation nurses, 150–179,
　　152–160
　　APNs (advanced practice
　　　nurses), 167–174
　　ONS position statement,
　　　154–160

primary nursing (job
　　description), 160–167
　research nurses, 174–175
job responsibilities for nurse practi-
　tioners. *See* oncology nurse practi-
　tioners, role and responsibilities of
job settings for nurse practitioners,
　66–69, 75. *See also* ambulatory care
　settings
　radiotherapy treatment centers,
　　145–148
　recruitment and retention, 111
　　radiation nurses, 176–178
　registered nurses in office settings,
　　93–95
justice (ethical principle), 335

K

kidney cancer, 52, 390
kidney-related side-effects, 191, 402,
　406

L

labor and delivery providers, salaries
　for, 28
laboratories in ICs, 104
laminar flow work stations, 104
language barriers to patient communi-
　cation, 186
Last Acts report, 265
late effects of cancer treatment, 399
law and legal issues. *See* legal issues
layout of outpatient facilities. *See*
　facility design
lead blocks for radiotherapy, 151, 205
leadership, 11, 16–17
learning. *See* entries at education
legal issues, 16
　authority and scope of practice, 73
　certification to practice, 74–77
　complementary and alternative
　　medicine (CAM), 371–373
　economics of care, 41
　licensing, 74–77
　　complementary and alternative
　　　medicine (CAM), 372
　　pharmaceutical care, 311
　　unlicensed assistive personnel.
　　　See UAP
　Medicare billing abuses, 70

outpatient surgery facilities,
　132–133
prescriptive authority. *See*
　prescriptions
reimbursement, 69–72
lesbians, support groups for, 388
leukemia
　oral infection, 299–301
　Web-based resources, 53, 384
levels of diagnostic codes, 92
levels of nursing care, radiation
　oncology, 160–167
liability with CAM therapies, 372–373
licensing, 74–77
　complementary and alternative
　　medicine (CAM), 372
　pharmaceutical care, 311
　unlicensed assistive personnel. *See*
　　UAP
Lied Transplant Center, 226
life expectancy, 4, 263–265. *See also* age
　and aging; palliative care
life insurance and survivorship, 392
lip moisturizing, 288
listservs. *See* mailing lists
liver cancer, websites about, 52
LMRPs (local medical review policies),
　37–38
local medical review policies. *See*
　LMRPs
logistical resources for survivor groups,
　395
long-term physical effects of cancer
　therapy, 406–407
longevity and death (U.S.), 4, 263–265.
　See also age and aging; palliative care
lung cancer, websites for, 53, 384
lung-related side-effects, 191
lymphoma
　side-effects management, 192
　Web-based resources, 53, 384

M

mailing lists
　for nurses, 59, 61
　to patients, 58
Make-A-Wish Foundation, 385
malpractice with CAM therapies, 372
mammography, 233. *See also* breast
　cancer
managed-care programs, 35–36

managerial responsibilities, ICs, 108–109

managing pain. *See* pain management

MAP (Medication Assistance Program), 41–42

marketing centers for outpatient surgery, 132

marketing survivorship programs, 395–396

maximizing payment for services, 39–43

medical calculators, 56

medical databases, Internet access to, 51

medical engineers, 151

medical errors, 10–11, 13, 196
  pharmaceuticals, 315–316
    automation in medication system design, 313–314
    guidelines for reducing errors, 322–323
    pain management, 253

medical group practices. *See* office practice settings

medical history. *See* patient records

medical insurance. *See* health and medical insurance

medical physicists, 151

medical prescriptions. *See* prescriptions

medical services, salaries for, 28

Medicare and Medicaid programs, 34, 36–40
  chemotherapy reimbursement, 112
  Medicare contractors, 37
  reimbursement from, 69–70

Medicare Cancer Coverage Improvement Act of 1993, 40

Medicare Managed Care, 36

Medication Assistance Program (MAP), 41–42

medications. *See* pharmaceuticals

melanoma, websites about, 53

memory requirements for PDAs, 57

men, treatment side-effects to, 403–404

menopause, premature, 403

mind-body medicine, 357

Mini-Mental State Exam, 270–271

minorities. *See* demographics

mixed-model CAM program, 367, 369

modality therapy, 181

models for outpatient care. *See also* ambulatory care settings
  ambulatory surgery facilities, 118–121
  complementary and alternative medicine (CAM), 366–370
  cooperative care, 226
  CRF (fatigue) clinics, 414–416
  e-consultations, 58
  hospice care, 271–273. *See also* palliative care
    continuity and coordination of care, 273–275
    underuse of, 264
  ICs (infusion centers), 106–107. *See also* ICs
  office practice settings, 81–97. *See also* ambulatory care settings
    economics and reimbursement, 90–92
    history of, 81
    patient classification systems, 89–90
    role of oncology nurses, 83–89
    surgical care in, 120
    trends and nursing shortages, 92–95
    types of, 82
  pain clinics and centers, 254–258
  pharmacy, 316–319
  radiotherapy treatment centers, 141–158, 160–179. *See also* radiotherapy treatment centers
    APNs (advanced practice nurses), 167–174
    nurse administration, 175–179
    primary nursing, 160–167
    role of radiation nurses, 152–160
  survivorship programs and support groups, 393–397
  symptom management, 351
  transplant therapy, 212–216. *See also* transplant therapy

moderated e-mail mailing lists, 60

moist desquamation, 193

moisturizing of lips, 288

mold technicians for radiotherapy, 151

money issues. *See* economics and finances

monitor size for waiting room computers, 59

monitoring CAM therapies, 363–365

mother ship model (CAM therapies), 367

motivation, patient. *See* psychosocial services

mouth care. *See* oral health and dental care

mouthrinses and -washes, 288–289, 300. *See also* oral health and dental care

movable equipment, defined, 131

MRI Simulator, 204

MSN (Masters of Science in Nursing) programs, 65–66

mucositis, 285, 291–298
  pain relief, 290
  transplant therapy, 223
  treatment for, 294–298

Multi-Leaf Collimator, 205

multidisciplinary collaboration, 142–143

multiphysician groups, 82–83. *See also* office practice settings

multiple myeloma, websites about, 53, 382

myelosuppression, oral care and, 283

N

narrative notes, 89. *See also* documentation

national care coverage, 37

National Research Act, 335

nausea and vomiting
  dental care and, 284
  transplant therapy, 223

NCCAM, 360–361

NCI (National Cancer Institute), 328

NCI-CTC score, for oral mucositis, 295

neck. *See* head and neck

network of providers. *See* managed-care programs

neutropenia, 221–222

NI (nursing informatics). *See* informatics

NIH (National Institutes of Health), 328

non-Hodgkin's lymphoma, side-effects related to, 192

nonmaleficence (ethical principle), 335

nonphysician providers (NPPs), 173

note-taking. *See* documentation

NPs. *See* oncology nurse practitioners

NPPs (nonphysician providers), 173
nurse administration, 175–179
    leadership, 11, 16–17
nurse education, 14, 26
    advocacy groups, 389–390
    clinical trials, 345
    complementary and alternative
        medicine (CAM), 365
    drug costs, 42–43, 45
    Internet-based learning, 59–62
    MSN (Masters of Science in
        Nursing) programs, 65–66
    office practice settings, 85
    patient education and, 51
    radiation therapy, 152
    recruitment requirements, 111,
        176–178
    self-development responsibilities,
        76
    survivorship programs, 382
    university hospital outpatient
        departments, 82
    validity of Web-based
        information, 51, 61–62
nurse practitioners. *See* oncology nurse
    practitioners
nurse researchers, 344. *See also* research
    nurses
nursing errors. *See* medical errors
nursing informatics (NI). *See*
    informatics
Nursing Informatics Working Group,
    18
nursing intensity classification systems.
    See patient classification systems
nursing leadership, 11, 16–17
nursing organizations, 2, 40. *See also*
    specific organization by name
nursing reimbursement. *See*
    reimbursement
nursing-sensitive outcomes
    (interventions), 15
    cognitive impairment, 400
    impact of cancer diagnosis,
        378–379
    infertility and reproductive effects,
        402–404
    mucositis, 293–294
    pain management checklist, 252
    psychosocial, 183
    survivorship programs, 393

nursing shortage (U.S.), 6–8, 43–44,
    111, 426–429
    effects on office practices, 92–95
    radiation nurses, 153, 176–178
nutrition and dietary counseling, 84
    alternative therapies, 359
    assessing for CRF (fatigue) clinics,
        418
    eating before surgery, 118
    ongoing physical assessment, 181
    oral health and dental care, 288
    post-treatment oral health, 287
    radiotherapy treatment centers,
        144
    standards for, 22
    survivorship and, 395
Nystatin rinses, 300

O

oasis model of CAM therapy, 368
office practice settings, 81–97. *See also*
    ambulatory care settings
    economics and reimbursement,
        90–92
    history of, 81
    patient classification systems,
        89–90
    role of oncology nurses, 83–89
    surgical care in, 120
    trends and nursing shortages,
        92–95
    types of, 82
OMAS score, for oral mucositis, 296
oncology infusion centers (ICs). *See* ICs
oncology nurse practitioners. *See also*
    unlicenced assistive personnel
    care requirements, 3
    history of ambulatory care, 1–2
    intensity classification systems. *See*
        patient classification systems
    position statements
        ambulatory oncology services, 3
        assistive personnel, use of, 20
        cancer care in older adults, 5
    medication error prevention and
        reporting, 13
        nurse education, 14
        radiation nurse responsibilities,
            154–160
        research and clinical trials, 24

recruitment and retention, 111,
    176–178. *See also* employment
    issues
reimbursement. *See* reimbursement
role and responsibilities of, 16,
    65–69, 75–77
    care settings and, 82
    clinical trials, 336, 342–345
    complementary and alternative
        medicine (CAM), 367–370
    CRF (fatigue) clinics, 415
    future issues, 78
    history of, 65, 81
    ICs (infusion centers), 108–111
    informed consent, 337–338
    job settings, 66–69. *See also*
        ambulatory care settings
    licensing and certification,
        74–77
    Medicare and Medicaid billing,
        39
    nurse administration, 175–179
    in office practice settings,
        83–89
    outpatient surgery facilities,
        132
    pain management, 249,
        257–258
    palliative care, 267–269,
        273–275
    pharmacy, 312–316
    pharmacy order reviews,
        316–317
    prescriptive authority, 72–74
    radiotherapy treatment centers,
        144, 147
    resources for patient education,
        377
    symptom management,
        351–353
    transplant therapy, 218–220
    trends and future issues, 78
salary. *See* salaries for service
    providers
    stress on, 44
Oncology Nursing Society. *See* ONS
oncology pharmacy. *See* pharmaceuticals
oncology providers, salaries for, 28
oncology staff nurses, 343–344
ongoing physical assessment, 180–181
online education. *See* distance education
OnLine Journal of Nursing Informatics, 20

ONS (Oncology Nursing Society), 40, 60, 85
  detailed job description for NPs, 75
  member demographics, 426–427
  position statements. *See* position statements, ONS
  radiation oncology nurses, 152–154, 196–197
open-membership support groups, 386–387
operating systems for PDAs, 57
Orahesive, 297
oral health and dental care, 279–302
  before, during, and after cancer treatment, 281–287
  chemotherapies, 4
  complications of cancer treatment
    GVHD (graft-versus-host disease), 281, 283, 286–287, 301–302
    infection, 299–301
    oropharyngeal mucositis, 223, 285, 290–298
    salivary function, 285–286, 288–290, 298
  differences among cancer patients, 280–281
  hygiene, 283, 287
  oral cancer, websites about, 53
  patient education, 287–291
organizational considerations
  breast cancer clinics, 241
  CAM therapy models, 366–367
  freestanding clinics, 148
  ICs (infusion centers), 101
organizations, professional nursing, 2, 40. *See also specific organization by name*
  survivorship programs and support groups, 383–385
orientation sessions for patients, 12–13, 146, 149
ORN (osteoradionecrosis), 286
oropharyngeal mucositis, 285, 291–298
  pain relief, 290
  transplant therapy, 223
  treatment for, 294–298
osteoradionecrosis, 286
out-of-pocket expenses of patients, 45–46
  advocacy groups, 389–390

alternative therapies, 356
e-consultations, 58
transplant therapy, 213, 216, 224–225
outflow, financial, 34–35, 43–45
  ambulatory surgery facilities, 118–121
  profitability, quantifying, 242
  transplant therapy, 224–225
outpatient allogenic transplants, 213
outpatient facility design. *See* facility design
outpatient models. *See also* ambulatory care settings
  ambulatory surgery facilities, 118–121
  complementary and alternative medicine (CAM), 366–370
  cooperative care, 226
  CRF (fatigue) clinics, 414–416
  e-consultations, 58
  hospice care, 271–273
    continuity and coordination of care, 273–275
    underuse of, 264
  ICs (infusion centers), 106–107. *See also* ICs
  office practice settings, 81–97
    economics and reimbursement, 90–92
    history of, 81
    patient classification systems, 89–90
    role of oncology nurses, 83–89
    surgical care in, 120
    trends and nursing shortages, 92–95
    types of, 82
  pain clinics and centers, 254–258
  pharmacy, 316–319
  radiotherapy treatment centers, 141–158, 160–179
    APNs (advanced practice nurses), 167–174
    nurse administration, 175–179
    primary nursing, 160–167
    role of radiation nurses, 152–160
  survivorship programs and support groups, 393–397
  symptom management, 351

transplant therapy, 212–216
outpatient surgery, 115–137
  advantages and disadvantages, 117–118
  discontinuous care model, 265
  history of, 115–116
  oral care and, 281
  patient care issues, 121–129
  planning and developing centers for, 129–135
    example of surgery center, 133–135
  providers, salaries for, 27–28
  trends, 116, 135
  types of facilities, 118–121
outreach, community, 89
ovarian cancer, websites about, 53, 384
ovaries and reproductive effects, 402–404
overhead costs, 45

P

PACU, 124, 127
pain management, 247–261
  assessing for CRF (fatigue) clinics, 418
  care settings for, 254–258
  integrating with clinical care, 249
  medication selection, 253, 268
  oral health and dental care, 290–291
    mucositis, 294
    during therapy, 283–284
  role of nurse practitioners, 257–258
  standards of care, 248–251
  transplant therapy, 223
palliative care, 263–277
  assessment tools, 269–271
  emotional issues, 273
  history of, 265–266
  hospice care, 271–273
    continuity and coordination of care, 273–275
    underuse of, 264
  integrating with total care, 266–269, 273–275
    medication selection, 268
  radiation therapy, 195
  role of nurse practitioners, 273–275
  symptom management, 351

pancreatic cancer, websites about, 53, 384

parents, support groups for, 389. *See also* caregivers

PAs (physician assistants), 173

patient admission criteria. *See* admission criteria for patients

patient advocacy, 87

patient assessment by nurses. *See* assessing patient health; triage nursing

patient choice model (CAM therapy), 368

patient classification systems, 56, 89–92

patient communication. *See* communicating with patients

patient costs for care, 45–46
   alternative therapies, 356
   ambulatory oncologic surgery, 117
   e-consultations, 58
   transplant therapy, 213, 216, 224–225

patient education, 11–14, 26, 87–88. *See also* communicating with patients
   advocacy groups, 389–390
   clinical trials, 336–338, 343
   complementary and alternative medicine (CAM), 363
   customized, 51, 54
   e-consultations, 58
   ethical right to, 198
   fatigue management, 419, 420
   financial assistance and counseling, 46–47, 145
   fluid and electrolyte imbalances, 21
   ICs (infusion centers), 105
   instructions for patients. *See also* documentation
     informed consent, 337
     outpatient surgery, 117–118
     postoperative instructions, 123
   misconceptions of radiation therapy, 181–182
   nurse education and, 51
   oral health and dental care, 281, 287–291
   orientation sessions, 12–13, 146, 149
   outpatient surgery, 117–118, 133

postoperative instructions, 123
radiotherapy treatment, 149, 187–188
recovery issues, 394
responsibilities of nurse practitioners, 77
survivorship, 377, 379, 392
   closed-membership support groups, 383
   Internet as resource, 397–399
transplant therapy, 217–218
validity of Web-based information, 51, 61–62
in waiting room, 58–59
websites for. *See* Web-based resources

patient evaluation. *See* assessing patient health

patient-focused clinical pharmacy services, 319

patient profiles and tracking, 56

patient records. *See also* documentation
   auditing, 72
   clinical trial documentation, 336–338
   CRF (fatigue) clinics, 417
   for dental provider, 281–282
   documentation of care, 16
   HIPPA. *See* HIPPA
   patient history, 67, 71, 182
   patient profiles and tracking, 56
   pharmaceutical care and, 310–311
     dedicated clinical pharmacy services, 318
     patient medication record form, 200–202

privacy. *See* privacy and confidentiality
   telephone and e-mail communication, 57–58

patient safety, 8–11, 198. *See also* medical errors
   complementary and alternative medicine (CAM), 363–365
   pain management, 253
   pharmaceuticals, 253, 314–315
   radiation safety officers, 151
   separating infectious patients from others, 102

patient self-care, 13–14
   fluid and electrolyte imbalances, 21

Home Care Assessment Tool, 270, 272

oral health and dental care, 286
side-effects management, 189
transplant therapy, 219

patient understanding. *See* evaluating patient understanding

patients, revenues from, 34–43
   billing software for PDAs, 56
   e-consultations, 58
   freestanding clinics, 148
   maximizing payment for services, 39–43
   outpatient surgery facilities, 132, 135
   profitability, quantifying, 242
   reimbursement. *See* reimbursement
   survivorship programs, 391–392

payments from patients. *See* inflow; patient costs for care

PBSCs, 220, 222. *See also* transplant therapy

PBSCT, ICs, 110

PDAs (personal digital assistants), 54–57

pediatric care
   birth and birthing defects, 403–404
   cognitive impairment, 400
   eligibility for outpatient surgery, 122
   IC waiting area, 104
   informed consent issues, 337
   mucositis, incidence of, 293
   oral health and dental care, 287
   outpatient transplants, 216
   radiotherapy treatment, 149
   survivorship programs and support groups, 388–389

peer-to-peer support groups, 383

performance improvement
   breast cancer clinics, 235–237
   clinical trials, 338
   ICs (infusion centers), 109
   pharmacy services, 320
   radiotherapy treatment centers, 195–196

Peridex, 289, 300

periodontium, 285. *See also* oral health and dental care

personnel costs, 43

personnel resources for survivor groups, 395

pharmaceuticals, 309–325. *See also* prescriptions
  clinical services, 316–319
  clinical trials. *See* research and clinical trials
  controlled substances, classifications for, 72
  costs to patients, 42–43
  CRF (fatigue) clinics, 419
  distribution of, 313–316
  documentation, 200
  drug reference software, 56
  education for pharmacists, 311, 321
  errors. *See* medical errors
  evaluating services, 319–320
  ICs and, 104
  MAP (Medication Assistance Program), 41–42
  maximizing billing for, 40–43
  oral health and dental care, 287, 290–291
    mucositis, 294
  oral infection, 300
  palliative care, 268
  patient safety, 314–315. *See also* medical errors
    pain management, 253
  prescriptive authority, 72–74
  role of pharmacists, 309–313
  supply costs, 45
  survivorship programs, 391–392
  symptom management, 353
  telemedicine systems, 353
  transplant therapy, 219
pharmacists, role of, 309–313
pharmacodynamics, 268
pharmacokinetics, 268–269
pharmacological therapies, 359
phase IV trials. *See* research and clinical trials
phases of clinical trials, 330–334
phone communications. *See* telephone-based communication
physical assessment of patients, 180–181
physical examination, 68, 71
physical layout of outpatient facilities. *See* facility design
physician assistants, 173
physician office settings. *See* office practice settings

physician's role in CRF clinics, 415–416
physicians in training, 38
physiological eligibility for outpatient surgery, 122
planning a care center. *See* facility design
plaque, dental, 287–290. *See also* oral health and dental care
policy adherence, 77
politics, 69, 78
population shifts, 4–6
position statements, ONS
  ambulatory oncology services, 3
  assistive personnel, use of, 20
  cancer care in older adults, 5
  medication error prevention and reporting, 13
  nurse education, 14
  radiation nurse responsibilities, 154–160
  research and clinical trials, 24
positioning, patient (radiotherapy), 151
postoperative care facilities, 121
postoperative communications, 122–123
post-traumatic stress disorder, 390
post-treatment recovery. *See* recovery from treatment
poverty and healthcare costs, 34. *See also* economics and finances
power requirements for PDAs, 57
PPO (Preferred Provider Organization), 36
  nurse practitioner reimbursement, 70
practice economics. *See* economics and finances
practice models. *See* models for outpatient care
practice standards and guidelines. *See* standards of practice
preadmission testing. *See* admission criteria for patients
precertification, 36
preclinical testing, 330–331
preconception, patient. *See* education, patient; evaluating patient understanding
preoperative testing and surveys, 124–126
prepaid health insurance, 35–36

prescriptions, 315, 316. *See also* pharmaceuticals
  guidelines for reducing errors, 322–323
  prescriptive authority, 72–74
  software for e-prescriptions, 56
pretreatment
  assessment during. *See* assessing patient health
  oral care during, 281–283
  oropharyngeal mucositis, 294
  vision and hearing evaluation, 401
prevention
  cancer, programs for, 26, 99
  dental demineralization, 299
  medical errors. *See* medical errors
  oral infection, 300
  pulmonary toxicity, 402
  symptom prevention programs, 353
  visual and hearing deficits, 401
primary care providers. *See* managed-care programs
primary nursing, 160–167
prioritizing medical attention. *See* triage nursing
privacy and confidentiality, 198
  complementary and alternative medicine (CAM), 371
  e-mail addresses, 58
  HIPPA. *See* HIPPA
  survivorship programs and support groups, 396, 398
PRN (Pain Resource Nurse) Program, 254
procedural terminology codes, 90–93
procedures in ICs, 105
professional associations
  nursing, 2, 40. *See also specific organization by name*
  survivorship programs and support groups, 383–385
professional discipline and CAM therapy, 373
proficiency level, radiation nurses, 160, 164–166
profitability, quantifying, 242
prognosis, impact of on patient, 182, 378–379
prostate cancer, 53, 403
protocol treatment nurses, 343–344

psychological effects of survivorship, 390

psychological eligibility for outpatient surgery, 122

psychosocial services, 23, 83. *See also* palliative care; quality of life
  CRF (fatigue) clinic operations, 417–419
  diagnosis, impact of on patient, 182, 378–379
  oral health and dental care, 281
  pain management. *See* pain management
  patient assessment by nurses, 181–185
  patient education and, 187
  radiotherapy treatment, 149
  survivorship programs, 377, 390, 399–405. *See also* survivorship programs
  transplant therapy, 216, 218

pulmonary side-effects to cancer therapy, 402, 406

Q

QOL. *See* quality of life

qualifications for nurse practitioners, 76–77

quality of care. *See* standards of practice

quality of information, 62. *See also* validity of Web-based information

Quality of Informed Consent questionnaire, 338

quality of life (QOL), 225
  complementary and alternative medicine (CAM), 371–373
  CRF (fatigue) clinics, 413–421. *See also* fatigue
  effects of survivorship, 390
  pain. *See* pain management
  palliative care. *See* hospice care; palliative care
  side-effects to treatment. *See* side-effects management
  stages of cancer experience, 378–379
  survivorship, 393

R

race. *See* demographics

radiation nurses, 150–179, 152–160. *See also* radiotherapy treatment centers
  APNs (advanced practice nurses), 167–174
  ONS position statement, 154–160
  patient education, 187–188
  primary nursing (job description), 160–167
  research nurses, 174–175

radiation oncologists, 150

radiation safety officers, 151

radiation therapy, 153
  oral care during, 283–285
  pulmonary side-effects, 402, 406
  transplant therapy with. *See* transplant therapy

Radiation Therapy Patient Care Record, 196–197

radioactive implant therapy, 150

radioimmunotherapy, 194

radiotherapy treatment centers, 139–209
  demographics, 142–143
  economic issues, 178–179
  history and trends, 139–144
  multidisciplinary collaboration, 150–179
    APNs (advanced practice nurses), 167–174
    basic roles of radiation nurses, 152–160
    nurse administration, 175–179
    primary nursing, 160–167
    research nurses, 174–175
  patient assessment (pretreatment), 179–186
  patient education, 187–188
  practice models and operational structures, 141–150
  services available, 148–150, 179–186, 204–206
  side-effects management, 188–194
  special considerations, 188–198
    ethics, 197–198
    quality assurance and documentation, 195–197
    treatment side-effects, 188–194

readiness of learn (patients), 88

readmission. *See* admission criteria for patients

recliners in waiting area, 102

records, patient. *See* documentation

recovery from treatment
  ICs (infusion centers), 105
  oral and dental care during, 285
  patient education, 394
  postanethesia recovery score form, 128
  postoperative care facilities, 121
  post-surgery, 124, 127–128
  survivorship programs, 392
  transplant therapy, 221

recruitment of nurses, 111, 176–178

recruitment of patients
  to clinical trials, 340–341
  survivorship programs, 396

referral form for CAM programs, 371

regional care coverage, 37

registered nurses. *See also* nursing shortage (U.S.)
  age of, 428
  employment settings for, 93–95
  radiotherapy treatment centers, 157–159
  trends, 426–429

registered pharmacists (RPh), 311

registries, nursing, 2. *See also* organizations, nursing

reimbursement, 69–72. *See also* economics and finances
  hospice care, 272–273
  ICs (infusion centers), 112
  maximizing payment for services, 39–43
  office practice settings, 90–92
  outpatient surgery facilities, 133
  survivorship programs, 391–392

reliability of websites, 51, 61–62, 397–398

religion. *See* spirituality

remote consultations, 58

renal cancer, 52, 390

renal side-effects to cancer therapy, 191, 402, 406

reporting patient services (coding), 90–93
  CAM therapies, 370
  medical errors, 13. *See also* medical errors
  outpatient surgery facilities, 130
  structures for, 66

reproduction dysfunction, 391, 402–404

research and clinical trials, 17, 24, 145, 327–346
  accrual and adherence issues, 339–342
  cognitive impairment, 400
  complementary and alternative medicine (CAM), 360–361
  ethics, 328, 334–339
  history and milestones, 328–329, 335
  nursing roles, 336, 342–345
  in oncology care, 333–334
  palliative and hospice care, 264
  phases of, 330–334
  responsibilities of nurse practitioners, 76
  role of radiation nurses, 159, 162
  treatment of oral mucositis, 296, 298
research nurses, clinical trials and, 342–343
research protocol, 335
resources for patient education, 88, 187. *See also* education, patient
survivorship programs and support groups, 377, 395
responsibilities of nurse practitioners, 16, 65–69, 75–77
  care settings and, 82
  clinical trials, 336, 342–345
  complementary and alternative medicine (CAM), 367–370
  CRF (fatigue) clinics, 415
  future issues, 78
  history of, 65, 81
  ICs (infusion centers), 108–111
  informed consent, 337–338
  job settings, 66–69. *See also* ambulatory care settings
  licensing and certification, 74–77
  Medicare and Medicaid billing, 39
  nurse administration, 175–179
  in office practice settings, 83–89
  outpatient surgery facilities, 132
  pain management, 249, 257–258
  palliative care, 267–269, 273–275
  pharmacy, 312–316
  pharmacy order reviews, 316–317
  prescriptive authority, 72–74
  radiotherapy treatment centers, 144, 147
  resources for patient education, 377

symptom management, 351–353
transplant therapy, 218–220
trends and future issues, 78
retention of nurse practitioners, 111, 176–178
retention of patients in clinical trials, 340
revenues from patient care, 34–43
  billing software for PDAs, 56
  e-consultations, 58
  freestanding clinics, 148
  maximizing payment for services, 39–43
  outpatient surgery facilities, 132, 135
  profitability, quantifying, 242
  reimbursement. *See* reimbursement
  survivorship programs, 391–392
reviewing orders for chemotherapy, 316–317, 322–323
rinsing teeth and mouth, 288–289, 300
role, nurse. *See* responsibilities of nurse practitioners
routine home care (hospice), 272
RTOG, radiation nurses, 174
RTTs (registered radiation therapists), 151
  job description, 157–159

S
safety of patients, 8–11, 198
  complementary and alternative medicine (CAM), 363–365
  pharmaceuticals, 253, 314–315
  radiation safety officers, 151
  separating infectious patients from others, 102
salaries for service providers, 27–28, 43–44. *See also* economics and finances; reimbursement
  office practice settings, 93–95
Salick Health Care, 133
saline rinse (mouth), 289
salivary function, 286. *See also* oral health and dental care
  fluoride applications, 288–290
  gland dysfunction, 298
  gland evaluation, 285
  mucositis and, 293
satellite facilities. *See* freestanding clinics
satisfaction, patient. *See* quality of life

scheduling
  CRF (fatigue) clinics, 417, 419
  patient care
    hospital-based outpatient surgery, 119
    ICs (infusion centers), 109
    office practice settings, 83–84
    systems for, 45
  radiotherapy treatment planning, 149–150
  survivorship program meetings, 396
  time for documentation, 197
scientific research, 15
scope of practice, 73, 372
screen size for waiting room computers, 59
screening services, 99
seating arrangements in waiting areas, 102
secondary malignancies, 405
security, waiting room computers, 59
self-care, 13–14
  fluid and electrolyte imbalances, 21
  Home Care Assessment Tool, 270, 272
  oral health and dental care, 286
  side-effects management, 189
  transplant therapy, 221
self-help groups for survivorship, 380
separating infectious patients from others, 102
services available in outpatient cancer care, 99–100
  ICs (infusion centers), 104
  radiation oncology centers, 148–150, 179–186, 204–206
sexuality-related side-effects to treatment, 402–404, 407
shortage of nurses. *See* nursing shortage
sialagogues, 298–299
siblings, support groups for, 388. *See also* caregivers
side-effects management, 188–194, 351–353
  clinical trials, 336–338
  fatigue. *See* fatigue
  long-term physical effects, 406–407
  survivorship programs and, 392
  transplant therapy, 221–222

simulation of radiotherapy treatments, 149

single-physician practices, 82. *See also* office practice settings

site-specific side-effects, 189, 193

skills required by nurse practitioners, 75, 77

Skin Cancer Foundation, The, 384

skin-related side-effects, 193, 201–202

sleep hygiene, 419

small equipment, defined, 131

social factors. *See* culture

social support. *See* psychosocial services

social workers, 144, 151

software for PDAs, 56, 57

sound requirements for waiting room computers, 59

space requirements in facility design, 23. *See also* facility design

outpatient surgery facilities, 130

specialties of pharmacy, 310, 312

specialty model of CAM therapy, 368

spirituality

assessing patient health, 186, 188–189. *See also* culture; psychosocial services

survivorship programs, 392

St. Vincent's Comprehensive Cancer Center, 133–135

staffing CAM therapy clinics, 367–370

staffing survivorship programs, 395

standardization of documentation systems, 196–197

standards of practice, 3, 85. *See also* performance improvement

ambulatory oncologic surgery, 117

APNs, critical issues for, 173–174

assistive personnel, use of, 20

breast cancer clinics. *See* breast cancer, clinics for

cancer care in older adults, 5

clinical trials, 338

complementary and alternative medicine (CAM), 363–365

current issues, 9–10

e-mail communication with patients, 55

freestanding clinics, 147

managed-care insurance programs, 36

medication error prevention and reporting, 13

nurse education, 14

nursing shortage and. *See* nursing shortage

nutrition, 22

outpatient surgery facilities, 132

pain management, 248–251, 257

pharmacy services, 320

psychosocial services, 23

quality of information, 62. *See also* validity of Web-based information

radiation oncology nurses, 152–154

radiation therapy, 195–196

research and clinical trials, 24

responsibilities of nurse practitioners, 76

safety in ambulatory care, 12

scheduling and, 84

side-effects management, 188–194

survivorship programs, 380–381

symptom management, 353

STOT (subtotal outpatient transplant program), 212, 224

stress

on nurse practitioners, 44

on patients. *See* emotional issues; psychosocial services

structured support groups, 383

students

as nurses, historically, 81

pharmacy, 311, 321

physicians in training, 38

recruiting as nurse practitioners, 111

responsibilities of nurse practitioners, 77

trends, 428

university hospital outpatient departments, 82

substance abuse and palliative care, 271

subtotal outpatient transplant program (STOT), 212, 224

supplies and equipment, 45

costs of, 45

ICs (infusion centers), 104

outpatient surgery facilities, 131

support groups, defined, 382, 386. *See also* survivorship programs and support groups

SUPPORT study, 264

supportive therapies in ICs, 105

surgery. *See* outpatient surgery

surveillance program for therapy services, 195

survivor groups, defined, 383, 386

survivorship programs and support groups, 377–405

characteristics of, 386–388

economic issues, 391–392

effectiveness of, 380–381

emergence of, 381–382

establishing support groups, 393–397

history of, 379

Internet-based resources, 384–385, 397–399

physiologic and psychological issues, 399–405

psychological effects of survivorship, 390

special populations, 387–390

types of, and definitions, 382–387

SWOT analysis, 237–238

symptom assessment. *See* assessing patient health

Symptom Distress Scale, 225

symptom management, 351–353

fatigue. *See* fatigue

survivorship programs and, 392

system resources for survivor groups, 395

systemic analgesics for oral pain, 290–291

T

talking with patients. *See* communicating with patients

taste change and dysfunction, 284, 300. *See also* oral health and dental care

teaching patients. *See* education, patient

technical procedures, 86

technology

accompanying cultural shifts, 424

breast cancer treatments, 233

chat rooms for support groups, 398

documentation, 196

growth of ambulatory care, 4

high-tech procedures in office settings, 88–89

informatics, 17–22
Internet. *See* Internet technologies
outpatient surgery, 116
pharmacy services, 313–315, 318
radiotherapy treatment centers,
    140–141
    history of, 142–144
    medical engineers, role of, 151
    quality assurance and documen-
        tation, 195–196
symptom management, 353
telemedicine systems, 353
transplant therapy, 211
teeth care. *See* oral health and dental
    care
telemedicine systems, 353
telemetry providers, salaries for, 28
telephone-based communication, 57–58
    documenting, 87
    ICs (infusion centers), 110
    office practice settings, 86–87
    pain management checklist, 252
    pre- and post-operative communi-
        cations, 122–123
terrorism, 425–426
tertiary settings, 147
testicular cancer, 403
testing for treatment eligibility. *See*
    admission criteria for patients
therapeutic options. *See* services
    available in outpatient cancer care
thinking problems. *See* cognitive
    impairment
thyroid dysfunction, 404, 407
time-limited support groups, 383
toilets, accessibility from waiting area,
    102
tooth care. *See* oral health and dental
    care
tooth extractions, 286. *See also* oral
    health and dental care
topical analgesics for oral pain, 290,
    295–297
total outpatient transplantation, 212
toxicities from transplant therapy, 221
toxicity, testing for (clinical trials),
    330–331
tracking patients, 56
training. *See* education, nurse
transplant therapy (HSCT), 211–227
    cooperative care vs., 226
    costs and charges, 224–225

criteria for patient admission, 217,
    223–224
mucositis and, 292
oral health and dental care,
    280–287
outpatient advantages and
    disadvantages, 216–217
patient and caregiver outcomes,
    225–226
patient models, 212–216
process of, 220–224
program for, 218–220
transportation. *See also* environment
    design
    after surgery, 118
    to care centers, 145
treatment area design, ICs, 102
treatment eligibility. *See* admission
    criteria for patients
treatment levels for infusion logs, 18
treatment modalities, 99–100
treatment planning, radiotherapy
    oncology, 149–150
trends. *See* future issues and trends
triage nursing, 15
    ICs (infusion centers), 107
    patient classification systems, 56,
        89–92
    telephone and e-mail communi-
        cation, 57–58, 86–87
trials. *See* research and clinical trials
Tricare insurance program, 70
trismus, 286
trust, 180
    effects of Internet on, 51–54,
        61–62
    survivorship programs and
        support groups, 394
    validity of Internet-based
        information, 51, 61–62
    validity of Web-based
        information, 397–398

U

UAP (unlicensed assistive personnel),
    84
    ICs (infusion centers), 108, 110
    responsibilities of, 86
understanding, patient. *See* evaluating
    patient understanding

uninsured patients. *See* health and
    medical insurance
United Ostomy Association, 5
universal side-effects, 189
university hospital outpatient
    departments, 82
University of Pennsylvania Clinical
    Practices, 38
unlicensed assistive personnel (UAP).
    See UAP
unmoderated e-mail mailing lists, 60
unscheduled office visits, 84
US TOO! International, 385

V

validity of Internet-based content, 51,
    61–62, 397–398
validity of Web-based information,
    397–398
vicarious liability with CAM therapies,
    373
viral infection, oral, 300, 301
viscous lidocaine, 297
vision-related side-effects to cancer
    therapy, 401, 407
Visual Analogue Scale, 284
Volunteers in Healthcare, 40
vomiting and nausea
    dental care and, 284
    transplant therapy, 223

W

waiting area
    design of, 102
    Internet access in, 58–59
watchful waiting, 378
Web-based resources. *See also* Internet
    technologies
    breast cancer clinics, 235–237
    cancer information, 52–54, 389,
        398
    clinical practice guidelines, 69
    financial assistance to patients, 47
    survivorship resources, 384–385,
        397–399
    validity of content, 51, 61–62,
        397–398
WHO score, for oral mucositis, 295
women, treatment side-effects to,
    403–404. *See also* demographics

workplace environment. *See* ambulatory
  care settings
World Wide Web. *See* Internet
  technologies
written documentation. *See*
  documentation

Z

Zilactin, 297